THE COMPLETE PCOA® REVIEW

Notice

The authors, editors, and publisher have made every effort to ensure the accuracy and completeness of the information presented in this book. However, the authors, editors, and publisher cannot be held responsible for the continued currency of the information, any inadvertent errors or omissions, or the application of this information. Therefore, the authors, editors, and publisher shall have no liability to any person or entity with regard to claims, loss, or damage caused or alleged to be caused, directly or indirectly, by the use of information contained herein.

The inclusion in this book of any product in respect to which patent or trademark rights may exist shall not be deemed, and is not intended as, a grant of or authority to exercise any right or privilege protected by such patent or trademark. All such rights or trademarks are vested in the patent or trademark owner, and no other person may exercise the same without express permission, authority, or license secured from such patent or trademark owner.

The inclusion of a brand name does not mean the authors, the editors, or the publisher has any particular knowledge that the brand listed has properties different from other brands of the same product, nor should its inclusion be interpreted as an endorsement by the authors, the editors, or the publisher. Similarly, the fact that a particular brand has not been included does not indicate the product has been judged to be in any way unsatisfactory or unacceptable. Further, no official support or endorsement of this book by any federal or state agency or pharmaceutical company is intended or inferred.

PCOA® is a trademark of the National Association of Boards of Pharmacy® (NABP®), and PCOA® in no way endorses, authorizes, or sponsors this guide.

THE COMPLETE PCOA® REVIEW

Bradley A. Boucher, PharmD, FCCP, FNAP, MCCM, BCPS
Editor-in-Chief
Professor of Clinical Pharmacy and Translational Science
Associate Dean, Strategic Initiatives and Operations
College of Pharmacy
The University of Tennessee Health Science Center
Memphis, Tennessee

Peter A. Chyka, BS Pharm, PharmD, DABAT, FAACT
Associate Editor
Professor Emeritus of Clinical Pharmacy and Translational Science
College of Pharmacy
The University of Tennessee Health Science Center
Knoxville, Tennessee

Andrea S. Franks, PharmD, BCPS
Associate Editor
Professor of Clinical Pharmacy and Translational Science and Family Medicine
Vice Chair for Education, Clinical Specialist, Family Medicine
College of Pharmacy and Graduate School of Medicine
The University of Tennessee Health Science Center
Knoxville, Tennessee

Robert B. Parker, PharmD, FCCP
Associate Editor
Professor of Clinical Pharmacy and Translational Science
College of Pharmacy
The University of Tennessee Health Science Center
Memphis, Tennessee

APhA
American Pharmacists Association
Washington, D.C.

Senior Director, Books and Digital Publishing: John Fedor
Director, Content Development: Janan Sarwar, PharmD
Acquisitions Editor: Janan Sarwar, PharmD
Editorial Services: Absolute Service, Inc.
Cover Design: Jane Debruijn, APhA Integrated Design and Production
Indexer: Jen Burton, Columbia Indexing Group

APhA was founded in 1852 as the American Pharmaceutical Association.

Published by the American Pharmacists Association
2215 Constitution Avenue, NW
Washington, DC 20037-2985
www.pharmacist.com
www.pharmacylibrary.com

To comment on this book by e-mail, send your message to the publisher at aphabooks@aphanet.org.

Library of Congress Cataloging-in-Publication Data

Names: Boucher, Bradley A., editor. | Chyka, Peter A., editor. | Franks, Andrea S., editor. | Parker, Robert B., PharmD, editor. | American Pharmacists Association, issuing body.
Title: The complete PCOA® review / Bradley A. Boucher, editor-in-chief ; Peter A. Chyka, associate editor, Andrea S. Franks, associate editor, Robert B. Parker, associate editor.
Description: Washington, D.C. : APhA Publications, [2020] | Includes bibliographical references and index. | Summary: "The objective of The Complete PCOA® Review is to provide a study guide on the knowledge necessary to perform well on the Pharmacy Curriculum Outcomes Assessment (PCOA®) examination developed and administered by the National Association of Boards of Pharmacy (NABP). Accordingly, the target audience are student pharmacists required by the Accreditation Council for Pharmacy Education effective 2016 to complete this assessment at their respective college or school of pharmacy. While not intended to be a comprehensive reference for all aspects of the basic sciences and pharmaceutical sciences, the goal is to address the four major pharmacy content areas as outlined within the PCOA® nationally uniform content competency statements. Material may be suitable as a study guide for current student pharmacists interested in a broad overview of the topics addressed as well as a resource following completion of the PCOA® in areas requiring attention. KEY FEATURES: Comprehensive review of basic pharmacy education Information summarized in user-friendly manner. Includes most important information in the respective areas covered on the PCOA® Key points summarized; Pertinent references included; Self-study questions and answers; Study tips"– Provided by publisher.
Identifiers: LCCN 2020025957 | ISBN 9781582123417 (paperback) | ISBN 9781582123646 (epub)
Subjects: MESH: Pharmacy | Technology, Pharmaceutical | Curriculum | United States | Examination Questions
Classification: LCC RM301.13 | NLM QV 18.2 | DDC 615.1076–dc23
LC record available at https://lccn.loc.gov/2020025957

How to Order This Book

Online: www.pharmacist.com/shop

By phone: 800-878-0729 (770-280-0085 from outside the United States)

VISA®, MasterCard®, and American Express® cards accepted.

Contents

Preface

I am honored to serve as editor-in-chief of the first edition of *The Complete PCOA® Review.* I would like to express my utmost appreciation to my area editors, Drs. Peter Chyka, Andrea Franks, and Robert Parker. These outstanding faculty members have worked in concert with colleagues largely at the University of Tennessee Health Science Center College of Pharmacy to develop a comprehensive review book that will help prepare student pharmacists for the Pharmacy Curricular Outcomes Assessment (PCOA) based on the published National Association of Boards of Pharmacy (NABP) content areas. The faculty of the University of Tennessee Health Science Center College of Pharmacy and I appreciate the confidence that the American Pharmacists Association (APhA) has demonstrated by allowing us this opportunity to assist student pharmacists in preparing for the PCOA.

The objective of this book is to provide a study guide on the knowledge necessary to perform well on the PCOA examination. This unique publication is one of the only resources currently available to student pharmacists completing the PCOA. The PCOA is a comprehensive tool developed and administered by the NABP. It was designed to provide an independent, objective, external measure of student performance in United States pharmacy curricula and was first launched by the NABP in 2009. At that time, many pharmacy programs chose to use it in various ways throughout their curricula (i.e., to different classes and with varying stakes attached), while many others chose not to use it at all. The Accreditation Council for Pharmacy Education mandated the use of the PCOA in their most recent accreditation standards revision, effective July 2016, requiring all pharmacy programs to administer the 3-hour examination to student pharmacists near the end of their didactic curriculum (typically the third professional year [P3] in a 4-year PharmD program). Pharmacy programs can use the PCOA data to review individual student pharmacist performance as well as a curricular continuous improvement tool from year to year. National comparison data are also available to each institution. Furthermore, some institutions administer the examination more than once (e.g., upon entry into a PharmD program and upon completion of the core didactic curriculum as a formative assessment).

The PCOA consists of 225 items encompassing four domains. Preparing for this exam is a daunting task when one considers the breadth of topics outlined within each of the four major competency areas—basic biomedical sciences; pharmaceutical sciences; social, behavioral, and administrative sciences; and clinical sciences—broken down into 28 subtopic areas. Furthermore, student pharmacists may be actively engaged in concurrent coursework at the time the PCOA examination is administered. Reviewing material from every course taken during a student pharmacist's formal pharmacy education would be an inefficient and nearly impossible task, as well as one that possibly contains dated information. Therefore, we have developed an up-to-date, succinct, comprehensive review of basic pharmacy educational information that reinforces material learned in the past for use as student pharmacists prepare to take the PCOA.

Furthermore, student pharmacists may identify areas that need additional reinforcement based on their level of success answering the self-study questions within the review book.

This study guide attempts to summarize the information in a user-friendly manner. Each chapter of the review book includes (1) educational material that synthesizes the most salient points, (2) key points (which further delineate the most important factors), (3) a study guide checklist, (4) self-study questions and answers, and (5) additional resources for further study as needed.

Importantly, this review book is not an exhaustive discussion of the topics presented; rather, it uses an abbreviated format to enable student pharmacists to review and organize the material in an efficient manner for easy recall and recognition. Student pharmacists should have confidence that their pre-pharmacy and pharmacy education has prepared them for the PCOA. In addition, a thoughtful review of the PCOA competency areas, especially in those subjects needing a refresher, may ensure greater success when taking the PCOA examination required by each student pharmacist's respective school or college of pharmacy. Finally, any student pharmacist interested in learning more about the PCOA examination should review the PCOA Information for Students on the NABP website (https://nabp.pharmacy/programs/pcoa/students/) or contact the NABP at 1600 Feehanville Drive, Mount Prospect, IL 60056 (telephone: 1-847-391-4406; fax: 1-847-375-1114; e-mail: help@nabp.pharmacy). Student pharmacist registration within NABP is coordinated through an administrator at each student's respective school or college of pharmacy. An optional 45-minute practice PCOA assessment consisting of 50 items is available following registration and within 14 days prior to the test day to help student pharmacists become more familiar with the types of questions on the examination as well as its format.

I wish to thank John Fedor, Senior Director, Books and Digital Publishing, and Janan Sarwar, PharmD, Director of Content Development, Books and Digital Publishing, both of the APhA Books and Digital Publishing Department, for their assistance with the editorial work on this book. The insight of APhA in recognizing the student pharmacists' need for this review book is a true service to the profession of pharmacy.

Bradley A. Boucher, PharmD, FCCP, FNAP, MCCM, BCPS
Editor-in-Chief

Contributors

Lucy J. Adkins, PharmD
Director of Pharmacy Practice Initiatives
Tennessee Pharmacists Association
Nashville, Tennessee

Hassan Almoazen, PhD
Associate Professor of Pharmaceutical Sciences
Director of PhD Program
University of Tennessee Health Science Center College of Pharmacy
Memphis, Tennessee

Katherine S. Barker, PhD
Research Specialist
Department of Clinical Pharmacy and Translational Science
University of Tennessee Health Science Center College of Pharmacy
Memphis, Tennessee

Gillian C. Bell, PharmD
Clinical Pharmacist, Personalized Medicine
Mission Health
Asheville, North Carolina

Nancy Borja-Hart, PharmD, BCPS
Associate Professor of Clinical Pharmacy and Translational Science
University of Tennessee Health Science Center College of Pharmacy
Clinical Pharmacist
St. Thomas Medical Partners, Internal Medicine Center
Nashville, Tennessee

Bradley A. Boucher, PharmD, FCCP, FNAP, MCCM, BCPS
Professor of Clinical Pharmacy and Translational Science
Associate Dean, Strategic Initiatives and Operations
University of Tennessee Health Science Center College of Pharmacy
Clinical Pharmacy Specialist, Critical Care
Regional One Health
Memphis, Tennessee

Michael L. Christensen, PharmD, BCNSP, FPPAG
Professor of Clinical Pharmacy and Translational Science and Pediatrics
University of Tennessee Health Science Center Colleges of Pharmacy and Medicine
Clinical Pharmacy Specialist, Pediatrics
Le Bonheur Children's Hospital
Memphis, Tennessee

Peter A. Chyka, BS Pharm, PharmD, DABAT, FAACT
Professor Emeritus of Clinical Pharmacy and Translational Science
University of Tennessee Health Science Center College of Pharmacy
Knoxville, Tennessee

Theodore J. Cory, PharmD, PhD
Assistant Professor of Clinical Pharmacy and Translational Science
University of Tennessee Health Science Center College of Pharmacy
Memphis, Tennessee

Micah J. Cost, PharmD, MS
Executive Director
Tennessee Pharmacists Association
Nashville, Tennessee

Brandon M. Edgerson, PharmD, MS
Vice President for Professional Services
Le Bonheur Children's Hospital
Memphis, Tennessee

Glen E. Farr, PharmD
Professor Emeritus of Clinical Pharmacy and Translational Science
University of Tennessee Health Science Center College of Pharmacy
Knoxville, Tennessee

Shannon W. Finks, PharmD, FCCP, BCPS (AQ-Cardiology), ASH-CHC
Professor of Clinical Pharmacy and Translational Science
University of Tennessee Health Science Center College of Pharmacy
Clinical Pharmacy Specialist, Cardiology
Veterans Affairs Medical Center
Memphis, Tennessee

Andrea S. Franks, PharmD, BCPS
Professor of Clinical Pharmacy and Translational Science and Family Medicine
Vice Chair for Education, Clinical Specialist, Family Medicine
University of Tennessee Health Science Center College of Pharmacy and Graduate School of Medicine
Knoxville, Tennessee

Justin Gatwood, PhD, MPH
Associate Professor of Clinical Pharmacy and Translational Science
University of Tennessee Health Science Center College of Pharmacy
Nashville, Tennessee

Bill J. Gurley, PhD
Professor of Pharmaceutical Sciences
University of Arkansas for Medical Sciences College of Pharmacy
Little Rock, Arkansas

Kirk E. Hevener, PharmD, PhD
Assistant Professor of Pharmaceutical Sciences
University of Tennessee Health Science Center College of Pharmacy
Memphis, Tennessee

Kenneth C. Hohmeier, PharmD
Associate Professor of Clinical Pharmacy and Translational Science
Director of Community Affairs
Residency Program Director, Community Pharmacy Residency Program
University of Tennessee Health Science Center College of Pharmacy
Nashville, Tennessee

S. Casey Laizure, PharmD
Professor of Clinical Pharmacy and Translational Science
University of Tennessee Health Science Center College of Pharmacy
Memphis, Tennessee

Kimberly C. Mason, PharmD
Executive Director, Pharmacy and Research
University of Tennessee Medical Center
Assistant Professor
University of Tennessee Health Science Center Colleges of Pharmacy and Medicine
Chair, Institutional Review Board
University of Tennessee Health Science Center Graduate School of Medicine
Knoxville, Tennessee

Bernd Meibohm, PhD, FCP, FAAPS
Professor of Pharmaceutical Sciences
Associate Dean of Graduate Programs and Research
University of Tennessee Health Science Center College of Pharmacy
Memphis, Tennessee

Annette M. Mendola, PhD
Director, Clinical Ethics
University of Tennessee Medical Center
Assistant Professor of Medicine
University of Tennessee Health Science Center Graduate School of Medicine
Knoxville, Tennessee

Robert B. Parker, PharmD, FCCP
Professor of Clinical Pharmacy and Translational Science
University of Tennessee Health Science Center College of Pharmacy
Memphis, Tennessee

A. Shaun Rowe, PharmD, MS, BCPS, BCCCP, FNCS
Associate Professor of Clinical Pharmacy and Translational Science
University of Tennessee Health Science Center College of Pharmacy
Pharmacist Specialist, Neurocritical Care
University of Tennessee Medical Center
Knoxville, Tennessee

Joseph M. Swanson, PharmD, BCPS, FCCM
Professor of Clinical Pharmacy and Translational Science and Pharmacology
University of Tennessee Health Science Center Colleges of Pharmacy and Medicine
Clinical Pharmacy Specialist, Trauma Intensive Care Unit
Regional One Health
Memphis, Tennessee

Jeremy Thomas, PharmD, CDE
Associate Professor of Pharmacy Practice
University of Arkansas for Medical Sciences College of Pharmacy
Little Rock, Arkansas

James W. Torr, PharmD
Associate Professor of Pharmacy Practice
Lipscomb University College of Pharmacy and Health Sciences
Nashville, Tennessee

Junling Wang, MS, PhD
Professor of Clinical Pharmacy and Translational Science
University of Tennessee Health Science Center College of Pharmacy
Memphis, Tennessee

James S. Wheeler, PharmD, BCPS
Assistant Professor of Clinical Pharmacy and Translational Science
Director of Continuing Professional Development
University of Tennessee Health Science Center College of Pharmacy
Nashville, Tennessee

La'Marcus T. Wingate, PharmD, PhD
Assistant Professor of Clinical and Administrative Science
Howard University College of Pharmacy
Washington, D.C.

G. Christopher Wood, PharmD, FCCP, FCCM, BCCCPS
Professor of Clinical Pharmacy and Translational Science
University of Tennessee Health Science Center College of Pharmacy
Clinical Pharmacy Specialist, Critical Care
Regional One Health
Memphis, Tennessee

C. Ryan Yates, PharmD, PhD
Principal Scientist in the National Center for Natural Products Research
University of Mississippi School of Pharmacy
Oxford, Mississippi

Study Guide for the PCOA 1

BRADLEY A. BOUCHER

1-1 KEY POINTS

- The Pharmacy Curriculum Outcomes Assessment (PCOA) is a computerized exam that is based on competencies established by the National Association of Boards of Pharmacy (NABP).
- Efficiency is important as you refresh the knowledge learned during your first three professional years with a strategic focus on those self-identified areas of weakness.
- Use the opportunity to take the PCOA practice exam available 14 days before the exam to become familiar with the computerized exam format and type of question items to expect.
- In reviewing the chapters of *The APhA Complete PCOA Review,* perform a self-assessment of your knowledge, especially less familiar topic areas.
- Be mindful of distractions and stress, and be efficient when preparing for the PCOA because you likely will have ongoing course demands to contend with during this time.

1-2 STUDY GUIDE CHECKLIST

- ☐ Determine the date that the PCOA will be administered at your school or college of pharmacy; this date is near the end of your didactic curriculum (typically during the spring of the third year in a 4-year PharmD program). Create and begin a routine studying schedule at least 4–6 weeks before the exam should you wish to be optimally prepared to do well on the exam.
- ☐ Review PCOA guidance and rules in the current NABP PCOA Information for Students (https://www.acpe-accredit.org/pdf/Standards2016FINAL.pdf).
- ☐ Practice answering easier questions quickly, allowing more time for challenging questions. (Note: The 3-hour PCOA has 225 questions.)
- ☐ Review the PCOA Content Areas on the NABP website (https://nabp.pharmacy/wp-content/uploads/2016/07/PCOA-Content-Areas-2016.pdf) to identify areas of relative strength and weakness.
- ☐ Review basic pathophysiology of common chronic diseases.
- ☐ Review names of commonly used prescription drugs, over-the-counter medications, and dietary supplements.
- ☐ Review specific medication counseling points.
- ☐ Review key nontherapeutic topic areas: biostatistics, pharmacoepidemiology, literature review, and pharmacoeconomic and pharmacogenomic principles.
- ☐ Study common pharmacy calculations and measuring system conversions; sterile compounding.

1-3 Introduction

The Pharmacy Curriculum Outcomes Assessment (PCOA) is a computerized exam that is based on competencies established by the National Association of Boards of Pharmacy (NABP). It is designed to provide an independent, objective, external measure of student performance in United States pharmacy curricula. The Accreditation Council for Pharmacy Education (ACPE) mandated the use of the PCOA, effective in 2016, in their most recent accreditation standards revision requiring all pharmacy programs to administer the 3-hour examination to students in their third professional year (P3). Pharmacy programs can use the PCOA data to review individual student performance as well as a curricular continuous improvement tool from year to year.

Think of yourself for a moment as an elite athlete or an accomplished musician. Would you wait until the week before a competition or performance to begin training or practicing? Would you focus only on your mind and not include your body? Would you neglect knowing the rule book or the sheet music? Would you check your smartphone periodically while practicing? Would you rely only on what you remember to do without the benefit of a coach or trainer? Successful athletes and musicians train for weeks and months, focus on mind and body, avoid distractions, and look to coaches to find strengths and weaknesses. You might still be competitive and accomplished with your natural abilities, but the odds are working against you without a proper conditioning and training period. This same attitude should translate to your preparation for the PCOA if you wish to perform optimally. Throughout your pre-pharmacy and profession education, you have gained experience and have learned facts and skills. In addition, you should have developed learning and study habits that have been successful for you. Now is the time to apply what you have learned about yourself to perform optimally on the PCOA by considering attitude, preparation, and practice.

1-4 Attitude

Begin with and maintain a positive attitude. Unlike most tests in an academic course that are like sprints of a discrete collection of knowledge, the PCOA is more like a marathon covering years and a large body of knowledge. Adjust your attitude and habits accordingly. Consider creating a schedule for study at least 4–6 weeks before the scheduled exam date at your school or college of pharmacy should you wish to be thoroughly prepared. Devote some of your best time of the day to studying; do not just fit your studying in whenever you feel like it. Like an athlete or musician, focus on the material during your study time, because studying is more efficient and effective without distractions or multitasking. Distractions and lack of focus make it easy to procrastinate. Develop a personal system and routine leading up to the exam, especially because you likely need to work around your regular coursework demands. Write down your goal for the next study session the night before. Positively look forward to reviewing material for the PCOA. You might be surprised by what you remember from your pharmacy curriculum and practice as well as areas that need some reinforcement. Furthermore, this can be a time of discovery of things that were not quite clear the first time; now you have an opportunity to put the pieces of the puzzle together. By keeping to a schedule to review several chapters a week beginning with your weakest topics and by maintaining a list of things to go over again, you will have time to address problem areas. Furthermore, consider the Key Points, Study Guide Checklist, and practice questions as a self-assessment and guide to focus your follow-up of the material.

1-5 Preparation

The Rule Book

Before you start studying, take time to review the guidance, rules, and description of the PCOA provided by the organization conducting the exam—the National Association of Boards of Pharmacy (NABP). The NABP website's section on its programs (https://nabp.pharmacy/programs/) has critical information about PCOA exam procedures and policies, content areas, question format, and other important information. Also on the website is the paperwork that needs to be completed if you are seeking testing accommodations. The deadline for this distinct accommodations paperwork will be on or before the deadline for PCOA registration. Information about registration is typically communicated by your school.

The Playing Field

The PCOA consists of 225 questions and lasts 3 hours, which averages 1.25 minutes per question. Some questions will take more or less time, but the time period is sufficient for you to answer all questions. Questions must be answered in sequence. Preparation and practice will allow you to answer the easier questions in less time so you may devote more time to more challenging ones.

There are several question formats on the PCOA. The questions vary in levels of difficulty.

1. Multiple-choice question with a single answer out of four possible responses, for example:

   Where is fat primarily stored in a middle-aged adult?

   A. *Adipose tissue*
   B. Connective tissue
   C. Skin tissue
   D. Vascular tissue

2. Multiple-response question, which is followed by a phrase similar to "Mark all that apply," for which there is no partial credit, for example:

   Which clinical laboratory test(s) would be useful to detect infection? (Mark all that apply.)

   A. Serum potassium
   B. Hematocrit
   C. *Sputum culture*
   D. Troponin
   E. *White blood cell count*

3. Constructed-response question, where a corrected rounded value is typically entered, for example:

   How much drug (in mg) would be contained in 12 mL of a 15% aqueous solution? (Answer must be numeric: Round the final answer to the nearest WHOLE number.)

1,800

4. Ordered-response question, where the choices are ranked by dragging an option to the appropriate rank position, for example:

Rank the following weights from least heavy to heaviest. (ALL options must be used.)

Unordered options	Ordered response
0.5 kg	*100 ng*
10 mcg	*10 mcg*
100 ng	*750 mg*
750 mg	*0.5 kg*

5. Hot-spot question, where the response is marked on a location of a diagram using the cursor to mark the spot or to select an option following the directions for doing so, for example:

Using the following diagram, identify the site of action of furosemide in the nephron by selecting the correct button.

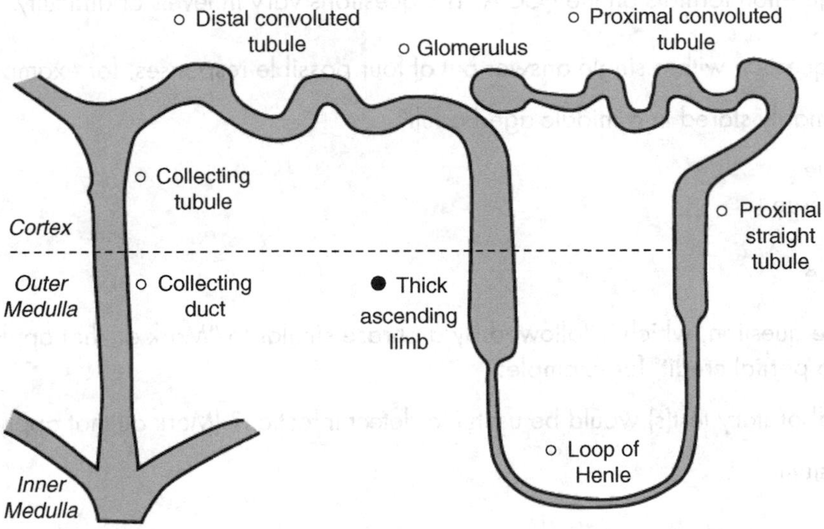

The Play Book

The PCOA tests within four major categories, referred to as the PCOA Content Ares, which is included in the *PCOA* outline (https://nabp.pharmacy/programs/pcoa/). The 2020 version of the four PCOA content areas are as follows:

- *Area 1:* Basic biomedical sciences (approximately 10% of exam)
- *Area 2:* Pharmaceutical sciences (approximately 33% of exam)
- *Area 3:* Social/behavioral/administrative sciences (approximately 22% of exam)
- *Area 4:* Clinical sciences (approximately 35% of exam)

General guidance on content: As noted, the PCOA is weighted toward clinical sciences (35%) and pharmaceutical sciences (33%) as indicated by the competencies. As a general guide, you should be familiar with the following information regarding drug therapy and should focus your study time on areas of weakness or unfamiliarity:

- What is the therapeutic category of this drug?
- What is the basic mechanism of action?
- What basic properties of a drug's chemistry could affect a medication's formulation and action?
- What type of patient counseling information should be provided?
- What are the major adverse effects of a drug class (side effects and toxic effects)?
- What are the major drug interactions and contraindications?
- What are the names (brand and generic) of commonly used prescription drugs, over-the-counter medications, and dietary supplements.

Priorities for Review

Student pharmacists within pharmacy curricula typically get inundated with therapeutic information and disease state management, which is a reason not to expend significant review time on these content areas. As such, review for the PCOA for many student pharmacists should be other areas such as general awareness of the elements of the U.S. health care system and contemporary pharmacy practice and the other content areas outlined below.

Chronic and common diseases: Focus on the more common and chronic diseases and their drug therapies. A general knowledge of the disease process is important, but avoid focusing the majority of study time on detailed disease characteristics, such as etiology, pathophysiology, diagnosis, and signs and symptoms, at the expense of drug therapy.

Nontherapeutic topics: Review of biostatistics, pharmacoepidemiology, literature, and pharmacoeconomic and pharmacogenomic principles should be a priority because these areas are sometimes topics of relative weakness for student pharmacists, who may be in need of a refresher.

Math: Pharmacy math is another fundamental area to review. Information to know includes conversion factors among the systems of measurement and math for compounding typical dosage forms such as ointments, solutions, and intravenous preparations. Be careful to take notice of the units of measure and decimal points in any math problem and calculation. Rounding as asked in the questions is necessary to earn points for a correct answer.

1.6 Exam Readiness

Self-Assessment

- As you review the chapters of *The APhA Complete PCOA Review,* perform a self-assessment of your knowledge by responding to the questions at the end of each chapter.
- To make your learning experience more effective, study the explanations for the correct responses. Also note the incorrect response options, and learn why they are incorrect.
- If you know the material well, progress to the next subject area in the spirit of efficiency.

PCOA Practice Exam

The NABP offers a tremendous opportunity to take a representative practice exam that simulates the PCOA testing experience; the practice exam is available to registrants 14 days before their scheduled exam. Although it is optional, the 50-question, 45-minute practice exam provides the chance to become familiar with the computerized format, experience the types of questions, and assess your stamina to be able to sit in front of a computer for test taking. The PCOA practice exam can be taken on any computer with an Internet connection. The specific practice exam questions will not be on the current version of the PCOA exam; regardless, the questions will provide a strong sense of questions that will likely be posed on the current exam.

Exam-Taking Advice

The following list contains suggestions for test taking:

1. Read directions carefully, and read questions at least twice to be sure of the nature of the question. Note any modifying terms such as *always, all, never, most,* or *usually;* any double negatives; and anything else about the way the question is worded that may change the meaning of the question and your response. In addition, formulating an answer prior to reading the answer options will decrease the likelihood of you being swayed by the available answer choices.
2. Read all the answer options thoroughly, and eliminate the obvious distractors or incorrect answers. Typically, two to three options can be eliminated for one or more reasons, and the final choice is between two answers. Select the *single best answer* for the multiple-choice format. Be cautious about reading multiple possibilities into questions because most questions should be straightforward. If you simply do not know the answer, eliminate any distractors and guess intelligently from the remaining options.
3. Pace yourself, but do not rush through the exam. The 3 hours scheduled for the PCOA should be more than adequate to complete the exam. Proceed at a reasonable pace, and answer approximately 75–80 questions per hour to finish comfortably in the time available. If only 40–50 questions are completed in the first hour, you should increase your speed. A timer is displayed on the computer screen, and an on-screen calculator is also available.
4. If you are definitely unsure of the correct response for a question, eliminate as many distractors as possible and make your best conclusion. Don't dwell on it; move on to the next question. As in musical performances, all musicians make mistakes in a performance, but they don't stop. They continue to the end of the song. A performance will not be judged by a few errors, and that will also be the case for your performance on the PCOA.

PCOA Examination Day

Avoid studying the day and evening before the exam—last-minute cramming may cause anxiety and affect your performance. On the evening before the exam, do something relaxing. Like an athlete, keep to your regular sleeping schedule and eating habits. On the day of the exam, eat breakfast (a healthy one). If your exam is scheduled in the afternoon, be on guard against fatigue by having a light lunch and adequate, but not excessive, hydration. (Hint: If you find that you are becoming tired during the exam, check your posture to ensure that you are sitting up straight—you may become more alert because your lungs can more effectively ventilate and oxygenate when you are not slouching.) Lastly, go to the location designated by your school or college arriving approximately 1 hour early and, like an athlete or musician, perform at your very best.

1-7 Conclusion

The PCOA examination is comprehensive in scope and will provide a solid assessment of your readiness to begin your experiential coursework. By adopting and maintaining a positive attitude, and steady preparation, the likelihood of success will be enhanced. This in turn will ideally provide a high degree of self-confidence relative to the progress that you have made during your professional journey. The many contributors to *The APhA Complete PCOA Review* hope that this publication will assist you in your preparation for the PCOA and your graduation as a pharmacist in the near future.

1-8 Additional Resources

Barker E. Most productive people: 6 things they do every day. Barking Up the Wrong Tree (blog), June 1, 2014. https://www.bakadesuyo.com/2014/06/most-productive people.

National Association of Boards of Pharmacy. *PCOA*. Mount Prospect, IL: National Association of Boards of Pharmacy; 2020. Accessed February 11, 2020. https://nabp.pharmacy/programs/pcoa/.

PCOA: The Pharmacy Curriculum Outcomes Assessment (PCOA), NABP: National Association of Boards of Pharmacy (NABP).

For important details, see the current *PCOA Information for Students*. Accessed February 11, 2020. Available at: https://nabp.pharmacy/programs/pcoa/students/.

1-9 Study Plan

BASIC BIOMEDICAL SCIENCES

area **1**

EDITOR: *ROBERT B. PARKER*

Anatomy and Physiology 2

JAMES S. WHEELER

2-1 KEY POINTS

INTEGUMENTARY SYSTEM

- The skin serves to cool and rid the body of toxic waste through the secretion, excretion, and evaporation of sweat from sweat glands. It also protects the body from desiccation and mechanical abrasion.

MUSCULAR SYSTEM

- The muscular system includes three types of cells: skeletal (voluntary), cardiac (involuntary), and smooth muscle (involuntary).

SKELETAL SYSTEM

- The bony skeleton provides protection from mechanical injury and attachment for muscles.

CARDIOVASCULAR SYSTEM

- The cardiovascular system is an enclosed entity including the heart, arteries, capillaries, and veins.
- The human heart consists of four primary chambers: the right and left atria and the right and left ventricles.

LYMPHATIC SYSTEM

- The lymph nodes, spleen, thymus gland, and tonsils produce lymphocytes, which contain macrophage-like, phagocytic lymphatic cells.

RESPIRATORY SYSTEM

- The function of the respiratory system is to filter, humidify, and transmit air to the lungs, where it oxygenates blood in the pulmonary alveoli and alveolar sacs.

DIGESTIVE SYSTEM PROPER

- Organs of the digestive system include the oral cavity, esophagus, stomach, small and large intestines, rectum, and anus.
- Accessory glands of digestion include the salivary glands, liver, gall bladder, and pancreas.

CENTRAL NERVOUS SYSTEM

- The nervous system consists of two types of cells: the neuron and neuralgia. Neurons are responsible for producing an action potential.

ENDOCRINE SYSTEM

- The endocrine system consists of ductless glands that secrete specific hormones directly into the bloodstream. They comprise the following glands: pituitary, thyroid, parathyroid, suprarenal, ovary, and testis.

URINARY SYSTEM

- Components of the urinary system include the kidneys, ureter, bladder, and urethra.
- The tubular nephron is the excretory part of the kidney (producing ultrafiltrate).

MALE REPRODUCTIVE SYSTEM

- Components of the male reproductive system include the testes, scrotum, and penis.

FEMALE REPRODUCTIVE SYSTEM

- The female reproductive system consists of the ovaries, fallopian (uterine) tubes, uterus, vagina, labia majora, labia minora, and clitoris.

2-2 STUDY GUIDE CHECKLIST

The following topics may guide your study of this subject area:

- ☐ Define the structure and function of each organ system
- ☐ Rank levels of anatomical structure
- ☐ List organs in each organ system and identify basic anatomical positions
- ☐ Explain basic concepts of biochemistry as it relates to the human body
- ☐ Discuss homeostatic control mechanisms
- ☐ Explain how drugs exhibit their action at the cellular level to affect each organ system

2-3 Introduction

Anatomy and physiology are fundamental, and they correlate with pharmacy by establishing the normal standard for structure and function of the healthy individual. This factual standard provides the basis for identifying the presence and degree of disease and pathology. It also provides a means of understanding the process of medicinal application, movement, absorption, and target organ and tissue action.

The body systems and focal topics reviewed in this chapter are the integumentary system; muscular system; skeletal system; cardiovascular system; lymphatic system; respiratory system; digestive system; central nervous system; endocrine system; urinary system; reproductive system; body fluids and electrolytes; and cell structure, organization, and physiology.

2-4 Integumentary System

The *integumentary system* consists of the skin and associated specializations such as nails, hair, and sebaceous and sweat glands.

Skin is the largest nonvisceral organ of the body and consists of the outer epithelial layer, called the *epidermis,* and an inner connective tissue, known as the *dermis.* Skin serves to cool and rid the body of toxic waste through the secretion, excretion, and evaporation of sweat from sweat glands. It also protects the body by serving as a barrier from mechanical abrasion.

The *epidermis* is a nonvascular layer and is made up of stratified squamous epithelium, which grows from the deeper basal layer to the outermost keratinized squamous cells of the corneum. Epidermis layers, from deep to superficial, are the stratum basale, stratum spinosum, stratum granulosum, and stratum corneum.

The *dermis* consists of dense, irregular connective tissue that is highly vascular and rich in lymphatics and cutaneous nerves.

The *hypodermis* is a looser connective tissue layer that facilitates movement of the overlying skin.

For clinical purposes, the skin is highly absorptive and facilitates the uptake of topically applied medications, such as salves and ointments. Also, subcutaneous medications may be administered to vascular-rich deep connective tissue through hypodermic injections.

2-5 The Muscular System

The function of the muscular system is to dynamically overcome gravity and to facilitate locomotion through movement of the skeleton and various organs of the body. Muscle cells are elongated to support contraction.

Types of Muscle Cells

Skeletal muscle cells are multinucleated, voluntary, and highly involved in the movement of the skeleton and the musculoskeletal system. Cardiac muscle cells are striated and involuntary and are found in the heart. They are responsible for contraction of the heart. Smooth muscle cells are uninucleated and involuntary. Smooth muscle is located in the walls of hollow organs, such as the stomach, intestines, bladder, blood vessels, and uterus.

Organelles of the Skeletal Muscle Cell

The cytoplasm of the muscle cell is filled with synchronously arranged and linearly organized protein strands called *myofilaments.* Mitochondria, Golgi, vesicles, lysosomes, and other organelles are randomly situated between myofibrils.

Myofilaments

Each myofibril contains cross-striated regions of alternating light and dark bands. The dark bands are called *A-bands.* A-bands consist of overlapping thin actin filaments and thick myosins. The light bands, or striations, are called *I-bands.* I-bands contain only thin actin filaments. *Z-lines* are places where adjacent thin filaments connect or abut to one another.

Myofibrils can be subdivided into smaller linear units called *microfilaments.*

The Sliding Filament Theory of Muscle Contraction suggests that thick and thin myofilaments interdigitate and slide between and with one another during muscle contraction. Calcium and adenosine triphosphate are vital in producing muscle contraction.

Origins, insertions, and action

Muscles attach to bones through tendons. The tendinous muscle attachment that moves the least during muscle contraction is called the *origin*; the attachment that moves the most is the *insertion.* The work that the muscle performs during its contraction is called the *action.*

Classifications and Types

Skeletal muscles are classified according to size (magnum), shape (rhomboid), function (levator), and number of tendinous attachments (digastricus). Types of skeletal muscle actions include flexion, extension, rotation, abduction, adduction, elevation, depression, protraction, retraction, dilation, and constriction.

Neuromuscular Junction

Skeletal muscle fibers require neuronal input to contract or act. Efferent axons terminate on skeletal muscle cells at specialized synaptic sites of contact called *motor end plates* or the *neuromuscular junction.*

The motor end plate synapse is where the axon terminal releases a neurotransmitter (usually acetylcholine) into the synaptic cleft. Specialized receptors are located on the plasma membrane of the muscle cell that can be energized by the neurotransmitter to produce an axon potential in the muscle cell.

2-6 The Skeletal System

The bony skeleton of the human body is internally located and provides protection from mechanical injury and attachment for muscles. It stores and, when necessary, releases calcium and other vital inorganic salts; is instrumental in blood formation through bone marrow; and acts as scaffolding in overcoming gravity.

Bone cell types include the following:

- ***Osteocytes:*** These mature melon-shaped bone cells are trapped in lacunae and maintain bone matrix.
- ***Osteoclasts:*** These multinucleated bone cells enzymatically digest and remodel bone matrix.
- ***Osteoblasts:*** These young bone cells actively build bone matrix.

Mature bone matrix consists of layers of helically organized connective tissue fibers (collagen, elastin, reticulin) that surround blood vessels in Haversian systems. The bone matrix is also infiltrated by calcium and phosphate crystalline salts, which are responsible for its rigidity and represent 65% of a bone's weight.

Flat bones consist of two tables of adult bone separated by an inner layer of red bone marrow called *dipolë.* Long bones contain an outer shell of mature lamellae bone and an inner and central core of bone marrow. The inner layer of bone marrow is separated from the innermost lamellae of bone by a delicate connective layer called the *endosteum.*

Bones are usually covered on the surface by a highly vascular, dense connective envelope called the *periosteum*. The periosteum also contains reserve or primitive bone cells that are capable of producing new bone cells and matrix. This layer is important in the healing and repair of bone fractures.

Classification of Bone

Bones can be classified as *short, long, irregular,* and *flat.* They are attached to one another by *joints.* Strong, dense regular connective tissue bands called *ligaments* generally hold joints together.

Joints are movable, semimovable, or nonmovable. Selected movable joints include *ball and socket, hinge, sliding,* and *peg in socket.*

Muscles attach to bone by *tendons.*

Red bone marrow contains *sinusoidal-line blood vessels* and *primitive blood-forming cells* that divide and differentiate into mature blood corpuscles.

Organization of the Skeleton

The skeleton proper can be subdivided into two units: the axial and appendicular skeleton. The *axial skeleton* consists of the skull and vertebral column. The *appendicular skeleton* contains the upper and lower extremities and the pectoral and pelvic girdles.

Selected bones of the cranium include the frontal, maxilla, mandible, sphenoid, parietal, temporal, occipital, nasal, and zygoma. Selected vertebrae and their number on the vertebral column are as follows: cervical (7), thoracic (12), lumbar (5), sacral (5), and coccygeal (4).

Vertebra components of the bony spine include the body, pedicles, lamina, transverse process, and posterior spine. The neural canal contains the spinal cord and is located between the lamina and pedicles.

Spaces between adjacent vertebrae are occupied by a fibrocartilaginous body called the *intervertebral disc.*

Vertebrae specializations and classification

The *cervical vertebrae* are the smallest vertebrae. They facilitate spinal movement (rotation, flexion, extension).

The *atlas,* which is the first cervical vertebra, contains no centrum or body and balances and supports the head. The *axis,* which is the second cervical vertebra, contains a cranially oriented projection from its centrum or body called the *dens.* The dens articulates with the anterior arch of the atlas, thus facilitating rotary movement.

Regional differences exist in the morphology of cervical through coccygeal vertebrae. Each of the 12 thoracic vertebrae is attached wholly or partially to a rib and provides protection to thoracic viscera and points of attachment for thoracic musculature. The five independent lumbar vertebrae are larger and are the strongest components of the vertebral column. The five sacral vertebrae are fused into a single, solid triangular mass of bone, which articulates with the iliac bones of the pelvic girdle as the *sacroiliac joint.* Coccygeal vertebrae are three to four in number and are small and vestigial.

Curvatures of the vertebrae and spine include the cervical curvature, thoracic curvature, lumbar curvature, and sacral curvature.

Ribs

Twelve pairs of ribs can be included with the axial skeleton, and they articulate with thoracic vertebrae posteriorly and the sternum anteriorly. The ribs and clavicle attach to the sternum anteriorly, and the sternum acts to limit the thorax ventrally.

Rib types are as follows:

- *True (1–7)* ribs link directly to the sternum via costal cartilages.
- *False (8–10)* ribs do not attach directly to the sternum but have costal cartilages that merge with the cartilage of the seventh rib.
- *Floating (11–12)* ribs have no costal cartilages and do not attach to the sternum.

Sternum

The sternum is located anteriorly in the thorax. It consists of the manubrium, body, and xiphoid process.

Appendicular Skeleton

The *appendicular skeleton* consists of the pectoral girdle and upper extremity and the pelvic girdle and lower extremity. Bones of the pectoral girdle are the clavicle and scapula.

Major bones of the upper limb include the humerus of the arm, radius and ulna of the forearm, carpal bones of the wrist, metacarpal bones of the hand, and phalanges of the digits.

Bones of the pelvic girdle include the ilium, pubis, and ischium.

Bones of the lower limb proper include the femur of the thigh, tibia and fibula of the leg, tarsal bones of the ankle, metatarsal bones of the foot, and phalanges of the digits.

2-7 Cardiovascular System

The cardiovascular system is an enclosed entity and includes the heart, arteries, veins, and capillaries.

Tissue Organization of Blood Vessels

The *intima* is the innermost epithelial layer of blood vessels. The flat, plate-like squamous cells of the intima facilitate the flow of blood and prevent clotting. Mechanical damage or the accumulation of calcium and fatty deposits in the intima may cause blood clots, which may cause cerebral accidents (strokes) or coronary artery heart disease.

The *media* is the middle layer of blood vessels and is the thickest layer in arteries. The media may contain several laminae of elastic fibers.

The *adventitia* is an outer layer of predominantly connective tissue. The adventitia of veins may contain one or more longitudinally arranged smooth muscle layers and may contain scant or rich laminae of elastic fibers.

Types of *arteries* include large arteries, medium arteries, small arteries, and arterioles. *Veins*, which accompany arteries, usually have larger diameters and thinner walls. Types of veins include large veins, medium veins, small veins, and venules.

Capillaries are the smallest blood vessels. They consist of an endothelial layer surrounded by connective tissue.

Oxygen and carbon dioxide readily diffuse from the blood cells and plasma across the thin, simple squamous endothelial layer of the intima into the connective tissue and the surrounding tissue fluid.

Heart

The heart is a modified blood vessel that functions to pump blood to various parts of the body. The heart contains three tissue layers in cross section:

- ***Epicardium:*** An outer layer of mesothelium and connective tissue
- ***Myocardium:*** A middle layer of several laminae of cardiac muscle
- ***Endocardium:*** An inner layer of simple squamous epithelium

Gross structure of the heart

The human heart consists of four primary chambers: the right and left atria and right and left ventricles. Each atrium has an antechamber called the *auricle*.

The great blood vessels of the heart include veins that bring deoxygenated blood to the right atrium and arteries that carry deoxygenated and oxygenated blood away from the heart. These veins include the superior vena cava, inferior vena cava, and coronary sinus.

The heart is located in the pericardial sac, in the central region of the thorax called the *middle mediastinum*. Components of the pericardial sac include the fibrous pericardium and the serous pericardium, with its visceral and parietal layers.

The right atrium receives deoxygenated blood from the head, neck, and upper extremities through the superior vena cava and from the thorax, abdomen, pelvis, and lower extremities through the inferior vena cava. Components of the right atrium include the pectinate muscles, crista terminalis, and fossa ovalis. The right atrium contracts to force blood to the right ventricle through the tricuspid valve.

The right ventricle is composed of the chordae tendineae, the papillary muscles, the trabeculae carneae, and the aortic vestibule. The right ventricle contracts to force blood through the pulmonary semilunar valve to the pulmonary trunk. The pulmonary trunk divides into right and left pulmonary arteries, which direct blood to the right and left lungs.

The left atrium consists of the left auricle, pectinate muscles, and openings for the four pulmonary veins. Oxygenated blood (from the lungs) is sent to the left atrium through the four pulmonary veins.

The left ventricle consists of the chordae tendineae, papillary muscles, trabeculae carneae, and aortic vestibule. Contraction of the left atrium propels oxygenated blood through the mitral or bicuspid valve to the left ventricle. Contraction of the left ventricle projects oxygenated blood through the aortic valve into the aorta and its branches. The cardiac musculature of the left ventricle is three times thicker than that of the right ventricle.

Components of the cardiac conducting system include the sinoatrial node, atrioventricular node, atrioventricular bundle (also known as the bundle of His), and Purkinje fibers. The sinoatrial node serves as the heart's natural pacemaker and is located in the right atrium.

The synchronous contraction of right and left atria before that of right and left ventricles is provided by the cardiac conduction system. The cardiac conduction system consists of modified cardiac muscle fibers that are specialized for conducting fast nerve-like impulses in cardiac tissue. These fibers facilitate the synchronous contraction of atria before ventricles.

Electrical activity of the heart

An electrocardiograph tracing has three components or waves: a *P wave,* which occurs with atria depolarization (contraction); a *QRS wave complex,* which represents depolarization of the ventricles (contraction); and a *T wave,* which represents electrical activity (repolarization) or relaxation of the ventricles.

2-8 The Lymphatic System

The lymph nodes, spleen, thymus gland, and tonsils produce lymphocytes, which contain macrophage-like, phagocytic lymphatic cells. These cells engulf and destroy invasive microbial cells. The thymus gland is the source of thymic lymphocytes (T-lymphocytes), which, after maturity, are distributed to other lymphatic organs. The spleen is the largest lymph organ of the body and also functions to store and destroy old red blood corpuscles.

Lymph fluid ultimately is returned to the venous system through the thoracic duct and right lymph duct. The excessive accumulation of lymphatic fluid in an extremity is a type of edema.

Lymph flow involves small lymph vessels in the extremities and other parts of the body that pick up tissue fluid from deep and superficial connective tissue, where it is conducted to larger vessels. These vessels empty the lymph into the thoracic duct and right lymphatic duct, which are the largest lymph vessels of the body. The thoracic duct empties lymph into the left brachiocephalic vein.

Lymph is composed of leukocytes and plasma-like tissue fluid. Lymph vessels consist of intima, media, and adventitia, which are highly disorganized tissues when compared with lamellae of arteries and veins.

Lymphatic tissue and organs include the diffuse lymph tissue (i.e., Peyer's patches of the small intestines), partially encapsulated tissue (i.e., tonsils), and totally encapsulated organs (i.e., the lymph nodes, which filter lymph fluid of microbes and cancerous cells).

The thymus gland is located in the anterior thorax and produces T-lymphocytes.

The spleen filters the blood, produces white blood cells, and stores blood for emergency perfusion resulting from hemorrhages. It contains concave and convex surfaces and is generally located deep in the 9, 10, and 11 ribs. An enlarged spleen may indicate the presence of infection.

2-9 Respiratory System

The function of the respiratory system is to filter, humidify, and transmit air to the lungs, where it oxygenates blood. The nasal cavity filters and conditions the inspired air.

The pharynx, larynx, trachea, bronchi, and bronchioles transmit air to the lungs, where the respiratory system oxygenates the blood through thin-walled pulmonary alveoli and alveolar sacs.

The trachea and bronchi contain a skeleton of C-shaped rings of hyaline cartilage, a mucosa of respiratory epithelium (pseudostratified ciliated columnar epithelium and goblet cells), and a submucosa that contains numerous mucous glands.

The lungs are bilateral organs containing hundreds of millions of alveoli and are located in the pleural cavity of the thorax. The left lung is divided into two lobes by the oblique fissure. The right lung is divided into three lobes by the horizontal and oblique fissures.

The pulmonary alveolus consists of a single layer of simple squamous epithelium (*pulmonary epithelium*), which is adjacent to a basement membrane and abuts against another layer of simple squamous epithelium (*endothelium*) of a capillary. This layer is referred to as the *blood–air barrier.*

Oxygen passes from a region of higher concentration in the pulmonary alveolus through the blood–air barrier to an area of less concentration in the blood of the capillary where hemoglobin is oxygenated. Carbon dioxide is more highly concentrated in the blood and travels by diffusion through the blood–air barrier to the lumen of the pulmonary alveolus, where it is exhausted.

The diaphragm is the major muscle of respiration and is located between the thorax and the abdomen. Contraction of this muscle causes an increase in thoracic volume and inhalation of air, whereas relaxation of the diaphragm forces carbon dioxide–laden air out of the lungs in exhalation.

2-10 Digestive System Proper

The *abdomen* is the region between the thorax (above) and the pelvic cavity (below). The diaphragm separates the abdomen from the thorax. No true muscular or connective partition demarcates the true pelvis from the abdominal cavity.

Selected organs of the abdomen include the liver, pancreas, kidney, suprarenal glands (adrenal), stomach, gall bladder, small intestines, and large intestines. The abdomen can be subdivided into four quadrants by the intersection of the vertically situated median plane and by a horizontally applied plane through the umbilical region.

The *parietal peritoneum* consists of a layer of simple squamous epithelium that lines the inner surface of the anterior and posterior abdominal walls. The *visceral peritoneum* is a similar epithelial layer that covers the outer surface of selected abdominal organs. The space located between visceral and parietal peritonea is called the *peritoneal cavity.* Several organs that are not entirely enclosed in the peritoneum but are located behind the peritoneum are referred to as *retroperitoneal structures.* They include the duodenum, pancreas, kidneys, ascending colon, and descending colon.

Intraperitoneal organs are enveloped by the visceral peritoneum on several sides and attach to the parietal peritoneum of the anterior or posterior abdominal walls by peritoneal reflections.

Organs of the digestive system include the oral cavity (teeth, tongue, salivary glands), esophagus, stomach, small and large intestines, rectum, and anus.

Accessory glands of digestion include the salivary glands, liver, gall bladder, and pancreas. The salivary glands produce saliva, which contains the enzyme amylase. They are anatomically associated with the oral cavity, where they project excretory ducts to the mouth. Consequently, the process of digestion begins in the mouth, where carbohydrates are initially broken down by amylase.

The liver is the largest visceral organ of the body and is important in detoxifying the blood of pathogens and toxins. It is shaped roughly like a pyramid lying on one side with its base on the right and its apex situated to the left. The liver receives blood from the portal vein. The blood contains nutrients absorbed from the stomach and intestines.

The liver is an important exocrine organ and secretes bile. Bile is a fatty emulsifier; after it is secreted from the liver, it is stored and concentrated in the gall bladder. Right and left hepatic ducts unite to form the common hepatic duct. The common hepatic duct from the liver joins the cystic duct of the gall bladder to form the common bile duct, which attaches to the descending portion of the duodenum. Other important functions of the liver include production of proteins, vitamin storage, control of carbohydrate metabolism, and removal of drugs and hormones from the blood.

The hepatic porta contains the portal vein, hepatic artery, and common bile duct. The liver gives off two excretory ducts, the right and left hepatic ducts, from hepatic lobes of the same name.

The liver possesses a dual blood supply through the portal vein and the hepatic artery. The portal vein is formed as a result of juncture of the superior mesenteric and splenic veins. The portal vein supplies venous blood from the small and large intestines to the liver as a component of the hepatic triad. The liver is also supplied with arterial blood through the proper hepatic branch of the celiac trunk.

The gall bladder is located in the right vertical groove of the H-shaped hepatic portal or root of the liver (on the visceral surface of the liver). It functions to concentrate and store bile.

The cystic duct is the excretory duct of the gall bladder, and it joins the common hepatic duct (which is formed from the union of the left and right hepatic ducts) to form the common bile duct. The common hepatic duct attaches and empties into the descending or second part of the duodenum.

The pancreas is composed of a head, neck, body, and tail. The pancreas is located in the C-shaped concavity of the duodenum, and the tail reaches the visceral surface of the spleen. It is centrally located and can be seen extending horizontally across the abdomen in the transpyloric region at approximately the first lumbar vertebra (L1).

The pancreas is both endocrine and exocrine in function, producing pancreatic enzymes as well as the hormone insulin. The islet pancreatic cells secrete insulin.

The pancreas contains both main and secondary pancreatic ducts, which empty pancreatic enzymes into the second part of the duodenum during digestion.

Hormones of the intestinal mucosa include secretin, gastrin, cholecystokinin, and enterocrinin.

Physiology of Digestion

Digestion is the process of breaking down large pieces of ingested food into simple molecules that can be absorbed by the mucosa and lymphatic and blood vessels of the gastrointestinal (GI) tract (stomach and small and large intestines).

Digestion begins in the oral cavity or mouth, where coarse and complex carbohydrates are broken down into smaller particles and mixed with saliva (containing salivary amylase), which transforms them into simpler carbohydrates. Mastication breaks down large chunks of animal and plant food materials (proteins, fats, carbohydrates) into smaller units. Food is forced into the stomach by smooth and skeletal arranged muscle, which lines the esophagus.

Stomach

The bolus of food is thoroughly mixed with gastric juices (primarily hydrochloric acid) in the stomach before it is released into the small intestine through the gastroduodenal sphincter. A major part of digestion occurs in the stomach, where hydrochloric acid is secreted through the gastric mucosal glands under the influence of the vagus nerve.

The regions of the stomach include the cardiac, fundic, corpus (body), and pyloric regions.

The mucosa consists of a lining of simple columnar epithelium and the lamina propria. It contains numerous regionally presented gastric and mucous glands.

The muscularis of the stomach contains three layers of smooth muscle. The lesser curvature of the stomach is connected to the visceral surface of the liver by a reflection of peritoneum called the *hepatogastric ligament* (lesser omentum). The greater omentum connects the greater curvature to the transverse colon.

For clinical purposes, the esophageal hiatus of the diaphragm is often the site of hiatal hernias of the fundus and cardiac regions of the stomach that project up into the posterior mediastinum, thereby facilitating gastric acid reflux into the esophagus and possible precancerous conditions. A vagotomy can be performed to alleviate excessive or uncontrolled hydrochloric acid secretion through the gastric glands.

Small Intestine

The small intestine is roughly two meters long and is composed of the duodenum, jejunum, and ileum.

Duodenum

The duodenum is the first part of the small intestine, and its name literally means 12 fingers. The C-shaped arrangement of the duodenum encloses the head of the pancreas.

The duodenum has four regional components: superior, descending, inferior, and ascending.

The second part of the duodenum receives both the common bile and the main pancreatic ducts through the hepatopancreatic ampulla. In contrast to the acidity of the stomach, the chemical environment of the duodenum is basic.

Jejunum

The jejunum is the second region of the small intestine. It contains numerous mucosal villi but no submucosal glands.

It occupies roughly two-fifths of the remaining small intestine. It is located in the upper right zone of the infracolic region.

Ileum

The ileum is the terminal three-fifths of the small intestine and is situated in the lower right region of the infracolic area, beyond the duodenum. Its submucosa contains numerous lymph nodules, which are referred to as *Peyer's patches.* It terminates at the ileocecal junction in the lower right quadrant of the abdomen.

Large Intestine

The large intestine is 1.5 meters long. It functions to remove water, store and compact fecal materials, and absorb vitamins. The large bowel contains no villi and the connective tissue between its numerous intestinal glands is filled with many lymphocytes. The large intestine also contains mucosa, submucosa, muscularis externa, and serosa.

Regions of the colon

Regions of the colon include the cecum; appendix; ascending, transverse, and descending colons; sigmoid; rectum; and anus.

The *cecum* is sac-like and is located in the lower right quadrant. It is continuous with the ileum at the slit-like ileocecal valve.

The vermiform appendix is a worm-like diverticulum of the cecum and is attached to the cecum's medial and posterior surface. It is filled with lymph nodules and lymphocytes.

The ascending colon is retroperitoneal and is located on the right side of the infracolic region, where it is directed cranially to its termination at the right colic flexure at about the third lumbar vertebra (L3). The right colic flexure is the location where the ascending colon makes an abrupt turn to the left to become the transverse colon.

The transverse colon is a horizontally directed continuation of the ascending colon at the right colic flexure. It forms an abrupt downward turn in the left upper abdominal quadrant as the left colic (splenic) flexure in the region of the spleen and left kidney. The transverse colon is connected to the greater curvature of the stomach by several layers of visceral peritoneal reflections called the *greater omentum*.

The descending colon is also retroperitoneal and directed inferiorly along the left wall of the abdominal cavity until it reaches the pelvic brim to become the sigmoid colon.

The sigmoid colon is sinuous (S-shaped) and descends to the pelvis. It enters the left aspect of the pelvic brim, where it ultimately terminates.

The terminal region of the large intestine consists of the rectum and anus.

Selected Blood Supply to the Abdominal Viscera

The descending abdominal aorta contains three unpaired branches:

- The *celiac trunk* supplies the stomach and part of the pancreas, liver, and duodenum.
- The *superior mesenteric artery* supplies part of the duodenum, jejunum, ileum, cecum, ascending colon, and transverse colon.
- The *inferior mesenteric artery* supplies the descending and sigmoid colons.

2-11 Central Nervous System

The central nervous system includes the brain and spinal cord. The nervous system consists of two types of cells: the neuron and the neuroglia. Neurons are responsible for producing an action potential. Types of neurons include *multipolar, pseudounipolar,* and *bipolar.*

Neuron and Nerve Cell Processes

Neurons contain a perikaryon (cell body of a mature neuron) and two types of cytoplasmic cellular extensions or processes—axons and dendrites.

Axons are long nerve cell processes of uniform diameter that generally carry efferent neuronal activity away from the cell body to other neurons or effector organs such as the muscle cell. Axons may be myelinated or unmyelinated. Myelin is a protein-fatty insulating material. The action potential of myelinated axons is faster than that of unmyelinated axons.

Dendrites are shorter, branching neuronal processes that generally receive nerve impulses from other cells through synaptic junctions.

The change of the resting potential to the action potential of the axon is facilitated by the movement of sodium and potassium ions through gated sodium and potassium channels on the surface of the plasma membrane of the axon.

Synapse

Related neurons make connections to one another through specialized cell-to-cell contacts called *synapses*. In general, the axon terminal of one neuron synapses on the cell body or dendrites of another neuron.

The *neuronal synapse* is the point of contact between neurons in which an action potential is transmitted from one nerve cell to another.

Neurotransmitters

The axon terminal of a given cell releases membrane-bound packages of chemicals called *neurotransmitters* into the synaptic cleft. The cell membrane of the adjacent, stimulated cell dendrite contains receptors that can be activated by the neurotransmitter to create an action potential in the second neuron, thus facilitating transneuronal action potential generation.

A large array of neurotransmitters exists in the nervous system, such as acetylcholine, GABA (γ-aminobutyric acid), and serotonin. Anesthetic function may be facilitated by blocking neurotransmitter release at the neuronal synapse.

Glial cells are generally smaller nerve cells. They are mechanically and metabolically supportive and protective of neurons. Types of glial cells include astrocytes, oligodendrocytes, microglia, and ependymal cells.

Brain

The brain, containing the left and right hemispheres, is that part of the central nervous system located in the cranium. It can be organized and subdivided into several developmental, morphological, and functional regions.

Telencephalon

Cerebral cortex

The cerebral cortex is made up of an outer layer of gray matter (neurons and glial cells) and an inner layer of deep white matter (glial cells and myelinated axonal fibers). The cerebral cortex is convoluted and has many bump-like gyri and shallow groove-like indentations referred to as *sulci*.

The cerebral cortex is divided into several lobes that are designated and named according to overlying cranial bone: the frontal, parietal, temporal, occipital, and limbic lobes. The various lobes are separated by regularly occurring sulci (shallow grooves) or fissures (deeper grooves). Each cerebral hemisphere contains a cerebrospinal fluid–filled cavity called a *lateral ventricle*.

Frontal lobe

The frontal lobe functions to provide higher cortical activity or mental integration.

Parietal lobe

The parietal lobe is located laterally on the cerebral cortex and is found between the vertically oriented central sulcus and the postcentral parieto-occipital sulci. Between the precentral and postcentral sulci are the similarly located precentral gyrus, central sulcus, and postcentral gyrus. The parietal lobe processes sensory information including taste, touch, and temperature.

The *precentral gyrus* is motor in activity and sends descending axonal fibers through the basal ganglia, internal capsule, tegmentum of the mesencephalon, ventral pons, and pyramids of the medulla, where they cross to the opposite side of the brain before terminating on the ventral horn gray matter of the spinal cord where they ultimately synapse on ventral horn lower motor cells. Ventral horn motor cells, in turn, send myelinated axons though spinal nerves to synapse on skeletal muscles of the body.

The *postcentral gyrus* is sensory (afferent) in function and receives the modalities of pain, temperature, and tactile (touch) from the skin, joints, and muscle and tendon spindles from peripheral nerve receptors. The peripheral nerve receptors send such sensations upward through the spinal nerve, dorsal roots, ascending tracts of the spinal cord, medulla, pons, mesencephalon, and internal capsule and finally to the cortex of the postcentral gyrus, where they synapse and are consciously appreciated.

Reading comprehension and auditory elucidation are also associated with the parietal lobe. The loss of such abilities is termed *dyslexia* and *aphasia*.

Temporal lobe

The temporal lobe functions in language, memory, and auditory information processing. It contains the deep gray matter amygdala nucleus. This structure is an important emotional center and is closely associated with the hippocampus, an important learning and memory module.

Occipital lobe

The occipital lobe is considered a primary and secondary visual center where light comes into consciousness.

Limbic lobe

The limbic lobe is closely related to the amygdala and is concerned with emotional expressions such as fear, aversion, and attraction.

Brain stem

The brain stem includes the diencephalon, mesencephalon, metencephalon, and medulla oblongata.

Diencephalon

The diencephalon (or in-between brain region) is located in the gray matter of the lateral wall of the third ventricle. It is subdivided into the dorsal thalamus and hypothalamus.

The *dorsal thalamus* is an important synaptic center that receives axons ascending from lower levels to the cerebral cortex. It also projects other cell fibers, which originate from the cerebral cortex, in descending pathways to lower levels of the brain stem and the spinal cord. Pain comes into consciousness at thalamic levels.

The *hypothalamus* is situated ventral to the dorsal thalamus; is closely related to the pituitary gland; and functions to regulate a plethora of hormones and several visceral activities such as appetite, thirst, sex drive, electrolyte balance, and blood sugar. Malfunctions of the hypothalamus have been suggested in anorexia nervosa, obesity, and precocious puberty.

Mesencephalon

The mesencephalon (or midbrain) is the region between the diencephalon and the pons. It contains a roof called the *tectum* (superior and inferior colliculi) and a floor called the *tegmentum* (cerebral peduncles).

Metencephalon

Pons

The word *pons* means bridge, and the pons connects the midbrain (mesencephalon) and the medulla oblongata. The trigeminal nerve connects to the lateral surface of the pons, and it has important connections to the cerebellum, mesencephalon, and medulla.

This region contains a mixture of ascending fibers of various origins called the *reticular formation* and major motor and sensory nuclei in addition to important ascending and descending axonal pathways.

Myelencephalon

Medulla oblongata

The medulla oblongata is the most caudal component of the brain stem. It contains nuclei that are related to control of cardiac function and respiration. Developmental defects of this nuclear complex have been implicated in sudden infant death syndrome.

The medulla oblongata contains many motor and sensory nuclei associated with cranial nerves. Ascending axons carrying sensory information from cervical and lumbar spinal cord levels synapse on the gracilis and cuneatus nuclei, and descending motor axons cross to the opposite side in the motor decussations.

The glossopharyngeal, vagus, and spinal accessory cranial nerves are attached to the medulla oblongata, which contains important sensory relay nuclei that send axons to the thalamus and cortex.

Cranial Nerves

Twelve pairs of cranial nerves are attached to the brain. Some are purely sensory and receive only afferent information. Other cranial nerves are all motor and provide efferent impulses to effector organs such as skeletal, cardiac, and smooth muscles and glands. Several cranial nerves are mixed and provide motor output to effector organs and receive sensory information from peripherally situated receptors.

Cranial nerves are designated by Roman numerals: olfactory (I), optic (II), oculomotor (III), trochlear (IV), trigeminal (V), abducens (VI), facial (VII), auditory (VIII), glossopharyngeal (IX), vagus (X), spinal accessory (XI), and hypoglossal (XII).

Spinal Cord

The spinal cord is connected cephalically to the brain by the medulla oblongata in the region of the foramen magnum and extends caudally to the level of the second lumbar vertebra. It consists of an outer layer of white matter and an inner core of gray matter.

Deep in the gray matter is a space housing cerebrospinal fluid called the *central canal*. The deeper gray matter can be organized physiologically into sensory dorsal horn and ventral motor horn regions. Thoracic regions of the spinal cord gray matter contain a lateral horn that contains motor cells involved in the sympathetic division of the autonomic nervous system. The spinal cord contains several reflex pathways for movement of the extremities.

Thirty-one pairs of spinal nerves are attached bilaterally to the spinal cord. More distally, each pair of dorsal and ventral roots unite to form a single mixed (sensory–motor) spinal nerve. Dorsal root fibers are efferent or sensory. In general, dorsal roots contain a dorsal root (sensory) ganglion. Ventral root fibers are motor or efferent.

2-12 Endocrine System

The endocrine system consists of ductless glands that secrete hormones directly into the bloodstream. The major endocrine glands are the pituitary gland, thyroid gland, parathyroid glands, suprarenal gland, and ovaries (testes in the male).

Pituitary Gland

The pituitary gland has classically been called the *master gland* because it releases hormones (releasing factors), which stimulate other ductless glands to increase or decrease their hormonal production.

Subdivisions of the pituitary gland include the adenohypophysis and the neurohypophysis. Hormones produced by the anterior pituitary (adenohypophysis) include follicular-stimulating hormone, thyrotrophic-stimulating hormone, growth hormone (somatotropic hormone), luteinizing hormone, interstitial cell-stimulating hormone, prolactin, and adrenocorticotrophic hormone. Hormones of the posterior lobe (neurohypophysis) include vasopressin and oxytocin.

Thyroid Gland

The thyroid gland is well encapsulated by connective tissue; is bowtie shaped; and consists of two lateral lobes and a connecting region, or isthmus. It is located in the anterior neck region anterior to the trachea. Thyroid-stimulating hormone is released from the anterior lobe of the pituitary into the bloodstream, where it travels to the thyroid gland and stimulates it to produce thyroxin and calcitonin.

The structural unit of the thyroid gland is the *thyroid follicle*. Thyroid follicle cells secrete thyroxin into the colloid substance, where it is stored for future release into the bloodstream. Thyroxin regulates general cell metabolism.

Parathyroid Glands

Parathyroid glands are located in the connective tissue capsule on the posterior aspect of the thyroid gland. Parathyroid glands (usually four) secrete parathyroid hormone, which regulates the amount of calcium in the bloodstream.

Suprarenal Gland

The suprarenal (adrenal) gland is triangular shaped and is situated on the cranial aspect of each kidney. It contains an outer cortical region and an inner medullary zone. The adrenal cortex secretes glucocorticoids, mineralocorticoids, and androgens. Glucocorticoids control the level of glucose in the blood plasma, mineralocorticoids regulate the concentration of electrolytes, and androgens influence sexual expression and drive. Cells of the adrenal medulla are neuronal in appearance and secrete the hormones epinephrine (adrenaline) and norepinephrine.

Ovaries

The ovary is an endocrine gland in that its cortex contains ovarian follicles, which are made up of thecal and follicular cells. The ovarian follicle secretes estrogen and progesterone during the ovarian cycle. Both estrogen and progesterone are functional in facilitating the uterine cycle. Estrogen is responsible for sexual maturity of the female body. Progesterone maintains the lining of the uterus during pregnancy.

At puberty, primary follicles develop into growing follicles, under the influence of follicle-stimulating hormone from the anterior lobe of the pituitary gland, and they release a mature ovum every 14 to 15 days of the ovarian cycle.

2-13 Urinary System

Components of the urinary system include the kidneys, ureter, bladder, and urethra.

The kidneys are bean-shaped organs that are located anterior to the 11 and 12 ribs of the posterior abdominal region within the extraperitoneal fatty connective tissue and deep to the peritoneum. Each kidney contains a medially directed, concave-like hilus, which receives the renal pelvis, renal veins, and branches of the renal artery.

Components of the renal cortex are the renal corpuscle, proximal convoluted tubules, and distal convoluted tubules. Components of the renal medulla include Henle's loop and collecting ducts.

The renal pelvis is funnel shaped, and its apex narrows and connects to the ureter. The ureter directs urine to the bladder, where it is stored and released through the urethra to the environment.

The tubular nephron is the excretory part of the kidney (producing ultrafiltrate). It consists of the following discernible subunits: renal corpuscles, proximal convoluted tubule, proximal straight tubule, thin segment of Henle's loop, thick ascending straight tubule, and distal convoluted tubule.

The kidneys are supplied bilaterally with blood through renal arteries from the descending abdominal aorta. The renal vein is a tributary of the inferior vena cava.

2-14 Reproductive System

Male Reproductive System

Components of the male reproductive system include the testes, scrotum, and penis. The testes are the primary sex organs of the male reproductive system, and they are housed in the scrotum. They serve to produce spermatozoa and the male sex hormone testosterone. Testosterone is responsible for the manifestation of secondary sex characteristics in the male and is produced and released by the interstitial cells of Leydig, which are located in the highly vascular connective tissue of the testes.

Accessory structures of the male reproductive system include the following:

- In the *vas deferens,* sperm cells migrate to the epididymis, where they mature and are activated.
- The *seminal vesicles* are glands that secrete sugars, which nourish the sperm in the male reproductive tract.
- The *ejaculatory ducts* are tubules that traverse the prostate gland and direct sperm into the urethra.
- The *prostate gland* is a mucous-secreting, pear-shaped structure that is located at the neck of the bladder, where it surrounds the urethra.
- The *Cowper's glands* are located in the perineum, where they produce an oily secretion.

Female Reproductive System

The female reproductive system consists of the ovaries, fallopian (uterine) tubes, uterus, vagina, labia majora, labia minora, and clitoris.

The ovaries are the primary organs of female reproduction. They are located internally in the pelvis and can be subdivided into an inner medulla and an outer cortex. The ovarian cortex contains germ cells, which are located in cellular enclosures called *follicles.*

The ovarian cycle can be summarized as follows:

- Mature follicular cells (and associated thecal cells) secrete female sex hormones in response to the presence of follicle-stimulating hormone from the anterior pituitary gland.
- Estrogen and progesterone are the primary female sex hormones produced by sexually mature ovaries.
- At puberty, primitive follicles begin to develop into mature follicles containing mature ovum or eggs.
- A mature ovum is released each month during the midpoint of the female ovarian–menstrual cycle of 28–30 days.

The buildup, subsequent deterioration, and final shedding of the uterine endometrium is called the *uterine cycle* and is facilitated and coordinated by the rise and fall of estrogen and progesterone in the ovarian cortex.

Hormonal contraception is based on the chronic presence of progesterone and estrogen hormones that prevent ovulation.

2-15 Body Fluids and Electrolytes

Electrolytes are charged minerals found in body fluids. Common electrolytes include sodium, potassium, calcium, chloride, and phosphate. Generally, electrolytes are obtained from foods and liquids that are ingested as part of the normal diet.

Normal electrolyte levels are maintained by the kidney (excretion) and the GI tract (absorption). The normal level for a given electrolyte can become elevated or depressed because of disease, medication, or abnormal diet.

Overhydration and Dehydration

The amount of body fluid and its electrolyte content constantly changes because of urination, sweating, vomiting, hormonal regulation, defecation, and hemorrhage.

Overhydration is a condition in which too much water is located in the body (blood vessels or connective tissue), resulting in swelling or edema.

Dehydration is the reverse condition of overhydration and is characterized by too little water in tissue fluid and blood vessels. Dehydration can lead to low blood pressure and can compromise the body's ability to sweat. It may lead to mental confusion and disorientation. It may be treated by the oral or intravenous provision of water and electrolytes.

Electrolyte Nomenclature

The following terminology is associated with electrolytes:

- The prefix *hypo-* indicates not enough or too little of a given electrolyte, and the prefix *hyper-* represents too much of a given electrolyte.
- *Kalemia* denotes potassium, and *natremia* denotes sodium.
- *Hyponatremia* is a low level of sodium, whereas *hypernatremia* is a high level of sodium.
- *Hypokalemia* is a condition in which the potassium level is low and may be the result of the use of diuretics, which cause the kidneys to excrete excess potassium.
- *Hyperkalemia* is a condition in which potassium is high. It is caused by the administration of medications that reduce the amount of potassium excreted by the kidneys or the overuse of potassium supplement medication.
- *Hypocalcemia* is a condition of low calcium. This condition can result from the low production of parathyroid hormone or low levels of vitamin D.
- *Hypercalcemia* is a condition of high calcium. It can result from a high level of parathyroid hormone or from bone cancer.

2-16 Cell Structure, Organization, and Physiology

There are three types of living units: prokaryotic cells, eukaryotic cells, and viruses.

Prokaryotic cells are those that lack a membrane-bound nucleus. This cell type contains deoxyribonucleic acid (DNA), which is organized into circular loops called *plasmids*. Bacteria and blue-green algae are examples of prokaryotic cells. They are generally round, rod shaped, or spiral shaped; divide by binary fission; and are only 1–2 micrometers in diameter.

Eukaryotic organisms have nuclear materials that are bound by membranes (nuclear membranes), and they can be subdivided into animal and plant cells. Eukaryotic cells also contain small intracellular, organ-like structures referred to as *organelles*.

Viruses consist of nucleic acids surrounded by a protein covering or shell.

Cellular organelles include the nucleus, mitochondria, endoplasmic reticulum (smooth and rough), vesicles, centrioles, lysosomes, and chloroplasts. Chloroplasts and the cell wall are found only in plant cells.

Cell Membrane

The *cell membrane* consists of a lipid bilayer studded by transmembrane proteins, which may be involved in the transportation of materials into and outside of the cell. *Integral proteins* are transmembrane proteins that may act as channels for the transportation of ions and water. *Peripheral proteins* are located on the cytoplasmic side of the cell membrane and may be involved in maintaining the cell shape.

Integral proteins are attached to carbohydrates that extend from the external surface of the cell membrane as a fuzzy coat or *glycocalyx*.

Nucleus

The *nucleus* is a porous, double-unit membrane-bound structure generally located at the center of the cell. It stores, transfers, and expresses genetic information required for protein synthesis necessary for the morphology and function of the cell. It contains DNA-protein strands called *chromatin*.

Chromatin may exist as euchromatin (active and thin) or heterochromatin (inactive and condensed). Chromatin condenses during cell division to form chromosomes.

Nucleolus

The *nucleolus* consists of ribonucleic acid (RNA), DNA, and protein and is involved in ribosome production. It is located within the nucleus and is not bound by a unit membrane.

Ribosomes

Ribosomes are special units of rRNA (ribosomal RNA) and protein that are formed in the nucleus but perform their activity in the cytoplasm. They are non-membrane-bound structures that are involved in the translation of mRNA (messenger RNA) into protein.

Free ribosomes are located in the cytoplasm and are not associated with the endoplasmic reticulum. Ribosomes also may be located on the surface of the endoplasmic reticulum.

Endoplasmic Reticulum

The *endoplasmic reticulum* is a single membrane structure that may or may not contain ribosomes on its surface. When its membranes are devoid of ribosomes, it is called the *smooth endoplasmic reticulum* and is often involved in lipid metabolism. When it contains ribosomes on its membranes, it is called *rough endoplasmic reticulum* and is involved with protein translation.

Golgi Complex

The *Golgi complex* consists of a stack of flattened membranes and vesicles that sort various protein and carbohydrate complexes.

Mitochondria

Mitochondria are round or elongated double-walled membrane structures involved in energy production as adenosine triphosphate. Mitochondria contain DNA in the form of mitochondrial genes.

Lysosomes

Lysosomes are enzyme-filled vesicles bound by a single membrane that facilitate intracellular digestion of proteins and carbohydrates.

Filaments

Filaments are protein strands or tubes that form the cytoskeleton and certain contractile elements of the cell (actin and myosin).

Microtubules

Microtubules form the mitotic spindle.

Vesicles

Vesicles are surrounded by a single membrane and are involved in storage and secretion.

Centrioles

Centrioles consist of several tubular structures that produce other microtubules and are highly active in cell division and maintenance of the cytoskeleton.

2-17 Questions

1. Which of the following is the outermost layer of the skin's epidermis?
   - A. Stratum corneum
   - B. Dermis
   - C. Stratum basale
   - D. Hypodermis

2. The I-band of skeletal muscle contains which of the following myofilaments?
   - A. Myosin
   - B. Actin
   - C. Tubulin
   - D. Collagen

3. Bones are usually covered on the surface by a highly vascular, dense connective envelope. Which of the following terms describes this envelope?
   - A. Periosteum
   - B. Endosteum
   - C. Dura mater
   - D. Synapse

4. Which of the following cells build bone matrix?
   - A. Osteocyte
   - B. Osteoblast
   - C. Osteoclast
   - D. Glial cell

5. The intervertebral disc is located in which of the following regions of the body?
   - A. Stomach
   - B. Sternum
   - C. Bony spine
   - D. Epidermis of the skin

6. The superior vena cava empties deoxygenated blood into which of the following regions of the heart?
   - A. Right atrium
   - B. Right ventricle
   - C. Left atrium
   - D. Left ventricle

7. The sinoatrial node (natural pacemaker) is located in which of the following regions?
   - A. Right atrium
   - B. Right ventricle
   - C. Left atrium
   - D. Left ventricle

8. Which of the following are lymphatic organs? (Mark all that apply.)
   - A. Spleen
   - B. Cecum
   - C. Tonsil
   - D. Thymus gland

9. Digestion of carbohydrates begins in which of the following regions?
   - A. Sigmoid colon
   - B. Stomach
   - C. Duodenum
   - D. Mouth

10. Which of the following is a large blood vessel that delivers deoxygenated blood to the liver?
    - A. Splenic artery
    - B. Portal vein
    - C. Thoracic duct
    - D. Celiac trunk

11. Which of these glands is both endocrine and exocrine in function?
    - A. Pancreas
    - B. Thymus gland
    - C. Adrenal gland
    - D. Pituitary gland

12. Which of the following kidney structures serves as the excretory function by producing ultrafiltrate?
    - A. Hilus
    - B. Renal pelvis
    - C. Tubular nephron
    - D. Renal cortex

13. Which of the following is a neurotransmitter that is released from the axon terminal of the neuromuscular junction?
    - A. Estrogen
    - B. Substance P
    - C. Acetylcholine
    - D. GABA

14. The ovarian follicle produces and secretes which of the following hormones?

A. Testosterone
B. Estrogen
C. Growth hormone
D. Follicle-stimulating hormone (FSH)

15. Which of the following regions of the brain is responsible for higher integration, planning, and thinking?

A. Frontal lobe
B. Occipital lobe
C. Thalamus
D. Medulla oblongata

16. Gaseous oxygen and carbon dioxide are exchanged in which level of the respiratory system?

A. Trachea
B. Bronchi
C. Pulmonary alveoli
D. Larynx

17. Which of the following has classically been called the *master gland*?

A. Adrenal gland
B. Thyroid gland
C. Pancreas
D. Pituitary gland

18. Which organ helps to maintain electrolyte levels by controlling excretion?

A. Colon
B. Liver
C. Kidney
D. Heart

19. Which of these organs is the largest visceral organ?

A. Colon
B. Liver
C. Kidney
D. Heart

20. Which of these cellular organelles is the main difference between prokaryotic and eukaryotic cells?

A. Mitochondria
B. Cytoplasm
C. Nuclear membrane
D. Endoplasmic reticulum

2-18 Answers

1. **A.** The stratum corneum is the outermost layer. The dermis, stratum basale, and hypodermis are all lower levels of the skin.

2. **B.** The protein actin is the main myofilament in the I-band of skeletal muscle.

3. **A.** The periosteum covers the surface of bones.

4. **B.** Osteoblasts actively build bone matrix. Glial cells are located in the brain and help maintain the other neuronal cells.

5. **C.** Intervertebral discs are a component of the bony spine. The sternum is also a component of the skeleton, but it is located in the chest and is a component of the rib structure.

6. **A.** Deoxygenated blood from the body is delivered to the right atrium by the superior vena cava.

7. **A.** The sinoatrial node is located in the right atrium.

8. **A, C, D.** The spleen, tonsils, and thymus gland are all part of the lymphatic system. The cecum is part of the colon.

9. **D.** The enzyme amylase is secreted in the mouth and begins the digestion of carbohydrates.

10. **B.** The portal vein delivers deoxygenated blood and nutrients from the GI tract to the liver.

11. **A.** The pancreas is both endocrine (secreting insulin) and exocrine (secreting digestive enzymes) in function.

12. **C.** The tubular nephron is the functional unit of the kidney producing urine and removing waste from the blood.

13. **C.** Acetylcholine is the neurotransmitter in the axon terminal of the neuromuscular junction. Estrogen and substance P are hormones. GABA is a neurotransmitter, but it is mostly localized to the brain.

14. **B.** Estrogen is a main female hormone and is secreted by the ovarian follicle. Testosterone is the primary male hormone. Follicle-stimulating hormone is released from the anterior pituitary gland.

15. **A.** The frontal lobe of the brain is responsible for higher integration, planning, and thinking.

16. **C.** The pulmonary alveoli are the smallest air-filled part of the lung and are the site of gas exchange between the lungs and the blood.

17. **D.** The pituitary gland releases hormones that stimulate the other ductless glands and has been called the *master gland.*

18. **C.** The kidney maintains normal electrolyte levels by controlling excretion and reabsorption.

19. **B.** The liver is the largest visceral organ and is important in detoxifying the blood of pathogens and toxins.

20. **C.** Prokaryotic cells lack a nuclear membrane. In eukaryotic cells, the nuclear materials are located within a nuclear double-walled membrane.

2-19 Additional Resources

Drake R, Vogl R, Mitchell A. *Gray's Anatomy for Students.* 3rd ed. Philadelphia, PA: Elsevier; 2015.
Moore K, Dalley A, Agur AMR. *Clinically Oriented Anatomy.* 8th ed. Baltimore, MD: Wolters Kluwer; 2018.
Schottelius B, Schottelius D. *Textbook of Physiology.* 18th ed. Saint Louis, MO: C. V. Mosby; 1978.
Shier D, Butler J, Lewis R. *Hole's Essentials of Human Anatomy and Physiology.* 12th ed. Boston, MA: McGraw-Hill; 2015.
Van De Graaff K, Fox S. *Concepts of Human Anatomy and Physiology.* 5th ed. Dubuque, IA: Wm. C. Brown; 1999.
Widmaier EP, Raff H, Strang KT. *Vander's Human Physiology: The Mechanisms of Body Function.* 14th ed. New York, NY: McGraw-Hill; 2016.

Biochemistry

3

MICHAEL L. CHRISTENSEN

3-1 KEY POINTS

- The cell has a highly complex, redundant, and regulated molecular set of machineries that maintain the complexity of life.
- Amino acids are the building blocks of proteins.
- Protein structures have four elements: primary (linear amino acid sequence), secondary (alpha helices and beta-pleated sheets), tertiary (folding protein into 3-D shape), and quaternary (multisubunit protein complex).
- Enzymes are proteins that function as catalysts for the myriad reactions necessary to carry out cellular development, metabolism, growth, differentiation, regulation, and apoptosis.
- Enzymes are characterized by specificity, high rate of activity, affinity for their specific substrate (K_m), and the maximal rate of reaction when substrate is present in excess concentration (V_{max}).
- The Michaelis–Menten equation, $v = (V_{max})/(1 + K_m/[s]) = V_{max}[s]/(K_m + [s])$, mathematically describes enzyme activity. Plotting $1/v$ on the y axis versus $1/[s]$ on the x axis is used to determine K_m and V_{max}.
- Most vitamins and certain metals act as coenzymes that facilitate enzyme catalytic activity.
- Carbohydrates are a major source of energy and are stored as glycogen in the liver and muscle.
- Fatty acids are major sources of energy and are critical components of cellular membranes as phospholipids.
- A single nucleotide polymorphism (SNP) can lead to an alteration in the amino acid sequence of the resulting protein. An SNP can be a silent mutation or cause a change that results in a disease such as sickle cell anemia.
- The nucleotide units of deoxyribonucleic acid (DNA) and ribonucleic acid (RNA) have three basic components: a purine or pyrimidine base molecule, a sugar molecule, and a phosphoric acid molecule.
- Protein synthesis occurs on the ribosome where messenger RNA (mRNA) carries the message and directs the order of amino acids in the protein, transfer RNA (tRNA) delivers each amino acid per the code, and ribosomal RNA (rRNA) catalyzes the assembly of amino acids into protein.
- The biochemical reactions in the nucleus include replication of DNA, repair of damaged DNA, transcription of DNA into RNA, and processing of RNA into a specific mRNA.
- Monoclonal antibodies produced by recombinant technology are one of the largest areas of new therapeutics currently in development.

3-2 STUDY GUIDE CHECKLIST

The following topics may guide your study of this subject area:

- ☐ Awareness of the four major biomolecules: carbohydrates, amino acids, fatty acids, and nucleotides
- ☐ Understanding that the biomolecules are building blocks for polysaccharides, proteins, lipids, and polynucleotides
- ☐ Description of the major groupings of amino acids
- ☐ Understanding of glucose metabolism
- ☐ Description of water and fat-soluble vitamin deficiencies or diseases
- ☐ Application of enzyme kinetic calculation as it relates to drug metabolism and clearance
- ☐ Description of the steps in carbohydrate metabolism and energy production
- ☐ Familiarity with nucleic acid metabolism

3-3 Introduction

Biochemistry is the study of the biological and chemical processes within living organisms. Life at the cellular level is highly complex and includes redundant processes that involve highly regulated macromolecular and molecular sets of machineries that give rise to the complexity of life. This chapter reviews the biomolecules, macromolecules, and macromolecular systems that are responsible for this machinery, regulation, and communication.

The major four groups of biomolecules are amino acids, fatty acids, carbohydrates, and nucleic acids. These building blocks, in turn, form the major macromolecules: proteins and enzymes, lipids, glycogen, ribonucleic acid (RNA), and deoxyribonucleic acid (DNA). Enzymes (proteins that form cellular machinery) have a primary role as catalysts of the myriad reactions necessary to carry out cellular growth, metabolism, differentiation, regulation, and ultimately, cell death (apoptosis). The critical metabolic pathways of energy production are from sugars and fatty acids metabolism. Nucleic acid metabolism includes DNA replication and repair; RNA production, control, degradation, and structural roles; and protein synthesis. The area of recombinant DNA technology is introduced as it relates to therapeutic protein production.

3-4 Chemistry of Biomacromolecules: Proteins, Carbohydrates, Fatty Acids and Lipids, and DNA and RNA

Proteins

Amino acids are the building blocks of proteins. After water, protein is the most abundant molecule in the body. Proteins form the structural backbone of cells and tissues and are responsible for enzymatic reactions, membrane transport, hormonal regulation of body function, immune system, and transmission of cell-to-cell messages. Table 3-1 lists the 20 amino acids encoded for mammalian DNA and incorporated into protein. The amino acids are listed by name, and their side-chain structure and three-letter and one-letter abbreviations are also included.

All amino acids contain an amino group and a carboxylic acid group and fall into two large groupings—primary and secondary amines—depending on the structure of the amine group. The nitrogen atom in primary amines has only one bond to a carbon atom, whereas for secondary amines, the nitrogen atom is bonded to two carbon atoms.

Amino acids can be placed into major groups on the basis of their side-chain structure or on the basis of whether they need to be acquired in the diet (essential), can be produced in the body from essential amino acids (nonessential), or become essential under certain conditions (conditional). Amino acids are classified as follows:

- ***Small:*** Glycine (Gly) and alanine (Ala)
- ***Branched-chain:*** Valine (Val), leucine (Leu), and isoleucine (Ile)
- ***Aromatic:*** Phenylalanine (Phe), tyrosine (Tyr), and tryptophan (Trp)
- ***Sulfur:*** Cysteine (Cys) and methionine (Met)
- ***Neutral:*** Asparagine (Asn), glutamine (Gln), serine (Ser), and threonine (Thr)
- ***Acidic:*** Glutamate (Glu) and aspartate (Asp)
- ***Basic:*** Lysine (Lys), arginine (Arg), and histidine (His)

The nine essential amino acids are His, Ile, Leu, Lys, Met, Phe, Thr, Trp, and Val. They cannot be synthesized from other amino acids or dietary constituents. Nonessential amino acids include Ala, Arg, Asn, Asp, Cys, Glu, Gln, Gly, Tyr, and Ser. Adults can produce Tyr from Phe and Cys from Met. However, infants and young children have only a limited ability to make these conversions. Hence, Tyr and Cys are considered conditionally essential in this population.

TABLE 3-1. Common Protein-Incorporated Amino Acids

Amino acid	Side chain	Three-letter abbreviation	One-letter abbreviation
General structure 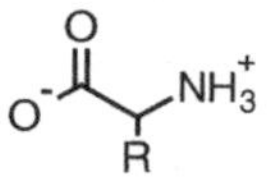	—R		
Alanine	$—CH_3$	Ala	A
Arginine	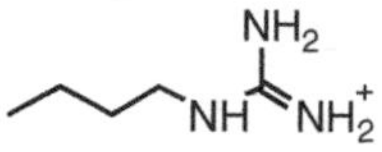	Arg	R
Asparagine	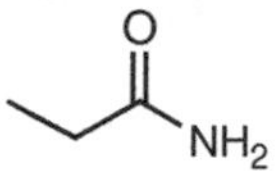	Asn	N
Aspartic acid (aspartate)	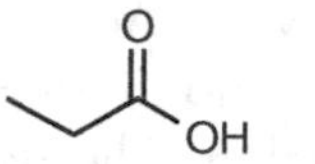	Asp	D
Cysteine	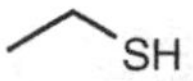	Cys	C
Glutamic acid (glutamate)	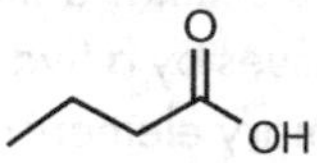	Glu	E
Glutamine	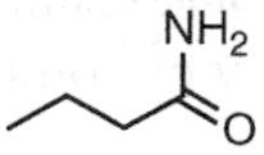	Gln	Q
Glycine	—H	Gly	G
Histidine	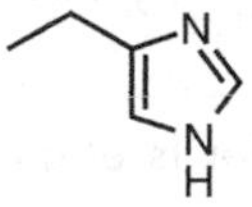	His	H
Isoleucine	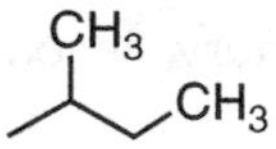	Ile	I
Leucine	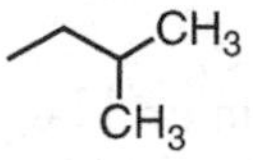	Leu	L
Lysine	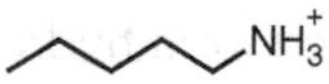	Lys	K
Methionine	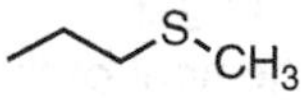	Met	M
Phenylalanine	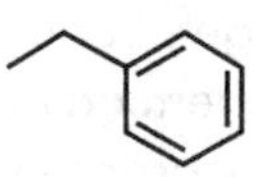	Phe	F
Proline[a]	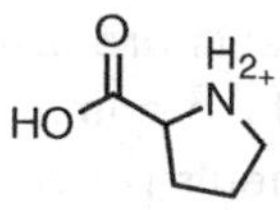	Pro	P
Serine	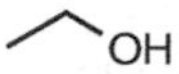	Ser	S
Threonine	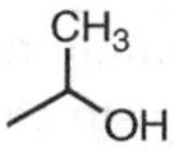	Thr	T

(continued)

TABLE 3-1. Common Protein-Incorporated Amino Acids *(Continued)*

Amino acid	Side chain	Three-letter abbreviation	One-letter abbreviation
Tryptophan	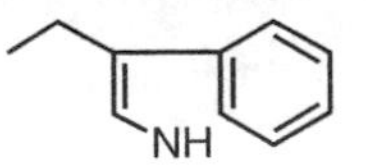	Trp	W
Tyrosine	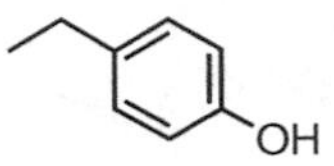	Tyr	Y
Valine	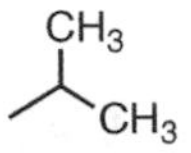	Val	V

a. For proline, the entire amino acid structure is shown.

Many amino acids are involved in critical metabolic pathways. Arginine, ornithine, and citrulline are the three amino acids of the urea cycle (conversion of ammonia to urea), which is the main pathway for excretion of nitrogen waste product from protein metabolism. The urea cycle is coordinated in the cytoplasm and in the mitochondria of the cell.

Another example is the tripeptide glutathione. It is a first-line cellular antioxidant formed from the amino acids glutamine, cysteine, and glycine. It is synthesized in all tissues by a two-step enzyme-mediated process.

A peptide bond formed between two amino acids is the primary element of peptide and protein structure. The formation of this bond is orchestrated at the cellular level by a very complex structure called the *ribosome* and involves several forms of RNA. However, the net chemistry of bond formation and hydrolysis can be easily depicted as

$$NH_2\text{-}CHR_1\text{-}COOH + NH_2\text{-}CHR_2\text{-}COOH \leftrightarrow NH_2\text{-}CHR_1\text{-}CONH\text{-}CHR_2\text{-}COOH + H_2O$$

Note that in the bond formation direction, a molecule of water is eliminated, whereas in the reverse (bond hydrolysis) direction, a molecule of water is inserted.

Protein and enzyme structure has four main elements: primary, secondary, tertiary, and quaternary (Figure 3-1 depicts these four elements of protein structure):

- *Primary structure* is the linear sequence of amino acids.
- *Secondary structure* is the first step in folding up the protein and begins with local groups of amino acids forming into two main structures: alpha helices are formed from predominantly hydrophilic amino acids, and beta-pleated sheets are largely formed from hydrophobic amino acids. These two sets of structures form largely through hydrogen bonding.
- *Tertiary structure* is the more complex folding and arrangement of these helices and sheets into a globular structure, which is held together through hydrogen bonds, ionic interactions, and disulfide bridges. Cysteine disulfide bonds provide some thermodynamic stability, but they mainly aid in proper protein folding. Tertiary structure may also incorporate non–amino acid components, such as metal ions, as a structural element. These elements are usually bonded to functional side-chain groups from amino acids in disparate parts of the primary sequence of amino acids. Thus, they can be structural elements or functional elements providing additional chemistry (in the case of enzymes and transport proteins).
- *Quaternary structure* is the combination of two or more individual protein chains to form a multisubunit protein complex. This structure is formed and maintained by hydrogen bonding, as well as by ionic and hydrophobic interactions. Quaternary structure of proteins allows greater regulation of transport function (i.e., hemoglobin and oxygen delivery) and enzyme activity (i.e., cooperativity and on–off control).

FIGURE 3-1. **Four Elements of Protein Structure**

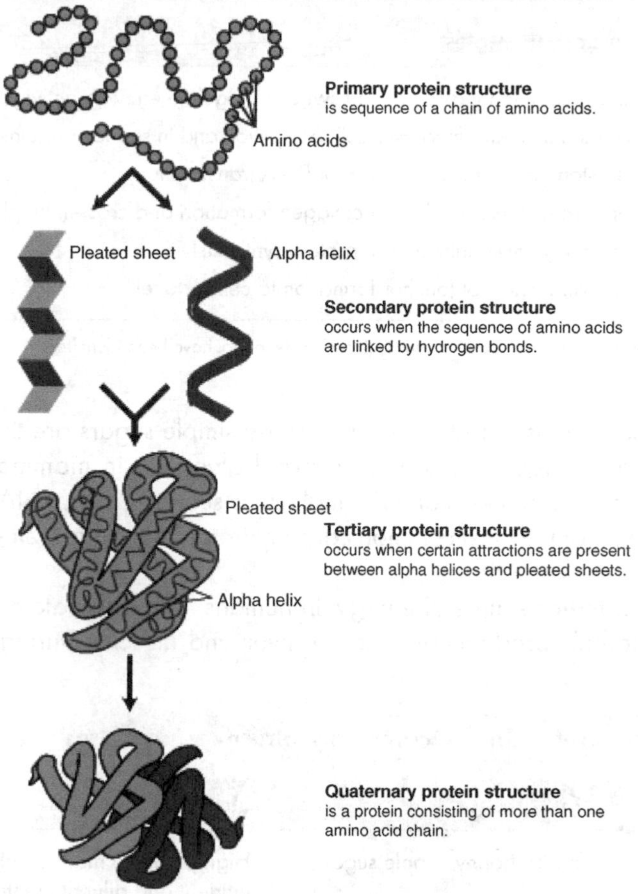
Primary protein structure
is sequence of a chain of amino acids.
Amino acids
Pleated sheet
Alpha helix
Secondary protein structure
occurs when the sequence of amino acids are linked by hydrogen bonds.
Pleated sheet
Tertiary protein structure
occurs when certain attractions are present between alpha helices and pleated sheets.
Alpha helix
Quaternary protein structure
is a protein consisting of more than one amino acid chain.

National Human Genome Research Institute (https://www.genome.gov/Glossary/Index.cfm?id=169).

Mutational changes in DNA can lead to abnormal proteins. Thus, a single nucleotide polymorphism (SNP) in the sequence of the coding DNA can lead to an alteration in the primary amino acid sequence of the resulting protein.

Sickle cell anemia is a good example of this type of alteration. Normal adult hemoglobin has a glutamic acid at the sixth position in the beta globin protein chain. Because of a single-point mutation (A–T), sickle cell patients have a valine at this position. This change in beta globin structure leads to a change in the overall hemoglobin (two alpha globin chains and two beta globin chains) structure, which leads to a "sickle" shape in the red blood cell and occasional blockage in the microvasculature (known as *sickle cell crisis*). Thus, a single change in a nucleotide in the DNA coding sequence can lead to a dramatic clinical effect.

In addition, many proteins undergo further modification after proper folding and assembly. These changes are termed post-translational modifications. Table 3-2 lists the most common of these modifications.

Although amino acids are the building blocks of protein, sugar molecules and fatty acids are the building blocks for other essential cellular components.

Carbohydrates

Carbohydrates (also called saccharides or sugars) are composed of only three elements—carbon, hydrogen, and oxygen—with the general chemical structure of $(CH_2O)_n$. The most common simple sugars are trioses ($C_3H_6O_3$, e.g., glyceraldehyde), pentoses ($C_5H_{10}O_5$, e.g., ribose and deoxyribose), and hexoses

TABLE 3-2. Common Post-Translational Modification of Specific Amino Acids[a]

Amino acids	Modification and examples
Ser, Thr, Tyr, Asp	Phosphorylation (commonly as an on–off switch to regulate enzyme activity)
Ser, Thr, Phe, Pro	Glycosylation (as a mechanism for cell–cell recognition and in surface proteins involved in signaling pathways)
His, Thr, Glu	Methylation (histone proteins and control of DNA transcription)
Lys, Asp, Pro, Tyr	Hydroxylation (Pro and Lys residues in collagen formation and cross-linking)
Amino terminus	Formylation or acetylation (initiation of protein synthesis)
Carboxyl terminus	Glycosylphosphatidylinositol (anchor formation to cell surface)

a. This list is only partial. To date, no post-translational modifications to Ala, Gly, Ile, or Val have been identified.

($C_6H_{12}O_6$, e.g., glucose, fructose, and galactose). These simple sugars are the building blocks for larger sugars used for cellular energy (starch in plants and glycogen in mammalians) or cellular structure (cellulose in plants), or as components of other molecules such as DNA, RNA, glycoproteins, and glycolipids. Table 3-3 lists some of the most common carbohydrates as well as their occurrence, gross structure, and uses.

Carbohydrates are a major source of energy. In humans, carbohydrate energy is stored as glycogen (the animal form of starch), predominantly in the liver and muscle. During fasting, glycogen can be

TABLE 3-3. Common Carbohydrates: Their Occurrences, Structures, and Uses

Carbohydrate	Occurrence	Structure and uses
D-glucose (dextrose), Glc	Fruits, honey, maple sugar	Highly soluble monosaccharide (MW = 180), used as nutrient and diluent in intravenous therapy
D-fructose, Fru	Fruits, honey, maple sugar	Soluble monosaccharide (MW = 180), some products for people with diabetes
Sucrose	Cane sugar, beet sugar	Soluble disaccharide of 1,2-linked Glc-Fru (MW = 360)
Lactose (milk sugar)	Milk and dairy products	Soluble disaccharide of 1,4-linked galactose-Glc
Amylose (plant starch)	Starchy plants and grains	Linear polymer of Glc units in 1,4 linkage (approximate MW = 10^5)
Amylopectin (plant starch)	Starchy plants and grains	Branched polymer of Glc units in 1,4 and 1,6 linkage (approximate MW = 10^4–10^5)
Glycogen (animal starch)	Liver, muscle	Branched polymer of Glc in 1,4 and 1,6 linkage (approximate MW = 10^5)
Cellulose	Plant cell walls, wheat bran	Linear polymer of Glc in 1,4 linkage, insoluble (approximate MW = 10^5–10^6)
Hemicellulose	Plant cell walls	Branched polymer of hexoses and pentoses, insoluble (approximate MW = 10^4)
Pectins	Fruits	Soluble linear polymers in 1,4 linkage of D-galacturonic acids, gel forming (MW = 10^4–10^5)
Carrageenan	Red seaweeds	Soluble linear polymer of disaccharides in 1,4 linkage, gel forming, component of many products (approximate MW = 10^4)
Maltodextrins	Usually corn	Partially hydrolyzed starch (corn or wheat), used in many medical foods
Corn syrup or corn syrup solids		Completely hydrolyzed starch (i.e., glucose units)

MW, molecular weight.

hydrolyzed to release glucose to maintain blood sugar levels. Fasting for 6–8 hours results in the body metabolizing glycogen stores, and then the body shifts to fat metabolism to meet energy needs.

Sugar molecules are also important in glycosylation, the post-translational modification of proteins. The specific scheme of glycosylation of cell surface proteins is essential to cell–cell recognition. A good example is the ABO human blood groups. Specific glycosylation of cell surface proteins (glycoproteins), as well as the same specific glycosylation of membrane lipids, is the base of the human blood groups. Figure 3-2 shows the specific groupings of carbohydrates that delineate the most common ABO human blood groups.

The glycosylation pattern shown is for red blood cell membrane proteins glycosylated at the Thr or Ser residues of specific membrane surface proteins. Glycosylation of membrane lipids also occurs.

Note that two genes control the addition of the last carbohydrate. Type A people express two copies of the gene that codes for A-pattern glycosylation. Type B people express two copies of the gene that codes for B-pattern glycosylation. AB people express one copy of A and one copy of B. Type O people express neither A- nor B-pattern genes.

Fatty Acids and Lipids

Lipids are water insoluble molecules that include fatty acids, cholesterol, essential vitamins, and glycerides. The glycerides are combinations of fatty acids esterified to a glycerol backbone. Monoglycerides have a single long-chain fatty acid attached by an ester linkage to a single hydroxyl group on glycerol, diglycerides have two long-chain fatty acids attached to glycerol, and triglycerides have all three hydroxyl positions on glycerol esterified to a fatty acid.

Lipids are structural components of cell membranes, the major storage form of energy (adipose tissue) and chemical messengers (steroid hormones). The basic unit of lipid is triglyceride, a glycerol backbone with three attached fatty acids. Fatty acids can be classified as short-chain (less than or equal to 5 carbons), medium-chain (6–12 carbons), long-chain (13–21 carbons), and very long-chain (greater than 22 carbons) fatty acids. Fatty acids are also classified on the basis of the number of double bonds—saturated (no double

FIGURE 3-2. Main Carbohydrate Elements of the Human ABO Blood Groups

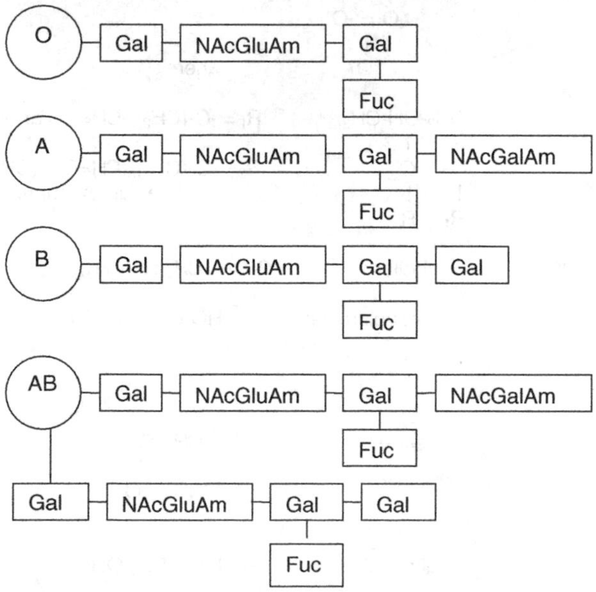

Adapted from Stamatoyannopoulos, Majerus, Perlmutter, Varmus, 2000.
Gal = galactose; NAcGluAm = N-acetyl-glucosamine; Fuc = fucose; NAcGalAm = N-acetylgalactosamine.

TABLE 3-4. Major Fatty Acids of Glycerophospholipids

Common names	Systemic names	Structural formulas
Myristic acid	n-tetradecanoic acid	CH_3-$(CH_2)_{12}$-COOH
Palmitic acid	n-hexadecenoic acid	CH_3-$(CH_2)_{14}$-COOH
Palmitoleic acid	cis-9-hexadecenoic acid	CH_3-$(CH_2)_5$-CH=CH-$(CH_2)_7$-COOH
Stearic acid	n-octadecanoic acid	CH_3-$(CH_2)_{16}$-COOH
Oleic acid	cis-9-octadecenoic acid	CH_3-$(CH_2)_7$-CH=CH-$(CH_2)_7$-COOH
Linoleic acid	cis, cis-9,12-octadecadienoic acid	CH_3-$(CH_2)_3$-$(CH_2$-CH=CH$)_2$-$(CH_2)_7$-COOH
Linolenic acid	cis, cis, cis-9,12,15-octadecatrienoic acid	CH_3-$(CH_2$-CH=CH$)_3$-$(CH_2)_7$-COOH
Arachidonic acid	cis, cis, cis, cis-5,8,11,14-eicosatetraenoic acid	CH_3-$(CH_2)_3$-$(CH_2$-CH=CH$)_4$-(CH_2)3-COOH

bonds), monounsaturated (1 double bond), and polyunsaturated (2 or more double bonds). Long-chain fatty acids, as phospholipids, are structural components of cell membranes. They are also the precursors for biologically active molecules important in cellular communication (prostaglandins and leukotrienes).

Phospholipids are diglycerides in which a phosphate group (plus other molecules) is linked to the glycerol backbone. For most phospholipids, the two fatty acid chains differ from each other. Table 3-4 lists the major fatty acids and Figure 3-3 depicts the structural elements of the most common phospholipids.

DNA and RNA

DNA contains the genetic code of the cell for the synthesis of specific proteins to build cells, tissues, and organs. The structure of DNA is a helical, double-stranded macromolecule in a complementary sequence.

FIGURE 3-3. Structure of Typical Phospholipids

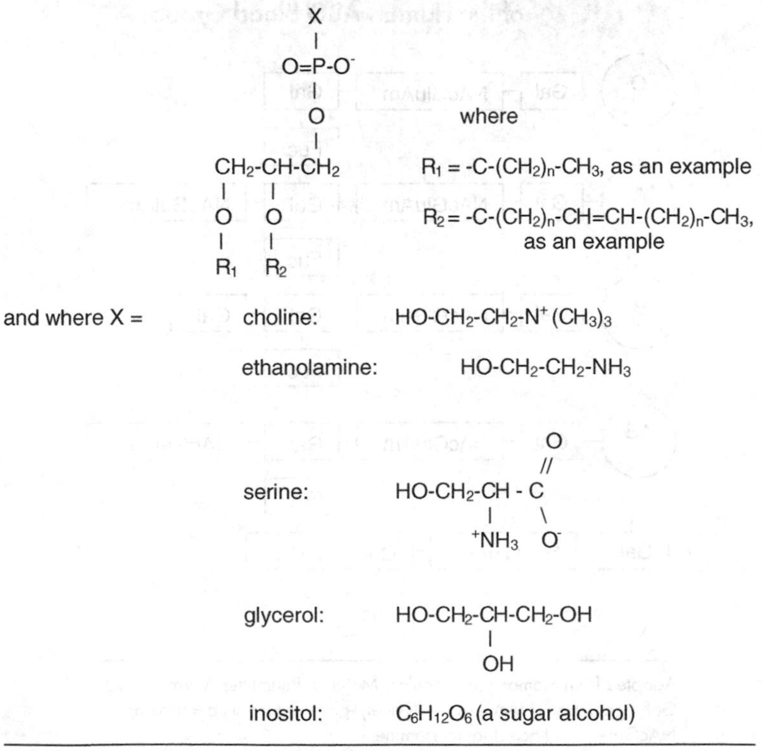

FIGURE 3-4. Chemical Structure of DNA and RNA Nucleotide Bases[a]

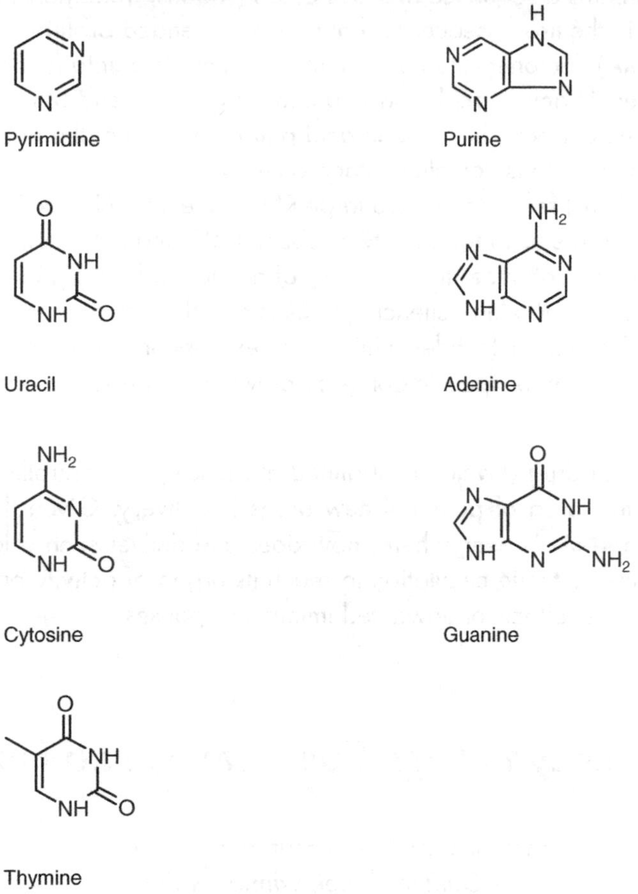

Based on Devlin 2010 and Metzler 2003.
a. Thymine (DNA) and uracil (RNA) differ only in a methyl group.

DNA consists of nucleosides that contain a pentose sugar (deoxyribose) and a nitrogenous base-pair (adenine–thymine [uracil in RNA], cytosine–guanine); when one to three phosphate groups are added, it is a nucleotide. Figure 3-4 shows the chemical structure of the DNA and RNA nucleotide bases. RNA has the pentose sugar ribose. During the process of gene expression, the genetic information stored in the base sequence of DNA molecules is transcribed into a base sequence of RNA; if this is messenger RNA, then the translation results in the amino acid sequence of a protein. Construction, maintenance, and transcription of the code (DNA → messenger RNA) as well as translation (messenger RNA → protein) involves polynucleotides (DNA and RNA).

DNA has the primary role of storing the information (genetic code) of the cell. The sections of DNA that carry specific genes are *exons*, while the sections of DNA that carry no genetic information are *introns*. Nearly all (99%) of the cell's DNA is found within the nucleus, and about 1% is found in the mitochondria.

The primary function of RNA is to transfer the genetic information in the nucleus to the cytoplasm where proteins are synthesized. About half of RNA is found in the ribosome, and only about 10% is in the nucleus. Three major types of unique structures perform specific functions in transcription and translation and control both transcription and translation. Following is a summary of the major groups of RNA and their functions:

- *Messenger RNA* (mRNA) is temporarily created for transferring a copy of the genetic information from DNA in the nucleus to the ribosome in the cytoplasm where it is translated into protein synthesis. Each gene produces a separate mRNA molecule when that specific protein is needed by the cell. In the formation of mRNA, DNA introns sequences have been eliminated, and the fused structure contains a sequence of triplet bases (codons) from the DNA exons, which code for each amino acid in the linear sequence that form the intended protein.

- *Transfer RNA* (tRNA) deciphers the code in mRNA. There is a unique tRNA for each amino acid. tRNA binds its specific amino acid, carrying it to the growing end of the polypeptide chain as mRNA instructs. The correct tRNA–amino acid pair is selected at the appropriate time because the tRNA three-base sequence is complementary to mRNA.
- *Ribosomal RNA* (rRNA) refers to the two large RNA molecules ($1–2 \times 10^6$ molecular weight) that bind a multitude of proteins to form the two subunit (30S and 50S) components of the ribosome. The ribosome complex catalyzes the assembly of amino acids into protein chains.
- *Small interfering RNA* (siRNA) or silencing RNA is a biological process in which RNA molecules that range from 18 to 25 nucleotides inhibit gene expression. siRNA can bind to mRNA, interfering with the expression of specific genes by preventing translation and enhancing mRNA degradation.

siRNA is an active area of drug development aimed at silencing or controlling genes. One of the main hurdles in developing this area of potential new drugs is delivery. Given that RNAse (the ubiquitous enzyme for hydrolyzing RNA) is everywhere, how does one deliver such a labile molecule and give it enough persistence in the systemic circulation to reach its organ of activity or target tissue? In addition, siRNA may induce off-target effects or unwanted immune responses.

3-5 Enzymes, Enzymology, Coenzymes, and Enzyme Kinetics

"Enzymes are the executors of the cell."
—*Günter Blobel, winner of the*
Nobel Prize in Physiology or Medicine, 1999

Enzymes are the macromolecular proteins that can catalyze chemical reactions; thus, they are the machinery of cellular metabolism. Enzymes are responsible for DNA synthesis and replication, they transcribe DNA into RNA, and they are essential to the process of translating the message of RNA into proteins.

Enzymes are also responsible for protein breakdown and for the conversion of substrate (carbohydrates and fatty acids) into cellular energy. They are responsible for the synthesis of hormones and hence for cell–cell communication.

Enzymes are indeed the machinery that makes cells work because they are also responsible for muscle contraction—the real work of an organism.

Enzymology

Enzymes are basically catalysts. They assist in chemical reactions but are not consumed in those reactions. They accelerate the chemistry of getting from substrate to product. They accomplish this (as do all catalysts) by lowering the activation energy (the energy barrier to get from substrate to product).

One of the characteristics of the chemistry of living things is that the chemistry must be done under relatively mild chemical conditions. Thus, most enzyme reactions must occur at reasonable temperatures, usually at one atmosphere of pressure, at relatively normal ionic concentrations (osmolarity), at reasonable ranges of pH (no harsh acid or base), and under a wide range of substrate (and product) concentrations. In addition, enzymes are very specific for the substrate on which they work and, hence, very specific in the products they help produce.

To accomplish these goals, enzymes work in a unique way. General catalysts (think of a platinum surface of a car's catalytic converter) do just that by assisting in a wide variety of reactions, such as breaking down a large hydrocarbon molecule into manageable pieces (i.e., octanes).

However, enzymes are very specific and have an optimal substrate and favored product. Although some enzymes (i.e., cytochromes) will work on a small number of substrates with very similar chemical makeup, many enzymes will work optimally on only a single substrate and produce only a single product. In the instances when an enzyme will work on two or more closely related chemicals, one reaction usually will be highly favored and the other reactions will occur at much slower rates.

The key elements of enzyme-assisted reactions are specificity (only one or a limited number of closely related substrates) and acceleration (reaction occurs manifold over what would normally occur).

How do enzymes accomplish these twin goals? Many explanations exist, but they fall into the following basic categories:

- ***Stearic or induced fit:*** The active site of the enzyme is spatially configured to accept only one substrate configuration or a very limited number. This model involves molecular size; orientation of reactive groups; ionic and hydrogen bonding; and possibly movement of the enzyme protein backbone or side-chain orientation (or "fit") during substrate binding, catalysis, or product release. This model has replaced the original lock-and-key model of enzyme activity.
- ***Localized chemistry:*** Some research suggests that the active site affords an environment for unique acceleration of the specific chemical reaction. As an example, the close, relatively nonsolvated interior hydrophobic core of an enzyme's active site might provide for unique acid–base chemistry.
- ***Transition state:*** The enzyme can form an intermediate with the substrate and, thus, lowers the energy barrier to the reaction of substrate going to product.

In addition, the enzyme can break down a relatively complicated chemical and change into relatively simple sequential steps (remove a hydrogen here, add a hydroxyl there, and so on). The proteolytic enzymes (trypsin and chymotrypsin) of normal digestion are good examples. They catalyze the hydrolysis of specific peptide bonds in the proteins of the diet.

The substrates, a water molecule and a peptide bond, are transformed into a free carboxylic acid group and a free amine group (i.e., two peptides). A reaction that normally would require 24 hours of strong acid at 110°C is accomplished in a microfraction of a second at physiological pH.

The rapid rate of the peptide bond hydrolysis (acceleration of the reaction) and the limitation to a small number of peptide bond types (specificity of the reaction) are the two hallmarks of enzyme catalysis. This miracle of catalytic chemistry takes place every day in the digestive tract.

Coenzymes

Coenzymes are small molecules that link with an enzyme and are required for the enzyme to express its catalytic activity. Coenzymes most often are associated with the active site of an enzyme or contribute to the chemistry of the enzyme-catalyzed reaction. The two major groups of coenzymes are vitamins and metals. An enzyme without its cofactor is an *apoenzyme* or *apoprotein*; an apoenzyme with its cofactor or cofactors is a *holoenzyme*.

In some instances—because the coenzyme binds to and then departs the enzyme after the catalyzed reaction—cofactors may appear to be more like substrates. In many cases, the coenzyme is covalently bound to the enzyme and functions in the chemistry at or near the active site. In a few cases, the actual role of the coenzyme seems to be as an intermediary between these two examples. For example, adenosine triphosphate (ATP), which behaves like a substrate in most cases, can act as a modulator of enzyme activity in some cases.

Many coenzymes are vitamins or are derived from vitamins. A good example is niacin (pyridine-3-carboxylic acid). Niacin can be converted into two key coenzymes, NAD and NADP. Each of these has a hydrogenated product (NADH and NADPH, respectively), and the respective ratios (NAD-to-NADH and

TABLE 3-5. Common Water-Soluble and Fat-Soluble Vitamins and Coenzymes

Vitamin[a]	Deficiency or disease	Good food sources	Coenzyme/reaction
Water soluble			
B_1 or thiamine	Beriberi	Seeds, nuts, legumes	TPP/oxidative decarboxylation
B_2 or riboflavin	Pellagra	Milks, eggs, organ meats	FAD/oxidation-reduction
B_3 or niacin (nicotinic acid)	Pellagra	Meats, nuts, legumes (but not corn)	NAD^+/oxidation-reduction
B_5 or pantothenic acid	n.a.	Yeast, grains, liver, egg yolk	Coenzyme A (CoA)/acyl group transfer
B_6 or pyridoxine	n.a.	Yeast, liver, wheat germ	PLP/decarboxylation, deamination
B_7 or biotin	n.a.	Tomato, egg yolk, yeast, soybeans	Biotin/carboxylation
B_{12} or cyanocobalamin	Anemia	Liver, eggs, cheese	Methylcobalamin/molecular rearrangements
Folic acid	Anemia	Yeast, liver, spinach	Tetrahydrofolate/one carbon transfer
C or ascorbic acid	Scurvy	Citrus fruits, cranberries, tomato	Reducing agent
Fat soluble			
A or retinoids	Night blindness	Fish liver oils, carrots, liver	Complexes with opsin
D or calciferols	Rickets	Fish liver oils, fortified milk	
E or tocopherols	n.a.	Green leafy vegetables, seeds, seed oils	
K or phylloquinones	Impaired blood clotting	Green leafy vegetables, egg yolk, cheese	Carboxylase/modified glutamate side chain

TPP, thiamine pyrophosphate; FAD, flavin adenine dinucleotide; NAD, nicotinamide adenine dinucleotide; PLP, pyridoxal phosphate; n.a., not applicable.
a. With the exception of vitamin D, all of these vitamins act as enzyme cofactors.

NADP-to-NADPH) are critical mediators of cellular energy production and indicators of oxidative-reductive capacity because of their role as coenzymes. Similarly, flavin mononucleotide and flavin adenine mononucleotide are the two coenzyme forms of the vitamin riboflavin.

Another form of coenzymes (although more appropriately labeled as *cofactors*) are the metals. Metals can be part of the active site or simply a stabilizing element of the enzyme tertiary structure. Metal ions as an element of the active site increase the type of chemistry available to facilitate reactions. The most common metals associated with enzymes as cofactors are zinc, copper, magnesium, manganese, and iron.

Table 3-5 lists the important water-soluble and fat-soluble vitamins, disease states associated with a deficiency in that vitamin, and coenzyme function. Table 3-5 also lists good food sources for that vitamin. Given the amount of processed foods in the typical Western diet, taking a daily multivitamin capsule is a reasonable recommendation.

Enzyme Kinetics

Although the chemistry (specificity and rate acceleration) of enzymes can be complicated and is not yet completely understood chemically, the kinetics of enzyme-catalyzed reactions can be easily expressed in mathematical terms.

Some of this same kinetic or mathematical treatment has important application to drug–receptor interactions and to the kinetics of drug metabolism and clearance. For example, the concept of K_m (first developed as the concentration of enzyme substrate that produces one-half of the maximal rate of enzyme activity) has direct application in the binding of drugs to cell surface receptors or to circulating proteins.

The velocity (V) or reaction rate of the enzyme-mediated reaction is expressed as

$$V = -d[s]/dt \text{ for the utilization of substrate, or}$$

$$V = -d[p]/dt \text{ for the production of product.}$$

The units of velocity are generally expressed as moles per liter per second (M s^{-1}) or more traditionally as moles per liter per minute (M min^{-1}). Obviously, they can be measured as substrate disappearance or product formation.

For a simple, first-order reaction (substrate goes to product without interaction of another molecule, except the enzyme), the velocity can be expressed as

$$V = -d[s]/dt = k[s]$$

where k is the rate constant and the velocity is proportional to the substrate concentration. Thus, the reaction rate (V) is maximal when the initial substrate concentration is in large excess over enzyme concentration and will decline as substrate is used up.

During the reaction, the concentration of substrate is constantly decreasing, so the $[s]$ at time $[t]$ can be expressed as any of the following equivalent expressions:

$$[s] = s_o^{-kt}, \ln[s_o]/[s] = kt, \text{ or } \log[s_o] - \log[s]$$
$$= kt/2{,}303$$

Enzyme Turnover Number and Specific Activity

If substrate molecules are in large excess over enzyme molecules, one can assume that all enzyme sites have substrate bound to the active site and that the reaction is proceeding at a maximal rate, V_{max}. Thus, $d[s]/dt = V_{max} = k[ES] = k[E_t]$, where E_t is the total amount of enzyme and consists of the total of free enzyme E plus enzyme–substrate complex ES.

Here, the constant k is known as the turnover number, or molecular activity. The enzyme activity is often expressed as units of activity per milligram of protein (specific activity). Also, the international unit of activity is defined as the amount of enzyme that produces, under optimal conditions of pH and temperature, 1 micromole of product per minute.

Relation of K_m and V_{max}, the Kinetic Parameters

Having defined V_{max} as the maximal rate (initial excess of substrate), we can now define K_m as that concentration of substrate where the rate of enzyme-mediated reaction is exactly one-half of V_{max}. K_m is also a measure of the affinity of an enzyme for the substrate. The Michaelis–Menten equation summarizes the initial reaction rate for a single substrate reaction as

$$v = (V_{max})/(1 + K_m/[s]) = V_{max}[s]/(K_m + [s])$$

The idealized plot of observed velocity versus initial substrate concentration is shown in Figure 3-5.

However, because of obvious experimental limitations (too many experiments at high substrate concentrations), this approach is never actually used. Instead, the Lineweaver–Burk (or double reciprocal) plot of $1/v$ versus $1/[s]$ is used to estimate K_m and V_{max}. The Michaelis–Menten equation is redone as shown in Figure 3-6.

FIGURE 3-5. Idealized Plot of Observed Velocity versus Initial Substrate Concentration

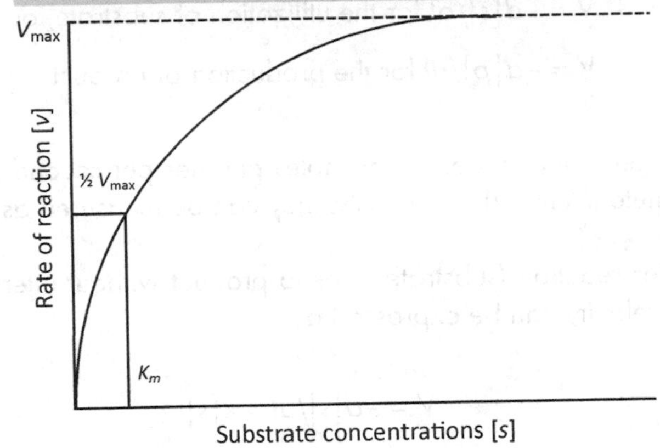

FIGURE 3-6. Revised Michaelis–Menten Equation

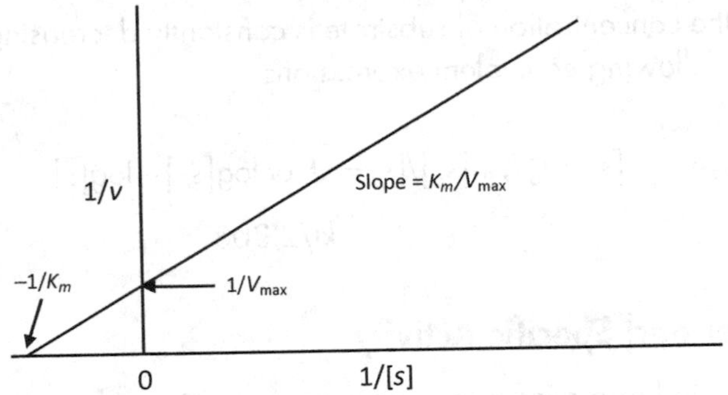

This revised equation is basically the familiar $y = mx + b$, where $b = 1/V_{max}$ (i.e., the y-axis intercept) and $m = K_m/V_{max}$ (i.e., the slope of the plot).

The Eadie–Hofstee plot improves the linearity of the enzyme kinetic plot approach by redoing the Michaelis–Menten equation as shown in Figure 3-7.

Note that the initial substrate concentration in each experiment can be chosen to give a more even spacing of data points and that both V_{max} and K_m can be estimated from intercept points and confirmed by the slope.

These concepts of enzyme kinetics can be applied directly to the kinetics of drug binding and drug clearance.

FIGURE 3-7. Michaelis–Menten Equation Incorporating Eadie–Hofstee Plot

$$v/[s] = (V_{max}/K_m) - v(1/K_m)$$

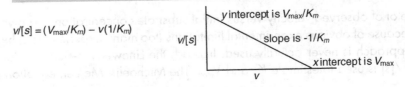

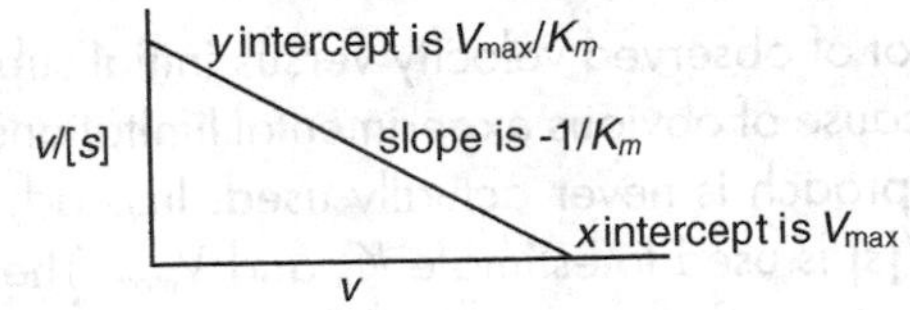

3-6 Metabolic Energy Production from Carbohydrates and Lipids

Metabolism is a cellular process of catabolism (extracting energy from nutrients) and anabolism (synthesizing new molecules from nutrients). ATP is the universal energy currency of the cell. The chemical energy stored in the phosphate bonds of ATP (ATP → ADP + Pi and ATP → AMP + PPi) drives mechanical work in muscle contraction, active cellular transport, and the synthesis and degradation of macromolecules. ATP, a nucleotide containing adenine, ribose, and triphosphate, is formed from the metabolism of carbohydrates, protein, and lipids.

Carbohydrate metabolism, or glycolysis, occurs in all human cells. The net reactions of glycolysis can be summarized as shown in Figure 3-8. Theoretically 38 moles of ATP are produced per mole of glucose by aerobic metabolism. This action generally does not happen because of ATP losses associated with moving pyruvate, phosphate, and ADP into the mitochondria as substrates for ATP synthesis. The likely maximum is about 30–32 ATP moles per mole of glucose.

Glucose can also be synthesized from noncarbohydrate precursors predominantly in the liver by a process known as gluconeogenesis. Precursor molecules include lactate, pyruvate, glycerol, and keto-acids from deaminated amino acids. Between eating, glucose levels are maintained by hydrolysis of glycogen. When liver glycogen becomes depleted, gluconeogenesis maintains glucose levels.

Fatty acids are oxidized in the matrix space of the mitochondria. The fatty acid is first primed with CoA-SH by an Acyl-CoA synthetase:

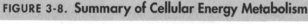

$$R\text{-}CH_2\text{-}CH_2\text{-}C(=O)\text{-}OH + ATP + CoA\text{-}SH \rightarrow$$

$$R\text{-}CH_2\text{-}CH_2\text{-}C(=O)\text{-}S\text{-}CoA + AMP + PPi$$

FIGURE 3-8. Summary of Cellular Energy Metabolism

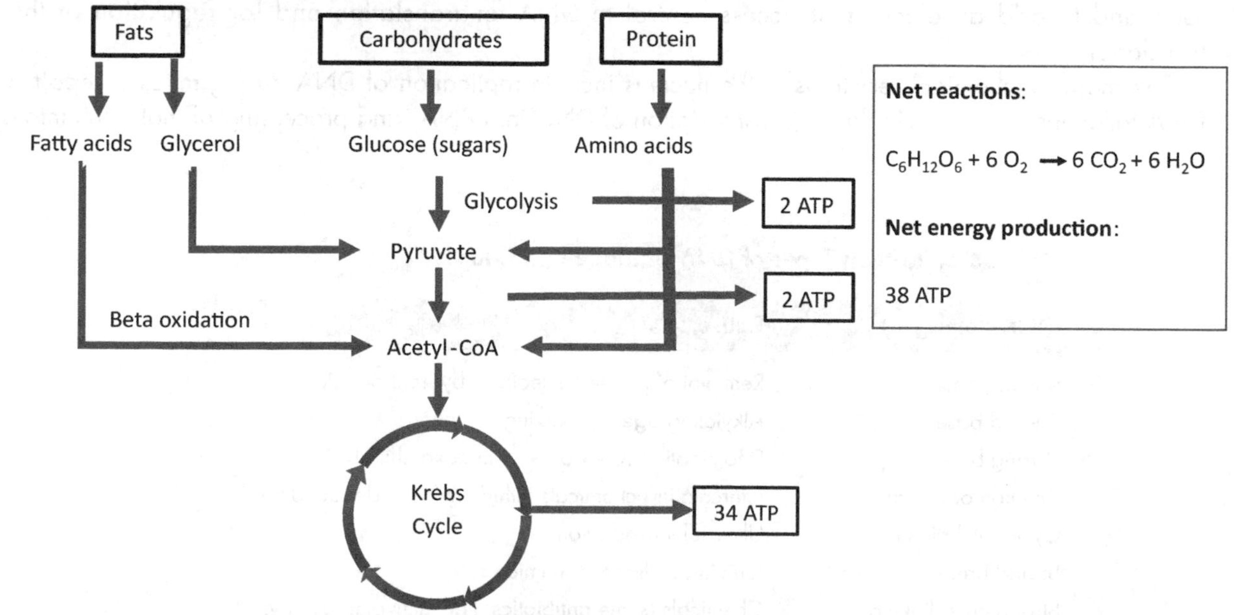

where ATP = adenosine triphosphate, AMP = adenosine monophosphate, PPi = inorganic diphosphate, and CoA = coenzyme A (derived from the vitamin pantothenic acid and cysteine). This product then enters the beta-oxidation cycle, where two carbon fragments are sequentially removed. Figure 3-8 summarizes this cycle. At each cycle, the original fatty acid is reduced by two carbons and the two carbon fragments (as acetyl-CoA units) are further oxidized in the citric acid cycle.

Long-chain fatty acids (C_{12} and larger) require carnitine for translocation into the mitochondrial matrix; medium-chain (C_6 and C_{10}) and short-chain (less than C_6) fatty acids are thought to be independent of carnitine for transport and metabolism.

If the original fatty acid molecule contains an even number of carbons, then acetyl-CoA is the only product. If the fatty acid chain contains an odd number of carbons, then the terminal product is propionyl-CoA.

Acetoacetate (4C), beta-hydroxybutyrate (4C), and acetone (from acetoacetate) are commonly listed as ketone bodies. Their concentrations can rise in ketosis or ketoacidosis in patients with diabetes mellitus. This condition can be life threatening. However, the brain and heart use ketone bodies as a direct energy source through reconversion to acetyl-CoA.

Acetyl-CoA plays a central role in energy production from amino acids, fatty acids, and carbohydrates. Acetyl-CoA can then be used to synthesize sterols, fatty acids, and ketone bodies, or it can be used in the tricarboxylic acid cycle to produce additional ATP.

3-7 Nucleic Acid Metabolism, DNA Replication and Repair, RNA Transcription, and Translation into Protein

A review of nucleic acid metabolism must begin with an understanding of the nucleus. The nucleus is the largest intracellular compartment and is surrounded by two membranes called the *nuclear envelope*. Within the nucleus is a subcompartment called the *nucleolus*.

DNA is contained within the nucleus as a highly organized and tightly coiled protein-RNA-DNA-containing complex called *chromatin*. The chromatin is further organized into chromosomes, which vary in number depending on the species.

The protein complex with DNA serves to compact the lengthy DNA molecules into a tighter, denser form and to add an element of access control to DNA for translation and for regulation of that translation.

The main biochemical reactions in the nucleus include replication of DNA during mitosis, repair of DNA following damage (Table 3-6), transcription of DNA into RNA, and processing of that RNA into a

TABLE 3-6. Known Types of DNA Damage and Causes

DNA damage	Cause
Missing base	Removal of purine nucleotides by heat or acid
Altered base	Alkylating agents, ionizing radiation
Wrong base	Deamination (C → U, A → hypoxanthine)
Deletion or insertion	Intercalating chemicals (ethidium bromide, acridine dyes)
Cyclobutyl dimer	Ultraviolet irradiation
Strand breaks	Ionizing radiation, chemicals
Strand cross-linking	Chemicals (some antibiotics, light-activated psoralens)

specific mRNA. Part of the processing of RNA occurs in the nucleolus. Translation of that message into protein (protein synthesis) occurs in the cytoplasm.

3-8 Recombinant DNA Technology

Synthesis of proteins occurs in the cytoplasm on a complex structure called a *ribosome*. The ribosome consists of two large lobes, termed 30S and 50S, formed of multiple proteins associated with ribosomal nucleic acids specific to each lobe. Ribosomes are usually attached to the rough endoreticulum.

Protein synthesis requires an mRNA, which specifies the sequence of amino acids, and a supply of charged tRNAs (the various aminoacyl tRNAs). Figure 3-9 depicts the transcription of DNA into an mRNA in the nucleus, the movement of the mRNA into the cytoplasm, and the translation of the mRNA sequence into a specific protein. Note the alignment of codons in the mRNA with the corresponding anticodon at the bottom of each tRNA.

FIGURE 3-9. Protein Synthesis

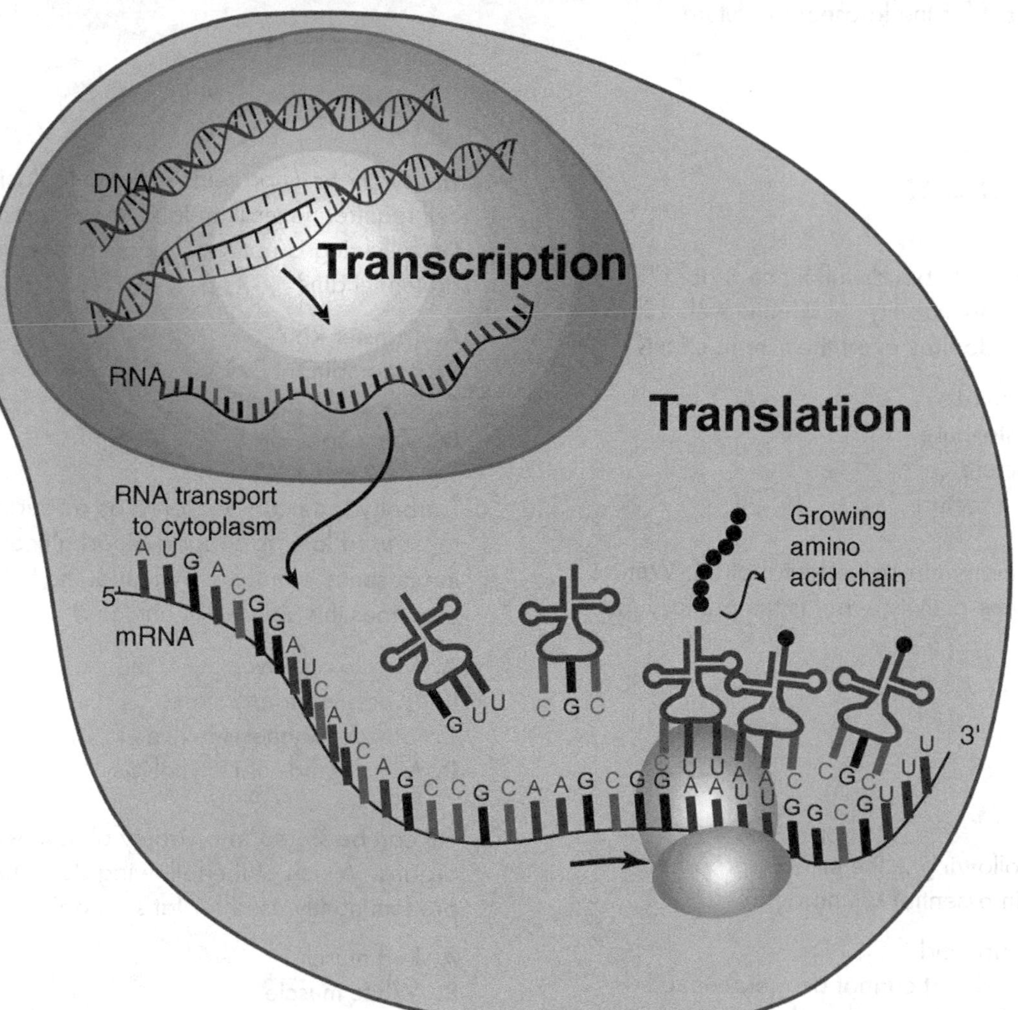

National Human Genome Research Institute (https://www.genome.gov/EdKit/pdfs/glossary_final-linked.pdf).

Thus, the specific sequence coded in the DNA is transcribed and then translated into a specific sequence of amino acids (a protein). The process is more complicated than shown in Figure 3-9 and requires initiation factors, elongation factors, energy, and a specific stop codon to complete the process of synthesizing one protein chain.

In vivo, many ribosomes act on the mRNA at the same time (but at varying points along the message). Thus, many protein molecules are being synthesized at the same time and are in various phases from initiation to completion.

In recombinant DNA technology, this process is adapted to overproduce a specific protein of interest in a microorganism (bacteria or yeast) or a cultured cell line. The process starts by identifying the DNA sequence of interest and then cloning that DNA sequence into the native DNA of the microorganism or cultured cell line. Using factors to promote or enhance the expression of the specific protein of interest, one can manipulate the system to overexpress the needed protein. Isolation of the protein of interest may be from the culture media (secreted protein) or may require cell lysis and purification of the protein of interest.

Obtaining a protein with the proper post-translational modification and glycosylation to match the original mammalian protein (from the cell culture or microorganism culture) is a significant challenge. Such recombinant therapeutic proteins are expensive to produce and are available in only limited quantities.

Monoclonal antibodies produced by recombinant technology are one of the largest groups of new therapeutics currently in the clinical trial arena and will continue to be an active area of new drug development for the foreseeable future.

3-9 Questions

1. The cysteine disulfide bonds influence proper protein folding and stability. At which level of protein structure do they exert their main effect?

A. Primary structure
B. Secondary structure
C. Tertiary structure
D. Quaternary structure

2. Vitamins have many effects on metabolism. With respect to enzyme activity, what is the primary role of vitamins?

A. Reactant
B. Cofactor
C. Substrate
D. Catalyst

3. Which of the following is the most appropriate definition for an essential amino acid?

A. A basic amino acid
B. An amino acid that cannot be metabolized
C. An amino acid that can be synthesized by humans
D. An amino acid that cannot be synthesized by humans

4. The synthesis of proteins in the cytoplasm of the cell requires several metabolic elements. Which of the following is *not* required to synthesize a new protein chain?

A. Transfer RNA
B. Recombinant DNA
C. Ribosome proteins
D. Messenger RNA

5. Carbohydrate can be stored as a source of energy to be used later to support blood glucose levels in the absence of intake. Which of the following best describes this storage in humans?

A. Muscle and liver glycogen
B. Liver and kidney starch
C. Gluconeogenesis in liver
D. Muscle and liver glycolysis

6. Fat can be stored in a variety of tissues and organs. Which of the following describes the tissue predominantly used for fat storage?

A. Red muscle
B. White muscle
C. Heart muscle
D. Adipose tissue

7. During fasting, humans can synthesize glucose from other carbon-chain precursors. Which of the following best describes this process?

A. Liver gluconeogenesis
B. Liver glycolysis
C. Muscle glycogen metabolism
D. Adipose lipolysis

8. Three amino acids in two cellular compartments are involved in the urea cycle (conversion of ammonia to urea). Which of the following correctly lists these three amino acids and the two cellular compartments?

A. Branched-chain amino acids (isoleucine, leucine, and valine) in the cytoplasm and mitochondria
B. Arginine, ornithine, and citrulline in the cytoplasm and mitochondria
C. Lysine, histidine, and arginine in the cytoplasm and mitochondria
D. Arginine, ornithine, and citrulline in the nucleus and the cytoplasm

9. Phospholipids are the main component of human cell membranes. In which category of glycerides do most cell membrane phospholipids fit?

A. Monoglycerides with a phosphate side chain
B. Triglycerides without a side chain
C. Diglycerides without a side chain
D. Diglycerides with a phosphate side chain

10. K_m and V_{max} are quantitative descriptors of enzyme activity. Which of the following is the best definition of V_{max}?

A. V_{max} is the rate of enzyme-mediated reaction when substrate is at the K_m concentration.
B. V_{max} is the number of active sites on the quaternary enzyme complex.
C. V_{max} is the rate of enzyme activity when all substrates are in excess concentration.
D. V_{max} is the initial rate of enzyme reaction when substrate is first bound.

11. Which of the following is the best working definition of K_m?

A. K_m is the concentration of substrate that produces one-half of the maximal rate (V_{max}) of enzyme activity.
B. K_m is the concentration of substrate that produces the maximal rate (V_{max}) of enzyme activity.
C. K_m is one-half the concentration of substrate that produces one-half of the maximal rate (V_{max}) of enzyme activity.
D. K_m is the concentration of coenzyme that produces the maximum rate of enzyme activity.

12. Which of the following are the two main groups of enzyme cofactors?

A. Minerals and trace metals
B. Water-soluble vitamins and minerals
C. Fat-soluble vitamins and minerals
D. Vitamins and metals

13. Which of the following best describes the two main hallmarks of enzyme-catalyzed reactions?

A. Specificity and accelerated rate of reaction
B. Rapid rate of reaction and wide range of substrates
C. Nonspecific higher activation energy
D. Specificity for substrate and cofactor

14. What is the main currency of cellular energy?

A. AMP
B. ADP + Pi
C. ATP
D. ATP + Pi

15. Corn syrup solids are used in a wide variety of processed food products. Which of the following best describes corn syrup solids?

A. Maltodextrins
B. Partially hydrolyzed starch
C. Soluble linear polymer of disaccharides
D. Completely hydrolyzed starch or glucose units

16. Beta oxidation of long-chain fatty acids occurs in which cellular compartment?

A. Nucleus
B. Cytoplasm
C. Mitochondria
D. Endoplasmic reticulum

17. Which part of protein synthesis involves rRNA?

A. The reading of the specific sequence of nucleotides in DNA
B. The assembly of amino acids into a protein chain in the ribosome
C. The provision of specific amino acids to be incorporated into the new protein
D. The specific sequence of amino acids to be incorporated into the new protein

18. What are the two main causes of DNA strand breaks?

A. Ionizing radiation and chemicals
B. Heat and acid
C. Intercalating chemicals and deamination
D. Antibiotics and light-activated psoralens

19. Which of the following best describes two problems associated with production of a therapeutic protein using recombinant DNA technology?

A. Obtaining the proper amino acid sequence and purifying it from the production media
B. Obtaining the proper post-translational modification of specific amino acids and glycosylation, if required
C. Obtaining a properly folded (i.e., native conformation) protein and eliminating impurities
D. Obtaining a protein of the correct molecular weight and achieving native conformation

20. Which of the following is the largest group of therapeutic proteins in development?

A. Endocrine proteins
B. Plasma proteins
C. Translation-regulating proteins
D. Monoclonal antibodies

3-10 Answers

1. C. Cysteine disulfide bonds help stabilize the overall native folded structure of proteins. Thus, their primary effect on protein stability is at the level of tertiary structure.

2. B. Although some vitamins can appear to be a substrate, the primary role of vitamins in metabolism is as an enzyme cofactor.

3. D. An essential amino acid is one that cannot be synthesized from another amino acid or metabolite by humans. Hence, essential amino acids must be contained in the diet for good nutrition.

4. B. Protein synthesis in the cytoplasm requires tRNA, and mRNA and takes place on the ribosome. Recombinant DNA is not an element of normal protein synthesis.

5. A. In humans, glycogen stored in muscle and liver is a primary source of stored carbohydrate to support blood glucose levels during fasting.

6. D. Although many tissues have a small amount of stored fat, adipose tissue is the main tissue for fat storage.

7. A. Gluconeogenesis is the process of synthesizing glucose from other carbon sources and takes place predominantly in the liver.

8. B. The amino acids arginine, ornithine, and citrulline are the main elements of the urea cycle. The urea cycle takes place in a coordinated process in both the cytoplasm and the mitochondria.

9. D. The most common cell membrane phospholipids are diglycerides with a phosphatidyl side-chain group such as phosphatidyl choline.

10. C. V_{max} is the initial rate of reaction when all substrates are in excess concentration over enzyme sites.

11. A. According to the mathematics that describes enzyme catalysis, K_m is the concentration of substrate that produces one-half of the maximal rate of enzyme catalyzed reaction. Because substrates are rarely present at excess concentration, this is a more realistic and practical measure of the enzyme affinity for substrate.

12. D. The two main groups of enzyme cofactors are vitamins (water and fat soluble) and metals such as zinc and iron.

13. A. The specificity for substrates and the rapid rate of reaction at physiological pH and temperature are the two main hallmarks of enzyme catalysis.

14. C. ATP is the main form of cellular energy. The release of energy in the ATP → ADP + Pi reaction or the ATP → AMP + PPi reaction provides the force to promote many metabolic reactions, including synthesis, degradation, and transport.

15. D. Despite the name, corn syrup solids are really just sugar (completely hydrolyzed starch or free glucose units). Products containing corn syrup solids may not be appropriate for all individuals (i.e., patients with diabetes).

16. C. Beta-oxidation of long-chain fatty acids occurs in the mitochondria and produces two carbon fragments (acetyl-CoA) for further metabolism and energy production.

17. B. Ribosomal RNA refers to the two specific RNA molecules that form the basis for the two subunits of the ribosome. mRNA contains the specific message that dictates the sequence of amino acids in the new protein, and tRNA refers to the family of RNA molecules that deliver the specific amino acid to the ribosome.

18. A. Ionizing radiation and chemicals are the two main causes of DNA strand breaks. Heat and acid can result in missing bases, deamination can result in an alteration to the wrong base, and antibiotics and light-activated psoralens can result in strand cross-linking. Fortunately, DNA repair mechanisms exist for most of these damages.

19. B. Achieving a native conformation and eliminating impurities are important in the production of a therapeutic protein. However, getting the proper glycosylation and post-translational modification (if required) can be the most challenging problems in production.

20. D. Monoclonal antibodies are the largest group of therapeutic proteins currently in clinical trials.

3-11 Additional Resources

Bender DA. *Introduction to Nutrition and Metabolism.* 5th ed. Boca Raton, FL: CRC Press; 2014.
Devlin TM. *Textbook of Biochemistry with Clinical Correlations.* 7th ed. New York, NY: John Wiley and Sons; 2010.
Metzler DE. *Biochemistry: The Chemical Reactions of Living Cells.* 2nd ed. Oxford, U.K.: Elsevier Press; 2003.
Schrödinger E. *What Is Life?* Cambridge, U.K.: Cambridge University Press; 1944.
Stamatoyannopoulos G, Majerus PW, Perlmutter RM, Varmus H. *The Molecular Basis of Blood Diseases.* 3rd ed. Amsterdam, The Netherlands: Elsevier; 2000.

Microbiology Related to Human Disease

4

BRADLEY A. BOUCHER

4-1 KEY POINTS

- Infectious diseases can affect virtually every body tissue and fluid in the presence of pathogenic microbes and a breakdown of host defenses.
- Prokaryotes are organisms lacking a nucleus and organelles. Among the prokaryotes that may cause infectious diseases are bacteria, rickettsiae, and chlamydiae.
- Viruses are fragments of nucleic acid that can replicate only in living cells.
- Fungi and protozoa are eukaryote microorganisms that can cause infectious diseases in humans. Fungi typically infect immunocompromised or malnourished individuals.
- Infectious diseases occur when a microbial pathogen gains access to host tissue and brings about physiologic or anatomic alterations in the host. The mere presence of microorganisms in the body is not synonymous with disease and may be normal in selected body areas, such as the skin and the intestinal tract.
- Transmission of microbes within the environment and between hosts can occur by several routes, including direct contact; airborne spread; contact with contaminated water, food, soil, and blood; sexual intercourse; and insect vectors.
- Infectious diseases of the upper respiratory tract, including the nose, paranasal sinuses, middle ear, pharynx, and tonsils, are most commonly caused by viruses.
- Infectious diseases of the lower respiratory tract, including the trachea, bronchi, and alveoli, can be caused by viruses as well as by numerous bacterial species.
- The number of patients infected with *Mycobacterium tuberculosis* is enormous worldwide. *M. tuberculosis* infection results in more deaths than any other bacterial cause.
- The majority of skin and soft-tissue infections are caused by normal skin flora (i.e., staphylococcal and streptococcal species).
- Sexually transmitted infectious diseases can be caused by bacteria, such as gonorrhea and syphilis, or by viruses, such as human immunodeficiency virus infection and genital herpes.
- Gastrointestinal infectious diseases can be caused by a wide variety of bacterial and viral pathogens as well as by toxins produced by invading bacteria.
- Recognition of characteristic patient signs and symptoms is essential for prompt treatment of infectious diseases.

4-2 STUDY GUIDE CHECKLIST

The following topics may guide your study of this subject area:

- [ ] Awareness of disease-producing microorganisms, their modes of transmission, and the principles of maintaining immunocompetence
- [ ] The typical four-phase growth curve that bacteria follow: lag, logarithmic, stationary, and decline
- [ ] The typical infection cycle periods: incubation, prodromal, acme, decline, and convalescent
- [ ] Elements of nonspecific host defense including physical barriers, pH, lysozymes, inflammation, complement, cytokines, neutrophils, macrophages, and the lymphatic system
- [ ] Elements of specific host defense including complement, T-lymphocytes, B-lymphocytes, antibody-mediated immunity, and cell-mediated immunity
- [ ] Types of infectious diseases including acute, chronic, local, systemic, communicable, contagious, endemic, epidemic, nosocomial, and opportunistic
- [ ] Principles of microbial invasion including penetration of physical barriers, nonspecific and specific immune dysfunction, virulence, inoculum, toxins, reservoirs, carriers, and vectors

4-3 Introduction

Infectious diseases are a major cause of morbidity and mortality in the world, which is not particularly surprising considering that humans live in a virtual sea of microorganisms. Despite their vast numbers, only a small percentage of microorganisms can cause an *infection,* which is defined as the multiplication of microbes in human tissue. Alternatively stated, humans and microorganisms generally exist harmoniously. However, when the complex interplay among (1) the invading microbe, known as the *pathogen* or *parasite;* (2) the person being infected, known as the *host;* and (3) the external environment is disrupted, the potential for disease exists. Understanding the role that each of these three principal variables has within this interplay is the key to understanding infectious diseases in humans.

4-4 Microbiology Fundamentals

Prokaryotes are organisms lacking a nucleus as well as organelles (e.g., endoplasmic reticulum, Golgi bodies, lysosomes, mitochondria, cytoskeleton). Among the prokaryotes are bacteria and the significantly smaller microbes known as mycoplasmas, rickettsiae, and chlamydiae. *Eukaryotes* have a well-defined nucleus, and they include fungi and protozoa of the microorganisms. All living things are prokaryotes or eukaryotes; they possess ribosomes that are ribonucleic acid (RNA)–protein bodies that participate in protein synthesis.

Cell walls are generally present in prokaryotes and may be present in eukaryotes. Cell walls protect the microorganism, thus enhancing its survival as well as determining the shape of the microorganism. Inherited characteristics of prokaryotes and eukaryotes are stored in deoxyribonucleic acid (DNA) molecules organized in chromosomes.

Viruses are extremely small microbes that are essentially fragments of nucleic acid (i.e., genome) packaged in a protein shell. Viral nucleic acid is either DNA or RNA but not both. According to the preceding definition, viruses are not living organisms. Their sole activity is replication, which can take place only in living cells. Among the microorganisms discussed, only the fungi can be seen with the unaided eye. Protozoa and the majority of bacteria can be seen with a light microscope. Viruses, mycoplasmas, and chlamydiae can be seen only with an electron microscope.

Bacteria have existed for billions of years. They are found in air, soil, and water and on the surfaces of plants and animals. Most bacteria can live independently given favorable conditions. Bacteria can exist in a mutually beneficial relationship with the host. For example, normal intestinal bacteria compete with pathogenic bacteria for nutrients. However, when the relationship is beneficial to one organism but harmful to the other, a *parasitic relationship* exists.

Bacteria are classified by genus and a species modifier. Bacteria can also be classified by their ability to retain a basic dye (crystal violet) after iodine fixation and alcohol decolorization, known as the *Gram reaction*. Specifically, Gram-positive bacteria retain the staining dye whereas Gram-negative bacteria do not. This difference likely is a consequence of variations in their respective cell wall content.

Bacteria exist in three basic shapes: rods, spheres, and spirals. Bacterial rods are known as *bacilli.* The rods may be single, but they can also form long chains. Spheres are known as *cocci* and may exist in pairs (diplococci), chains (e.g., streptococci), or clusters (e.g., *Staphylococci* species). Spiral bacteria are curved rods that resemble commas or may be corkscrew in shape (e.g., spirochetes). Bacteria may also possess tail-like features known as *flagella,* for motion, or hair-like structures (*pili*), for attachment to host cell surfaces.

A capsule may surround bacteria, making them less susceptible to destruction by host organism defenses. Bacteria can also possess plasmids (e.g., R-factor plasmids) in their cellular cytoplasm. *Plasmids* are small circular molecules of DNA that can replicate independent of the chromosomal DNA. Plasmids have implications relative to conveying resistance to other bacterial strains through the transfer of genetic information. Some bacteria may produce spores that are highly resistant to environmental changes. Noteworthy among the spore-producing bacteria are the *Clostridium* and *Bacillus* species.

Mycoplasmas are the smallest free-living microbes. They lack the bilayered cytoplasmic membrane found in other bacteria, although they do not require host cells for replication, a feature that distinguishes them from viruses. Mycoplasmas do not have a cell wall but are bounded by a limiting lipid membrane. Mycoplasmas can be identified under a microscope by their resistance to an acid-staining technique that differentiates them from bacteria that do not retain the stain. Mycoplasmas have a characteristically longer incubation time than do other bacteria or viruses. Mycoplasmas also differ from the vast majority of bacteria in that they are obligate intracellular parasites. Other "small bacteria" include the *Rickettsiae* and *Chlamydiae* species. Unlike other prokaryotes, rickettsiae and chlamydiae require hosts for metabolic and reproductive activities.

Bacteria flourish under varying environmental conditions. Most pathogenic bacteria grow at temperatures between 35°C and 42°C. Oxygen is essential for many bacteria, known as *aerobic bacteria.* Anaerobic bacteria grow in oxygen-free environments such as dead tissue. Facultative bacteria can grow in either oxygen state. Most bacterial species grow best under a neutral pH condition, which explains why the very low pH found in the human stomach deters growth of most bacteria and why most acidic foods are rarely contaminated with bacteria. Bacteria also have nutritional needs, including an absolute necessity for water and organic matter such as that found in living tissue. Other environmental factors influencing cell growth include salinity and light.

Bacteria typically follow a four-phase growth curve. The first phase is the *lag phase,* in which bacteria adapt to their new environment. The second phase is the *logarithmic phase*, in which bacteria double during each reproductive period involving chromosomal duplication and binary fission. During this period, symptoms begin to appear in the host. In this phase, a host's susceptibility to some antibiotics is greatest through the antibiotics' interference with cell wall synthesis, cellular metabolism, and the like. Mutations or alterations in the bacterial DNA on the chromosome during the replication process may weaken the strain compared to the parent strain but may impart resistance to host defenses. Mutations are generally random and unpredictable events but may be induced using various disinfectant techniques, such as ultraviolet light or nitrous oxide gas. The third phase is the *stationary phase,* when reproduction and death rates equalize. The latter is influenced by host defense systems being engaged in destruction of the bacterial pathogen as well as by nutrients becoming scarce, accumulation of bacterial waste products, and shortages of oxygen and water. The last phase is the *decline phase,* during which an exponential decline in bacterial numbers is observed. Quantification of bacteria is possible in microbiologic laboratories using a variety of techniques.

Viruses are the smallest agents known to cause disease in living things and exist in many sizes and shapes. More than 400 distinct viruses infect humans. Their shape is determined by the shape of the viral protective protein shell known as the *capsid.* In addition to particles of nucleic acid and protein, viruses may possess a covering membrane known as the *lipid envelope.* Because of their very small size, viruses are much more complex and time consuming to detect than bacteria. No uniform classification system exists for viruses. Thus, viruses are sometimes classified by the body tissue affected or, alternatively, by whether they are DNA or RNA viruses.

Viruses are obligate, intracellular parasites that require host cell structural and metabolic components for replication. Alternatively stated, viruses lack the machinery for producing energy or synthesizing large molecules. After commandeering the host cells, which are thousands of times larger or more, the virus replicates exponentially, often destroying the host cells in the process. The typical virus replication cycle within a host is attachment and penetration followed by biosynthesis, maturation, and release. In some instances, however, the viruses may be integrated into the host cells' DNA, rendering them immune to the normal host cell defenses. This relationship, known as *lysogeny,* may establish a latent or dormant state for the virus within cells that can result in later reactivation of the virus.

Fungi are classified into two broad groups referred to as *yeasts* and *molds.* They form long chains of intertwined filaments known as *hyphae.* Both are larger than bacteria. Fungi possess a rigid cell wall that distinguishes them from bacteria. *Pneumocystis jiroveci* (previously *Pneumocystis carinii*)—originally thought to be a protozoan—is now believed to have characteristics more like a yeast. Fungi are normally not pathogenic. However, they may cause infectious diseases in patients who have defects in their immune system or who are malnourished. In these instances, fungi and other microorganisms are referred to as *opportunistic pathogens.* Most fungi prefer acidic conditions and grow best at temperatures close to room temperature. Regardless, fungal pathogens can thrive at body temperature. Fungi are aerobic organisms, except that facultative yeasts can grow in both aerobic and anaerobic conditions. Fungi can reproduce by both asexual and sexual processes. The former may involve the formation of spores on the fungal hyphae that are capable of germinating new hyphae. Spores can also develop following sexual reproduction by fungi.

Protozoa are single-cell eukaryotes that belong in the animal kingdom, unlike bacteria, viruses, and fungi. They lack cell walls, ingest food particles, and move about freely. Most protozoa are harmless except for several notable pathogens (e.g., *Plasmodium* species, *Giardia lamblia*). These pathogens can multiply in mammalian hosts like other microorganisms.

Metazoans, such as the helminths (flukes, flatworms, tapeworms), are multicellular organisms with well-developed organ structures. They cannot multiply within their host, thus requiring reexposure for spread of disease.

4-5 Principles of Host Resistance

Humans are able to coexist without invasion by microbial pathogens because of both nonspecific (innate) and specific (acquired) host defenses that have evolved over millions of years. Disease develops when the effects of the invading organism override these host defenses.

Nonspecific Immunity

The most important nonspecific barrier preventing entry of microorganisms into the body is the skin. The various mucosal surfaces within the respiratory, gastrointestinal, and vaginal tracts are also important physical barriers to microbial invasion. Lysozyme, which is a nonspecific destructive enzyme found in human saliva and tears, is another nonspecific host defense mechanism in the mouth and eyes, respectively. The low pH found within the stomach, bile, and digestive enzymes and peristalsis are other defenses from ingested microbes and colonizing organisms within the gastrointestinal tract. The low pH of the urine and vaginal tracts are nonspecific host defenses within the urinary tract and vagina, respectively.

More than 30 proteins circulating in the blood, known generally as *complement,* are involved in both nonspecific and specific host immunity. On invasion, complement can bind to microbial proteins and enhance ingestion of the microbes through a process referred to as *phagocytosis.* Interferons are another nonspecific group of proteins in the human body that have the ability to trigger the immune system and inhibit viral reproduction. Among the various body cell lines, natural killer cells function independently of the specific immune system, destroying foreign cells while sparing host cells.

Last, inflammation is a nonspecific host defense mechanism. On microbial invasion or injury, the blood vessels at the site dilate, thereby increasing capillary permeability. This action is followed by plasma flow and migration of leukocytes (white blood cells) into the tissue and fluid accumulation. Complement and low-molecular-weight glycoproteins known as *cytokines* also are integrally involved in the inflammatory response, including fever development. *Fever,* which is controlled by the hypothalamus, is defined as a body temperature above normal (37.5°C) and is considered by some authorities to be a form of nonspecific resistance. Examples of proinflammatory cytokines include the interleukins (e.g., interleukin-1, interleukin-6) and tumor necrosis factor-α. Leukocytes, of which approximately 55–60% are neutrophils and 5–8% are monocytes, contain enzymes that digest foreign materials after engulfing the invader. On maturation in the tissue, monocytes are referred to as *macrophages.* Macrophages are constantly patrolling tissues for evidence of microbial invasion. On activation, macrophages may initiate the inflammatory response, release of cytokines, and neutrophil recruitment.

Macrophages also function as phagocytes within the lymphatic system. The lymphatic system carries a fluid (i.e., lymph) that surrounds cells throughout the body and eventually empties into the vena cava. Pockets of tissue along the circulatory path of the lymphatic system are known as *lymph nodes;* they contain phagocytes. Specialized lymph nodes in the body include the tonsils, adenoids, spleen, thymus, and Peyer's patches in the small intestine.

Specific Immunity

Specific immunity is an extraordinarily complex system within humans that protects against foreign substances, including microorganisms. Recognition of foreign substances versus host cells is critical to specific immunity. Chemicals referred to as *antigens* trigger specific immunity. Typical antigens are large protein or polysaccharide molecules (i.e., greater than 10,000 daltons) and can be thought of as the fingerprint to which the immune system responds on exposure, thus providing specific resistance to infection and disease.

Lymphocytes (approximately 30–35% of circulating leukocytes) are the foundational cell line relative to specific immunity. B-lymphocytes are largely responsible for antibody-mediated immunity (AMI), whereas T-lymphocytes are responsible for cell-mediated immunity (CMI). B-lymphocytes are produced in the bone marrow and colonize the lymphoid system along with the T-lymphocytes. B-lymphocytes produce antibodies that become highly specific proteins after presentation of circulating antigens to these lymphocytes by macrophages. The term *immunoglobulin* is used interchangeably with antibody. Subsequent interaction of the antibodies with the antigen results in eventual destruction of the latter by inactivating the antigen or by increasing its susceptibility to other body defense processes (e.g., phagocytosis). Enhancement of phagocytosis by antibodies or complement is known as *opsonization*. Importantly, after acute exposure, some B-lymphocytes become memory B-lymphocytes, which have the long-term capability of rapidly producing antibodies on reexposure to the same antigen.

T-lymphocytes originate in the thymus and populate lymph nodes, the spleen, the tonsils, and other lymphoid tissue. Four distinct types of T-lymphocytes exist, each having a specialized function. Cytokines also have a role in regulating CMI processes. After exposure to selected antigens as presented by macrophages, cloned cytotoxic T-lymphocytes leave the lymphoid tissue, migrate to the infection site via the lymphatic and blood vessels, and initiate the process of targeted cell lysis. As with B-lymphocytes, some T-lymphocytes become memory cells, thereby providing long-term immunity.

In general, AMI is involved with both bacterial and viral host defense, whereas CMI is essential to viral host defense. Specific immunity is one of the primary mechanisms used by vaccines to prevent viral and bacterial infections. In essence, vaccines stimulate antibody production as well as T-lymphocytes within the immune system, thereby providing a defense against the invading pathogen under exposure. Specific immunity is also a means to neutralize toxins produced by pathogens through the administration of pharmaceuticals known as *toxoids*. Again, this reaction is accomplished by stimulation of antibodies to these known toxins before or after exposure.

4-6 Host–Pathogen Relationships

Infection and *infectious diseases* are not synonymous—that is, individuals may be infected without disease. This state is most apparent with normal body flora whereby microorganisms infect the body without causing disease. Body areas where microorganisms are found in healthy individuals include the skin, the oral cavity, the small and large intestines, and the vagina.

In contrast, blood, lymph, cerebral spinal fluid, and most internal organs are free of microorganisms (sterile); presence of microbes in these fluids or spaces typically indicates infection. Disease occurs when a microbial pathogen gains access to host tissue and brings about physiologic or anatomic alterations in the host. In such instances, the normal defense mechanisms that are in place to ward off pathogens have been compromised.

Infectious diseases can be acute or chronic. Acute diseases tend to be serious but of relatively short duration. Chronic infectious diseases tend to be milder but may persist for months or years. Furthermore, infectious diseases can be local (i.e., restricted to one body area) or systemic, which signifies spread of the pathogen into deep organs or more than one body system. In some instances, infections are extracellular. In other instances, microorganisms replicate intracellularly.

Communicable infectious diseases refer to those diseases that can be transmitted from host to host. All communicable diseases are infectious, but not all infectious diseases are communicable; if an infectious disease is highly communicable, it is said to be *contagious*. Communicable infectious diseases can be *endemic,* which refers to a low level of disease within a select geographic area. An *epidemic* refers to an explosive outbreak of a disease within a population, while the term *pandemic* indicates a disease that is worldwide.

Infectious diseases can also be referred to by their geographic site of onset. For example, some infectious diseases may be community acquired whereas others develop after admission to a health care institution (e.g., hospital-acquired infection). The latter frequently are referred to as *nosocomial infections.* Infections are classified as primary if the initial disease is caused by the invading organism. Secondary infectious diseases generally occur because of a weakened immune system or because of the use of antimicrobials. Opportunistic infections may be primary or secondary.

Microbial Invasion

Before disease can occur, the microorganism must first gain access to the host, penetrate the host tissue, and grow at that location. For example, cuts or scrapes, burns and other types of wounds, tooth extractions, intravenous injections, or insect bites are mechanisms by which the nonspecific defense of the skin can be compromised. Mechanical obstruction of body passages resulting in stasis of body fluids is another means by which normal defenses can be overcome. Common sites of obstruction include the lung, urinary tract, biliary tract, and Eustachian tubes. Placement of foreign bodies, such as indwelling catheters, can also circumvent normal host defense and allow microbial growth. Under certain conditions, normal body flora can be overgrown by pathogenic organisms, predisposing the host to infection. This last type of infection can occur in the skin and gastrointestinal tract.

Both nonspecific and specific immune defenses may be dysfunctional as a result of genetic defects, noninfectious disease states, or immunosuppressive therapies. Examples include altered phagocytosis secondary to neutropenia, malignancies, cytotoxic drug therapy, and radiation therapy. Individuals who are at an increased risk of infection because of congenital or acquired host defense are referred to as *compromised hosts*. Virtually any microorganism can become pathogenic in such individuals. Overall, the likelihood of a particular infectious pathogen causing disease is a function of the level of host resistance; the aggressiveness of the invading organism, which is known as *virulence;* and the absolute number of the microbes in some instances. This last variable is known as the *dose* or *inoculum* of the pathogen. Toxins produced by the pathogens can also increase their virulence. In actuality, such toxins may cause disease without invasion of body tissues.

Environments or hosts that support growth of infectious organisms are known as *reservoirs*. Reservoirs can be water, soil, or animals. The most common reservoir for human pathogens, however, is other humans. A *carrier* is a host that has recovered from an infectious disease but continues to shed the pathogen. Transmission of microbes within the environment and between hosts can occur by several routes. These routes include direct contact; airborne spread, which includes inhalation of respiratory droplets, dust, and spores; contaminated water, food, or soil; contaminated blood and blood products; sexual transmission; and insect vectors.

Vectors do not cause infectious diseases but carry pathogens from one host to another. Examples of vectors and the respective diseases they cause in humans are mosquitoes and malaria, yellow fever, West Nile virus, and Dengue fever; ticks and Lyme disease, Rocky Mountain spotted fever, and Q fever; and fleas and the plague.

Understanding infectious disease transmission is a key component in preventing disease. Universal precautions include thorough hand washing before and after patient contact; proper disposal of contaminated needles; and use of masks, gloves, and gowns for selected patients and procedures.

General Infectious Disease Manifestations

On invasion, the pathogen may be confined to the portal of entry. In other instances, the pathogens, their toxins, or both may be transported to distant body sites by the circulating blood.

The time between the entry of the microorganism into the body and the appearance of symptoms is known as the *incubation period.* The incubation period can range from days to years.

The period when general infectious symptoms, such as nausea, fever, headache, muscle aches, or malaise, manifest is referred to as the *prodromal period.*

The *acme period* is when specific symptoms occur. During this period, patients may have a high fever and chills as well as a change in skin color. In addition, patients may experience blood pressure changes, increased heart rate, swollen lymph glands, and a rash. Pain, tenderness, and redness may also be present at sites of inflammation. Laboratory findings may include an elevation in leukocytes and increases in immature neutrophils. Collectively, these physiologic changes are referred to as the *acute phase response.* During the acute phase response, selected plasma proteins may be produced in the liver (e.g., C-reactive protein, serum amyloid A protein). Elevations in these proteins and globulins may be useful as an indicator of disease and are responsible for increases in the laboratory test known as the *erythrocyte sedimentation rate.*

The *period of decline* is when fever begins to subside, sweating may occur, and the skin color returns to normal. Last, the *convalescent period* is when the body systems return to normal.

4-7 Infectious Diseases and Pathogenic Microorganisms in Humans

Diseases of the Upper Respiratory Tract

The upper respiratory tract includes the nose, paranasal sinuses, middle ear, pharynx, and tonsils. Viruses are the most common cause (90%) of upper respiratory infections (URIs). Rhinoviruses; influenza type A and B; parainfluenza viruses type 1, 2, and 3; coronaviruses; and adenoviruses are the most frequent causes of the common cold in humans and can cause pharyngitis. A vaccination exists only for the influenza virus.

The viruses are transmitted by water droplets and typically cause headache; cough; dry, scratchy throat; sneezing; and a runny nose. Often these viruses have a seasonal variation. Respiratory syncytial viruses can also cause URIs, particularly in infants and young children, but in adults as well.

Included among the bacterial causes of URI are group A streptococcus and *Streptococcus pyogenes* (see Table 4-1). These microbes are also transmitted via airborne droplets expelled during coughing or sneezing. *S. pyogenes* is responsible for a condition known as *strep throat,* characterized by high fever, coughing, swollen lymph nodes and tonsils, and a bright red appearance of the pharyngeal tissues. *Scarlet fever* is strep throat accompanied by a skin rash; it can lead to rheumatic fever. *Rheumatic fever* is inflammation of the small blood vessels in the body and may result in rheumatic heart disease and glomerulonephritis.

TABLE 4-1. Selected Airborne Bacterial Diseases of the Upper Respiratory Tract

Disease	Causative pathogen	Description of pathogen	Characteristic signs and symptoms
Strep throat	*Streptococcus pyogenes*	Gram-positive encapsulated streptococcus	Sore throat
Scarlet fever	*Streptococcus pyogenes*	Gram-positive encapsulated streptococcus	Skin rash
Diphtheria	*Corynebacterium diphtheriae*	Gram-positive rod	Pseudomembrane
Pertussis (whooping cough)	*Bordetella pertussis*	Gram-negative rod	Mucous plugs and cough (seal bark)
Epiglottitis	*Haemophilus influenzae*	Gram-negative rod	Severe throat pain, fever, muffled voice
Sinusitis	Indigenous microbiota	Various	Pain, tenderness, swelling

Adapted from Pommerville, 2014.

The majority of bacterial cases of otitis media involve *S. pneumonia,* which is also known as *pneumococcus. Haemophilus influenzae* type b and *Moraxella catarrhalis* also frequently cause otitis media. Less common bacterial URIs are pertussis (whooping cough), caused by *Bordetella pertussis,* and diphtheria, caused by *Corynebacterium diphtheriae,* which may involve a pathogenic toxin. Both are rare because of vaccination programs.

Lower Respiratory Tract Infections

The lower respiratory tract consists of the trachea, bronchi, and alveoli. Approximately 50% of lower respiratory tract infections involve viral pathogens. For example, all of the viruses previously listed as causes of URI can cause tracheobronchitis and, less commonly, pneumonia in adults. *Pneumonia* refers to an inflammation of the bronchial tubes and lungs. Symptoms can present abruptly and include sudden chills, severe cough, fatigue, headache, high fever, chest pain, back and leg pain, and a tight chest. Viruses also cause acute viral laryngitis, especially parainfluenza types 1, 2, and 3, as well as croup, which involves inflammation of the larynx, trachea, and bronchi. The latter condition is associated with a distinctive cough known as a seal's bark.

Many bacteria can cause pneumonia (see Table 4-2). The majority of community-acquired pneumonia cases involve pneumococcus. Pneumococcus typically afflicts immunocompromised individuals and is associated with a high mortality in the elderly. In addition to having the signs and symptoms just discussed,

TABLE 4-2. Selected Airborne Bacterial Diseases of the Lower Respiratory Tract

Disease	Causative pathogen	Description of pathogen	Characteristic signs and symptoms
Pertussis	*Bordetella pertussis*	Gram negative	Malaise, low-grade fever, severe cough
Tuberculosis (TB)	*Mycobacterium tuberculosis*	Acid-fast rod	Active TB: cough, weight loss, fatigue, fever, night sweats, chills, breathing pain
Infectious bronchitis	*Streptococcus pneumoniae*	Gram-positive diplococcus in chains	Runny nose, sore throat, chills, general malaise, slight fever, dry cough
	Haemophilus influenzae	Gram-negative rod	
	Mycoplasma pneumoniae	Mycoplasma	
	Chlamydophila pneumoniae	Chlamydia	
Community-acquired pneumonia (CAP)	*Streptococcus pneumoniae*	Gram-positive diplococcus in chains	High fever, sharp chest pains, difficulty breathing, rust-colored sputum
Atypical CAP	*Mycoplasma pneumoniae*	Mycoplasma	Headache, fever, fatigue, dry hacking cough
	Legionella pneumophila	Gram-negative rod	
Health care-acquired pneumonia	*Streptococcus pneumoniae*	Gram-positive diplococcus in chains	Chills, high fever, sweating, shortness of breath, chest pain, cough with thick greenish or yellow sputum
	Staphylococcus aureus	Gram-positive coccus in clusters	Chills, high fever, sweating, shortness of breath, chest pain, cough with thick greenish or yellow sputum
	Klebsiella pneumoniae	Gram-negative rod	
	Pseudomonas aeruginosa	Gram-negative rod	
Chlamydial pneumonia	*Chlamydophila pneumoniae*	Chlamydia	Headache, fever, dry cough

Adapted from Pommerville, 2014.

patients may have difficulty breathing and produce rust-colored sputum. Individuals at high risk should receive a pneumococcal vaccine. *Staphylococcus aureus* is another common cause of community-acquired pneumonia. Patients within hospitals can be afflicted by a large array of bacteria. Common nosocomial pathogens are *Klebsiella pneumoniae, Serratia marcescens, Enterobacter* species, *Proteus* species, *Haemophilus influenzae* type b, *Acinetobacter baumannii, Escherichia coli, Pseudomonas aeruginosa,* and *S. aureus.* Many of these pathogens are normal inhabitants of the gastrointestinal and respiratory tracts.

Atypical pneumonia is a term to describe a nonclassic bacterial lower respiratory tract infection. This condition is sometimes referred to as "walking pneumonia." The bacterium often associated with atypical pneumonia is *Mycoplasma pneumoniae.* Typical symptoms are a dry, hacking cough; sore throat; headache; fever; and fatigue. Other atypical pneumonia pathogens include viruses, *Chlamydia pneumoniae,* and *Legionella pneumophila.*

Mycobacterium tuberculosis is a pathogen that most commonly affects immunocompromised hosts, including, most prominently, patients infected with the human immunodeficiency virus (HIV). The number of patients infected with this pathogen is enormous worldwide and results in more deaths than any other bacterial cause. *M. tuberculosis* enters the respiratory tract through airborne droplets. Its spread is exacerbated by crowded conditions and poverty, leading to malnutrition and homelessness. Signs and symptoms of tuberculosis include coughing, weight loss, fatigue, fever, night sweats, chills, and breathing pain. Spreading to other organs, including the kidneys, liver, bone, and meninges, is a complication of pulmonary tuberculosis. Other pulmonary infections observed in immunocompromised patients include the fungi *Coccidioides immitis, Cryptococcus neoformans, Histoplasma capsulatum, Aspergillus fumigatus,* and *Pneumocystis jiroveci* (see Table 4-3).

Skin and Soft-Tissue Infections

Although a major nonspecific barrier to microbial invasion, the skin and its underlying soft tissue can also be the site of a variety of infections, both primary and secondary. As primary infections, they usually affect normally healthy tissue and involve a single pathogen. Examples include impetigo, a superficial skin infection typically seen in children; cellulitis, an infection of the epidermis, dermis, and superficial fascia; and severe infections of the subcutaneous tissue and muscle known as *necrotizing fasciitis* and *myonecrosis,* respectively.

Alternatively, secondary infections occur in areas of previously damaged skin. These infections include diabetic foot ulcers, pressure sores, penetrating trauma, animal and human bite wound sites, and burns. The number of bacteria that can cause these respective skin and soft-tissue infections is extensive and includes both aerobic and anaerobic bacteria. The majority of these infections involve normal skin flora,

TABLE 4-3. Summary of Selected Fungal Diseases of Humans

Disease	Organism	Transmission	Affected organ or body area
Cryptococcosis	*Cryptococcus neoformans*	Airborne yeast cells	Lungs, spinal cord, meninges
Candidal vaginitis	*Candida albicans*	Sexual contact	Vagina
Thrush	*Candida albicans*	Skin contact	Mouth
Athlete's foot	*Trichophyton* species	Contact with hyphal fragments	Feet
Histoplasmosis	*Histoplasma capsulatum*	Airborne spores	Lungs and various other organs
Blastomycosis	*Blastomyces dermatitidis*	Airborne spores	Lungs and various other organs
Coccidioidomycosis	*Coccidioides immitis*	Airborne arthrospores	Lungs
Aspergillosis	*Aspergillus fumigatus*	Airborne spores	Lungs
Pneumocystis pneumonia	*Pneumocystis jiroveci*	Airborne droplets	Lungs

Adapted from Alcamo, 2001.

with staphylococcal and streptococcal species being the most common. However, violated skin can be infected with soil where pathogens such as *Clostridium tetani* and *C. perfringens* reside. The former causes the disease known as *tetanus,* and the latter is responsible for gas gangrene.

The eye may be the primary site of infections as well. For example, bacterial conjunctivitis—more commonly referred to as "pink eye"—is most often caused by *Haemophilus aegyptius.* Fungi can also infect the skin, mouth, and nails. These infections include such common conditions as tinea pedis (athlete's foot), caused by fungi called *dermatophytes,* and oral candidiasis (thrush), caused by *Candida albicans.* Fungal infections involving only the skin are referred to as *cutaneous* or *superficial mycoses.*

Viruses cause many skin and soft-tissue diseases. Herpes simplex type 1 virus is responsible for cold sores on the lips, gums, and mouth. This virus spreads through direct contact. The herpes simplex viruses may remain dormant for long periods and be reactivated by numerous factors. Varicella zoster is the virus responsible for chicken pox and shingles. Chicken pox manifests as fever, headache, malaise, and eruption of fluid-filled vesicles on the skin that itch intensely. Shingles occurs when the virus multiplies in nerve roots on reactivation from its dormant state. This condition, which can be excruciatingly painful, presents as blotchy, red patches that circle the trunk of the body.

Although the manifestation of varicella zoster involves the skin, transmission occurs through respiratory droplets in addition to direct contact. Similar transmission occurs with the viruses causing measles. Patients with measles develop a characteristic rash, hacking cough, sneezing, nasal discharge, and an aversion to bright light. Mumps is another virus contracted only via respiratory droplets. With the exception of herpes simplex, all of these conditions can be prevented through the use of vaccines. Warts are small benign skin growths and another condition caused by viruses.

Genitourinary Tract Infections and Sexually Transmitted Diseases

Infections of the bladder rank among the most common infections in humans. Patients' symptoms include abdominal discomfort, pain on urination, and the urge to urinate frequently. *Proteus mirabilis* and *Escherichia coli* are among the most common pathogens related to bladder infections. Women are affected far more commonly than men because of the much shorter urethra and the location of the urethra relative to the vaginal canal and anus. These anatomic differences allow bacteria to migrate much more readily into the bladder.

Infections of the kidneys are more uncommon than bladder infections and are typically caused by a broader array of bacteria originating in the intestinal tract, including Gram-positive organisms. The prostate gland in men can also become infected with pathogens similar to other urinary tract infections.

Diseases that spread from human-to-human contact, particularly sexual intercourse, are generally referred to as *sexually transmitted diseases* (STDs). Among the common STDs caused by bacteria are gonorrhea, syphilis, and chancroid.

Gonorrhea is caused by the bacterium *Neisseria gonorrhoeae* and is characterized by urethral discharge and painful urination. Long-term complications in women include sterility and spontaneous abortions.

Syphilis is an STD caused by the spiral bacterium *Treponema pallidum.* After the bacteria penetrate the body through mucous membranes during intercourse, a three-stage disease can develop. Primary syphilis manifests as painless ulcers known as *chancres* on the external genitalia and perianal area, and the mouth if oral intercourse has occurred. Secondary syphilis involves many bodily organs spread through the lymphatic system and the circulating blood, accompanied by flu-like symptoms. The third phase, or tertiary syphilis, can slowly produce an inflammatory reaction in virtually any organ of the body. Most notable are involvement of (1) the heart and cardiovascular system and (2) the central nervous system.

Chlamydia trachomatis is a bacterium that can cause an STD that manifests as purulent discharge from the urethra or vagina. Patients may be asymptomatic other than this prominent sign.

Chancroid, which is caused by the bacterium *Haemophilus ducreyi,* presents as shallow ulcers, often on the penis in males or the labia or clitoris in females.

Among the nonbacterial STDs is trichomoniasis, caused by the protozoan *Trichomonas vaginalis.* Trichomoniasis typically produces a vaginal discharge. In addition, vaginal candidiasis, caused by *Candida albicans,* may be contracted as an STD but may also develop independent of sexual intercourse.

Unquestionably, the most feared viral STD is that caused by HIV (types 1 and 2) and the potential of these retroviruses to cause acquired immune deficiency syndrome (AIDS). Although the most common means of transmission of HIV is through sexual intercourse, it can also spread through contaminated blood (e.g., shared needles of intravenous drug users); contaminated blood products; and perinatal contact (in utero, labor and delivery, breast-feeding). The primary target of HIV in humans is the helper T-lymphocyte known as *CD4*. Failure of this fundamental cell line within the CMI line of defense places the host at risk for opportunistic infections.

Symptoms of HIV infections can be numerous and include an ever-weakening state, fever, diarrhea, rash, lymph node swelling, night sweats, malaise, depression, and muscle wasting. In addition, all of the signs and symptoms associated with secondary opportunistic infections may be present in the HIV-infected patient. These latter pathogens include fungi (see Table 4-3); protozoa (e.g., *Pneumocystis jiroveci*); bacteria (e.g., *Mycobacterium tuberculosis*); and other viruses (e.g., cytomegalovirus).

Another less serious, but highly prevalent, viral STD is genital herpes. This condition is caused by the herpes simplex type 2 virus and typically presents as itching and throbbing in the genital area resulting from the formation of painful blisters. As is true of herpes simplex type 1 infections, genital herpes can be a recurrent problem on reactivation of the latent virus.

Gastrointestinal Infections and Enterotoxigenic Poisonings

A wide of array of pathogens can invade the gastrointestinal tract (see Table 4-4). Often these infections are the result of ingestion of contaminated food and water. In addition to proliferation of the microorganisms, toxins produced by these pathogens may cause disease. An example is the toxin produced by *Clostridium botulinum;* this toxin can induce flaccid paralysis in its victims. *Staphylococcus aureus* can also produce a toxin and is a common cause of food poisoning. Symptoms typically include nausea, vomiting, abdominal cramping, and diarrhea.

A particularly deadly waterborne gastrointestinal pathogen is *Vibrio cholerae,* which is responsible for the infection known as cholera. This organism produces an enterotoxin that stimulates massive water loss

TABLE 4-4. Summary of Selected Foodborne and Waterborne Bacterial Diseases

Disease	Causative pathogen	Description of pathogen	Toxin	Characteristic signs and symptoms
Botulism	*Clostridium botulinum*	Gram-positive spore-forming rod	Yes	Difficulty swallowing, slurred speech, blurred vision, trouble breathing, flaccid paralysis
Staphylococcal food poisoning	*Staphylococcus aureus*	Gram-positive coccus in clusters	Yes	Abdominal cramps, diarrhea, vomiting, nausea
Typhoid fever	*Salmonella typhi*	Gram-negative rod	Unknown	Bloody stools, abdominal pain, fever, lethargy, delirium
Salmonellosis	*Salmonella* serotypes	Gram-negative rod	Not established	Fever, diarrhea, vomiting, abdominal cramps
Shigellosis	*Shigella sonnei*	Gram-negative rod	Yes	Diarrhea
Cholera	*Vibrio cholerae*	Gram-negative curved rod	Yes	Severe, watery diarrhea; nausea; vomiting; muscle cramps; dehydration
Enterotoxigenic *E coli.* (ETEC), Enteropathogenic *E. coli* (EPEC)	*Escherichia coli* serotypes	Gram-negative rod	Yes	Diarrhea, vomiting, cramps, nausea, low-grade fever

Adapted from Pommerville, 2014.

from severe diarrhea. Another pathogen found in contaminated water is *Salmonella typhi*. The disease caused by this organism is typhoid fever and is characterized by deep ulcers in the intestinal tract, bloody stools, lethargy, delirium, and fever.

Salmonella species can also cause disease following ingestion of contaminated food, most notably poultry and dairy products. *Shigella* species can cause nausea, fever, vomiting, watery diarrhea, and abdominal cramping after ingestion of contaminated water or food. *Escherichia coli* produces a toxin that can cause infantile diarrhea and what is known as *traveler's diarrhea*. *Clostridium difficile* is yet another bacteria that produces a toxin resulting in severe diarrhea and a condition known as *pseudomembranous colitis*.

Although all of the previously mentioned gastrointestinal pathogens are bacteria, viruses are responsible for the majority of cases of gastroenteritis, especially in children. Viruses that can cause acute viral gastroenteritis include rotavirus, calicivirus, enteric adenovirus, and astrovirus.

A unique gastrointestinal infection found in humans is a common cause of peptic ulcers. The pathogen, *Helicobacter pylori,* is transmitted by contaminated water and food. The association between *H. pylori* and peptic ulcers is a relatively recent discovery. This infection could not occur except for the ability of *H. pylori* to withstand the high acidity in the stomach through the indirect production of the neutralizing base, ammonia.

Central Nervous System Infections

Neisseria meningitidis, Haemophilus influenzae type b, and pneumococcus are bacteria that invade the respiratory system and cause meningitis (inflammation of the brain lining). A vaccination is available for each of these pathogens. Meningococcal meningitis can be particularly dangerous and involves a circulating toxin produced by *N. meningitidis*. This condition is most prevalent in people living close to one another. Adenoviruses may also cause meningitis.

Inflammation of the brain tissue is generally referred to as *encephalitis*. It can be caused by a number of viruses, including those causing the diseases mumps and polio. Vaccines for these two conditions have resulted in a dramatic decline in their incidence. Fever, headache, stiff neck (as in meningitis), altered mental status, and muscle paralysis (as in polio) characterize central nervous system infections.

Intra-Abdominal Infections

Intra-abdominal infections can affect organs (e.g., liver) or the abdominal cavity. The latter condition is referred to as *peritonitis* and can be caused by spread of bacteria from the blood but more commonly involves a perforation of the intestinal tract. Thus, pathogens are typically those residing in the intestinal tract, including various Gram-negative rods, Gram-positive cocci, and anaerobic bacteria (e.g., *Bacteroides fragilis*).

Hepatitis is an inflammation of the liver that can be caused by viral pathogens. Hepatitis A is an acute form transmitted by feces-contaminated food or water, whereas hepatitis B and C are transmitted by direct or indirect contact (e.g., sexual intercourse) with contaminated blood. Hepatitis B has both an acute and a chronic form, whereas hepatitis C tends to be chronic in nature. Vaccines currently exist for hepatitis A and B.

Mononucleosis is an acute infectious disease caused by the Epstein–Barr virus and is transmitted through contact with infected saliva. Symptoms typically include fever, sore throat, enlargement of the lymph nodes and spleen, and a high leukocyte count.

Miscellaneous Infections

Other serious infections include those affecting the lining of the heart (i.e., endocarditis); bones (i.e., osteomyelitis); and joints (e.g., infectious arthritis).

4-8 Questions

1. Which of the following microorganism classes are prokaryotes? (Mark all that apply.)

A. Protozoa
B. Viruses
C. Bacteria
D. Rickettsiae

2. Which of the following general shapes exist for bacteria? (Mark all that apply.)

A. Rods
B. Spirals
C. Cubes
D. Spheres

3. Which of the following is *not* a component of the normal bacterial growth curve?

A. Release phase
B. Stationary phase
C. Logarithmic phase
D. Lag phase

4. The most important nonspecific barrier to microorganism invasion in humans is

A. lysozyme.
B. interferons.
C. low pH in the stomach and urine.
D. skin.

5. Which of the following circulating white blood cell types is referred to as a macrophage on maturation within body tissues?

A. Neutrophils
B. Eosinophils
C. Lymphocytes
D. Monocytes

6. Which of the following cell lines is most important relative to specific defense against bacteria?

A. Natural killer cells
B. B-lymphocytes
C. Helper T-lymphocytes
D. Cytotoxic T-lymphocytes

7. In which of the following anatomic areas can bacteria normally be located? (Mark all that apply.)

A. Large intestine
B. Liver
C. Vagina
D. Lungs

8. Which of the following human defense mechanisms is essential for viral host defense?

A. Cell-mediated immunity
B. Phagocytosis
C. Antibody-mediated immunity
D. Inflammation

9. A communicable disease that is present at a low level within a select geographic area is referred to as

A. pandemic.
B. endemic.
C. hospital acquired.
D. epidemic.

10. Disease caused by pathogens is generally a function of which of the following variables? (Mark all that apply.)

A. Inoculum of the pathogen
B. Level of host resistance
C. Climatic conditions of the host
D. Virulence of the microorganism

11. Which is the most common reservoir for human pathogens?

A. Soil
B. Other humans
C. Pets
D. Tap water

12. Which of the following infectious diseases involve vectors? (Mark all that apply.)

A. Measles
B. Rocky Mountain spotted fever
C. Malaria
D. Yellow fever

13. Which of the following is the period when specific signs and symptoms are at their highest intensity during the course of an infectious illness?

A. Prodromal period
B. Incubation period
C. Convalescent period
D. Acme period

14. Which of the following microorganisms are the most common cause of upper respiratory tract infections?

A. Gram-positive bacteria
B. Viruses
C. Molds
D. *Mycoplasma* species

15. The majority of community-acquired lower respiratory tract infections are caused by which of the following microorganisms?

A. *Klebsiella pneumoniae*
B. *Mycobacterium tuberculosis*
C. Parainfluenza viruses
D. *Streptococcus pneumoniae*

16. Which of the following viruses is responsible for the condition known as shingles?

A. *Varicella zoster*
B. Herpes simplex type 1
C. Cytomegalovirus
D. Epstein–Barr virus

17. Which of the following pathogens routinely infect immunocompromised hosts? (Mark all that apply.)

A. *Pneumocystis jiroveci*
B. *Mycobacterium tuberculosis*
C. *Helicobacter pylori*
D. *Treponema pallidum*

18. Which of the following are transmission routes for the human immunodeficiency virus? (Mark all that apply.)

A. Contact with contaminated blood
B. Breast-feeding
C. Mosquito vector
D. Sexual intercourse

19. Which of the following bacteria can cause gastric ulcers?

A. *Escherichia coli*
B. *Helicobacter pylori*
C. *Staphylococcus aureus*
D. *Salmonella typhi*

20. Which of the following transmission routes is associated with the hepatitis A virus?

A. Sexual intercourse
B. Contact with contaminated blood
C. Feces-contaminated food or water
D. Inhalation of respiratory droplets

4-9 Answers

1. **B, C, D.** Viruses, bacteria, and rickettsiae are prokaryotes and are all correct answers. Protozoa are eukaryotes.

2. **A, B, D.** Bacteria exist in three basic shapes: rods, spirals, and spheres. They do not exist as cubes.

3. **A.** Bacteria typically follow a four-phase growth curve: lag phase, logarithmic phase, stationary phase, and decline phase.

4. **D.** The most important nonspecific barrier preventing entry of microorganisms into the body is the skin.

5. **D.** On maturation in the tissue, monocytes are referred to *macrophages*.

6. **B.** B-lymphocytes are largely responsible for antibody-mediated immunity, whereas T-lymphocytes are responsible for cell-mediated immunity. Natural killer cells are part of nonspecific immunity in humans.

7. **A, C.** Bacteria are normally located in the large intestine and vagina. Bacteria are not normally found in the liver or lungs.

8. **A.** CMI is essential to viral host defense. AMI is also involved in bacterial host defense. Phagocytosis is a process through which complement binds to microbial proteins and enhances ingestion of microbes. Inflammation is a nonspecific host defense mechanism that involves dilation of blood vessels at the site of microbial invasion or injury, followed by plasma flow and migration of leukocytes into the tissue and fluid accumulation.

9. **B.** An endemic infection is a low-level disease within a select geographic area. An *epidemic* refers to an explosive outbreak of a disease within a population, while the term *pandemic* indicates a disease that is worldwide. Hospital-acquired, or nosocomial, infections develop after admission to a health care institution.

10. **A, B, D.** The likelihood of a pathogen causing a disease is a function of the inoculum of the pathogen, the level of host resistance, and the virulence of the microorganism. The climatic conditions of the host are generally not important.

11. **B.** Reservoirs can be water, soil, or animals. The most common reservoir for human pathogens, however, is other humans.

12. **B, C, D.** Rocky Mountain spotted fever is caused by a tick vector. Malaria and yellow fever are caused by mosquitoes as a vector. Measles is caused by a virus and does not involve a vector.

13. **D.** The incubation period is the time between the entry of the microorganism into the body and the appearance of symptoms. General infectious symptoms appear during the prodromal period. The acme period is when highly intense specific symptoms occur. These periods are followed by the period of decline, when symptoms begin to subside, and the convalescent period, when body systems return to normal.

14. **B.** Viruses cause 90% of upper respiratory infections.

15. **D.** The majority of community-acquired lower respiratory tract infections are caused by *Streptococcus pneumoniae*.

16. **A.** *Varicella zoster,* which is responsible for chicken pox, also causes shingles.

17. **A, B.** *Pneumocystis jiroveci* and *Mycobacterium tuberculosis* are microbes that generally infect immunocompromised hosts. *Helicobacter pylori* is a bacterium that can cause gastric ulcers, and *Treponema pallidum* is a spirochete that causes syphilis—host immune status is not a factor for either microbe.

18. **A, B, D.** HIV can be transmitted by contact with contaminated blood, breast-feeding, and sexual intercourse. It is not transmitted by mosquitoes.

19. **B.** *Helicobacter pylori* can cause gastric ulcers.

20. **C.** Hepatitis A virus is spread through feces-contaminated food or water.

4-10 Additional Resources

Alcamo IE. *Fundamentals of Microbiology.* 6th ed. Boston, MA: Jones and Bartlett; 2001.

Bergquist LM, Pogosian B. *Microbiology: Principles and Health Science Applications.* Philadelphia, PA: W. B. Saunders; 2000.

Goering RV, Dockrell HM, Zuckerman M, et al., eds. *Mims' Medical Microbiology.* 5th ed. Philadelphia, PA: Elsevier Saunders; 2013.

Greenwood D, Barer M, Slack R, Irving W. *Medical Microbiology.* 18th ed. Edinburgh, NY: Churchill Livingstone/Elsevier; 2012.

Levinson W, ed. *Review of Medical Microbiology and Immunology.* 14th ed. New York, NY: McGraw-Hill Education; 2016.

Murray PR, Rosenthal KS, Pfaller MA, eds. *Medical Microbiology.* 8th ed. Philadelphia, PA: Elsevier; 2016.

Pommerville JC. *Fundamentals of Microbiology.* 10th ed. Burlington, MA: Jones and Bartlett; 2014.

Ryan KJ, Ray CG. *Sherris Medical Microbiology.* 6th ed. New York, NY: McGraw-Hill; 2014.

Immunology

5

KATHERINE S. BARKER

5-1 KEY POINTS

- Immune cells can be categorized as lymphoid (B-lymphocytes, T-lymphocytes, NK [natural killer] cells) or myeloid (monocytes, macrophages, eosinophils, neutrophils, basophils).
- Innate immunity refers to a primitive immune response driven by monocytes, macrophages, and neutrophils, which recognize pathogens through cell surface interactions and phagocytize them.
- Adaptive immunity involves specific recognition of antigens by B- and T-lymphocytes and provides immune "memory."
- B-lymphocytes produce immunoglobulin, also known as antibodies, which can possess one of five different "classes" of heavy chains (alpha, gamma, delta, epsilon, mu) and either kappa or lambda light chains. Two identical light chains and two identical heavy chains comprise a single antibody molecule.
- B-lymphocytes produce IgM (immunoglobulin M) in a primary antibody (humoral) response and then can produce any one of the five classes of antibodies in subsequent humoral responses, depending on the types of cytokine molecules detected by the B-lymphocyte.
- Antibodies recognize and bind epitopes, a discrete portion of an antigen, through specific intermolecular interactions between the epitope and a combination of the variable regions of the heavy and light chains of the antibody.
- Antibody–epitope binding leads to B-lymphocyte activation involving internalization, processing, and subsequent presentation of antigen with major histocompatibility complex (MHC) surface molecules, as well as production of cytokines, cytokine receptors, and secreted antibodies.
- B-lymphocytes present antigens in the context of MHC surface receptors to T-lymphocytes, which become activated when the antigen–MHC complex interacts with the T-cell receptor in conjunction with additional signals through various receptor–ligand engagement between the T- and B-lymphocyte.
- In addition to antigen recognition, antibodies also have an effector function in which they bind fragment crystallizable (Fc) receptors on the surface of monocytes, macrophages, neutrophils, mast cells, and T-lymphocytes. These receptors are bound by the Fc region of the antibody, comprised of the constant and class-specific region of the heavy chains.
- There are four types of hypersensitivity, each of which requires a presensitized host: type I (immediate hypersensitivity or allergy), type II (cytotoxic or antibody-dependent [tissue antigen] hypersensitivity), type III (antibody-dependent [soluble antigen] hyper-sensitivity), and type IV (delayed-type hypersensitivity).

5-2 STUDY GUIDE CHECKLIST

The following topics may guide your study of this subject area:

- ☐ Characteristics of innate and adaptive immunity
- ☐ The structure of an antibody, the different classes of heavy chains, and the functional domains of an antibody molecule
- ☐ B-lymphocyte activation involving engagement of antigen with antibody versus mitogen-mediated B-lymphocyte activation
- ☐ T-lymphocyte activation involving engagement of T-cell receptor
- ☐ Various tests measuring antibody titers and antigen reactivity
- ☐ The difference between active and passive immunizations
- ☐ Different antigen preparations for active immunizations
- ☐ Key differences between the four types of hypersensitivities
- ☐ Types of transplants and the factors involved in graft rejection

5-3 Introduction

The environment in which we live is filled with microorganisms such as bacteria, viruses, protozoa, and fungi. Some of these microorganisms, collectively termed *pathogens,* can infect the human body and cause disease. In turn, the human body's immune system has evolved to counteract these pathogens and protect us from infection.

Historically, the understanding of the immune system has evolved with medicine's understanding of microorganisms. However, even though vaccines were developed as early as the late 18th century and the use of sterilization and disinfection followed in the late 19th century, a modern understanding of the immune system and immune processes was not initiated until the mid-20th century.

This chapter gives an overview of some of the key components of the immune system and immune function. Included are discussions on the differences between innate and adaptive immunity, the structure and functions of antibodies, the basis of immunization, and differences in the four types of hypersensitivities. The last sections of the chapter deal with applications of our understanding of the immune system, such as immunizations, antibody-based laboratory testing, and transplants and graft rejection.

5-4 Components of the Immune System

The immune system consists of natural barriers as well as specific immune cells. The first line of defense of the immune system consists of the external barriers of the body, such as the skin, tears, digestive tract, and bronchi. Because the skin covers nearly the entire body, it acts as a potent physical shield against entry of pathogenic organisms. Tears contain lysozymes and antibodies that help protect the eyes from infection. The digestive tract—namely, the gut—is awash with acid and digestive enzymes that are quite effective in ridding the body of many potential pathogens ingested with food and drink. Likewise, the bronchi guard against infection by airborne pathogens by being equipped with mucous and cilia. The mucus traps microorganisms and particulates, and the cilia coordinately move the trapped material away from the lungs and out of the respiratory tract.

Many of these barriers—particularly the skin and the gut—harbor commensal organisms that help guard against infection by at least two modes: (1) secretion of defense molecules that lyse or neutralize pathogens and (2) colonization of the site to the point where conditions, such as available nutrients necessary for growth, are unsustainable for pathogens. Because human pathogens live in the external environment, they gain entry into the body by bypassing these barriers. Therefore, maintaining the integrity of these body parts is crucial to the success of the immune system.

Critical to any immune response is the normal function of immune cells. Immune cells arise from progenitor cells, which, in turn, arise from hematopoietic stem cells and can be categorized as lymphoid or myeloid in nature. Lymphoid cells differentiate from lymphoid progenitor cells into natural killer (NK) cells, B-lymphocytes (also called B-cells), or T-lymphocytes (also called T-cells). The maturation of B- and T-lymphocytes in primary and secondary lymphoid tissues will be discussed later in this section. Myeloid cells are different from myeloid progenitor cells; myeloid cells are either antigen-presenting cells (APCs), such as monocytes and macrophages, or granulocytes, such as eosinophils, neutrophils, and basophils. Table 5-1 lists types of immune cells, their functions, and the receptors they express.

Lymphocyte development and selection are crucial in specific immune responses. Internally, several organs participate in the immune response; these organs can be classified as primary and secondary lymphoid organs. The *primary lymphoid organs*—bone marrow and thymus—produce naive B- and T-lymphocytes and NK cells. Within these primary lymphoid organs, cells obtain their repertoire of specific cell surface antigen receptors required to recognize foreign organisms throughout the body. Also during this time of development, these cells undergo selection for tolerance to self-antigens within the primary

TABLE 5-1. The Most Common Human Leukocytes, Their Functions, and Other Characteristics

Cell type	Function	Cell surface markers expressed
Lymphoid		
B-lymphocytes:		
Memory B-cell	Antibody production, antigen presentation	CD19, CD20, Igα, Igβ, CD40, MHC I and II
Plasma cell	Antibody production	
T-lymphocytes:		
Cytotoxic	Killing of infected cells	CD8, TCRα, TCRβ, CD3, CD28, MHC I
T_H1 (T-helper 1)[a]	B-cell activation	CD4, TCRα, TCRβ, CD3, CD28, MHC I
T_H2 (T-helper 2)[a]	B-cell activation	CD4, TCRα, TCRβ, CD3, CD28, MHC I
Suppressor	Reduction of B- and T-cells' immune responses[b]	TCRγ, TCRδ, CD3, MHC I
NK cells	Killing of tumor cells and virus-infected cells	CD11b, CD2, CD8, CD56, IL-2R, KIR, MHC I
Myeloid		
Eosinophils	Granule-mediated killing of extracellular pathogens (parasites)	FcεR, CD11a, CD11b, VLA-4, FcγR, MHC I
Monocytes and macrophages	Antigen presentation, phagocytosis	CD11a and CD18, CD11b and CD18, CD14, FcγR, IL-2R, MHC I and II
Neutrophils	Phagocytosis, granule-mediated killing	Complement receptors, CD11a, CD11b, VLA-4, FcγR, MHC I
Mast cells	Inflammation, allergy	FcεR, CD11a, CD11b, VLA-4, FcγR, MHC I
Basophils	Inflammation, allergy	FcεR, CD11a, CD11b, VLA-4, FcγR, MHC I
Platelets	Blood clotting, inflammation	MHC I, FcεR, FcγR

FcεR, fragment crystallizable receptor for IgE; FcγR, fragment crystallizable receptor for IgG; Igα, immunoglobulin α; Igβ, immunoglobulin β; IgG, immunoglobulin G; IL-2R, interleukin-2 receptor; KIR, killer cell immunoglobulin-like receptor; MHC I, major histocompatibility complex class I; MHC II, major histocompatibility complex class II; TCRα, T-cell receptor α; TCRβ, T-cell receptor β; TCRγ, T-cell receptor γ, TCRδ T-cell receptor δ; VLA-4, very late antigen–4.

a. Other types of T-helper cells have been identified, but their roles are still to be elucidated.

b. The role of suppressor T-cells is still a matter of debate.

lymphoid organs so that they recognize and react only to non-self-antigens in the periphery. The bone marrow houses hematopoietic stem cells, which differentiate into B-lymphocytes or NK cells. The thymus is the primary lymphoid organ in which T-lymphocytes mature from hematopoietic stem cells and undergo selection. Once these cells are differentiated in the bone marrow or the thymus, they are released into the bloodstream, where some migrate to secondary lymphoid tissues.

The *secondary lymphoid organs and tissues* consist of the spleen, lymph nodes, and mucosa-associated lymphoid tissues, such as tonsils and Peyer's patches. These sites encompass an environment in which naive lymphocytes can interact with antigens, other lymphocytes, and accessory cells. The immune reactions that occur within these secondary lymphoid tissues serve to prime or activate these immune cells for future immune responses. In general terms, once a naive lymphocyte enters the secondary lymphoid tissue, it recognizes a specific antigen presented by an APC such as a macrophage. This antigen is presented in the context of a cell surface receptor called a *major histocompatibility complex (MHC) molecule* (discussed later in this chapter). This antigen–MHC complex is bound by an antigen receptor on the lymphocyte—namely, the T-cell receptor (TCR) on T-lymphocytes and the membrane antibody in conjunction with accessory cell surface molecules called the B-cell receptor (BCR) on B-lymphocytes. This engagement of antigen–MHC complex with the antigen receptor causes a cascade of events involving production and secretion of cytokines and chemokines. The lymphocytes will begin to activate and differentiate by expressing new cytokine and chemokine receptors on the cell surface; they also will begin to proliferate in response to some of these chemical signals. This process, called *clonal selection,* is necessary for the full maturation of lymphocytes that can migrate to sites of infection in the periphery. Because clonal selection requires the recognition of specific antigens, and each lymphocyte in the repertoire of millions of lymphocytes in the body recognizes a particular antigen, some lymphocytes in the repertoire may never mature in a person's lifetime.

5-5 Innate and Adaptive Immunity

In general, immune responses can be classified as innate or adaptive. Innate and adaptive immunity work together to protect the body against a vast array of pathogenic organisms. *Innate immunity* refers to the action of mononuclear phagocytes (monocytes and macrophages) and polymorphonuclear neutrophils (PMNs, or simply neutrophils), which circulate throughout the body. These cells possess a primitive, somewhat nonspecific recognition system; this critical recognition occurs through the interaction of receptors on the surface of phagocytes and PMNs with receptors, other cell surface molecules, or structural components of pathogens. Once these cells bind pathogenic organisms, phagocytes internalize them by physically enveloping the pathogen with projections of the phagocyte, thus forming a *phagosome.* The phagosome then merges with a specialized compartment of the phagocyte called a *lysosome,* which contains enzymes that digest the microorganism. These bits of digested pathogen can then be combined with MHC molecules, after which the antigen–MHC complex can be expressed on the cell surface of the phagocyte. Similarly, PMNs will bind and ingest extracellular pathogens in phagolysosomes, but they do not present antigen on their cell surface. These cells also contain granules filled with antibiotic and lytic molecules. On specific interaction of certain cell surface molecules, the neutrophil can release the contents of its granules outside the cell. Although PMNs are the most abundant immune cell types present in the blood, they are extremely short lived.

Another type of immune response is *adaptive immunity.* Two features of adaptive immunity distinguish it from innate immune responses. First, unlike innate immunity, adaptive immunity involves specific recognition of antigens. Second, adaptive immune responses involve immune "memory," which provides lifelong protection of the body against the same pathogens. B- and T-lymphocytes participate in adaptive immune responses. The concepts of specificity and memory in adaptive immunity will be explained further.

Adaptive immunity refers to immune responses that have two phases: a primary and a secondary immune response. The primary phase of an adaptive immune response, which usually occurs in lymphoid tissue as described previously, occurs when specific recognition and binding of a foreign antigen occur; this antigen–antibody interaction is described in more detail in a later section of this chapter. The B-lymphocyte binds extracellular antigen through the B-cell receptor, which activates the B-lymphocyte to produce and release soluble antibody, to express new receptors (including cytokine receptors on its cell surface) and to secrete cytokines. The BCR activation also causes the B-lymphocyte to proliferate. Some of the activated B-lymphocytes become memory B-cells; these long-lived cells circulate throughout the body and are primed to recognize their specific antigens through antigen–antibody interaction as before. This secondary or memory response results in further proliferation of this B-lymphocyte clone. The B-lymphocytes that do not become memory cells mature into antibody-producing cells known as *plasma cells;* plasma cells are terminally differentiated, meaning that they do not proliferate, and the function of these short-lived cells is to produce and release large amounts of antibody.

Adaptive immune responses from T-lymphocytes are similar to those of B-lymphocytes but involve interactions of TCR and MHC molecules. A T-lymphocyte's TCR specifically recognizes and binds antigen that is associated with an MHC molecule. Two classes of MHC molecules are referred to as *MHC class I* and *MHC class II.* MHC class I molecules are found on the cell surface of nearly every cell in the body. These molecules present intracellular antigens—that is, antigens from pathogens that live and reproduce *inside* a host cell, such as viruses and obligate intracellular bacteria. MHC class II molecules are found on the cell surface of APCs and present phagocytosed or internalized antigens from extracellular pathogens.

Antigens may be internalized by B-lymphocytes through specific binding of antigen and BCR; after this binding occurs, the antigen–BCR complex is internalized, and the antigen is processed and presented in the context of an MHC class II molecule.

Once the specific TCR–MHC interaction takes place, the T-lymphocyte is activated. The nature of this activation differs according to the type of T-lymphocyte (see Table 5-1). Three main subsets of T-lymphocytes exist: T-helper cells, cytotoxic T-cells, and T-suppressor cells. T-helper cells express CD4 cell surface markers in conjunction with the TCR and recognize antigens in the context of MHC class II molecules on APCs. Cytotoxic T-cells express CD8 cell surface markers in conjunction with the TCR and recognize antigens in the context of MHC class I molecules on infected cells. Whether T-suppressor cells represent a true subset of T-lymphocytes is still debatable, mainly because T-suppressor cells can be either $CD4^+$ or $CD8^+$ T-cells; however, T-suppressor cells do respond to antigen binding by secreting cytokines that suppress immune responses. Like B-lymphocytes, the T-lymphocyte clone that responds to a specific antigen will proliferate and differentiate, with some of the proliferating cells circulating in the periphery as memory T-cells.

5-6 Antibody Structure

The antibody is composed of four chains linked together by covalent bonds: two antibody heavy chains and two antibody light chains (Figure 5-1). Both heavy and light chains have globular variable regions at the N-terminus of the polypeptides; the variable region of the heavy chain is termed *V_H domain,* and the variable region of the light chain is termed *V_L domain.* The V_L domain of one light chain and the V_H domain of one heavy chain form an antigen-binding site (also known as the *antibody-combining site*); therefore, each intact antibody molecule has two antigen-binding sites. The light chain also has one globular constant region at the C-terminus of the polypeptide (C_L), while the remainder of the heavy chain is composed of three globular constant regions (C_H1, C_H2, and C_H3). As the V_L and V_H domains interact to form the antigen-binding site, similarly the C_L and the C_H1 domains interact in the antibody structure. Between the C_H1 and C_H2 domains on the heavy chain is the hinge region, which provides the antibody flexibility of

FIGURE 5-1. Structure of an Antibody[a]

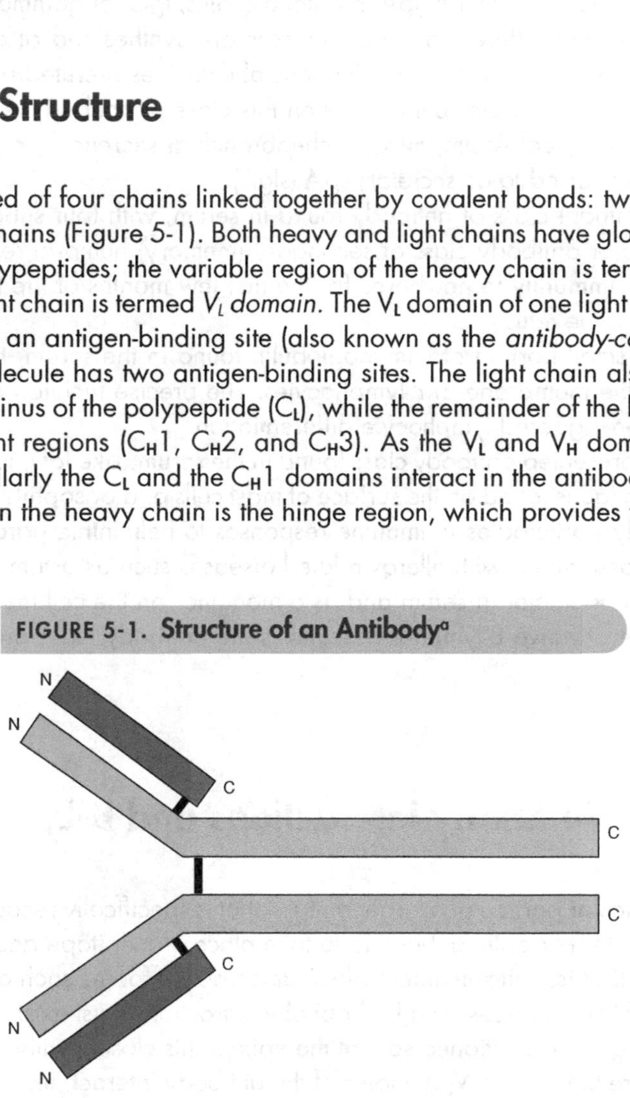

a. The antibody is composed of two heavy-chain polypeptides (shown in light gray) and two light-chain polypeptides (shown in dark gray). They are held together covalently by disulfide bonds (shown in black). The N-terminal regions of the heavy and light chains together form antigen-binding sites, whereas the C-terminal regions of the two heavy chains together form the Fc region, the ligand for Fc receptors found on the surface of several types of leukocytes.

movement so the antigen-binding sites operate independently. Finally, between the hinge region and the C-terminus of the heavy chain, the C_H3 domains of each heavy chain interact with each other.

The antibody molecule can be fragmented into functional domains. Cleavage of an antibody molecule with the cysteine protease papain yields two antigen-binding (Fab) fragments, each consisting of one light chain, the V_H and C_H1 domains of one heavy chain, and one fragment crystallizable (Fc) fragment consisting of the hinge region and C_H2 and C_H3 domains of the heavy chains. Not surprisingly, the Fab fragments function to bind antigen because they contain an intact antigen-binding site. The Fc fragment functions as an effector portion of the antibody, as discussed later in this section.

Antibodies can be composed of one of two types of light chains: *kappa* (κ) or *lambda* (λ) chains, which differ from each other by sequence. Additionally, antibodies can be composed of one of five different types of heavy chains—alpha (α), gamma (γ), delta (δ), epsilon (ϵ), and mu (μ)—which differ from each other by sequence, charge, size, and carbohydrate content. The type of heavy chain in an antibody determines its function and superstructure, and therefore, antibody name designations correspond to the heavy chain they possess: immunoglobulin A (IgA) for alpha chains, IgG for gamma, IgD for delta, IgE for epsilon, and IgM for mu. The five different antibody classes are synthesized at different times in the humoral response and in response to different combinations of cytokines secreted by effector (accessory) cells.

IgA can be found in the serum, but most often this class of antibody is found as a dimer in mucosal secretions such as saliva, colostrum, milk, tracheobronchial secretions, and urogenital secretions. In its dimerized form, it is referred to as *secretory IgA* (sIgA).

IgG is the predominant class of antibody found in serum, with four subclasses of IgG molecules. IgG collectively is the major antibody class of secondary (memory) humoral responses. It plays a major role in imparting passive immunity to newborns for the first few months of life because maternal IgG passes across the placenta to the fetus.

IgD constitutes a small portion of immunoglobulin found in the serum; however, it is usually found in large quantities on the membrane of B-lymphocytes. The precise function of IgD is unknown, but it may play a role in antigen-triggered lymphocyte differentiation.

IgE is the least represented antibody class found in the serum. Like IgD, it is overwhelmingly membrane associated, although IgE is found on the surface of mast cells and basophils. Some evidence indicates that this class of antibody participates in immune responses to helminthic parasites; however, in developed countries, it is most associated with allergy-related diseases such as asthma and hay fever.

IgM is found as a pentamer in serum and as a monomer on the cell membrane of B-lymphocytes. It is found on the surface of naive B-lymphocytes and is the antibody class produced in a primary humoral response.

5-7 Epitope–Antibody Interactions and B-Lymphocyte Activation

The *epitope* is a particular portion of a larger antigen that is specifically recognized by an antibody through the antigen-binding site. For optimal binding to take place, the epitope and the antigen-binding site must be complementary; that is, suitable intermolecular attractive forces such as hydrogen bonding, electrostatic forces, van der Waals forces, and hydrophobic attractions must exist. These intermolecular attractive forces must be arranged or positioned so that the epitope fits closely within the "groove" of the antibody-combining site, where the V_H and V_L domains of the antibody interact, like a hand in a glove (Figure 5-2). An antibody that has high attractive and low repulsive forces for a particular epitope is said to have high *affinity*. In addition, an antibody can be characterized by its *avidity*, which measures the combined affinities of each paratope for all of its corresponding available epitopes on an antigen. For example, a pentameric IgM antibody that can bind a complex antigen with multiples of the same epitope, such as an epitope present on a highly represented cell surface marker on a pathogen where all 10 antigen-binding sites can be simultaneously bound, has a higher avidity than a monomer form of the same IgM antibody or of a pen-

FIGURE 5-2. Antigen–Antibody Interaction[a]

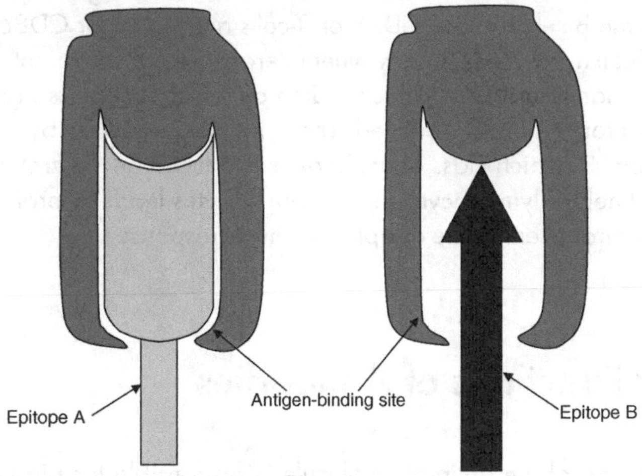

a. The antigen-binding site of an antibody is epitope-specific. Epitope A (at left) is bound optimally by the antibody because maximal interaction exists between the epitope and the antigen-binding site. Epitope B (at right) has minimal interaction with the antigen-binding site, is not bound by the antibody, and would therefore not be recognized by this antibody.

tameric IgM antibody that binds a less plentiful cell surface marker (where fewer than 10 antigen-binding sites can be simultaneously bound).

B-lymphocyte activation can occur by two different types of antigens: T-dependent and T-independent antigens. T-independent antigens include mitogens and large extracellular antigens. *Mitogens* are large, non-antigen-specific molecules; they can activate B- and T-lymphocytes by binding and cross-linking the antigen receptors *outside* the antigen binding site. Mitogens are molecules that typically cause extremely high cytokine production from the lymphocytes they activate. They include pokeweed mitogen, derived from pokeweed; phytohemagglutinin, derived from red kidney beans; and concanavalin A, derived from castor beans. Pokeweed mitogen is a B-cell mitogen, whereas all three are T-cell mitogens. Lipopolysaccharide, also called *endotoxin,* is a component of the outer membrane of Gram-negative bacteria and is a potent mitogen of murine B-cells and of mammalian monocytes and macrophages. Large, extracellular antigens can be considered a T-independent antigen only when membrane antibody on the B-lymphocyte is cross-linked, meaning that more than one BCR is able to bind the antigen simultaneously or that the BCR and a co-receptor on the cell surface become bound simultaneously. These non-mitogen, T-independent antigens include not only pathogens, but also large polymeric molecules such as Ficoll and dextran. T-dependent antigens are classic antigens that require action and activation of both T- and B-lymphocytes to elicit specific antibody production.

B-lymphocyte activation requires several key steps to occur. The initial step involves antigen binding the BCR, where it is internalized in an intracellular compartment and degraded and where antigenic peptides are combined with MHC class II molecules. At the same time, once the BCR is cross-linked during antigen binding, the co-receptor molecules Igα and Igβ become activated, which results in a cascade of phosphorylation events, ultimately leading to the activation of transcription factors and subsequent induced expression of cytokines, cytokine receptors, and other co-stimulatory molecules that are transported to the cell surface for expression or for secretion. In the case of stimulation by T-independent antigens, B-lymphocytes will also secrete antibody almost exclusively of the IgM class.

As the B-lymphocyte becomes activated through this signaling cascade, T-helper lymphocytes bind antigen–MHC class II complexes presented by the B-lymphocyte and experience a similar signaling cascade through the activation of the co-receptor molecule CD4 by the tyrosine kinase lck (p56) and TCR-associated tyrosine kinase fyn. This engagement of TCR and MHC molecules causes polarization, or clustering of many cell surface molecules on both the B- and the T-lymphocytes, to facilitate receptor binding between the cells. These interactions include CD40 on B-cells and CD40 ligand (CD40L) on T-cells, which send additional signals to the B-cell nucleus; CD28 on T-cells and CD80 or CD86 on B-cells, which send additional signals to the T-cell nucleus; and many other interactions. Engagement of these receptors and ligands enhances the intracellular signaling and, depending on which receptors are engaged, modifies the types of cytokines and receptors that are produced. The cytokines produced by T-cells go on to further activate B-cells and help determine which class of antibody is produced and secreted by the B-cell. Ultimately, the interaction between T-helper lymphocytes and B-lymphocytes leads to proliferation and differentiation of the B-cells and is a central event in the adaptive immune response.

5-8 Effector Functions of Antibodies

Whereas the Fab portion of the antibody molecule is responsible for binding antigen, the Fc portion of the antibody molecule drives the effector functions. The Fc portion elicits these effector functions through the binding of Fc receptors (FcRs) on the cell surface of leukocytes such as monocytes, macrophages, T-cells, neutrophils, and mast cells. Each class of heavy chains has separate FcRs, with several members of each FcR class; however, the two most prominent classes are the FcγRs (receptors for IgG) and the FcεRs (receptors for IgE). The three FcγRs function—once bound by the Fc domain of an antibody molecule—to enhance phagocytosis through opsonization, aid in antibody-dependent cellular cytotoxicity, facilitate mediator release, and enhance antigen presentation. There are two FcεRs: the high-affinity FcεRI and the low-affinity FcεRII. The high-affinity receptor is present primarily on mast cells and basophils, and the low-affinity receptor is present on most leukocytes. Because both of these receptors trigger degranulation, the FcεRs figure prominently in allergic reactions (this topic is discussed further in Section 5-12).

5-9 Cytokines and Chemokines

Cytokines and chemokines are key signal transducers between leukocytes. The signals they transduce to cells are complex, because a cytokine can elicit a different outcome depending on the magnitude of cytokine secretion and the type of additional cytokines secreted. These molecules activate or repress the actions of other cells. They can act as chemoattractants; that is, they can signal other cells to move toward a site of infection or inflammation. They can influence the differentiation of nearby leukocytes. As previously mentioned, they can influence the type of immunoglobulin class that is synthesized by nearby B-lymphocytes. Because of the influence of cytokines on the cells in their microenvironment, production of individual cytokines is transient and tightly regulated.

There are several different groups of cytokines, which were named according to their originally discovered function. Generally, these groups are the interleukins (ILs), tumor necrosis factors (TNFs), interferons (IFNs), growth factors, chemokines, and colony-stimulating factors (CSFs). Each of these groups can be subdivided according to its structure or the structure of its receptors, but these subgroupings are beyond the scope of this chapter. To date, nearly 40 different ILs have been found, and they consist of molecules that originate from a variety of leukocytes and have many different functions. Alternatively, TNF-α and TNF-β each have the same functions, including activating macrophages, granulocytes, and cytotoxic cells; inducing cell adhesion; and enhancing the production of MHC class I molecules. However, TNF-α is produced by macrophages and lymphocytes, whereas TNF-β is produced only by lymphocytes.

There are three IFN molecules: IFN-α, IFN-β, and IFN-γ. IFN-α and IFN-β are produced primarily by leukocytes and act on tissue cells to induce MHC class I expression, stimulate NK cells, induce an antiviral state, and inhibit proliferation in those target cells. IFN-γ is produced by T-cells and NK cells to act on both tissue cells and leukocytes to induce expression of both MHC class I and class II molecules, activate macrophages, induce cytokine synthesis in macrophages, induce an antiviral state, and inhibit the action and proliferation of T_H2 cells.

Several growth factors are secreted by, or act on, leukocytes, including fibroblast growth factor (FGF), which promotes angiogenesis; platelet-derived growth factor (PDGF), which promotes angiogenesis; transforming growth factor–α (TGF-α), which promotes endothelial development; transforming growth factor–β (TGF-β), which inhibits the activation of lymphocytes and monocyte-derived phagocytes and can induce apoptosis; and vascular endothelial growth factor (VEGF), which promotes angiogenesis and is chemotactic for macrophages.

The name *chemokine* is derived from "chemotactic cytokine"; not surprisingly, therefore, chemokines' overall function is the ability to promote chemotaxis. Chemokines are integral to the process of *inflammation*—that is, a series of responses to increase the migration of leukocytes (namely, lymphocytes, phagocytes, and PMNs) to the site of infection. This group of cytokines is rather large, comprising nearly 50 members.

Colony-stimulating factors, as suggested by the name, promote proliferation of leukocytes, primarily myeloid cells. These factors are produced mainly by macrophages but are occasionally produced by T-cells and fibroblasts. CSFs include macrophage colony-stimulating factor (M-CSF), granulocyte colony-stimulating factor (G-CSF), and granulocyte–macrophage colony-stimulating factor (GM-CSF).

5-10 Basis of Immunization

Immunizations, or vaccinations, provide a way to administer prepared antigen or antibody to an individual to strengthen that individual's immune response to an infection or toxin. *Passive immunization* is the direct injection of antibody against an antigen; it is an uncommon vaccination but is done, for example, to combat exposure to tetanus toxin. Most immunizations are *active immunizations*—the administration of prepared antigen so the individual develops a strong memory B-cell response. In this way, an individual immunized against a particular antigen or pathogen will have the memory B-cells that will react to infection by that pathogen with rapid and robust production of protective antibodies.

Vaccines for active immunization can be made with a variety of antigen preparations. Live, natural organisms can be used, as in the case of the smallpox vaccine, but this antigen preparation is rarely used. Live, attenuated organisms can be used. Attenuation involves impairing the pathogen so that it loses its virulence; for example, it can no longer infect cells but still has its antigens intact. Live, attenuated vaccines include the MMR (measles, mumps, rubella) and oral polio vaccines. Killed, intact organisms can be used as antigen preparations in vaccines such as the typhoid vaccine, the Salk polio vaccine, and some preparations of influenza vaccines. Prepared fractionated antigen can be used as a vaccine; such vaccines take into account the fact that cell surface proteins are the most antigenic portions of the pathogen. Vaccines using this preparation include pneumococcal vaccines, Hib (*Haemophilus influenzae* type b) vaccine, and HBV (hepatitis B virus) vaccine. More experimental preparations involve recombinant deoxyribonucleic acid (DNA) technology and take advantage of the fact that the genomes of several human pathogens have been fully sequenced. Therefore, genes encoding immunogenic proteins (proteins that can elicit a strong immune response) can be cloned and expressed in order for proteins synthesized in a laboratory to be injected, can be cloned into a viral genome so the attenuated virus can express the proteins upon injection, or can be injected as "naked DNA" so that the protein can be synthesized by the immunized individual and then serve as antigen.

An immune response to a vaccine can be strengthened by combining an adjuvant with the prepared antigen. Adjuvants are typically inorganic salts that are emulsified with antigen and (1) serve to concentrate the antigen at the injection site in order for B-cell activation and antibody production to be more effective or (2) serve to elicit a strong cytokine or chemokine response to enhance the immune response to the antigen.

5-11 Measurement of Immune Responses Using Laboratory Tests

From the extensive studies and subsequent discoveries of immune mechanisms and characterization of components of the immune system, researchers have devised laboratory tests to examine and measure immune reactions in patients. These tests can predict immunodeficiencies or provide insight into the nature of a patient's immune response. A few of these tests are highlighted here.

A complement fixation test measures the presence of antibody in serum. The test is performed by placing a standard amount of antigen in tubes. Then the antiserum to be tested is added at different dilutions to the experimental tubes while saline is added to the control tube. A standard concentration of complement is then added to all tubes. If the antiserum contains specific antibody for the antigen present in the tubes, then antigen–antibody complexes will form, and all complement will be fixed in those immune complexes. As a point of comparison, the control tube, which contains no antibody, will have free complement present. Finally, an indicator cell, such as sheep red blood cells (SRBCs), and a small amount of anti-SRBC antibody are added to all of the tubes. In the tubes in which the antiserum contained antigen-specific antibody, the SRBCs will collect at the bottom of the tube and there will be no cell lysis. In the control tube and in the tubes in which antiserum did not contain any antibodies specific for the antigen, the complement will be able to bind SRBCs, thus leading to cell lysis.

A hemagglutination test detects antibodies to red blood cell (RBC) antigens; similarly, in a modification of the test where the RBCs are bound and coated by an antigen, the test detects antibodies to that particular antigen. In short, this test is performed by adding a standard amount of RBCs to tubes or wells of a multiwell plate and then adding increasing dilutions of the antiserum to be tested to the wells. If antigen-specific antibody is present at a high enough concentration, the antibodies will cross-link with the RBCs and form a mat-like complex that settles to the bottom of the well as a diffuse-looking circle. If too little or no antigen-specific antibody is present in the antiserum, the RBCs will collect in a tight pellet at the bottom of the well. Positive control wells and negative control wells are always included in these assays to ensure that the reagents are working properly.

A precipitin, or *immunodiffusion,* test detects the presence of different antibodies in an antiserum and their reactivity toward different epitopes of an antigen. This test is performed by punching three holes, arrayed like the points of a triangle, in a Petri dish containing solidified agar. The antiserum to be tested is placed in one hole, and peptide epitopes or different antigens are placed in the remaining holes. The solutions of antiserum and antigen are allowed to diffuse through the agar. When the antibody and antigen reach each other in the agar, either they will bind to form a complex and precipitate, or they will continue to diffuse. If more than one epitope or antigen that the antiserum binds is in one well, then separate precipitates corresponding to each antigen–antibody complex will form.

An enzyme-linked immunosorbent assay (ELISA) is a test performed in a multiwell plate to measure quantitatively the amount of antigen-specific antibody in an antiserum or to measure the amount of a particular factor, such as a cytokine, present in serum. Measurement of antibody concentration is achieved by plating serial dilutions of serum to be tested into a multiwell plate coated with a particular antigen. Then a fluorescent-labeled antibody that is specific for Fcγ is added to the wells; this antibody will bind in the Fc domain of the antibodies that are bound to the antigen. The multiwell plate is then analyzed, or read, in a luminometer to detect and quantify the amount of fluorescence compared to the positive control wells in which a specific amount of antigen-specific antibody was added.

An ELISA to measure cytokine concentration can be performed one of two ways. The antiserum can be plated in the wells of a multiwell plate and the serum proteins allowed to bind to the plastic. Then the antigen-specific antibody is added. If this antibody is directly labeled with a fluorescent tag, then the plate is read in the luminometer; if the antibody is not labeled, then a fluorescent-tagged Fc-specific antibody is added to detect antigen–antibody complexes. Alternatively, cytokine concentration can be measured by antibody capture or sandwich ELISA, where antigen-specific antibody is coated in the wells. The serum samples are added, and whatever does not bind the antibody is washed away. Then a second fluorescent-labeled, antigen-specific antibody is added that recognizes a different epitope of the antigen. The fluorescence signals are then detected by luminometer.

5-12 Hypersensitivities and Histamine Release

Hypersensitivity can be defined as an exaggerated immune response that is often harmful to the individual. It can be classified as one of four types: I, II, III, or IV. Each type of hypersensitivity requires a presensitized (previously exposed) host. Type I hypersensitivity is also known as *immediate hypersensitivity* or *allergy* and includes atopy (allergic rhinitis or hay fever, food allergies, eczema); asthma; and anaphylaxis. Type I hypersensitivity is mediated by elevated IgE production, IgE being bound by Fc epsilon receptor on the surface of mast cells, and the bound IgE being cross-linked by antigen-allergen, leading to degranulation and release of other mediators such as histamine. Forms of atopy are sometimes treated by *hyposensitization,* which is repeated injection of controlled doses of allergen, or by avoidance of the allergen. Asthma is treated by administration of inhaled bronchodilators and corticosteroids to ease inflammation of bronchial passages. Individuals known to have anaphylactic reactions to allergens should avoid contact with the allergen to prevent attacks; however, such individuals also should carry a dose of epinephrine (EpiPen), diphenhydramine (Benadryl), or dexamethasone (Decadron) in case they unexpectedly encounter the allergen. Epinephrine acts as a bronchodilator, diphenhydramine is an effective antihistamine, and the steroid dexamethasone is anti-inflammatory. These drugs act to ease the inflammation symptoms directly or to counteract the histamine release by mast cells.

Type II hypersensitivity is also referred to as *cytotoxic* or *antibody-dependent hypersensitivity* and is a reaction to tissue or membrane antigens (not soluble antigens). Reactions occur when antibodies to surface antigens bind and cause destruction of the cell or tissue. Examples of type II hypersensitivity include transfusion-related reactions caused by incompatible blood type (either the blood-typing antigens [A, B, or O] or the Rh+ or Rh– Rhesus antigens [Rh< or Rh–]), newborn hemolytic disease (where maternal antibodies destroy the fetal RBCs because of incompatible blood type), and autoimmune diseases such as Goodpasture syndrome (caused by antibodies to the basement membrane of the kidney) or myasthenia gravis (caused by antibodies to acetylcholine receptors at nerve–muscle junctions).

Type III hypersensitivity involves antibody-dependent reaction to soluble antigens. Type III reactions occur because of the formation of immune complexes between antibody and the soluble antigen. Examples include serum sickness (injection of foreign antigen leading to formation and deposition of immune complexes in blood vessels), Arthus reaction (subcutaneous immune complex formation occurring at a local site in and around the walls of small blood vessels), and systemic lupus erythematosus (caused by antibodies to DNA, histones, and antigens of the nucleus).

Type IV hypersensitivity is also called *delayed-type hypersensitivity* (DTH) and is mediated by a memory T-cell response. T-cells that have been sensitized to an allergen by a previous contact recruit other leukocytes to the site of the allergen upon a later encounter. Because of the cell recruitment, a delay occurs in the allergic reaction. Examples of DTH include contact dermatitis (allergen contact with the epidermis resulting in inflammation and redness caused by infiltration of leukocytes and cytokine release), tuberculin reaction (local reaction of inflammation and redness at the site of subcutaneous injection of prepared antigen from *Mycobacterium tuberculosis*), and granulomatous reactions (stimulation from a foreign body or particulate such as talc or silica resulting in a granuloma, which is a mass of lymphocytes and macrophages surrounding an allergen too large to be phagocytized). DTH reactions can be prevented simply by avoiding contact with the offending allergen.

5-13 Autoimmune Diseases and Immunodeficiencies

Autoimmune diseases are simply immune reactions directed against self-antigens. These diseases can be directed to specific organs or can be systemic, depending on the nature and location of the self-antigen. A few autoimmune disorders have been described in the previous discussion of hypersensitivities. Autoimmunity tends to have a hereditary component. For example, relatives of individuals with Hashimoto's thyroiditis also have higher antibody titer (concentration) of thyroid-specific antibodies. Also, the relative risk for developing certain autoimmune diseases, such as Addison's disease, type 1 (juvenile) diabetes, or rheumatoid arthritis, is increased in individuals possessing certain alleles of MHC class II genes. Certain infectious agents may trigger autoimmunity in some individuals in a phenomenon referred to as *molecular mimicry.* This phenomenon occurs when antigens from a pathogen share epitopes with self-antigens; therefore, infection with this pathogen can result in activation of B-cells producing self-reactive antibodies, and subsequent production of the self-reactive antibodies leads to immune reactions to self-antigens. For example, development of rheumatic fever (immune reactions to self-antigens in the heart valve) sometimes occurs several weeks after an individual has recovered from a streptococcal infection. Autoimmune diseases are chronic diseases because self-antigens and the self-reactive leukocytes or antibodies are continuously present; however, in certain cases, autoimmunity can be controlled by immunosuppressive therapy.

Immunodeficiencies are, as the name suggests, conditions or disorders in which all or only a portion of the immune system is absent in an individual. They can be hereditary (primary) or acquired (secondary). Immunodeficiencies leave the individual vulnerable to particular types of infections, depending on the portion of the immune system that is lacking.

B-cell immunodeficiencies include X-linked agammaglobulinemia (no B-cell maturation and little detectable serum antibody); common variable immunodeficiency, or CVID (defective T-cell signaling to B-cells resulting in defective B-cell maturation and little detectable serum antibody); and various deficiencies in different antibody isotypes (caused by defects in class switching). All of these B-cell deficiencies are hereditary except CVID, which is a rare defect potentially acquired from a previous Epstein–Barr virus infection.

T-cell deficiencies include severe combined immunodeficiency, or SCID (a chromosomal defect in IL-7 receptor expression that leads to no T-cell maturation, or a separate defect of purine degradation enzymes leading to accumulation of nucleotides, which is toxic to lymphocytes); MHC class II deficiency (which leads to impaired T_H cell development, resulting in poor B-cell activation and differentiation and in poor antibody response); acquired immune deficiency syndrome, or AIDS (caused by infection with human immunodeficiency virus, which infects $CD4^+$ T-cells and leads to severe immunodeficiency caused by impaired T_H cell function); and ataxia telangiectasia, or AT (a defect in DNA repair enzymes, which leads to chromosomal breaks in the immunoglobulin or TCR loci, resulting in impaired antibody production and severe cell-mediated immune responses).

Complement protein deficiencies exist in which one or all of the complement proteins are not expressed in an individual. Defects in phagocyte function also occur, such as chronic granulomatous disease, or CGD (a defect in an oxygen reduction enzyme resulting in faulty pathogen killing in the phagolysosome).

In addition to the acquired immunodeficiencies that have been described, there are other secondary immunodeficiencies, which can be caused by a number of other factors, including steroid use, immunomodulatory drugs and cancer chemotherapy, nutrient deficiencies, and malnutrition.

5-14 Transplant and Graft Rejection

Certain instances necessitate transplanting organs, tissue, or cells from a donor individual into a recipient individual. Some examples are kidney transplantation into a recipient with end-stage renal disease, pancreatic islet cell transplantation into a recipient with diabetes, skin graft in a severely burned recipient, and bone marrow transplantation in a recipient who is immunodeficient. The most important consideration in performing a transplant is the genetic relatedness between donor and recipient, which can be described using a series of terms: autograft, isograft, allograft, and xenograft. An *autograft* occurs when the donor and the recipient are the same person, as in the case of a skin graft from one part of the body to a different part of the body. An *isograft* is rare because it involves a graft from a donor who is genetically identical to the recipient, which would be the case for identical twins. An *allograft* is the most common transplantation situation, in which the donor is genetically related to the recipient; the individuals do not have to be familial relatives, but the more closely related they are, the better the chance of success. A *xenograft* occurs when the donor is a different species than the recipient, as in the case of a monkey donor and human recipient. Graft rejection and success depend on the histocompatibility of the donor and recipient. Because MHC molecules are responsible for the strongest reactions of alloantigens, matching the MHC haplotype of the donor and recipient is crucial. The MHC genes are codominant, meaning that all of the MHC genes are equally expressed in an individual.

T-cells play a major role in graft rejection because T_C cells interact with MHC class I molecules, which are present on the surface of all nucleated cells, and T_H cells interact with MHC class II molecules, which are present on the surface of APCs. During graft rejection, APCs from the graft (which express the foreign MHC class II molecules), from the host (which process and present graft antigens that were shed from the graft tissue), or both activate T_H cells, which in turn secrete IL-2 and IFN-γ as well as other cytokines such as TNF-β, IL-4, and IL-5. This secretion leads to a robust immune activation in which B-cells become activated to secrete graft-specific antibodies, macrophages and other phagocytes become activated, T_C cells become activated, and expression of MHC molecules on APCs and the graft itself is upregulated. All this activity results in antibody-dependent cell-mediated cytotoxicity through cooperation among phagocytes, T-cells, and B-cells; cell-mediated cytotoxicity by T_C cells; and cell damage and lysis through complement activation and secretion of inflammatory mediators by macrophages.

Although exact tissue matching of MHC haplotypes is the most direct way to ensure a successful transplant, it is impossible in allograft transplantation because more than 100 different HLA (human leukocyte antigen) specificities are known to be reactive. Therefore, allograft transplant recipients undergo immunosuppressive therapy to prevent transplant rejection. Common immunosuppressive drugs include steroids, cyclosporine and other macrolides, and azathioprine. Steroids are anti-inflammatory and suppress MHC expression and macrophage activation. Cyclosporine, FK506, and rapamycin are fungal macrolides that interfere with the production of IL-2 and IFN-γ and, therefore, profoundly suppress the activation of lymphocytes and macrophages. Azathioprine, a nucleotide analog, is an antiproliferative drug that incorporates quickly into newly synthesized DNA in rapidly dividing cells; therefore, if leukocytes become activated and start proliferating, they will quickly die once azathioprine becomes incorporated into the genome.

5-15 Questions

1. Innate immune responses involve phagocytosis of extracellular pathogens by

A. T_C and T_H cells.
B. B-cells and plasma cells.
C. macrophages and PMNs.
D. platelets and mast cells.

2. Antigen-presenting cells such as macrophages present antigen in the context of MHC class II molecules to

A. neutrophils.
B. T_H cells.
C. B-cells.
D. eosinophils.

3. Adaptive immune responses in which B-cells are activated and produce antibody without any involvement of T-cells involve what kind of antigens?

A. T-independent antigens
B. T-dependent antigens
C. Self-antigens
D. Cytokines

4. B-lymphocytes become activated by engagement of antigen with

A. CD8.
B. the cell membrane.
C. TCR.
D. BCR.

5. B-lymphocytes that do not mature as memory B cells instead become

A. plasma cells.
B. antibody-producing cells.
C. macrophages.
D. both A and B.

6. T-lymphocyte activation takes place by interaction between the TCR and

A. BCR.
B. CD8.
C. MHC with antigen.
D. HIV.

7. The V domains of one heavy chain and one light chain of an antibody comprise

A. the Fc region.
B. the antigen-binding site.
C. the hinge region.
D. the BCR.

8. The predominant class of antibody present in the serum is

A. IgA.
B. IgG.
C. IgD.
D. IgM.

9. The MMR vaccine is an example of what type of antigen preparation?

A. Prepared fractionated antigen
B. "Naked DNA"
C. Live, attenuated organisms
D. Killed organisms

10. Passive immunizations involve injection of

A. antigen-specific antibody.
B. cytokines.
C. B-cells.
D. antigen.

11. Which of the following is an example of a suitable antigen preparation used in vaccinations? (Mark all that apply.)

A. Attenuated pathogen
B. Heat-killed pathogen
C. Fully virulent pathogen
D. Preparations of a portion of the pathogen

12. Type I hypersensitivity is mediated by

A. IgM.
B. IgA.
C. IgE.
D. IgG2b.

13. Type II hypersensitivity is directed toward

A. soluble antigens.
B. membranes and tissues.
C. mast cells.
D. antibodies.

14. An example of type III hypersensitivity is

A. tuberculin test.
B. serum sickness.
C. asthma.
D. anaphylaxis.

15. Type IV hypersensitivity is also called

A. serum sickness.
B. atopy.
C. hay fever.
D. delayed-type hypersensitivity.

16. Autoimmunity arises because of reactivity of leukocytes or antibodies to

A. allografts.
B. pathogens.
C. vaccinations.
D. self-antigens.

17. Which of the following is an example of an immunodeficiency? (Mark all that apply.)

A. Rheumatic fever
B. AIDS
C. SCID
D. X-linked agammaglobulinemia

18. Which of the following is the most common type of transplant?

A. Isograft
B. Xenograft
C. Autograft
D. Allograft

19. The most important determination in tissue typing is

A. MHC haplotype.
B. complement fixation.
C. isotype determination.
D. cell adhesion.

20. Which of the following is *not* an immunosuppressive drug used in transplant patients?

A. FK506
B. Antihistamine
C. Azathioprine
D. Cyclosporine

5-16 Answers

1. **C.** Macrophages and PMNs are phagocytes that use a nonspecific system for recognition of foreign objects.

2. **B.** T_H cells recognize antigen peptides in the context of MHC class II through interaction with T-cell receptors.

3. **A.** T-dependent antigens require T-cell help. In non-self-reactive individuals, self-antigens are not recognized by mature B-cells, and although cytokines are involved in adaptive responses, they do not trigger adaptive immune responses.

4. **D.** Naive B cells become activated by binding antigen with their BCR. The CD8 molecule and TCR are not found on B-lymphocytes. Antigens do not engage with the cell membrane of B cells to cause B-cell activation.

5. **D.** B-lymphocytes can mature to memory B cells and plasma cells. Plasma cells are also known as antibody-producing cells; therefore, both A and B are correct. Macrophages are in the myeloid lineage and are unrelated to B-lymphocytes.

6. **C.** The T-cell receptor on the T-lymphocyte cell surface engages with processed antigen presented in the context of MHC molecules on the surface of APCs.

7. **B.** The variable regions (V domains) of the heavy and light chains possess sequences that recognize and bind discrete epitopes of antigens. The Fc region is composed of the constant region of the heavy chains of an antibody and binds Fc receptors. The hinge region of an antibody is found between the V and C domains of the heavy chains. The BCR is not an antibody.

8. **B.** IgG is the predominant antibody type in serum because it constitutes approximately 75% of total immunoglobulin in serum.

9. **C.** The MMR vaccine is an example of a live, attenuated vaccine.

10. **A.** Passive immunization refers to the idea that one individual's antibodies raised against a particular pathogen are introduced into another individual to provide immediate immunologic protection.

11. **A, B, D.** Immunization with a fully virulent pathogen would allow the pathogen to infect the individual and cause disease. The other preparations listed either inactivate the pathogen (attenuated or heat-killed) or only include a portion of the pathogen, all of which are strategies used for effective vaccine development.

12. **C.** Type I, or immediate, hypersensitivity is mediated by IgE, which can become cross-linked on mast cells and lead to histamine release.

13. **B.** Examples of type II hypersensitivity are ABO incompatibility, Rhesus factor incompatibility, and Goodpasture syndrome because each of these

involves the reaction of the host to molecules on membranes and tissues.

14. **B.** By definition, type III hypersensitivity is directed toward soluble antigens such as those found in serum.

15. **D.** Choice A is an example of type III hypersensitivity, and choices B and C are examples of type I hypersensitivity.

16. **D.** Autoimmune reactions occur when leukocytes or antibodies react to self-antigens.

17. **B, C, D.** Rheumatic fever is an example of an autoimmune disorder. AIDS, SCID, and X-linked agammaglobulinemia are all examples of immunodeficiencies.

18. **D.** Although xenografts, isografts, and autografts are all valid transplants, allografts are the most common.

19. **A.** Determination of MHC haplotypes is done to investigate histocompatibility between donor and recipient of cell and tissue transplants.

20. **B.** Antihistamine is a type of allergy medication.

5-17 Additional Resources

Cancro MP, Kearney JF. B cell positive selection: road map to the primary repertoire? *J Immunol.* 2004;173(1):15–19.

DeFranco AL. Structure and function of the B cell antigen receptor. *Annu Rev Cell Biol.* 1993;9:377–410.

Lim MS, Elenitoba-Johnson KS. The molecular pathology of primary immunodeficiencies. *J Mol Diagn.* 2004;6(2):59–83.

Lopes-Carvalho T, Foote J, Kearney JF. Marginal zone B cells in lymphocyte activation and regulation. *Curr Opin Immunol.* 2005;17(3):244–250.

Mosmann TR, Coffman RL. Different patterns of cytokine secretion lead to different functional properties. *Annu Rev Immunol.* 1989;7:145–173.

Roitt I, Brostoff J, Male D, eds. *Essential Immunology.* 13th ed. London: Mosby; 2017.

Romagnani S. Immunological tolerance and autoimmunity. *Intern Emerg Med.* 2006;1(3):187–196.

Rose NR, Hamilton RG, Detrick B, eds. *Manual of Clinical Laboratory Immunology.* Subsequent ed. Washington, DC: American Society for Microbiology; 2002.

Wadia PP, Tambur AR. Yin and yang of cytokine regulation in solid organ graft rejection and tolerance. *Clin Lab Med.* 2008;28(3):469–479.

PHARMACEUTICAL SCIENCES

area

2

EDITORS: *ROBERT B. PARKER (6, 7), AND ANDREA S. FRANKS (8–13)*

Medicin

KIRK E. HEVENER

6-1 KEY POINTS

- Most drugs are weak aci a drug molecule is depen and the pH of the physiol is located.
- The pH-partition theory rel compartment's (i.e., stomo ionization and the resulti excretion of the drug.
- Drug binding to a recept chemical interactions, inc hydrogen bonds, and hy
- Many drugs are chiral, a bind. The stereochemistry bind to a receptor and p
- *Prodrugs* are chemically n form in which they are ad to the biologically active
- A *pharmacophore* is the features of a drug that is

6-2 STUDY GUIDE CH

The following topics may g

- ☐ Understand the nomen the organic functional
- ☐ Describe the physicoch organic functional gro the overall properties water solubility).
- ☐ Know the common aci as well as their relative absorption, distributio
- ☐ Discuss the basic bioc (protein, nucleic acids

6-3 Physicochem Absorption,

Acid–Base Properties of Dru

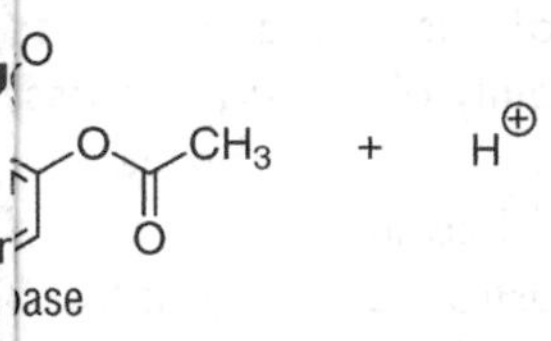

Most drugs can be grouped of drugs influence their absor groups (Table 6-1) in a drug

An acidic drug (e.g., aspi a basic drug (e.g., amphetai

Resonance stabilization o electrons from the nitrogen a strength [pK_a] = 4–5) are less

Amphoteric drugs contain

TABLE 6-1. Common Functional G

Acidic functional groups	Conjugate
R–SO₂–OH Sulfonic acid (0–1)	Sulfonate
R–COOH Carboxylic acid (5–6)	Carboxylat
R–SO₂–NH₂ Sulfonamide (9–10)	Sulfonamic
Thiophenol (9–10)	Thiopheno
Phenol (9–11)	Phenolate

a. The conjugate bases and conjugate acids of acidic and basic funtional groups. The neutral fu

are neutral (i.e., nonelectrolytes). e 6-1) as a part of their chemical , pyrrolidine and piperidine) are ible to serve as a proton acceptor. nolecules because the lone pair of not available to accept a proton. weak bases. In pyridine, unlike pyr- natic sextet. Thus, an unshared pair lable to serve as a proton acceptor. gth of organic functional groups. It asic. It can be used to calculate the ng a derivation of the Henderson– er solubility of a drug, which is an

d formations with water molecules of a drug in water. The aqueous , distribution, and excretion. ates for parenteral administration assive diffusion. method that relates the solubiliz-) to the number of carbon atoms of 5 to 6 carbons, while phenols ed in detail in the Lemke resource

Partition Coefficient (Log *P*)

The *partition coefficient (P)* of a drug is the ratio between the fraction of the drug (un-ionized) that dissolves in an organic phase (typically octanol) and the fraction that distributes into an aqueous phase (water). The ratio is typically expressed as the log *P* value of the drug. The log *P* value can be used to estimate the ability of a drug to cross biological membranes, which can aid in prediction of a drug's distribution.

Biological membranes are lipid bilayers with a lipophilic interior. Thus, drugs with high log *P* values cross biological membranes more easily and tend to be rapidly absorbed through passive diffusion from the gastrointestinal (GI) tract.

Nonetheless, drugs must have some degree of aqueous solubility because the availability of the drug molecule in solution form is necessary for drug absorption. Furthermore, the biological fluids at the absorption site are aqueous in nature. Therefore, the chemical nature of the drug molecule must maintain a desirable log *P* to facilitate drug absorption.

Polar functional groups (e.g., OH [hydroxyl], NH_2 [amine], and COOH [carboxylic acid]) increase the hydrophilic character of drugs, whereas nonpolar groups (e.g., halogens, sulfur, and aliphatic and aromatic hydrocarbons) increase their lipophilicity.

pH-Partition Theory

The pH-partition theory relates the effect of a biological compartment's pH and a drug's pK_a to the extent the drug is ionized or un-ionized and its resulting absorption, distribution, or excretion. The theory is governed by factors such as the dissociation constant, lipid solubility, and pH of the fluid at the site of absorption. It influences drug absorption from the GI tract and drug transport across biological membranes. The ratio of un-ionized to ionized fractions of a drug in solution is influenced by the pK_a of the drug and the pH of the solution at the biological site or compartment.

Generally, if the pK_a of a weakly acidic drug is greater than the pH of its environment (e.g., gastric fluid), the drug exists predominantly in the un-ionized state, which facilitates absorption. In contrast, if the pK_a of the acidic drug is less than the pH of its environment, the drug exists mostly in the ionized state, which limits absorption.

A similar relationship applies to basic drugs. Thus, for weakly basic drugs, if the pK_a of the drug is greater than the pH of its environment (e.g., gastric fluid), the drug will exist mostly in the ionized state, which limits absorption. However, if the pK_a of the weakly basic drug is less than the pH of its environment (e.g., the duodenum), the un-ionized form of the drug will predominate, which promotes absorption.

6-4 Chemical Basis for Drug Action

Drug–Receptor Interactions

Most drugs produce their effects by binding to specific *receptors*. In the context of this section, we refer to "receptor" as the biological macromolecule to which a drug binds to exert its action, whether that is a membrane-bound protein receptor, an enzyme, RNA (ribonucleic acid), or DNA (deoxyribonucleic acid). The affinity of a drug for its receptor and the resulting pharmacological outcome may be influenced by the type of chemical interactions the drug makes with the receptor, the conformation of the drug, and the stereochemistry of the drug molecule.

Chemical interactions

A drug molecule binds to its receptor through complementary chemical interactions. During the drug binding process, the functional groups of the drug molecule interact with corresponding functional groups of the receptor by a combination of chemical interactions (Figure 6-2). The outcome of these drug–receptor

FIGURE 6-2. Examples of Potential Multiple Drug–Receptor Interactions of Pindolol with Adrenergic Receptors

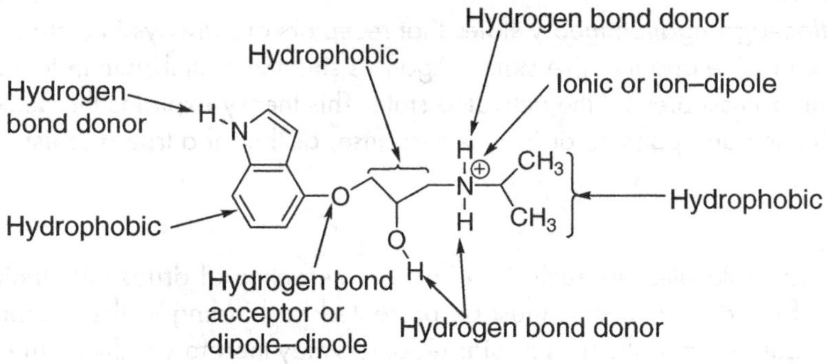

interactions may be agonism (activation) of the receptor or antagonism (inhibition) of the receptor to produce the desired therapeutic effect. Changes in the chemical composition of the drug molecule (caused by metabolism or degradation) may eliminate a desired drug–receptor interaction, which may result in loss of therapeutic efficacy. The chemical interactions that may occur between a drug and its receptor include the following:

- A covalent bond (50–150 kcal/mol) is the strongest of these interactions. Sharing of electrons between an atom from the drug and an atom from the receptor results in the covalent bond formation. Covalent bonding is usually irreversible and can lead to destruction of the receptor. A new receptor must often be synthesized for full recovery of cellular function.
- An ionic bond (5–10 kcal/mol), also known as a *salt bridge,* is a type of electrostatic interaction that occurs between oppositely charged functional groups on the drug and the receptor.
- A hydrogen bond (2–5 kcal/mol) is another type of electrostatic interaction in which a hydrogen atom serves as a bridge between two electronegative atoms, one from the drug and the other from the receptor.
- A hydrophobic interaction (0.5–1 kcal/mol) is also referred to as *van der Waals forces* or *London forces.* The interaction occurs between nonpolar regions of the drug and the receptor. The drug must be close to the receptor for this interaction to occur.

Receptor theory

Several theories have been formulated to explain the observed effects of the binding of a drug molecule to its receptor, including the following:

- The *occupancy theory* states that the binding of a drug (agonist) to its receptor results in a conformational change in the receptor that initiates a pharmacological response with a magnitude directly proportional to the number of receptors bound by the drug.
- The *rate theory* states that the number of drug–receptor interactions per unit time determines the magnitude of the pharmacological response.
- The *induced fit theory* states that a receptor undergoes conformational change near a drug molecule to allow effective binding of the drug to the receptor. Unlike an agonist, an antagonist does not induce the correct conformational change to induce a response.
- The *macromolecular perturbation theory* combines the rate and induced fit theories. It suggests that two types of conformational changes occur, and the rate of their existence determines the observed pharmacological response. Agonists produce the required conformational change for pharmacological response, but antagonists produce a nonspecific conformational change, which fails to induce pharmacological response. This theory partly explains the

activity of partial agonists, which elicit only a partial response, regardless of drug concentration.

- The *activation–aggregation theory* states that receptors are always in a state of dynamic equilibrium between active and inactive states. Agonists shift the equilibrium in favor of the active state, whereas antagonists prevent the activated state. This theory explains the activity of inverse agonists, which elicit an opposite, or inverse response, as that of a true agonist.

Stereochemistry

Receptors are chiral molecules. As such, for effective interaction of drugs with their target receptors, the pharmacophore of the drug molecule must be presented for binding to the receptor in a specific three-dimensional arrangement. Enantiomers or diastereomers may therefore induce different receptor perturbations. Enantiomers are nonsuperimposable mirror images that possess the same physical and chemical properties. They typically have one or more stereocenter. Diastereomers are not mirror images; they possess different configurations at one or more, but not all, stereocenters. Diastereomers can have different physical and chemical properties. For example, the drug labetalol (Figure 6-3) has two stereocenters. R,R-labetalol is the enantiomer of S,S-labetalol; but a diastereomer of R,S-labetalol.

The *R,R*-diastereomer of labetalol binds best to the β-adrenergic receptor; the *S,R*-diastereomer binds best to the α-adrenergic receptor; the *S,S*-diastereomer has some α-adrenergic receptor blocking activity but no activity at β-adrenergic receptors; and the *R,S*-diastereomer has practically no activity at the α- and β-adrenergic receptors. These differences in pharmacological activities may be attributable to the spatial orientation of the groups at the chiral centers of the drug in relation to the receptor (Figure 6-3).

Geometric (configurational) isomers are another type of stereoisomer. They are characterized by a specific orientation of functional groups around a chemical feature of a molecule (e.g., a double bond or ring substituents). Cis-trans isomerism and E/Z isomerism are examples of geometric isomers. Like enantiomers and diastereomers, geometric isomers can have different receptor affinities and activities.

Drug Stability

Drugs may undergo chemical reactions that result in loss of therapeutic efficacy, generation of toxic molecules, or both. Drugs can undergo decomposition by several chemical pathways, but the most common are oxidation and hydrolysis.

Molecular oxygen promotes drug oxidation, which may be catalyzed by light, heat, metal ions, and peroxides. Examples of drugs that are prone to oxidation include phenolic drugs (e.g., morphine, acetaminophen, salbutamol); catecholamines (e.g., epinephrine); and polyunsaturated oils (e.g., vitamins A and E). These drugs undergo decomposition by a free radical chain reaction.

FIGURE 6-3. Effect of Stereochemistry on the Interaction of Diastereomers of Labetalol with Adrenergic Receptors[a]

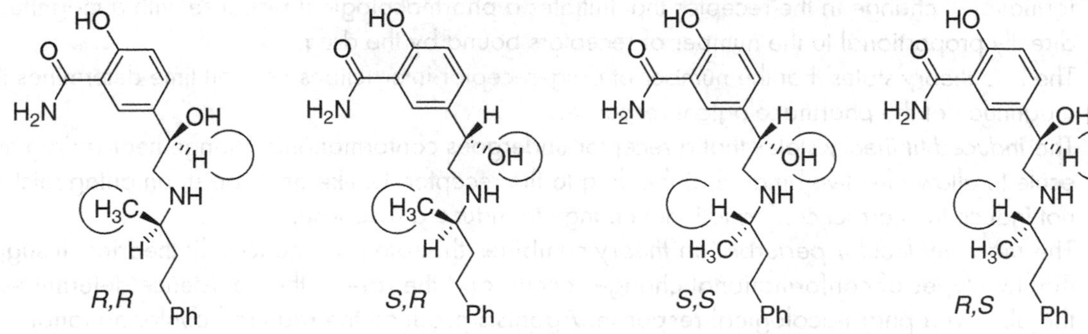

a. The OH and CH3 groups at the chiral centers may make bonding interactions with the different adrenergic receptors depending on their stereochemical orientation. These interactions may influence the pharmacological activities of the diastereomers.

Decomposition of drugs through oxidation may be prevented by the following:

- Packing the drug under an inert gas atmosphere to exclude oxygen
- Packaging the drug in amber-colored containers to exclude light
- Adding chelating agents to remove metal ions
- Adding antioxidants

Several functional groups (especially esters and amides) in drug molecules are susceptible to hydrolysis. The process is slow but is accelerated in the presence of acids and bases. Examples of drugs prone to hydrolysis include aspirin, procaine, and the penicillins. Amides are usually hydrolyzed at a much slower rate than esters, and this is often taken advantage of in drug design to extend the activity of a drug. A notable example is local anesthetic agents. The ester-based procaine has an anesthetic duration of 15 to 30 minutes because of its rapid inactivation by hydrolysis. The amide-based lidocaine can last up to 3 hours when given locally.

Prodrugs

Prodrugs are chemically modified drugs that are inactive in the form in which they are administered but are converted in vivo to the therapeutically active drug. The prodrug concept has been used to improve therapeutic outcome of drugs by improving their pharmacokinetic properties or improving patient compliance (Figure 6-4), as in the following examples:

- Tenofovir disoproxil is a phosphoester prodrug with improved absorption over the di-anionic parent compound. The two phosphoester bonds are cleaved in vivo to give the parent monophosphate drug, which is then phosphorylated to the active compound, tenofovir diphosphate.
- Enalapril is an ester prodrug of enalaprilat with enhanced bioavailability because of its higher affinity for the peptide carrier.
- Depot prodrugs of neuroleptics such as fluphenazine decanoate have significantly improved the therapy of schizophrenia because these intramuscular injections have very slow absorption and can be administered only once or twice a month.
- The bad taste of the drug sulfisoxazole, an antibacterial commonly used in pediatrics, has been masked by attaching an acetyl group to the sulfonamide nitrogen to improve patient compliance.

FIGURE 6-4. Examples of Prodrugs[a]

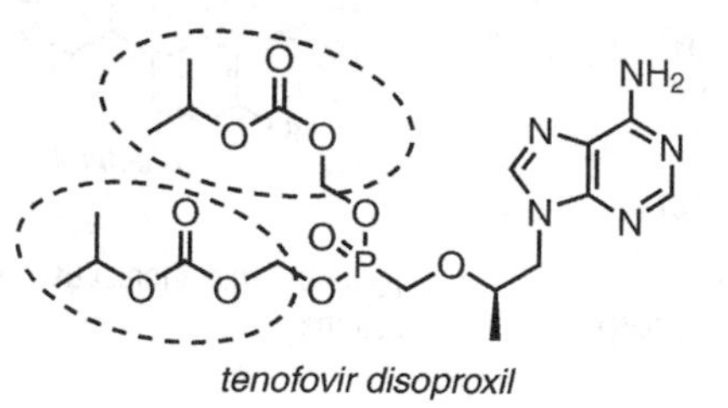

tenofovir disoproxil

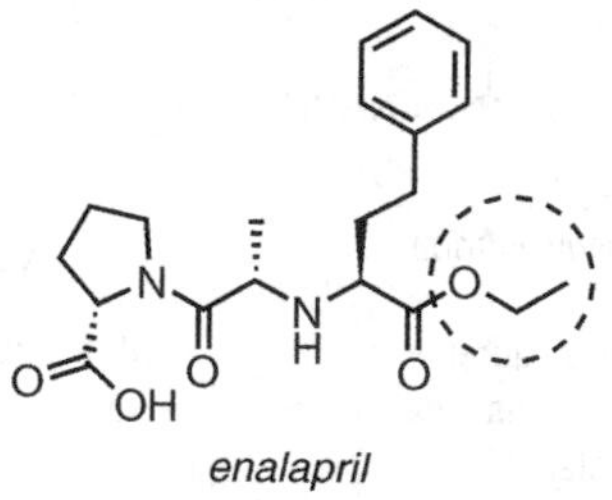

enalapril

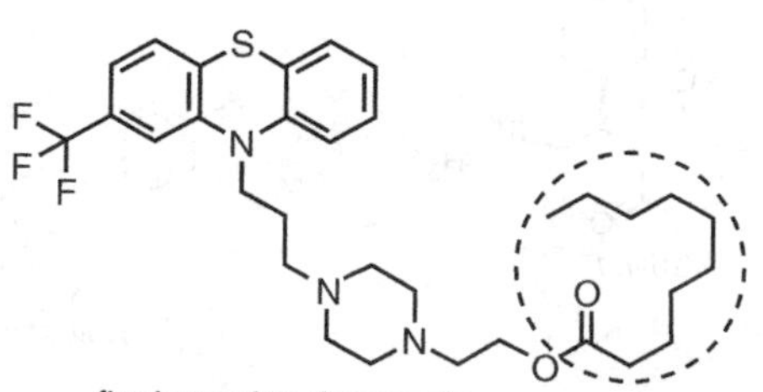

fluphenazine decanoate

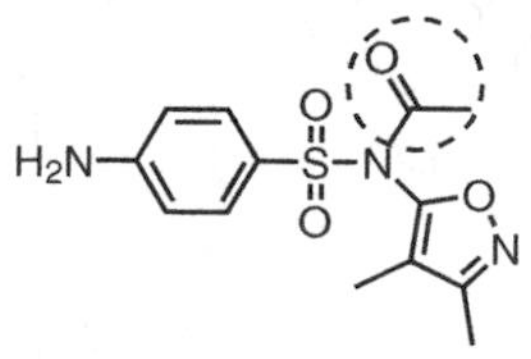

acetyl sulfisoxazole

a. Prodrug moieties are shown circled in dashed lines.

6-5 Fundamental Pharmacophores for Drugs Used to Treat Disease

A *pharmacophore* may be defined as a set of structural features in a molecule that is recognized at a receptor site and is responsible for the molecule's biological activity. These features can include ionizable groups, hydrogen bond donors or acceptors, lipophilic features, aromatic ring systems, and other features typically arranged in a specific three-dimensional orientation that imparts a high degree of affinity for a given receptor. A pharmacophore can be considered the minimal set of features in a molecule required to produce a biological or pharmacological effect. Figure 6-5 lists the pharmacophores of selected drugs used to treat disease.

FIGURE 6-5. Pharmacophores of Selected Drugs in Clinical Use

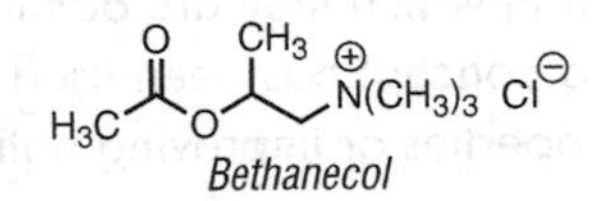
Bethanecol

Selective muscarinic agonist used to treat postoperative urinary retention and abdominal distention

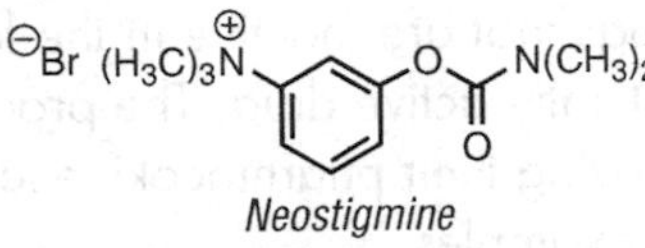
Neostigmine

Reversible acetylcholine esterase inhibitor used to treat postoperative abdominal distention, urinary retention, and myasthenia gravis

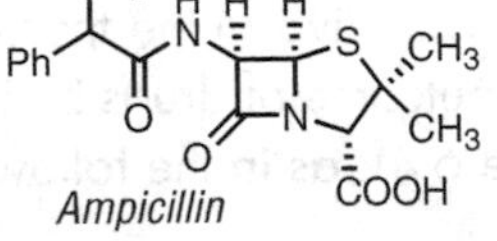
Ampicillin

Penicillin antibacterial agent

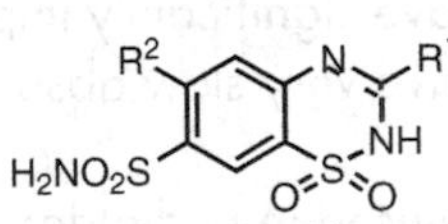
Benzothiazide

Thiazide diuretics

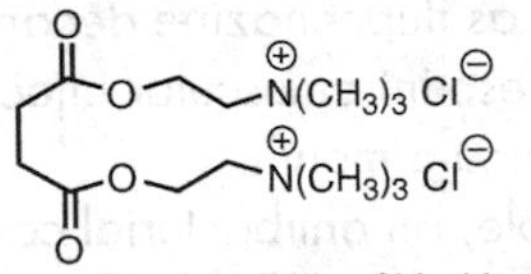
Succinylcholine Chloride

Nicotine antagonist used as a depolarizing neuromuscular blocking agent

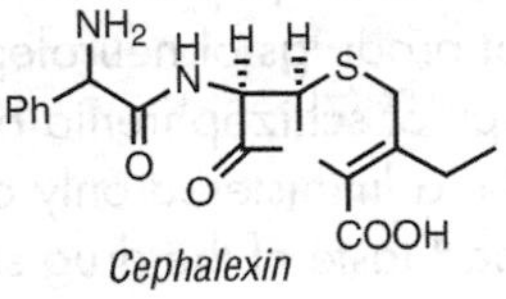
Cephalexin

Cephalosporin antibiotic

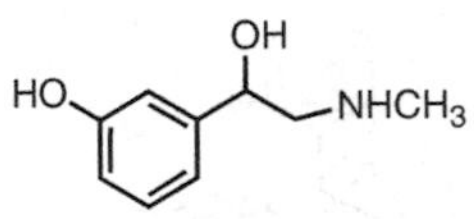
Phenylephrine

Selective α_1-adrenergic agonist used as a nasal decongestant

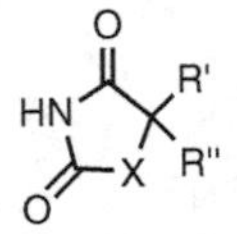
X = NH, O, or CH_2

Antiepileptic agents (e.g., phenytoin [*X = NH*])

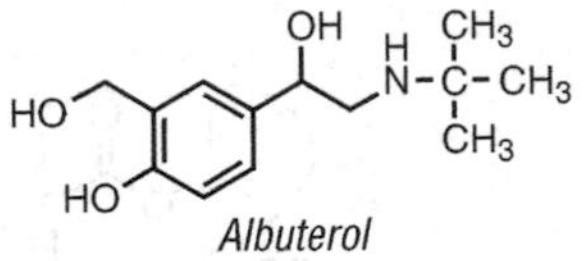
Albuterol

β_2-adrenergic agonist used to treat asthma

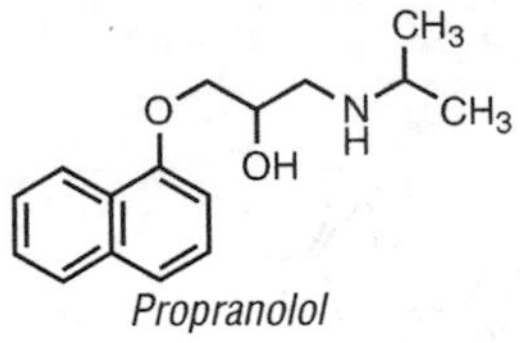
Propranolol

Nonselective β_2-adrenergic antagonist used to treat hypertension and arrhythmias

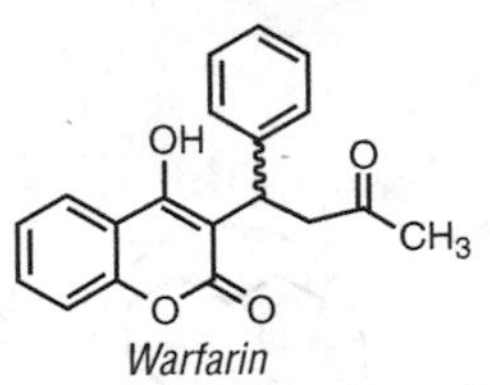
Warfarin

4-hydroxycoumarin oral anticoagulant

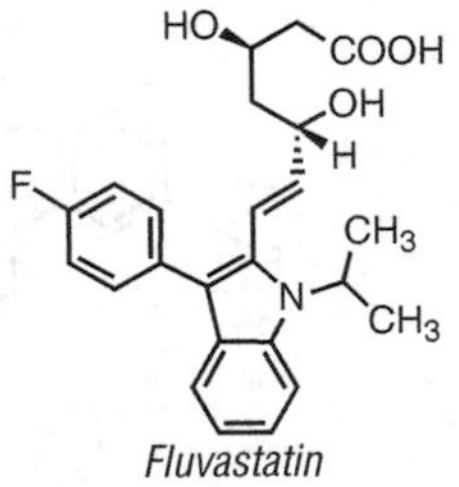
Fluvastatin

Statin used to treat primary hypercholesterolemia

FIGURE 6-5. Pharmacophores of Selected Drugs in Clinical Use *(Continued)*

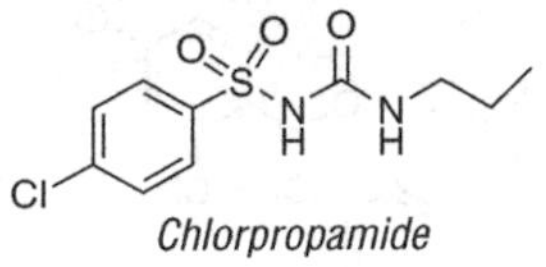

Chlorpropamide

Sulfonylurea hypoglycemic agent used to treat diabetes

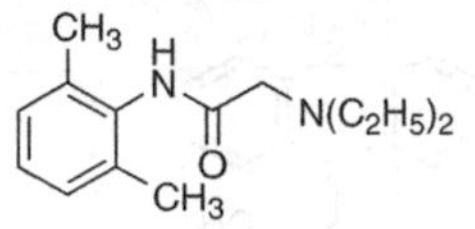

Lidocaine

Local anesthetic agent

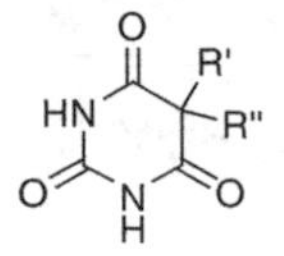

Barbiturates

Agents used as sedative-hypnotics, antiepileptics, or anesthetics

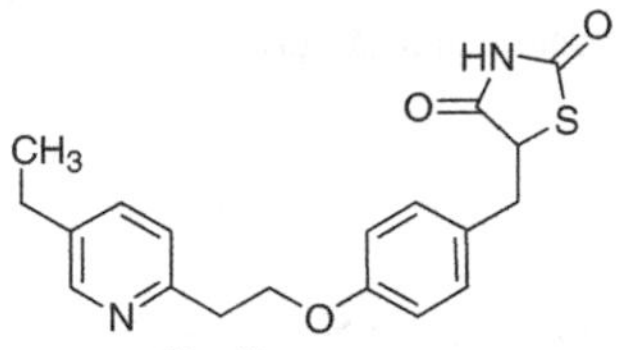

Pioglitazone

Member of the glitazone antidiabetic agents

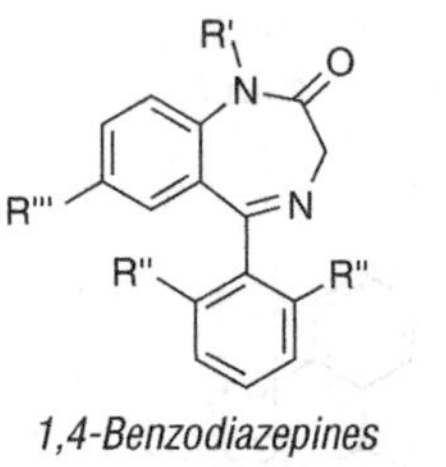

1,4-Benzodiazepines

Agents used as anxiolytics, antiepileptics, or muscle relaxants

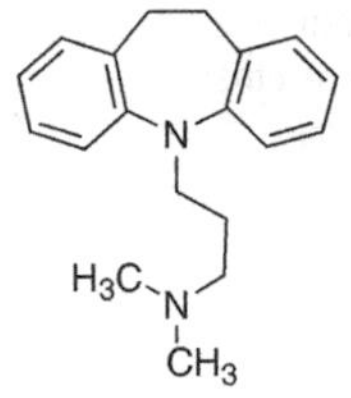

Imipramine

Tricyclic antidepressant

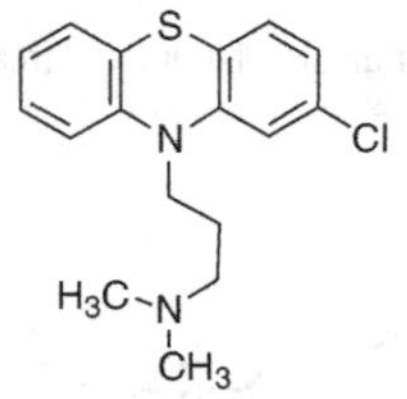

Chlorpromazine

Phenothiazine antipsychotic agent

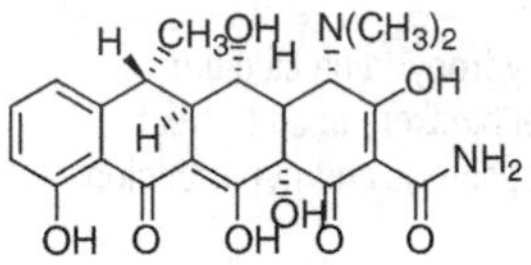

Doxycycline

Tetracycline antimicrobial agent

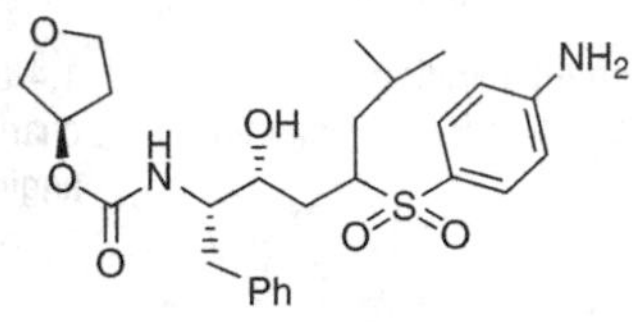

Amprenavir

Antiviral agent and HIV protease inhibitor

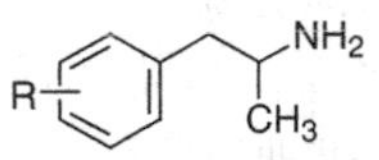

Phenylisopropylamines

Central nervous system stimulants (e.g., amphetamine)

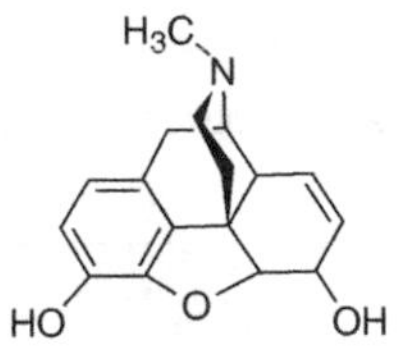

Morphine

μ-opioid receptor agonist

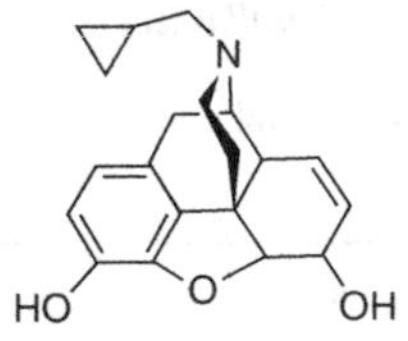

Naltrexone

μ-opioid receptor antagonist

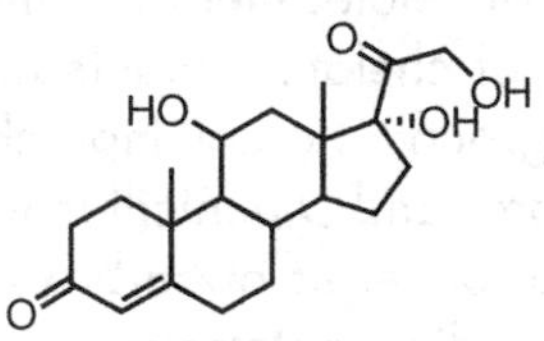

Hydrocortisone

Member of the adrenocorticoids

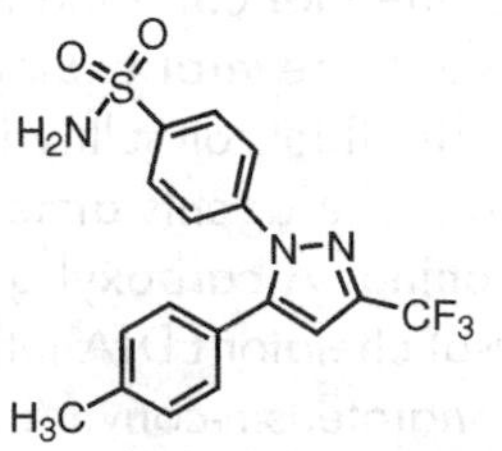

Celecoxib

Selective COX-2 inhibitor

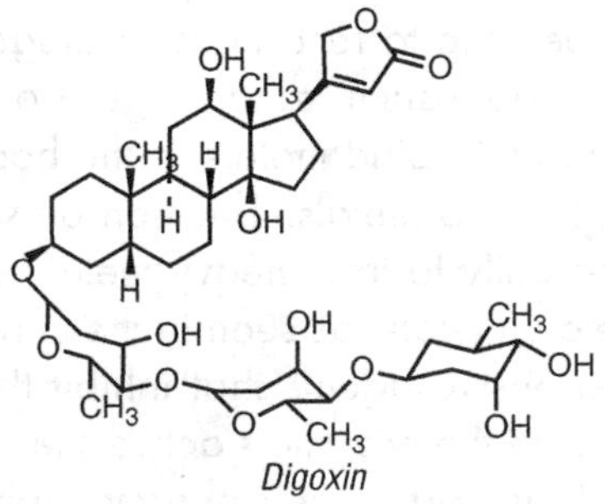

Digoxin

Cardiac glycoside

(continued)

FIGURE 6-5. Pharmacophores of Selected Drugs in Clinical Use *(Continued)*

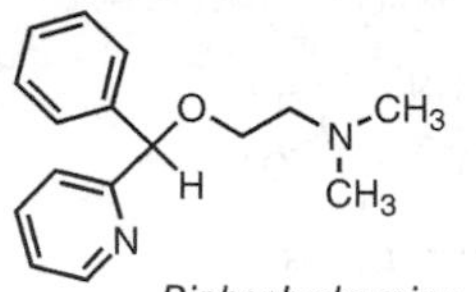

Diphenhydramine

First-generation ethanolamine ether antihistamine

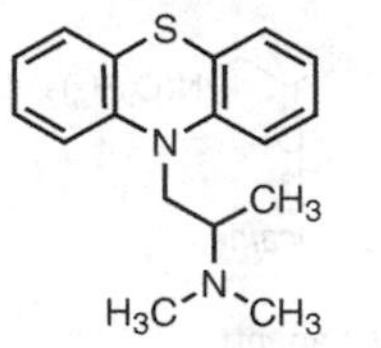

Promethazine

First-generation tricyclic antihistamine, H_1 antagonist

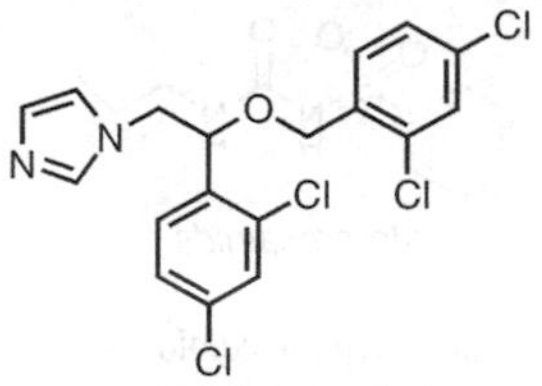

Miconazole

Imidazole antifungal agent

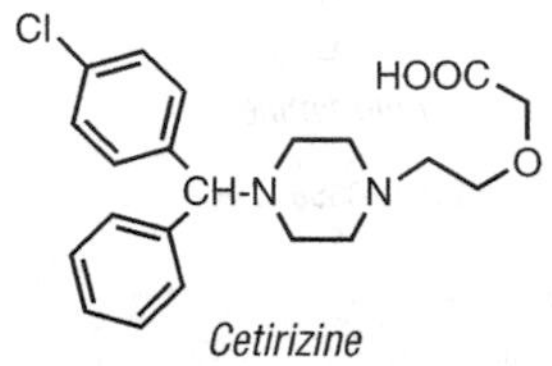

Cetirizine

Second-generation nonsedating H_1 antihistamine

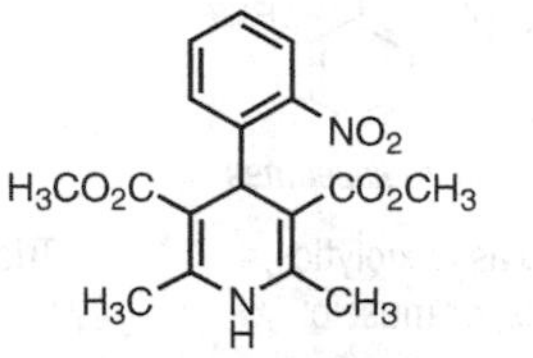

Nifedipine

1,4-dihydropyridine calcium channel blockers used to treat angina pectoris and hypertension

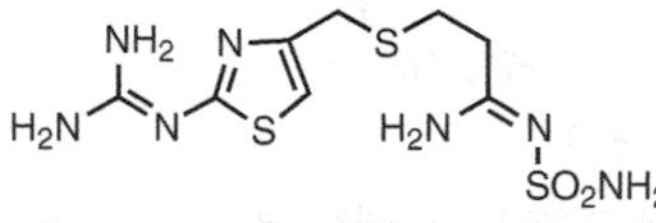

Famotidine

H_2 receptor antagonist used to treat peptic ulcers

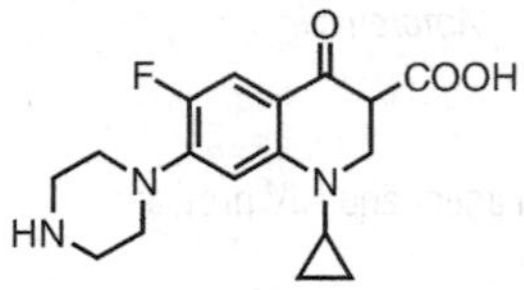

Ciprofloxacin

Quinolone antimicrobial agent

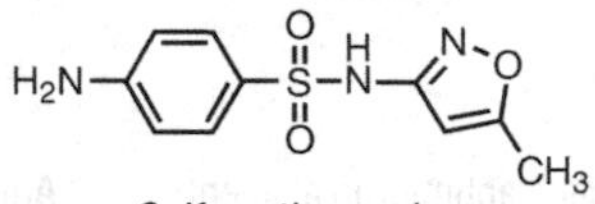

Sulfamethoxazole

Sulfonamide antimicrobial agent

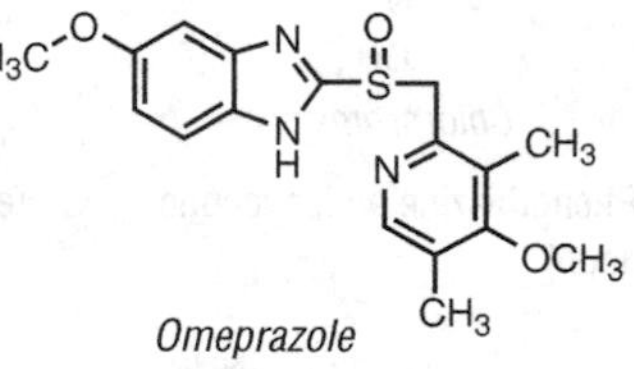

Omeprazole

H^+/K^+-ATPase proton pump inhibitor used to treat peptic ulcers

HIV, human immunodeficiency virus.

Some functional groups or parts of drug molecules can possess specific activity in the body not necessarily associated with receptor binding; these are known as *chemical motifs*. An important chemical motif to be able to recognize in drugs is one that can bind to, or chelate, metals in the body (e.g., calcium, magnesium, zinc). Figure 6-6 shows several examples of chelating motifs on agents and drugs known to bind metals in the body. The thiol, or sulfhydryl group, is a common chelating motif that can bind to metals. This can be seen in the agents dimercaprol and D-penicillamine, which are used medically to treat heavy metal poisoning. A carboxyl group, or series of carboxyl groups, can also chelate metals, as seen in the universal chelator EDTA (ethylenediaminetetraacetic acid). Certain antihypertensive agents that inhibit the angiotensin-converting enzyme do so by interacting with a zinc metal in the enzyme's active site. These drugs possess either a thiol (captopril) or carboxyl group (lisinopril) as part of their pharmacophore.

Last, 1,3-dicarbonyl or 1-carbonyl, 3-hydroxyl groups are known to chelate divalent metals such as calcium or magnesium, as shown with calcium and the drugs tetracycline and ciprofloxacin in Figure 6-6. This can have a negative effect on both the absorption of the drugs themselves and the body's use of the metals, particularly in growing children. For these reasons, drugs possessing this chemical motif are often contraindicated for pediatric use and co-administration with metal salts (e.g., antacids) is strongly discouraged.

FIGURE 6-6. Examples of Drugs and Functional Groups That Can Chelate Metals[a]

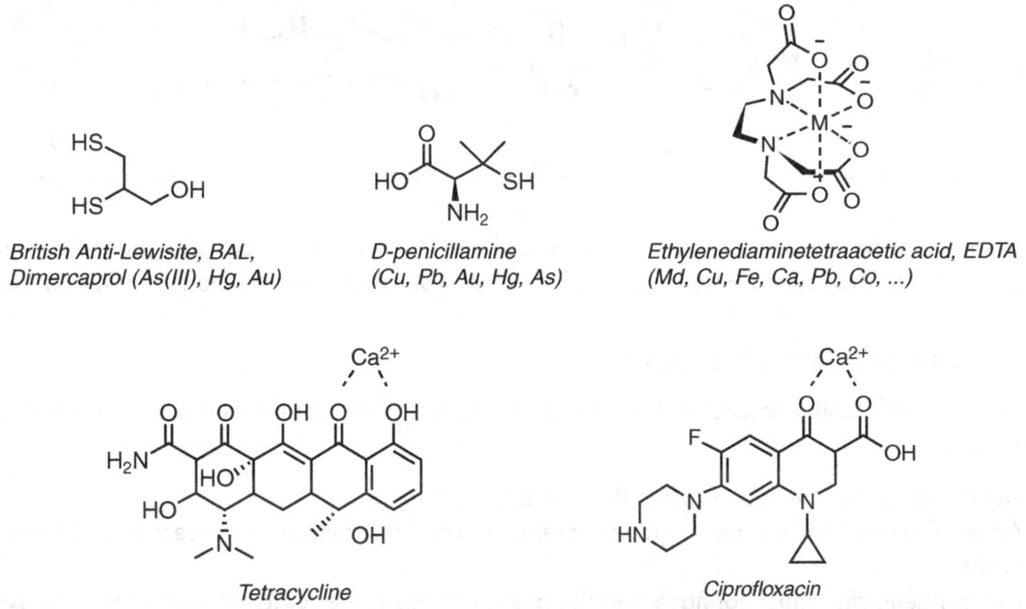

a. Most common metals acted upon by given chelating agents (top row) are given in parentheses.

6-6 Structure–Activity Relationships in Relation to Drug–Target Interactions

Drugs are generally discovered after structural modification of a lead compound. The lead compound may be discovered serendipitously (e.g., the benzodiazepines) or from endogenous sources (e.g., insulin); exogenous sources (e.g., opium alkaloids); rational drug design (e.g., HIV [human immunodeficiency virus] protease inhibitors); clinical observation (e.g., sildenafil); high-throughput screening programs; and genomics and proteomics. The *lead* is a prototype compound with a desired pharmacological activity, but it may also have undesirable features such as toxicity, limited in vivo metabolic stability, and other pharmacokinetic or pharmacodynamic problems.

To address these problems, structure–activity relationship (SAR) studies are usually undertaken. These studies involve the synthesis and biological evaluation of several analogues of the lead compound with the goal of enhancing the desirable properties of the compound while minimizing or eliminating undesirable characteristics.

The SAR study may include homologation (e.g., increasing or decreasing the length of alkyl chains), chain branching, ring–chain transformations, functional group modifications, and bioisosteric replacements. A bioisosteric replacement is the replacement of a functional group in a drug with a similar functional group that may produce the same physiological effect. This is often done to improve the physicochemical properties of a drug or to mitigate pharmacokinetic liabilities. Classical bioisosteres typically possess the same valence or are ring equivalents (e.g., methylene and ether), whereas nonclassical bioisosteres may not retain valence or may have significantly different structures (e.g., tetrazole ring and carboxyl group).

Selected examples are discussed in the following sections to illustrate SAR studies in relation to drug–target interactions.

Sulfonamides

The discovery that the antibacterial activity of the first sulfonamide, Prontosil, was due to its reduction product, sulfanilamide, initiated the first SAR studies. These studies led to the observation that compounds of the

FIGURE 6-7. General Structures of Drugs Derived from SAR of the Sulfonamides

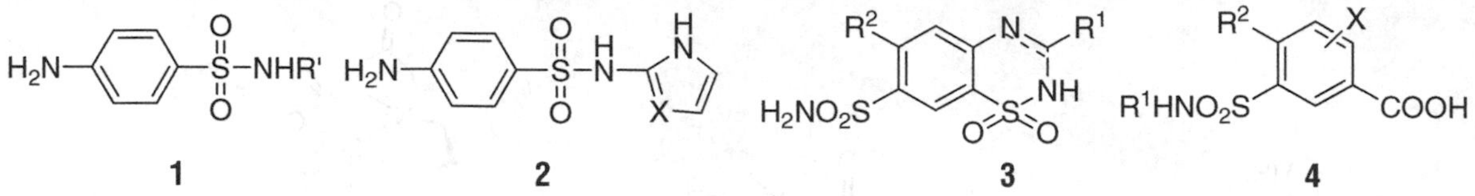

general sulfonamide structure displayed diuretic and antidiabetic activities in addition to their antibacterial activity and led to the sulfonylurea drugs used to treat hyperglycemia and the thiazide diuretic agents.

SAR for antimicrobial activity of sulfonamides

Sulfonamides with antimicrobial activity have structure 1 (Figure 6-7) and must satisfy the following requirements:

- The amino group must be para to the sulfamoyl group.
- An unsubstituted anilino amino group is preferred, but if a substituent is present, it must be removable in vivo.
- The benzene ring must not have additional substituents or be replaced with other ring systems.
- Monosubstitution on the sulfonamide nitrogen enhances activity, especially if the substituent is a heteroaromatic group, but disubstitution results in loss of activity.
- The acidity of the sulfonamide group is key to the receptor binding and activity of these agents. Electron-withdrawing substituents (e.g., heteroaromatic ring systems) at the R′ position improve activity by enhancing the acidity of this group.

SAR for antidiabetic activity of sulfonamides

Compounds with structure 2 (Figure 6-7), where X = O, S, or N and forms a part of a heteroaromatic system (e.g., thiadiazole or pyrimidine) or an acyclic structure (e.g., urea or thiourea), demonstrate antidiabetic activity.

SAR for diuretic activity of sulfonamides

Two classes of diuretics were discovered because of SAR studies of sulfonamides. They are the thiazide diuretics of general structure 3 (Figure 6-7) (e.g., hydrochlorothiazide) and the high-ceiling diuretics of general structure 4 (e.g., furosemide).

Phenylethanolamines

Agents in the phenylethanolamine class act upon the α- and β-adrenergic receptors in the sympathetic nervous system to produce a variety of physiological effects. The physiological neurotransmitter that acts upon these receptors is norepinephrine, which acts equally upon both α- and β-receptors, and several analogs with clinically useful activity have been developed (Figure 6-8).

FIGURE 6-8. SAR of the Phenylethanolamines

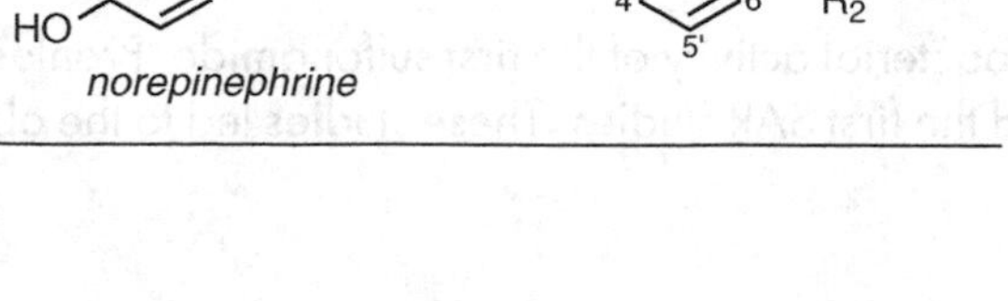

SAR for adrenergic activity of phenylethanolamines

The hydroxyl group at the 1-position must be in the R-configuration for maximum activity:

- As the R_1 substituent increases in size, α-receptor activity (agonism) decreases. A *t*-butyl group gives maximum β-receptor activity (agonism). Groups larger than *t*-butyl (4 carbons) lead to α-receptor antagonism.
- Small alkyl groups at the R_2 position (methyl or ethyl) slow metabolism and increase the duration of activity. Ethyl groups at this position afford some β-receptor selectivity. The 1R, 2S-isomers are preferred for maximum activity.
- For the R_3 position, 3′,4′ hydroxyl groups produce activity at both α- and β-receptors, but are rapidly metabolized by COMT (catechol-O-methyl transferase). 3′,5′ hydroxyl groups or 3′ hydroxymethyl, 4′ hydroxyl substitutions are poor COMT substrates (increased duration of activity) and afford β-receptor selectivity.

1,4-Benzodiazepines

The serendipitous discovery of chlordiazepoxide (Librium) initiated SAR studies, which led to the discovery of several 1,4-benzodiazepines that are used as anxiolytics, hypnotics, antiepileptics, and muscle relaxants.

After many benzodiazepines were synthesized and studied for biological activity, several SAR conclusions were reached. These conclusions are summarized in Figure 6-9, which is an example of a *SAR (or molecular activity) map* (a structural drawing of a lead compound annotated to show where in the molecule specific structural changes affect activity or potency).

Fluoroquinolones

The fluoroquinolone drugs were discovered fortuitously in the 1960s when the compound nalidixic acid, a byproduct of chloroquine production, was found to possess antibacterial activity. The compounds are now known to interfere with the activity of topoisomerase enzymes in bacteria, which maintain correct supercoiling states of DNA during transcription and translation. Several decades of research and hundreds

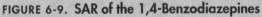

FIGURE 6-9. SAR of the 1,4-Benzodiazepines

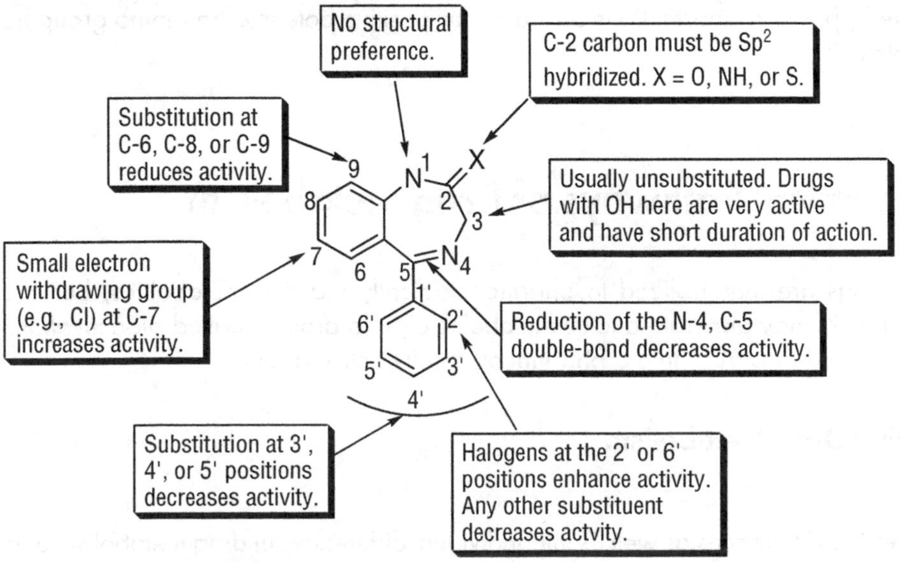

FIGURE 6-10. SAR of the Fluoroquinolones

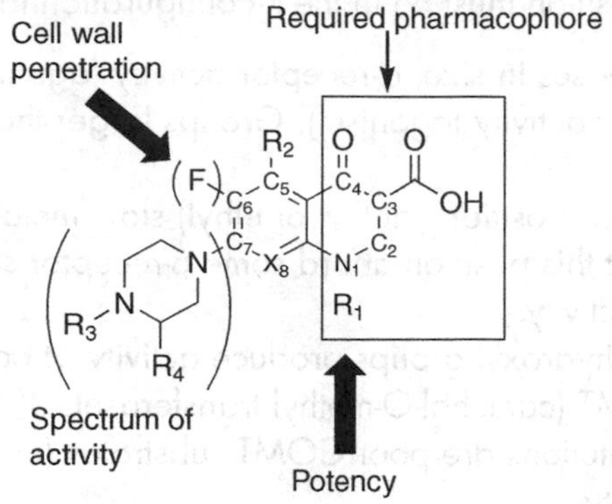

of synthesized compounds have led to a very clear understanding of the SAR of this antibacterial drug class, as shown in Figure 6-10.

SAR for antibacterial activity of fluoroquinolones

- The minimum pharmacophore required for activity is the 4-pyridone ring with a 3-carboxylic acid group (shown in box in Figure 6-10).
- Activity is nearly eliminated if the 2,3-double bond is reduced.
- A fluorine substituent at the C_6 position enhances activity, likely because of increased lipophilicity and cell penetration.
- Heterocyclic substituents at the C_7 position improve Gram-negative activity. A basic nitrogen is required at this position for oral activity.
- Piperazine rings at the C_7 position can cause central nervous system (CNS) effects because of off-target binding to GABA (γ-aminobutyric acid) receptors; this can be decreased by adding methyl or ethyl groups at the R_3 and R_4 positions or a bulky substituent at the R_1 position.
- Nitrogen at the X_8 position increases bioavailability. Methoxy group instead of halogen or hydrogen at this position increases stability to ultraviolet light and decreases phototoxicity.
- For the R_1 position, alkyl groups affect Gram-positive potency and half-life.
- For the R_2 position, substitutions control Gram-positive potency. An amino group here reduces phototoxicity.

6-7 Chemical Pathways of Drug Metabolism

Generally, drugs are metabolized to pharmacologically inactive metabolites, but in some cases, the metabolic process may generate a toxic metabolite or, in a process called *bioactivation,* may convert an inactive compound (prodrug) into a pharmacologically active agent.

Factors Affecting Drug Metabolism

Genetic factors

Racial and ethnic differences as well as interindividual differences in drug metabolism and disposition may be due to genetic polymorphisms (mutations) in drug-metabolizing enzymes. For example, cytochrome

P450 (CYP) 2D6 is involved in the metabolism of more than 30 cardiovascular and central nervous system drugs. Mutations in the gene encoding for CYP2D6 generate three phenotypic subgroups of metabolizers (i.e., poor, extensive, or ultrarapid metabolizers). Thus, patients on drugs that use the CYP2D6 pathway as the major metabolic route may experience different responses ranging from severe toxicity to complete lack of efficacy.

Physiological factors

Age, gender, pregnancy, nutritional status, and disease (especially liver disease) can affect drug metabolism. The livers of very young patients, such as newborns, are not fully developed, so these patients, as well as geriatric patients whose liver function has declined, metabolize drugs more slowly than the normal adult population. Differences in drug metabolism between men and women and between pregnant and nonpregnant women have also been observed.

Pharmaceutical factors

Dose amount, dose frequency, dosage form, and route of administration may affect the rate and extent of drug metabolism.

Environmental factors

Inhibition of drug-metabolizing enzymes by environmental toxicants and competition with other xenobiotics for these enzymes may affect the rate of drug metabolism. Co-administration with other drugs that are inducers or inhibitors of CYP enzymes also influences metabolism. Tobacco, alcohol, and recreational drug use may also interfere with the extent, and possibly the route, of metabolism of certain drugs.

Phase 1 and Phase 2 Drug Metabolism Reactions

Many enzymes are involved in drug metabolism, but the various isoforms of the CYP450 mixed-function monooxygenases located in the liver are the most important enzymes involved in drug metabolism. The two major groups of metabolic reactions in the body are termed *phase 1* and *phase 2 reactions.*

Phase 1 reactions include oxidation, hydroxylation, reduction, and hydrolysis (see Table 6-2 for examples). The reactions generally introduce a nucleophile (e.g., OH [hydroxyl], NH_2 [amine], and COO^- [carboxylate]) into the drug molecule.

In phase 2 reactions, a nucleophile in the drug molecule reacts with a masking group (e.g., glucuronic acid, sulfate, and acetyl and certain amino acids) to give a conjugate that typically possesses enhanced water solubility. In glucuronic acid conjugation, the drug (or its phase 1 metabolite) is appended to an activated glucuronic acid (uridine diphosphate glucuronic acid) to give the glucuronide metabolite (Figure 6-11, panel a). Sulfate conjugation involves the transfer of a sulfate group from PAPS (3′-phosphoadenosine-5′-phosphosulfate) to the drug (Figure 6-11, panel b). Compounds that contain an amino group may undergo acetylation as a phase 2 reaction (Figure 6-11, panel c). Drugs containing carboxylic acid functional groups (e.g., nonsteroidal anti-inflammatory drugs [NSAIDs]) usually undergo conjugation with amino acids (e.g., glycine and glutamine).

Metabolism of some drugs (e.g., acetaminophen) generates reactive intermediates that are detoxified by conjugation with glutathione. Several oxygen-, sulfur-, and nitrogen-containing drugs are metabolized by methylation under the catalysis of methyltransferases (e.g., catechol-O-methyltransferase). Acetylation and methylation reactions generate lipophilic compounds that are generally not pharmacologically active because of decreased affinity for the target receptor. Most drugs undergo phase 1 and phase 2 reactions sequentially, but drugs that are highly polar or resistant to drug-metabolizing enzymes are excreted mostly unchanged.

TABLE 6-2. Selected Examples of Phase 1 Reactions Catalyzed by CYP450 Enzymes

Drug	Metabolite	Drug	Metabolite
Side-chain oxidation		*Ring oxidation*	
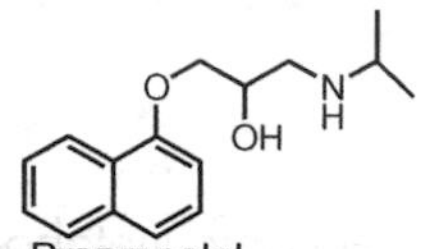 Propranolol	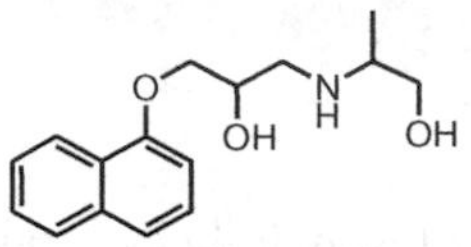	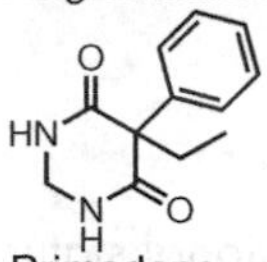 Primadone	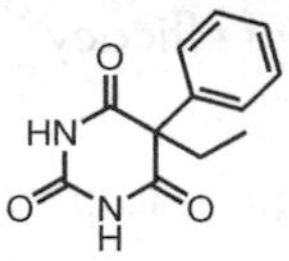 Phenobarbital
Sulfoxidation		*Deamination*	
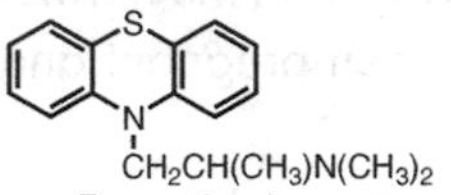 Promethazine	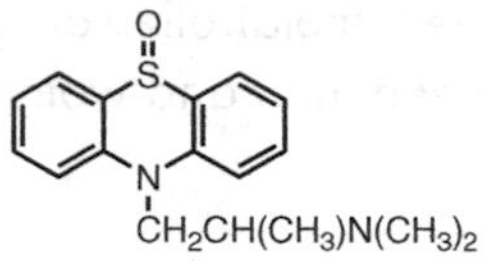	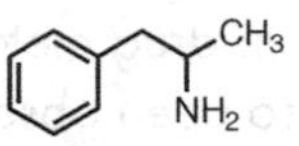 Amphetamine	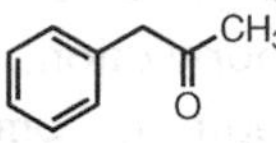 + NH_2
N-Dealkylation		*Aromatic hydroxylation*	
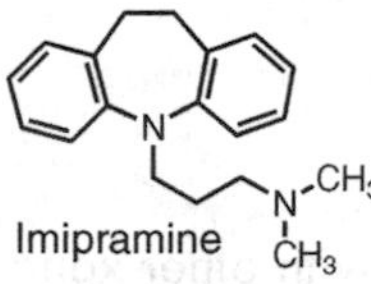 Imipramine	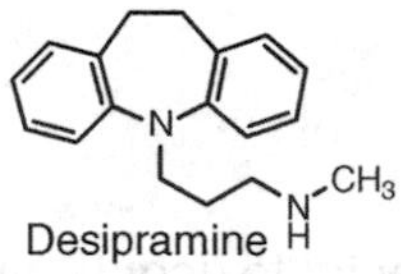 Desipramine	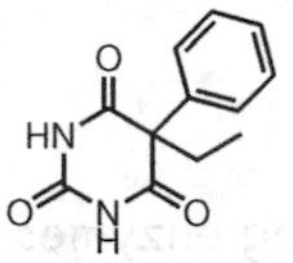 Phenobarbital	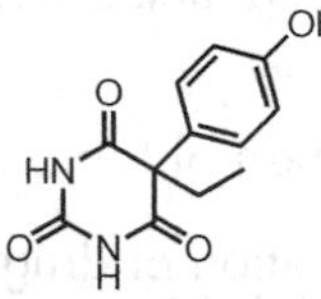
O-Dealkylation		*Desulfuration*	
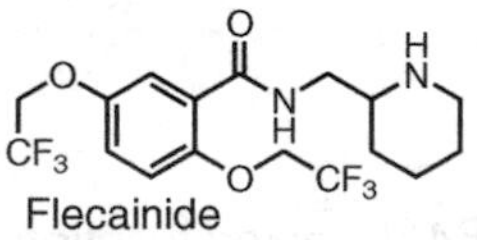 Flecainide	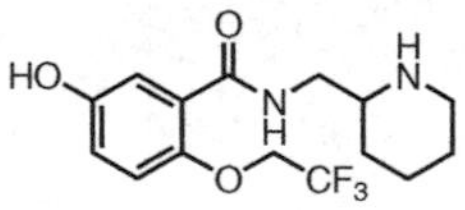	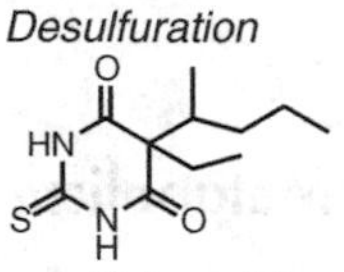 Thiopental	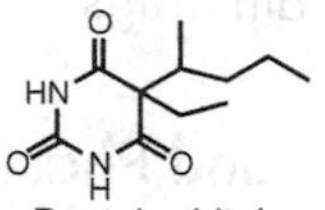 Pentobarbital

6-8 Applicability to Making Drug Therapy Decisions

The pharmacist's role as a member of the health care team is to help improve patients' quality of life by ensuring the responsible use of pharmaceuticals. To adequately meet this responsibility, the pharmacist must be able to integrate concepts in the basic sciences, including the medicinal chemistry of drug molecules, with the clinical sciences. This section presents examples of situations in which chemical knowledge of pharmaceutical agents aids in making drug therapy decisions.

Drug–Drug Interactions

A common clinical problem is one in which the efficacy or toxicity of a drug is affected because of co-administration of two or more drugs.

Drugs that are potent inducers or inhibitors of the CYP enzymes may influence the metabolism and elimination of other drugs on co-administration. Cimetidine is a potent inhibitor of several CYP isozymes and, therefore, can increase the risk of toxicity when co-administered with drugs metabolized by the CYP isozymes such as CYP1A2 (e.g., clozapine); CYP2C9 (e.g., phenytoin); CYP2D6 (e.g., antidepressants); and CYP3A4/5/7 (e.g., lovastatin).

FIGURE 6-11. Examples of Phase 2 Reactions

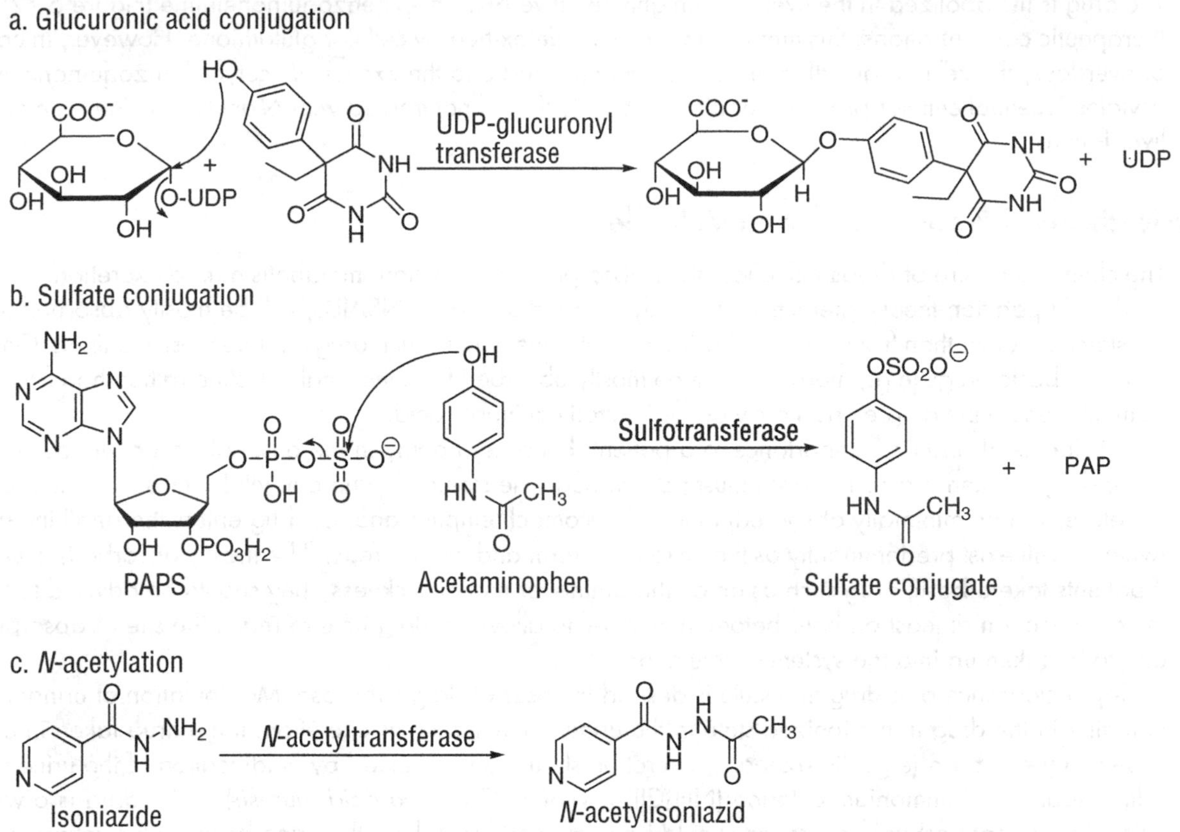

Phenytoin and rifampin are examples of CYP isozyme inducers. Drugs that are substrates of CYP3A4 and CYP2C9 are generally very susceptible to enzyme induction, which leads to rapid elimination of such drugs, resulting in decreased pharmacodynamic activity.

Co-administration of drugs with opposing mechanisms of action should be avoided because it will make one or both drugs ineffective. For example, vitamin K stimulates the synthesis of clotting factors, and warfarin inhibits the synthesis of clotting factors. Co-administration of these drugs may diminish the effectiveness of warfarin.

The chemistry of drugs must also be considered when coformulating medications, such as placing two drugs in the same intravenous (IV) bag or running them together in the same IV line. Coformulation or co-administration of a basic drug with an acidic drug may result in the formation of an insoluble precipitate, which may harm the patient directly or lack therapeutic efficacy. Unless documentation exists that two drugs are compatible, the pharmacist must exercise caution when combining them, particularly if the pK_a values of the two drugs are significantly different.

Drug Metabolism

Drugs with amino groups generally undergo *N*-acetylation (Figure 6-11, panel c). Because of a mutation in the gene encoding for one of the major enzymes involved in *N*-acetylation, *N*-acetyl transferase-2 (NAT2), some individuals have a reduced activity of NAT2. They are termed *slow acetylators,* compared to the *fast acetylators* with normal NAT2 activity. Fast acetylators terminate the activity of amine-containing drugs (e.g., procainamide and isoniazid) much faster than slow acetylators, who cannot metabolize such drugs quickly and so tend to accumulate the drug, which can lead to toxicity (e.g., liver damage with isoniazid).

Acetaminophen is a popular over-the-counter analgesic that is safe if taken in recommended doses. The drug is metabolized in the liver to the highly reactive *N*-acetyl-*p*-benzoquinoneimine (Figure 6-12). At therapeutic concentrations, this metabolite is rapidly detoxified by cellular glutathione. However, in cases of overdose, the cellular glutathione pool is overwhelmed and the excess *N*-acetyl-*p*-benzoquinoneimine arylates essential cellular proteins, leading to toxicity that, if not treated with *N*-acetylcysteine, can cause liver failure.

Physicochemical Properties of Drug Molecules

The chemical nature of drugs influences their absorption, distribution, metabolism, and excretion.

The pH partition theory predicts that weakly acidic drugs (e.g., NSAIDs) will be mostly absorbed from the stomach rather than from the more basic small intestine, where such drugs will be mostly ionized. On the contrary, basic drugs (e.g., morphine) will be mostly absorbed from the small intestine rather than from the stomach, where the drug exists mainly as the ionized conjugate acid.

This fact is of practical importance to a patient, because a delay in the onset of action will occur if a basic drug is taken orally. The drug must pass through the stomach (where it will be mostly ionized and, therefore, will be minimally absorbed) before the stomach empties and the drug enters the small intestine (where it will exist predominantly as the un-ionized form and, therefore, will be mostly absorbed). Hence, if patients take a basic drug such as an antihistamine for motion sickness, they should be advised to take their medication at least an hour before they travel to allow the drug time to reach the site of absorption and to be taken up into the systemic circulation.

Rapid clearance of a drug molecule is desired in cases of drug overdose. Manipulation of urinary pH to maintain the drug in the ionized state in the urine will enhance its excretion. If the drug taken in overdose is a weak base (e.g., flurazepam), excretion should be enhanced by acidification of the urine with administration of ammonium chloride (NH_4Cl) or vitamin C (*forced acid diuresis*). If the drug is a weak acid (e.g., phenobarbital), excretion should be enhanced by making the urine basic with administration of sodium bicarbonate ($NaHCO_3$) (*forced alkaline diuresis*).

Antacids such as TUMS will neutralize stomach pH to approximately 3.5. Therefore, patients must be counseled on the effect of combining acidic or basic drugs with antacids because the presence of the antacid may enhance or diminish the rate of absorption of the drug.

Antacids also should not be taken with tetracyclines because the antibiotic will form a chelate with metal ions in the antacid, which will diminish the extent of absorption of the tetracycline. Tetracyclines should not be taken concomitantly with foods that are rich in calcium for this same reason. The drug will form a complex with calcium ions and may be deposited in developing teeth, leading to discoloration of the teeth. For this reason, tetracyclines should not be given to children (6–12 years old) who are forming their permanent set of teeth.

FIGURE 6-12. Metabolism of Acetaminophen

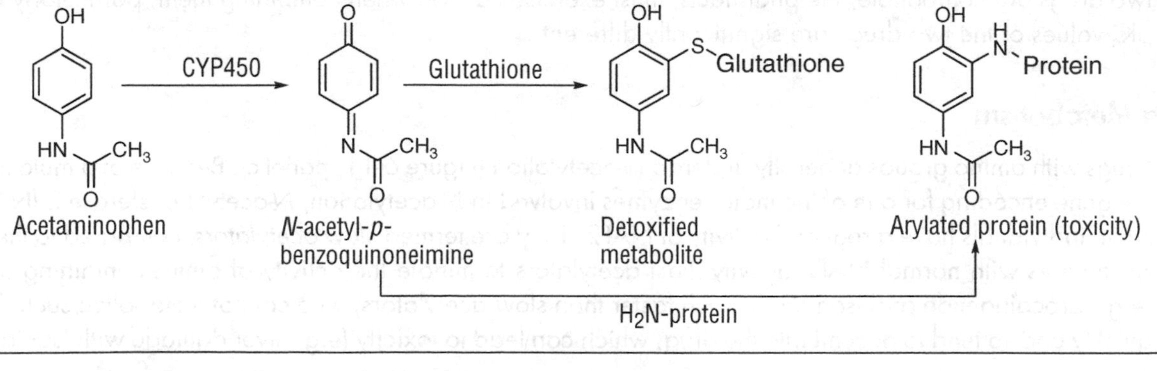

FIGURE 6-13. Oxidation of Epinephrine

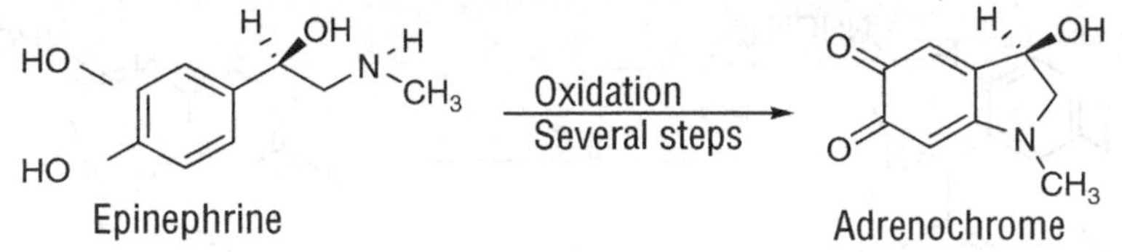

Adapted with modification from Cairns, 2012:224.

Drug Stability

Drug decomposition can result in loss of efficacy, generation of toxic products, or both. Therefore, drugs administered to patients must meet standards of desirable purity.

Oxidation

Drugs with phenolic groups, such as epinephrine, norepinephrine, and isoproterenol, are very susceptible to oxidation. These drugs are white crystalline solids, which change color (darken) on exposure to air. As shown in Figure 6-13, epinephrine is, on oxidation, converted to adrenochrome (a red-colored compound), which can polymerize to give black-colored compounds. Therefore, parenteral solutions of epinephrine that develop a pink color or contain crystals of black compound must be discarded.

Hydrolysis

Many functional groups in drug molecules (especially esters and amides) are susceptible to hydrolysis during storage. For example, aspirin is very susceptible to hydrolysis (Figure 6-14). The reaction produces salicylic acid and acetic acid, which are responsible for the smell of vinegar when a bottle of aspirin is opened.

The lactam ring of penicillin and cephalosporin antibiotics is also prone to hydrolysis (Figure 6-14). For this reason, these drugs are supplied as dry powder for reconstitution by the pharmacist before dispensing. The reconstituted drug must be stored in a refrigerator to limit hydrolysis.

When exposed to light, some drugs undergo decomposition and so must be packaged in amber-colored containers. For example, chlordiazepoxide undergoes a light-catalyzed cyclization reaction to generate an inactive compound (Figure 6-15).

FIGURE 6-14. Hydrolysis of Aspirin and Ampicillin

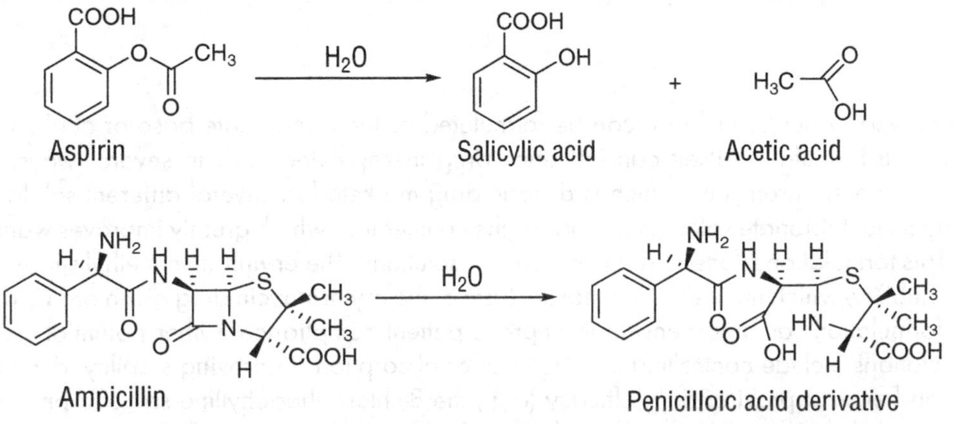

FIGURE 6-15. Light-Catalyzed Decomposition of Chlordiazepoxide

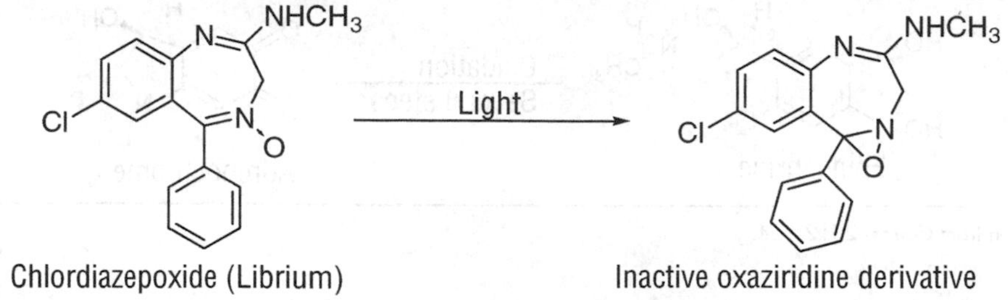

Adapted with modification from Cornelissen, Beijersbergen Van Henegouwen, Gerritsma, 1979.

Phototoxicity

Some drugs can absorb light in the visible and ultraviolet range, which can lead to the generation of free radicals. In susceptible patients, these drugs can cause skin irritation, erythema, and extreme sensitivity to strong sunlight. These photoreactive drugs are notable for their aromatic rings, often substituted with electron-withdrawing groups (e.g., halogens). Examples include some tetracyclines, fluoroquinolones, certain tricyclic antidepressant agents, NSAIDs of the propionic acid class, and amiodarone. Management of drug phototoxicity can include the use of sun blocks, avoidance of prolonged exposure to sunlight, or discontinuation of the drug itself.

Plasma Protein Binding

Another key factor in therapeutic decision making that is influenced by medicinal chemistry is the ability of a drug to bind to plasma proteins in vivo. The plasma proteins most relevant to binding drugs are human serum albumin and alpha-1 acid glycoprotein. Because these proteins are large, they do not distribute well from the plasma into tissues, meaning that bound drugs may not reach their sites of activity, metabolism, or excretion. Thus, only the unbound "fraction" of drug produces the biological activity. An example is the drug warfarin, an anticoagulant, which is 97% bound to plasma proteins.

The binding of drugs to plasma proteins is influenced by their physicochemical features. Albumin is a slightly basic protein and tends to bind drugs that are acidic or neutral. Lipophilic drugs also tend to show a higher albumin-binding potential. Alpha-1 acid glycoprotein is slightly acidic and tends to bind basic drugs.

Changes in the amount of a drug bound to plasma proteins can be influenced by the total amount of the drug in the body, the amount of plasma proteins circulating (certain disease states can affect plasma protein levels), and the administration of another drug that can displace the bound drug from the plasma protein. The latter is a potential drug–drug interaction mechanism.

Salts

Drugs that are weakly acidic or basic can be formulated as their conjugate base or acid salts, and the choice of the salt formulation itself can influence drug therapy decisions in several ways. A notable example is the drug erythromycin, which is a basic drug marketed in several different salt formulations. The erythromycin lactobionate salt uses a sugar as the counter ion, which greatly improves water solubility of the drug. This formulation is often used in parenteral solutions. The erythromycin ethyl succinate salt has poor water solubility, which masks the unpleasant taste of the erythromycin drug given orally. This is useful in pediatric formulations as a suspension to improve patient compliance. Other potential uses of differing salt formulations include controlling drug release or absorption, improving stability, decreasing pain of injection, and even improving drug efficacy (e.g., the 8-chloro theophylline salt of diphenhydramine, dimenhydrinate, reduces the sedative effect of diphenhydramine because theophylline is a stimulant).

6-9 Questions

Use Drug Illustration 6-1 to answer Questions 1–5.

DRUG ILLUSTRATION 6-1.

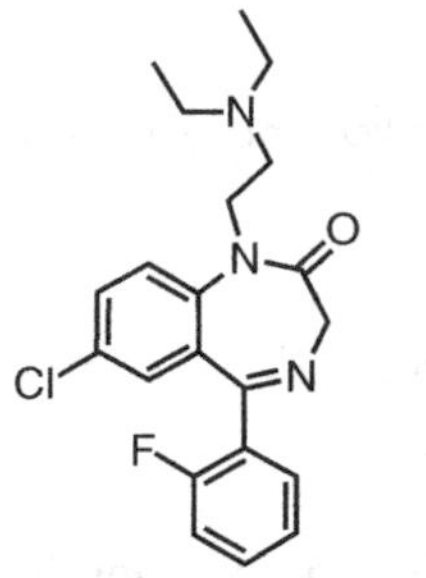

Drug 1 ($pK_a = 8.2$)6-

1. At what site of the GI tract will drug 1 be *least* absorbed?

A. Stomach (pH 2)
B. Duodenum (pH 6)
C. Colon (pH 8)
D. Absorption of drug from the GI tract is pH independent.

2. Drug 1 and others of similar pharmacophore are used as

A. diuretics.
B. anticancer agents.
C. anxiolytic agents.
D. anticoagulants.

3. The chemical bonding interaction that is *not* likely to occur between drug 1 and its target receptor is

A. covalent bonding.
B. ionic bonding.
C. hydrogen bonding.
D. hydrophobic interaction.

4. The tertiary amine group of drug 1 may form an ionic bond with which amino acid at the drug's target receptor?

A. Arginine
B. Lysine
C. Glycine
D. Glutamic acid

5. The best way to promote urinary clearance of drug 1 is to

A. administer water for injection.
B. administer a solution of $NaHCO_3$.
C. administer 5% dextrose.
D. administer a solution of NH_4Cl.

Use Drug Illustration 6-2 to answer Question 6.

DRUG ILLUSTRATION 6-2.

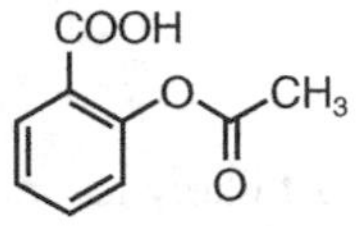

Aspirin

6. Drugs such as aspirin should not be stored in the bathroom because of the likelihood of decomposition through

A. hydrolysis.
B. hydrogenolysis.
C. dehydration.
D. reduction.

Use Drug Illustration 6-3 to answer Question 7.

DRUG ILLUSTRATION 6-3.

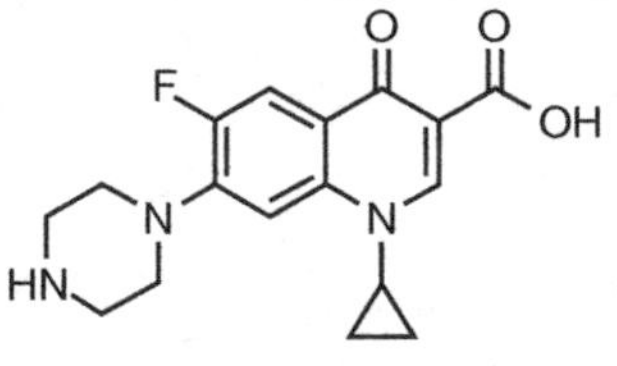

ciprofloxacin

7. Ciprofloxacin (Cipro) is used clinically as

A. an anticoagulant.
B. an antihistamine.
C. an antibacterial.
D. a sedative-hypnotic.

Use Drug Illustration 6-4 to answer Questions 8–13.

DRUG ILLUSTRATION 6-4.

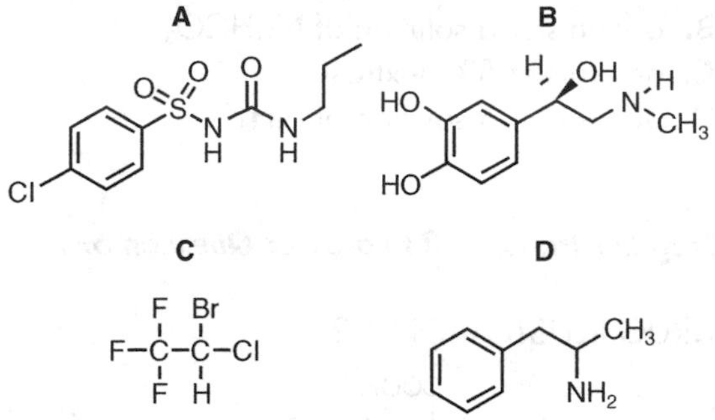

8. Which drug is most likely to undergo decomposition via oxidation?

A. Drug A
B. Drug B
C. Drug C
D. Drug D

9. Which drug contains a sulfonylurea functional group?

A. Drug A
B. Drug B
C. Drug C
D. Drug D

10. Which drug will undergo *N*-demethylation in vivo?

A. Drug A
B. Drug B
C. Drug C
D. Drug D

11. Which drug has a primary amine functional group?

A. Drug A
B. Drug B
C. Drug C
D. Drug D

12. Which drug is *not* ionizable?

A. Drug A
B. Drug B
C. Drug C
D. Drug D

13. Which drug will be predicted to have the highest log *P* value?

A. Drug A
B. Drug B
C. Drug C
D. Drug D

14. Which of the following is a phase 2 reaction?

A. Acetylation
B. Oxidation
C. Demethylation
D. Deamination

15. The drug that is a potent inhibitor of several CYP isoforms and therefore must be used with caution in combination therapy is

A. aspirin.
B. cimetidine (Tagamet).
C. gabapentin (Neurontin).
D. levetiracetam (Keppra).

16. How would you treat an overdose of acetaminophen?

A. Use forced alkaline diuresis.
B. Use forced acid diuresis.
C. Administer an osmotic diuretic.
D. Administer *N*-acetylcysteine.

Use Drug Illustration 6-5 to answer Questions 17–20.

DRUG ILLUSTRATION 6-5.

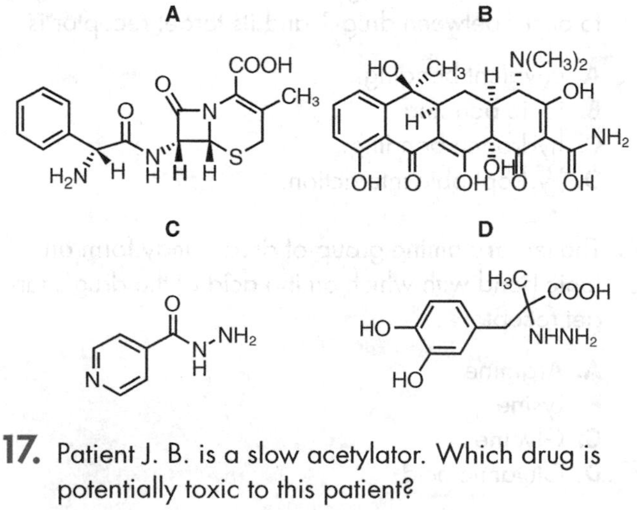

17. Patient J. B. is a slow acetylator. Which drug is potentially toxic to this patient?

A. Drug A
B. Drug B
C. Drug C
D. Drug D

18. Which drug must be reconstituted just before use to prevent decomposition?

A. Drug A
B. Drug B
C. Drug C
D. Drug D

19. Which drug must *not* be co-administered with antacids?

A. Drug A
B. Drug B
C. Drug C
D. Drug D

20. Which drug has a single pair of enantiomers?

A. Drug A
B. Drug B
C. Drug C
D. Drug D

6-10 Answers

1. A. Most drugs are absorbed from the GI tract as the un-ionized form by passive diffusion. Drug 1 (flurazepam) is a basic drug, so its ionization will be greatest in the stomach, which will limit absorption.

2. C. Drug 1 belongs to the group of drugs known as 1,4-benzodiazepines. Drugs in this class may be used as anxiolytics, hypnotics, antiepileptics, or muscle relaxants.

3. A. Covalent bonding involves the sharing of electrons between an electrophilic center (usually in the drug molecule) and a nucleophilic center (usually in the receptor). Drug 1 does not possess an electrophilic center capable of such an interaction with its receptor.

4. D. The tertiary amine of drug 1 will be protonated at physiologic pH and so can form an ionic bond with a glutamate of the receptor if it is close to the protonated amine.

5. D. Administration of NH_4Cl will decrease urinary pH to about 6, which will promote ionization of drug 1. The ionized form of the drug will not undergo passive diffusion back into systemic circulation but will readily dissolve and be excreted in the urine.

6. A. Aspirin is the acetyl ester derivative of salicylic acid. In the presence of moisture, the ester group can be hydrolyzed.

7. C. Ciprofloxacin is a fluoroquinolone drug. These drugs are used as antibacterial agents.

8. B. Phenolic drugs and drugs with the catechol group (e.g., epinephrine) are prone to decomposition through oxidation when exposed to air.

9. A. Drug A is chlorpropamide, which is a first-generation sulfonylurea antidiabetic agent.

10. B. Drug B has an *N*-methyl group, so it is a candidate for *N*-demethylation.

11. D. Drug D has a primary amine functional group. Drug B has a secondary amine group. Drugs A and C do not contain amine functional groups.

12. C. Drug C cannot donate a proton or accept a proton. It is therefore not ionizable. Drug A is an acidic drug because of the presence of the sulfonylurea group in its structure. Drugs B and D are basic drugs because of the amine group in them.

13. C. Halogens are lipophilic in character and so will increase the log *P* values of drugs, whereas polar groups are hydrophilic in character and so will decrease log *P* values of drugs. Drug C is the only drug in the illustration without polar residues; hence, it should have the highest log *P* value.

14. A. Acetylation is a phase 2 reaction that occurs in drugs with amine groups. All of the other reactions are phase 1 reactions.

15. B. Cimetidine is an antipeptic ulcer agent that inhibits several CYP450 isoforms. For example, it inhibits CYP1A2, CYP2C9, CYP2D6, and CYP3A4.

16. D. Acetaminophen is metabolized in the liver to a reactive quinoneimine intermediate, which is detoxified by glutathione. In overdose, the body's supply of glutathione is overwhelmed, which could result in hepatotoxicity. *N*-acetylcysteine reacts with the quinoneimine just like glutathione to detoxify it.

17. C. Slow acetylators are prone to having high plasma levels of drugs, such as drug C (isoniazid), that possess an amine group because such drugs are metabolized by acetylation. Drug D has a basic group (the hydrazine), but it can also be metabolized by glucuronide conjugation or methylation. Because of the multiple routes of metabolism, drug D is unlikely to be toxic to J. B.

18. **A.** Drug A is a cephalosporin. The cephalosporin and the penicillin antibiotics have a β-lactam ring, which may undergo ring opening in aqueous media. These drugs must be reconstituted just before dispensing and must be stored in the refrigerator.

19. **B.** The tetracyclines will chelate metal ions, which will lower their bioavailability.

20. **D.** Drug D (carbidopa) has only one chiral center, so it has only a single pair of enantiomers. Drugs A and B have multiple chiral centers, so they have diastereomers and multiple enantiomers. Drug C does not have a chiral center.

6-11 Additional Resources

Beale JM Jr, Block JH, eds. *Wilson and Gisvold's Textbook of Organic Medicinal and Pharmaceutical Chemistry.* 12th ed. Baltimore, MD: Lippincott, Williams & Wilkins; 2011.

Cairns D, ed. *Essentials of Pharmaceutical Chemistry.* 4th ed. Chicago, IL: Pharmaceutical Press; 2012.

Cornelissen PJG, Beijersbergen Van Henegouwen GMJ, Gerritsma KW. Photochemical decomposition of 1,4-benzodiazepines: chlordiazepoxide. *Int J Pharm.* 1979;3(4–5):205–220.

Harrold MW, Zavod RM, eds. *Basic Concepts in Medicinal Chemistry.* 1st ed. Bethesda, MD: American Society of Health-System Pharmacists; 2013.

Lemke TL, ed. *Review of Organic Functional Groups: Introduction to Organic Medicinal Chemistry.* 5th ed. Philadelphia, PA: Lippincott, Williams & Wilkins; 1992.

Lemke TL, Williams DA, Roche VF, et al., eds. *Foye's Principles of Medicinal Chemistry.* 7th ed. New York, NY: Lippincott, Williams & Wilkins; 2013.

Nogrady T, Weaver DF. *Medicinal Chemistry: A Molecular and Biochemical Approach.* 3rd ed. New York, NY: Oxford University Press; 2005:108–128.

Pharmacology

7

BERND MEIBOHM

7-1 KEY POINTS

- Most drugs exert their effects by interacting with molecular targets such as receptors, enzymes, transporters, ion channels, and nucleic acids.
- Receptor theory is the underlying principle for drug–receptor interactions. Drug–receptor interactions entail the consecutive processes of binding, recognition, and signal transduction.
- Ligands for receptors can be differentiated into full agonists, partial agonists, antagonists, and inverse agonists.
- The rational use of drugs and the design of effective dosage regimens are determined by the two pharmacological subdisciplines pharmacokinetics and pharmacodynamics.
- Selectivity of a drug toward the desired therapeutic effect rather than the undesired side effects largely determines a drug's therapeutic range and benefit-to-risk ratio.
- Integrated pharmacokinetic–pharmacodynamic relationships allow the description of the continuous profile of drug effect intensity over time in response to a given dose or dosing regimen.
- Functional tolerance is the consequence of time-dependent drug–receptor interactions such as receptor desensitization or receptor downregulation.
- Adverse drug reactions (ADRs) can be differentiated into type A (dose-dependent, predictable ADRs) and type B (non-dose-related, unpredictable ADRs). The frequency and severity of type A ADRs are directly related to a drug's therapeutic range and selectivity.
- Drug–drug interactions can originate from interactions in pharmacokinetic and pharmacodynamic processes. Inhibition or induction of drug-metabolizing enzymes and drug transporters are the most important pharmacokinetic drug–drug interactions.
- The U.S. Food and Drug Administration (FDA) has the authority to regulate development, manufacturing, use, and marketing of drugs and medical devices to ensure their safety and efficacy.
- Preclinical drug development is aimed at the evaluation and optimization of new chemical entities and biologics in in vitro and in vivo animal models with regard to efficacy and safety and the provision of sufficient data for an investigational new drug application filing.
- Clinical drug development can be differentiated in phase I, II, III, and IV studies and is intended to establish efficacy and safety in the intended indication in humans.

7-2 STUDY GUIDE CHECKLIST

The following topics may guide your study of the subject area:

- ☐ Differentiation of molecular targets of drugs
- ☐ Explanation of receptor theory and the concepts of binding and recognition
- ☐ Comparison and contrast of the concepts of agonism and antagonism
- ☐ Explanation of the concepts of selectivity, risk-to-benefit, and therapeutic range
- ☐ Explanation of the pharmacodynamics of drug action through concentration–effect relationships and the concepts of potency and intrinsic activity
- ☐ Relation of drug action and concentration–effect relationships to quantitative drug–target interactions
- ☐ Mechanistic rationalization of time-dependent changes in concentration–effect relationships
- ☐ Differentiation of dose-related from idiosyncratic adverse drug reactions
- ☐ Explanation of drug–drug-interactions based on pharmacokinetic or pharmacodynamic processes, or both
- ☐ Description of the drug development process and the role of the FDA in this context

7-3 Mechanism of Action of Drugs of Various Categories Including Biologics

The effects of drugs can be described on four different levels:

- ***The system level:*** An effect occurs on an integrated body system, such as the cardiovascular or the respiratory system.
- ***The tissue level:*** An effect occurs on tissue function, such as secretion, proliferation, or metabolic activity.
- ***The cellular level:*** Signal transduction occurs within a cell, such as the cascade of a biochemical signaling pathway (e.g., the Raf kinase pathway).
- ***The receptor level:*** Interaction takes place with a drug's molecular target, such as the β_2-adrenergic receptor.

Knowledge about a drug's effect at all four levels is necessary to assess the drug's potential effectiveness, synergistic or antagonistic effect with other medications, and potential interactions with other drugs.

Molecular Targets of Drugs

To exert an effect, either desired or undesired (side effect or adverse effect), drugs need to interact with molecular targets. Depending on the availability of its molecular targets in tissues and cells, a drug may profoundly affect one type of tissue but not affect other types of tissues. Examples of frequent molecular targets of drugs follow.

Receptors of endogenous hormones or neurotransmitters

A drug can act either as an agonist or as an antagonist on a receptor system. An agonist at a receptor system triggers the action, which is also produced by the receptor's natural, endogenous ligand. An antagonist blocks the effect of the natural endogenous agonist on the receptor system. Examples include loperamide, which is an agonist for the μ-opioid receptor, and propranolol, which is an antagonist for β-adrenergic receptors.

Enzymes

Enzyme activity can be modulated by blocking the normal enzymatic reaction either through direct binding to the enzyme or through competitive inhibition by serving as a false substrate, thereby inhibiting the enzymatic processing of the natural substrate. For example, atorvastatin inhibits the enzyme HMG-CoA (3-hydroxy-3-methylglutaryl coenzyme A) reductase in the endogenous synthesis pathway of cholesterol.

Transporters

The exchange of ions or other molecules across biomembranes can be stimulated or inhibited, for example, for antiporters (exchange of ions across biomembranes) or for symporters (cotransport of ions across biomembranes). For example, cardiac glycosides such as digoxin inhibit the Na^+/K^+-ATPase.

Ion channels

Transmembrane ion channels can be blocked, or their probability of opening can be increased or decreased. The former is usually the case for voltage-operated ion channels; the latter is the case for receptor-operated ion channels. For example, voltage-operated sodium channels are blocked by lidocaine, and the GABA (γ-aminobutyric acid)–gated chloride channel (a receptor-operated ion channel) is modulated by benzodiazepines.

Nucleic acids

Drugs can inhibit the expression of genes (1) by directly binding to deoxyribonucleic acid (DNA) and, thus, modulating their transcription; or (2) by binding to messenger ribonucleic acid (mRNA) and, thus, modulating the translation of the gene. For example, fomivirsen binds to viral mRNA, thereby inhibiting viral replication in case of cytomegalovirus infection in the eye.

Drugs that act without specific molecular targets

Although most drugs require a molecular target to exert their effects, the following drugs act without interaction with specific molecular targets:

- Buffers, used as antacids
- Gaseous and volatile general anesthetics
- Osmotic diuretics or laxatives

The previously outlined concepts are largely applicable to traditional small molecule drugs, chemically defined compounds that are chemically synthesized with defined chemical structure and purity. Recently, many biologics have been added to the pharmacopeia as medications. Most biologics, except for blood, blood products, and vaccines, are products that are produced by recombinant technologies in genetically modified organisms, either bacteria or mammalian cell lines. Biologics are usually defined by their production process rather than their chemical structure because of their inherent complexities as large therapeutic proteins. Currently approved biologics comprise mainly three groups:

- ***Monoclonal antibodies and antibody constructs:*** Antibody-based drugs usually serve as antagonists for receptors or inactivate ligands to natural receptors. Some antibody-based drugs, however, may have agonistic activity.
- ***Hormones and growth factors:*** These factors usually serve as ligands for endogenous receptor systems. Insulin or erythropoietin are examples.
- ***Enzymes:*** Recombinantly produced enzymes are mainly used as enzyme replacement therapy in situations where endogenous enzyme activity is insufficient for homeostasis.

Receptor Theory

The majority of drugs exert their effects by interaction with receptors. Four major classes of receptor superfamilies exist:

- ***Receptor-operated channels:*** An extracellular binding domain is coupled with multiple transmembrane domains that form an ion channel. An example is the nicotinic acetylcholine receptor.
- ***Receptor-operated enzymes:*** The receptor has an extracellular ligand-binding domain that is linked by a transmembrane region to an intracellular catalytic domain that has either tyrosine kinase activity or guanylyl kinase activity when the binding site is activated. An example is the epidermal growth factor receptor.
- ***G-protein-coupled receptors:*** These receptors have a transmembrane protein with extracellular and intracellular domains. The intracellular domain is coupled with G-proteins, which facilitate signal transduction after stimulation of the receptor by second-messenger pathways. The drug-binding domain lies within one of the transmembrane domains. An example is the α_1-adrenergic receptor.
- ***DNA-linked receptors:*** DNA-linked receptors are intracellular receptors, in contrast to the other three receptor types discussed, which are transmembrane receptors. The ligand-binding domain is linked to a DNA-binding domain. An example is the androgen receptor.

Several prerequisites for receptor-mediated drug effects must be fulfilled:

- ***Binding:*** For receptor-mediated drug effects, binding of the drug to a specific region in the three-dimensional structure of the receptor is a prerequisite to exert a biological response.
- ***Recognition:*** The receptor protein must exist in a conformational state that allows recognition and binding of a compound. It must satisfy the following criteria:
  - *Saturability:* Receptors exist in finite numbers.
  - *Reversibility:* Binding must occur noncovalently because of weak intermolecular forces (H-bonding, van der Waals forces).
  - *Stereoselectivity:* Receptors should recognize only one of the naturally occurring optical isomers of a drug.
  - *Agonist specificity:* Structurally related drugs should bind well, whereas dissimilar compounds should bind poorly.
  - *Tissue specificity:* Binding should occur in tissues known to be sensitive to the endogenous ligand. Binding should occur at physiologically relevant concentrations.
  - *Transduction:* Binding of an agonist must be translated into some type of functional response (biological or physiological).

Receptor Interaction

Receptors are large proteins that contain a site that recognizes drugs and binds them similarly to the way a key fits a lock. Most cells harbor many different receptor types and many receptor molecules of each type.

Binding of a ligand (e.g., a drug) results in a conformational (allosteric) change in the three-dimensional structure of the receptor, creating an active agonist–receptor complex that activates a signal transduction system. Drug–receptor complexes are repeatedly and randomly created by collision of drug molecules with unoccupied receptors. The formed drug–receptor complexes also dissociate into their components, so a dynamic equilibrium exists between the two states.

Agonist–receptor complexes fluctuate between inactive and active conformations. The active conformation results in signal transduction and subsequent cellular response.

The number of drug receptors on a cell is not necessarily constant. It can change under prolonged stimulation or lack thereof by receptor up- or downregulation, which is frequently observed during chronic drug therapy.

Ligands for receptors can be differentiated according to their ability to trigger the signal transduction (Figure 7-1):

- *Full agonists* bind to receptors and produce a molecular response (conformational change and subsequent cellular responses) that results in maximum tissue response.
- *Competitive antagonists* bind to receptors without initiating a molecular response. Their effect is produced by denying endogenous agonists access to the receptor.
- *Partial agonists* bind to receptors and produce a molecular response, but even at high concentrations, the maximum cellular response is not achieved. Thus, the maximum tissue response for a partial agonist is less than that for a full agonist. Because partial agonists can compete with full agonists in binding to the receptor, they can act as antagonists to full agonists.
- *Inverse agonists* bind to receptor molecules that are in an activated state in the absence of a ligand (basal activation). Thus, inverse agonists decrease the basal activation level of a receptor by stabilizing its inactive form.

Tissue responses are not necessarily directly proportional to molecular responses resulting from agonist–ligand interactions. In most cells, the maximum cellular response to an agonist is already reached when only a small fraction of receptors is occupied. Thus, the number of receptors is much higher than necessary

FIGURE 7-1. Concentration–Activity Relationships for Agonists and Antagonists

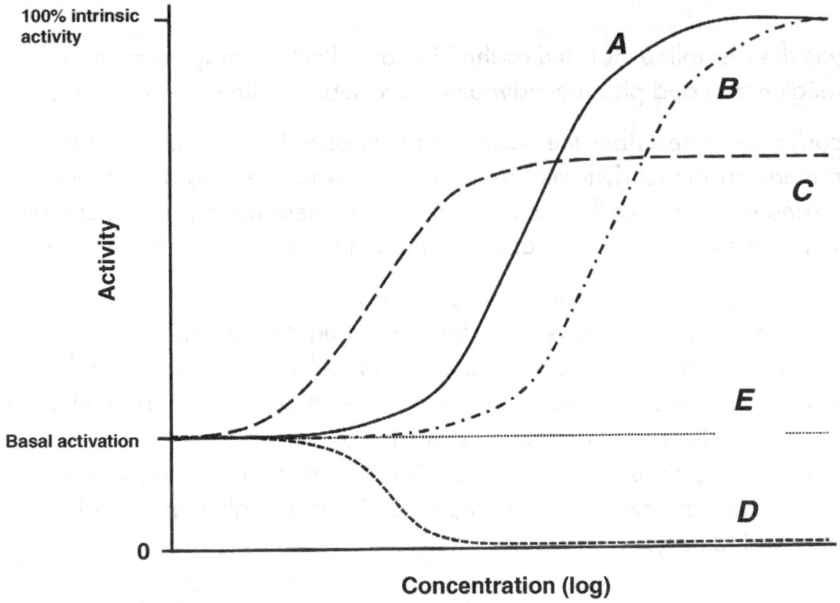

The figure shows concentration–activity relationships for full agonists (*A* and *B*), a partial agonist (*C*), an inverse agonist (*D*), and a competitive antagonist (*E*). *A* and *B* reach the full intrinsic activity but have different potency (EC_{50}). *C* has a lower intrinsic activity (and, in this example, also a lower potency). *D* reduces basal activation. *E* inhibits competitive ligand binding to the receptor and results in no intrinsic activity.

for achieving the maximum response. This so-called receptor reserve (spare receptors) increases the sensitivity toward small changes in agonist concentration. For example, the skeletal neuromuscular junction has 30 million nicotinic acetylcholine receptors. Activation of 40,000 of these receptors already elicits an action potential followed by full twitch of the muscle fiber.

Partial agonism results from an inefficient activation of the receptor by a drug. The subsequent cellular response depends on the presence or absence of spare receptors:

- If there are no spare receptors, the maximum cellular response is less for a partial agonist than for a full agonist, and the partial agonist does not achieve the same maximum cellular response as the full agonist.
- If there are spare receptors (as in most cells), the partial agonist needs to interact with more receptors of the receptor pool to achieve the maximum cellular response; thus, a higher dose is required to achieve this response. If the dose is high enough, the partial agonist may achieve the same maximum cellular response as the full agonist.

For antagonism, two main mechanisms can be distinguished:

- *Competitive antagonists* bind to the site normally occupied by the agonist, thereby reducing the number of receptors available for agonist binding.
- *Noncompetitive antagonists* bind to a different ligand-binding site on the receptor (allosteric site). This binding to the allosteric site results in a conformational change of the receptor that leads to reduced or no agonist binding and, thus, no signal transduction.

Antagonism at the molecular level—that is, at the receptor–interaction level—must be distinguished from physiologic antagonism. In physiologic antagonism, the effects of two drugs are opposite on the level of the organ system or whole body but are mediated through different receptor systems and signaling pathways. The opposing effect of acetylcholine and noradrenalin on arterioles is an example of physiologic antagonism.

7-4 Pharmacodynamics of Drug Binding and Response

Pharmacology is the discipline that studies the biologic effects of drugs and the ways they produce such effects. Pharmacokinetics and pharmacodynamics are subdisciplines of pharmacology:

- *Pharmacodynamics* describes the desired and undesired actions of drugs in qualitative and quantitative manners. Pharmacodynamics thus describes what the drug does to the body.
- *Pharmacokinetics* describes the uptake, distribution, metabolism, and excretion of drugs in the body—that is, their disposition. Pharmacokinetics thus describes what the body does to the drug.

The rational use of drugs and the design of effective dosage regimens are facilitated by an appreciation of the relationships among the administered dose of a drug, the resulting drug concentrations in various body fluids and tissues, and the intensity of the pharmacologic effects caused by these concentrations. These relationships—and thus the dose of a drug required to achieve a certain effect—are determined by the drug's pharmacokinetic and pharmacodynamic properties.

By interacting with target structures in different tissues and by interacting with more than one molecular target, drugs may have not only desired therapeutic effects, but also undesired effects, which may lead to adverse effects and toxicity.

Selectivity

Selectivity describes a drug's property to interact with one molecular target as opposed to others. Selectivity depends on the chemical structure of the drug, the drug dose, the route of drug administration, and patient factors such as physiologic or pathophysiologic conditions and genetically determined susceptibility.

An ideal drug has a high selectivity toward the desired therapeutic effect rather than toward undesired side effects at the therapeutically used dose level and administration pathway. The latest generations of inhaled corticosteroids, such as fluticasone propionate, have a high selectivity toward anti-inflammatory activity in the lung (e.g., for the treatment of asthma) as compared to undesired systemic effects such as growth retardation. This selectivity of fluticasone propionate is accomplished by its high metabolic instability after being absorbed into the systemic circulation.

Benefit-to-Risk Ratio

The *benefit-to-risk ratio* is a formal approach to comparing the therapeutically desired effect of a drug with its health risks related to adverse effects and toxicity. The therapeutic acceptance of a benefit-to-risk ratio depends on the nature and severity of the treated disorder. In a life-threatening condition, a higher risk may be tolerable for therapeutic benefit than would be acceptable, for example, in prophylactic drug treatment.

In cancer chemotherapy, potent drugs with limited selectivity and high adverse effect potential are often administered at the maximum tolerable dose to achieve high efficacy of tumor kill. In contrast, the same benefit-to-risk ratio would not be tolerable for the chronic pharmacotherapy of a nonacute life-threatening condition, such as hypercholesterolemia.

Therapeutic Range

For many drugs, a therapeutic range of concentrations can be defined in which a high likelihood of efficacy exists (that is, desired therapeutic response), with limited toxicity. The *therapeutic range* is a range of drug plasma concentrations within which the probability of desired clinical response is relatively high and the probability of unacceptable toxicity is relatively low (Figure 7-2). As such, the therapeutic range is a leveraging of the selectivity of a drug between therapeutic and toxic activity.

A therapeutic range should never be used as an absolute concentration outside of which drug concentrations are either ineffective or toxic, but rather as a therapeutic guidance. Because pharmacodynamic param-

FIGURE 7-2. Therapeutic Range

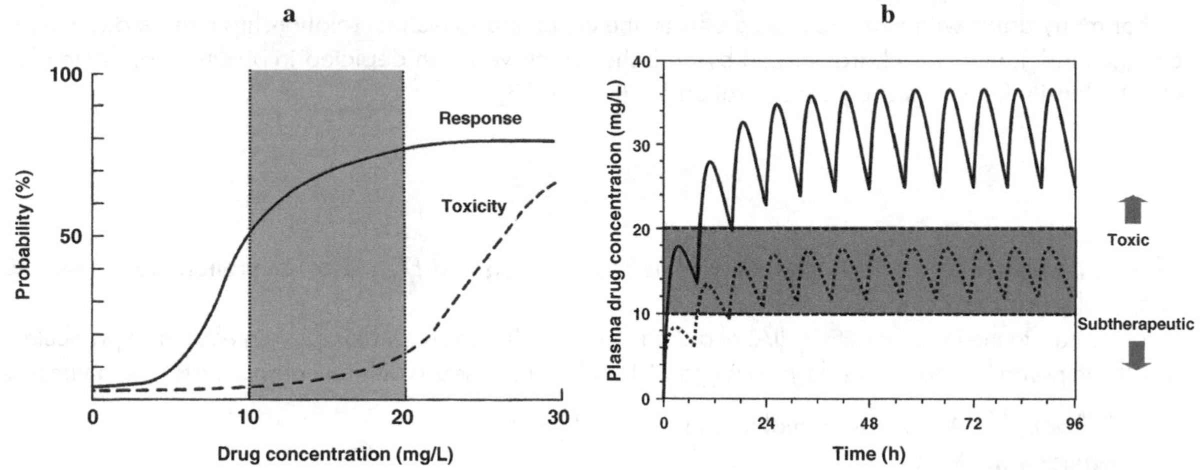

Panel a shows a drug concentration–probability of effect relationship. The probability of achieving the desired response is very low when drug concentrations are less than 5 mg/L (as is the chance of observing toxicity). As drug concentrations increase from 5 to 20 mg/L, the probability of desired effect (response) increases significantly, while the probability of toxicity increases more slowly. One could select a therapeutic range of 10 to 20 mg/L, where the minimum probability of a therapeutic response is at least 50% and the probability of therapeutic failure (in this case, toxicity) is less than 10%.

Panel b demonstrates an optimal dosage regimen that maintains the plasma concentration of the drug within the therapeutic range. The dosing interval (time between doses) is the same, but the dose given in regimen 2 (bold line) is twice as large as that given in regimen 1 (dotted line). As shown, drug accumulates in the body during multiple dosing. Regimen 1 results in plasma concentrations within the therapeutic range. For regimen 2, the therapeutic range is reached quickly, but the dosage regimen ultimately results in a high likelihood of toxicity.

eters and, thus, concentration–effect relationships, are variable among different patients, the therapeutic range can indicate only a high probability of therapeutic response in a patient population; it cannot predict the response in an individual patient.

Drugs with a wide therapeutic range have a large margin between concentrations necessary to achieve therapeutic activity and concentrations that will result in toxicity. β-lactam antibiotics are an example of drugs with a wide therapeutic range.

Drugs with a narrow therapeutic range have only a small margin between drug concentrations necessary for efficacy and those that have a high likelihood of toxicity. Digoxin is a drug with a narrow therapeutic range; it has an upper limit of 2 ng/mL, which is less than threefold higher than its lower limit of 0.8 ng/mL.

Drugs with a narrow therapeutic range often require individualization of dosing to keep plasma concentrations in the therapeutic range despite differences in pharmacokinetic parameters among different patients. *Therapeutic drug monitoring* is an approach that measures drug plasma concentrations of a patient receiving drugs with a narrow therapeutic range and adjusts the patient's dose and dosing interval in such a manner that concentrations remain in the therapeutic range throughout the whole therapy.

Pharmacodynamics of Drug Action and Relationship to Drug Disposition

For most drugs, therapeutic response and toxicity are related to their free concentration at the site of action. However, drug concentrations at the site of action (e.g., brain tissue for benzodiazepines) often cannot be practically measured. Thus, drug concentrations in accessible body fluids such as plasma are often related to the observed effect under the assumption that the drug concentrations in the measured body fluid and at the site of action are in a constant relationship.

Pharmacodynamic models characterize the concentration–effect relationship of a drug. Whereas the pharmacokinetics of most drugs exhibits linear behavior (i.e., doubling the dosing rate results in doubling the systemic exposure), the pharmacodynamics is usually characterized by nonlinearity (i.e., the relationship between plasma concentration and effect is nonlinear and levels off at a maximum effect being reached with a specific dosing regimen).

For many drugs with reversible drug effects, the concentration–effect relationship can be described by an E_{max} model, which is characterized by an S-shaped curve when depicted in a semilogarithmic plot of effect intensity (E) versus drug concentration (C) (Figure 7-3):

$$E = \frac{E_{max} \times C}{EC_{50} + C}$$

where E_{max} is maximum effect possible with the specific drug and EC_{50} is concentration that causes 50% of E_{max}, the half-maximum effect.

E_{max} refers to the intrinsic activity (IA) of a drug. The IA is the relative maximal drug effect in a particular tissue. If compared to a natural endogenous ligand, the IA can be used to differentiate agonists from antagonists:

- ***Full agonist:*** IA = 1 (i.e., equal to endogenous ligand)
- ***Antagonist:*** IA = 0
- ***Partial agonist:*** 0 < IA < 1 (produces less than the maximal response of the natural, endogenous ligand, despite maximal binding to the receptors)
- ***Inverse agonist:*** IA = −1 (i.e., reduction below baseline level)

EC_{50} refers to the potency of a drug. The *potency* is the ability to cause a functional change at a certain concentration. It is related to the affinity of the drug for its target structure (e.g., a receptor). A more potent drug needs a lower concentration to cause the same functional change in a target structure (i.e., it has a smaller EC_{50}).

FIGURE 7-3. E_{max} Model

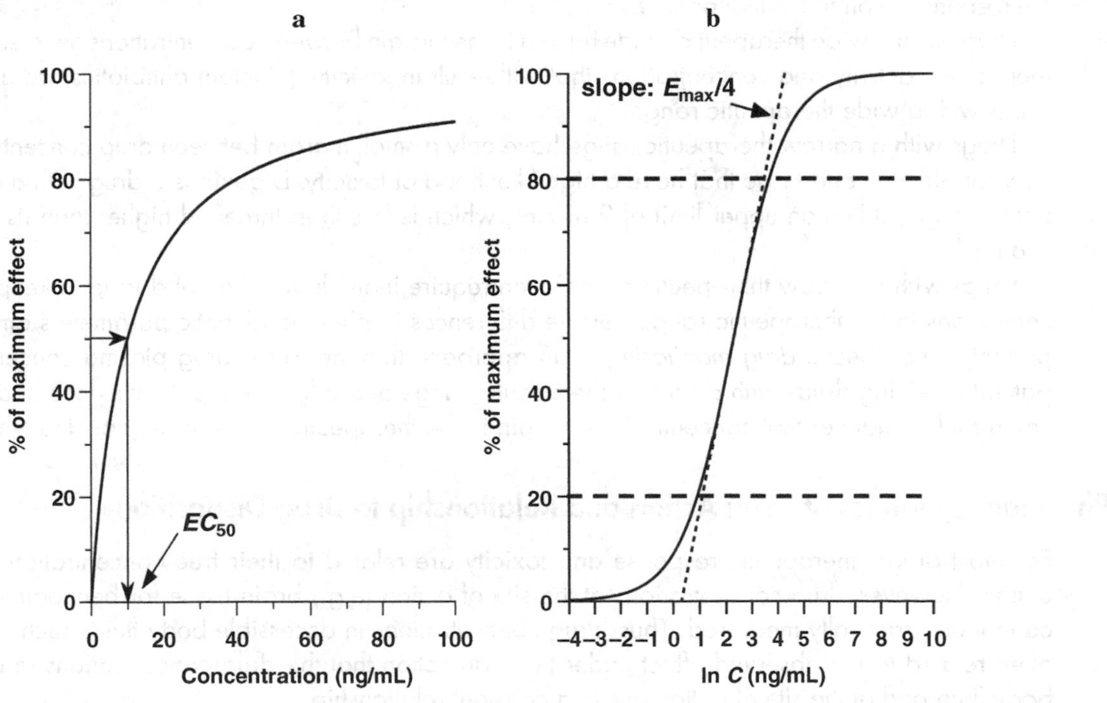

~~Adapted with modification from Meibohm, Derendorf, 1997:404.~~
The figure depicts the effect versus concentration relationship defined by an E_{max} model, depicted in a linear (panel a) and a semilogarithmic (panel b) plot. EC_{50} denotes the concentration that produces one-half the maximum effect. In the range between 20% and 80% of the maximum effect, the effect is directly proportional to the logarithm of the concentration, with a slope of $E_{max}/4$.

Although the E_{max} model is an empirical relationship, its value lies in the fact that it can be related to the receptor theory of drug action. Under the assumption that the observed effect E is directly proportional to the number of occupied receptors, E_{max} is equivalent to the number of receptors available and EC_{50} is equivalent to the affinity constant of the drug to the receptor (i.e., the concentration at which half the receptor sites are occupied).

The E_{max} model describes the concentration–effect relationship over a wide range of concentrations, from zero effect in the absence of drug to maximum effect at concentrations much higher than EC_{50} ($C >> EC_{50}$). Three characteristic phases can be distinguished:

- ***Linear phase:*** For concentrations much smaller than EC_{50} ($C << EC_{50}$), the E_{max} model simplifies to a linear model:

$$E = m \times C$$

where slope $m = E_{max}/EC_{50}$

- ***Constant phase:*** For concentrations much larger than EC_{50} ($C >> EC_{50}$), the effect is essentially constant:

$$E \approx E_{max}$$

- ***Log-linear phase:*** For E between ~20% and ~80% of E_{max}, the E_{max} model follows a log-linear relationship, where the effect is proportional to the logarithm of the concentration:

$$E \approx \ln C$$

Pharmacokinetic–Pharmacodynamic Relationships

Pharmacokinetic–pharmacodynamic (PK–PD) relationships integrate a pharmacokinetic model component that describes the time course of drug in plasma and a pharmacodynamic model component that relates the plasma concentration to the drug effect. Thus, PK–PD models allow the description of the continuous profile of drug effect intensity over time in response to a given dose or dosing regimen. The general concept of PK–PD relationships is presented in Figure 7-4.

Drug–Target Interactions

When drugs interact with their molecular targets, the resulting drug–target binding can be reversible or irreversible:

- *Reversible* drug–target interaction is mediated by ionic bonding, hydrogen bonding, or hydrophobic interaction.
- *Irreversible* drug–target interaction is mediated by covalent bonding.

For reversible interaction with a molecular receptor, binding of the ligand (drug) to the receptor occurs when ligand and receptor collide with the proper orientation and energy. The binding process follows the law of mass action, if one assumes that all receptors are equally accessible, no partial binding occurs (receptors are either free of ligand or bound with ligand), and the ligand is not altered by binding. The relationship can be described as follows:

$$[\text{drug}] + [\text{receptor}] \underset{k_{off}}{\overset{k_{on}}{\rightleftharpoons}} [\text{drug} \circ \text{receptor}]$$

where [drug], [receptor], and [drug · receptor] are the concentrations of the free drug, the free receptor, and the drug–receptor complex, respectively. k_{on} and k_{off} are rate constants for the association and dissociation process, respectively.

FIGURE 7-4. PK–PD Modeling

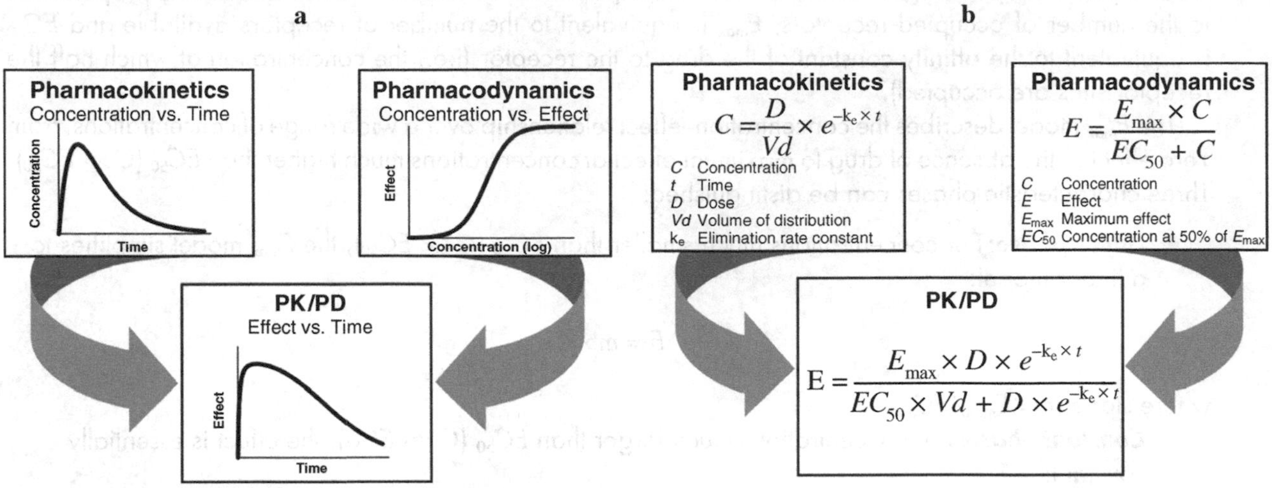

Adapted with modification from Meibohm, Derendorf, 1997:177.
Panel a shows the general concept of integrated PK–PD modeling. Pharmacokinetics describes the time course of drug concentration resulting from a dosing regimen. Pharmacodynamics describes the relationship between drug concentration and effect intensity. The integrated PK–PD model describes the time course of effect intensity resulting from a dosing regimen. Panel b depicts a simple, integrated PK–PD model where the pharmacokinetics is described by a one-compartment model with instantaneous drug input and the pharmacodynamics is described by an E_{max} model. The integrated PK–PD model describes the effect intensity over time based on the PK parameters elimination rate constant k_e and volume of distribution Vd as well as the PD parameters maximum achievable effect (E_{max}) and concentration that produces the half maximal effect (EC_{50}).

The rate of association or number of binding events per time is equal to

$$[\text{ligand}] \times [\text{receptor}] \times k_{on}\ ;\ [k_{on}] = M^{-1}\text{min}^{-1}$$

The rate of dissociation or number of dissociation events per time is equal to

$$[\text{ligand} \circ \text{receptor}] \times k_{off}\ ;\ [k_{off}] = \text{min}^{-1}$$

Thus, the rates of association and dissociation depend solely on the number of receptors, the concentration of ligand, and the rate constants k_{on} and k_{off}.

At equilibrium, the rate of formation equals that of dissociation:

$$[DR] \times k_{off} = [D] \times [R] \times k_{on}$$

$$K_D = \frac{k_{off}}{k_{on}} = \frac{[D] \times [R]}{[DR]}$$

where $[D]$ and $[R]$ are the concentrations of free drug and free receptor, respectively, and $[DR]$ is the concentration of the drug–receptor complex. The dissociation constant K_D is an inverse measure of receptor affinity. It is the drug concentration that produces 50% of receptor occupancy.

Although EC_{50} is related to K_D, it is often not identical because K_D solely characterizes the drug–receptor interaction, whereas EC_{50} also represents the efficiency of signal transduction pathways subsequent to receptor interaction.

The drug–target interaction can be time variant if, for example, the potency or intrinsic activity of a drug and its target structure are changing. Functional tolerance development is a prime example of a time-variant drug–target interaction. Functional tolerance is characterized by a reduction in effect intensity over time despite constant effect-site concentration. This diminishing response with rechallenging stimulus may be caused by a decrease in the number of receptors, called *receptor downregulation*, or by a decrease in the signal transduction efficiency, called *receptor desensitization*.

Functional tolerance results in a clockwise hysteresis loop in the plot of effect intensity versus target-site concentration.

Receptor downregulation entails internalization or proteolytic degradation of receptors in response to prolonged ligand-induced stimulation, resulting in a net loss of available receptors in the cell. In this situation, intrinsic activity (E_{max}) of the drug typically decreases while potency (EC_{50}) remains unchanged.

Receptor desensitization entails loss of agonist signal transduction efficiency, for example, by the uncoupling of G-protein for G-protein-coupled receptors in response to prolonged ligand-induced stimulation, resulting in less efficient signal transduction by the receptor. In this situation, intrinsic activity (E_{max}) of the drug remains typically unchanged because the receptor number remains unchanged, whereas EC_{50} increases because more receptors need to be stimulated to produce the same drug response.

7-5 Adverse Effects and Side Effects of Drugs

Because any xenobiotic may interact not only with the intended target structure (e.g., a receptor in a specific tissue), but also with the same, similar, or unrelated receptors or other target structures in the same or other tissues, the intended or beneficial effects of pharmacotherapy are usually also accompanied by side effects, often termed adverse drug reactions (ADRs) when they lead to unintended effects. Investigation of these potential off-target effects constitutes a major effort during the drug development process.

ADRs are defined as any response to a drug that is noxious and unintended and that occurs at doses used in humans for prophylaxis, diagnosis, or treatment.

- A type A ADR, also called a *side effect,* is a dose-related, predictable reaction to a drug. Side effects are expected on the basis of the pharmacologic activity of the drug, and depending on their severity, they are accepted as occurring in a certain fraction of treated individuals.
- A type B ADR is a non-dose-related, unexpected ADR, also called an *idiosyncratic reaction.* Examples of type B ADRs include allergic reactions as well as carcinogenic and teratogenic effects.

Pharmacovigilance is a systematic approach to collecting, monitoring, researching, assessing, and evaluating ADR-related information from health care providers and patients. The U.S. Food and Drug Administration (FDA) has established a national ADR reporting system, the MedWatch system.

The frequency and severity of type A ADRs is directly related to a drug's therapeutic range and selectivity (see Section 7-4). The more selective a drug is with regard to its receptor interactions, the larger its therapeutic range will be and the less likely the occurrence of type A ADRs.

The phosphodiesterase type 5 (PDE-5) inhibitor sildenafil, for example, is approved for the treatment of erectile dysfunction. Sildenafil has only limited selectivity toward some other phosphodiesterase families, particularly phosphodiesterase type 6 (PDE-6). PDE-6 is expressed only in the retina and is relevant for visual transduction. Partial inhibition of PDE-6 by therapeutic sildenafil doses has been associated with the relatively high frequency of visual disturbances under sildenafil therapy. Tadalafil, another PDE-5 inhibitor with much higher selectivity for PDE-5 than PDE-6, has a substantially lower frequency of visual side effects than sildenafil.

7-6 Mechanisms of Drug–Drug Interactions

Drug–drug interactions can occur on the pharmacokinetic level, the pharmacodynamic level, or both simultaneously.

Pharmacokinetic drug–drug interactions occur if a drug interferes with the absorption, disposition, and elimination of another drug. Most frequent sources of pharmacokinetic drug–drug interactions are inhibition or induction of the activity of drug-metabolizing enzymes and drug transporters, such as the following examples:

- Ketoconazole is a strong inhibitor of the drug-metabolizing enzyme cytochrome P450 (CYP) 3A4 and has the potential to substantially increase the systemic exposure of drugs primarily metabolized by CYP3A4, such as the immunosuppressants cyclosporine and tacrolimus.
- Rifampin is a strong inducer for the drug-metabolizing enzymes CYP2D6 and CYP3A4 and results in reduced systemic exposure of drugs that are predominantly metabolized by these enzymes, such as tamoxifen.
- Quinidine is a strong inhibitor of the drug efflux transporter P-glycoprotein. Quinidine coadministration results in increased exposure to digoxin, most likely through reduced renal elimination and increased gastrointestinal uptake of digoxin secondary to inhibition of P-glycoprotein.

The reader is referred to the constantly updated pharmacokinetic drug–drug interaction database at Indiana University (http://medicine.iupui.edu/clinpharm/ddis/) for more examples and detailed information. Although often cited in the pharmaceutical literature, pharmacokinetic drug–drug interactions based on protein binding-site displacement have, for most drugs, only limited or no clinical relevance.

Pharmacodynamic drug–drug interactions can occur on the levels of the receptor or the organ or functional system. Pharmacodynamic interactions on the molecular level occur when drugs interact with the same receptor system:

- Competitive interaction of two agonists for a receptor will enhance the response by resulting in more occupied, activated receptors.
- Competitive interaction of an agonist and an antagonist will reduce the response as antagonist molecules compete with agonist molecules for the same binding sites. Competitive antagonism can be overcome by increasing the agonist concentration.
- Noncompetitive interaction of an agonist and an antagonist will reduce the response as the antagonist interacts with an allosteric binding site that reduces the affinity of the agonist for the receptor or reduces signal transduction efficiency. Noncompetitive antagonism cannot be overcome by increasing the agonist concentration.
- For example, naloxone is a μ-opioid receptor competitive antagonist and antagonizes the effect of the μ-opioid receptor-ligand morphine. Buprenorphine is a partial agonist for the μ-opioid receptor. Buprenorphine acts as a competitive antagonist for morphine if co-administered because it competes with morphine for μ-opioid receptors and has a lower IA than morphine.

Pharmacodynamic drug–drug interactions occur on the organ or system level if two drugs do not interact with the same molecular structure but enhance or diminish each other's effect through different molecular pathways that affect the same response system. For example, the potentiating effect of coadministration of aspirin (acetylsalicylic acid) and warfarin is likely the consequence of an inhibition of blood coagulation by two separate pathways.

7-7 Drug Discovery and Development

The approval and marketing of drugs in the United States is regulated by the Federal Food, Drug, and Cosmetic Act of 1938 and its amendments, particularly the Kefauver–Harris amendments of 1962, which established requirements for drugs to be efficacious and safe. The act gives the FDA the following dual missions:

- Protecting the public health by ensuring the safety, efficacy, and security of human and veterinary drugs, biological products, medical devices, foods, cosmetics, and products that emit radiation

- Advancing the public health by helping speed innovations that make medications and foods more effective, safer, and more affordable and by helping the public obtain the accurate, science-based information it needs to use medications and foods to improve health

The Federal Food, Drug, and Cosmetic Act provides the FDA with the authority to regulate development, manufacturing, use, and marketing of drugs and medical devices to ensure their safety and efficacy:

- Permission for marketing a drug in the United States requires prior submission and approval of a new drug application (NDA) to the FDA. Biologics require submission and approval of a biologics license application (BLA).
- Generic versions of a small molecule brand-name drug can be approved by a process with reduced requirements. In such cases, an abbreviated new drug application (ANDA) is submitted. At the core of an ANDA is the requirement to show bioequivalence between an approved reference drug and the generic version of the drug.
- Biologics that are highly similar to and have no clinically meaningful differences from an existing FDA-approved reference product can be approved as a biosimilar with reduced requirements. Biosimilarity is established in an extensive comparability exercise that includes critical quality attributes and preclinical and clinical comparisons.
- The first use in humans of a drug that is a new molecular entity or a biologic requires submission of an investigational new drug (IND) application.

Drug Discovery and Preclinical Development

The drug discovery process is aimed at identifying a lead compound and ideally several backup compounds that target a specific biochemical pathway or receptor that interferes with pathogenesis, disease progression, or the symptoms of a disease. The process usually entails understanding the molecular mechanism of the disease, selecting a target, designing compounds that interact with the target in the desired fashion (hits), and then optimizing the initial hits to obtain leads for further development. Enabling techniques in this process include high-throughput screening, combinatorial chemistry, quantitative structure–activity relationships, structure-based design, and computer-based molecular modeling.

Preclinical drug development entails the evaluation and optimization of chemical leads in in vitro assays and in vivo animal models with regard to efficacy and safety.

In vitro preclinical studies frequently include cell-line-based assays as well as cell-free systems (e.g., isolated receptor systems). These studies are usually aimed at identifying the mechanism of action of a drug and assessing its potential for off-target effects, such as interaction with pharmacologic targets or mechanisms other than the one required to elicit the desired effect.

In vivo preclinical studies in animal species are aimed at the following:

- Establishment of drug efficacy in animal models of the targeted disease
- Establishment of pharmacokinetic and pharmacodynamic relationships, including oral bioavailability, penetration into different organs and tissues, and the dose-concentration-effect relationship.

Tested species usually include rodent (rat, mouse) and nonrodent species (rabbit, dog, pig, monkey), including nonhuman primates.

Drug manufacturing and formulation development efforts at this stage of development are aimed at scaling up drug substance and drug product manufacturing for producing materials for further preclinical testing, especially toxicology, and for clinical testing. Manufacturing of pharmaceutical products for clinical testing and use must be conducted under current Good Manufacturing Practice (GMP) guidelines that have been established by the FDA.

Toxicology studies performed during preclinical development include acute toxicity, multidose (long-term) toxicity, reproductive toxicity, mutagenicity, and carcinogenicity. Acute and repeat-dose toxicology studies must be performed in at least two species, one of which must be a nonrodent species. All studies submitted to the FDA for regulatory decisions (e.g., IND, NDA decisions) must be performed under Good Laboratory Practice (GLP) conditions.

Preclinical-to-Clinical Transition

Animal scale-up is used to extrapolate results from preclinical development to humans, thereby defining the first-in-human dose to be used initially in human studies. Allometric approaches are frequently used to scale pharmacokinetic and pharmacodynamic properties across animal species and humans.

Before a new drug can be studied in humans, an IND application needs to be filed with the FDA. The IND application is intended to ensure that the product is reasonably safe for initial use in humans. The application must contain information in three broad areas:

- ***Animal pharmacology and toxicology studies:*** It must include preclinical data to permit an assessment about whether the product is reasonably safe for initial testing in humans.
- ***Manufacturing information:*** It must include information pertaining to the composition, manufacturer, stability, and controls used for manufacturing the drug substance and the drug product.
- ***Clinical protocols and investigator information:*** It must include detailed protocols for proposed clinical studies to assess whether the initial phase trials will expose subjects to unnecessary risks.

The FDA has 30 days to object to an IND after it has been filed.

Research in human subjects is regulated by several federal laws, and each investigational study in humans requires approval by an institutional review board or ethics committee that ensures adequate protection of the human subjects involved and ethical considerations in their use for research purposes. Written, informed consent must be obtained from all research subjects before enrollment in clinical studies.

Clinical Drug Development

Clinical drug development usually comprises four major phases.

Phase I studies usually comprise small numbers of healthy subjects (less than 100 subjects). Phase I studies are intended solely to establish the tolerability and safety of a new drug product. Secondary aims include characterizing the pharmacokinetics in humans. Efficacy is not an objective in phase I studies. For drugs that have inherent toxicity, such as cytotoxic anticancer medications, phase I studies are performed in patients with the targeted disease instead of healthy individuals. Nevertheless, establishing tolerability and safety remain the primary objectives in these studies.

Phase II studies are performed in patients with the illness to be treated and usually comprise between 24 and 300 subjects. Early phase II (phase IIa) studies are proof-of-concept studies that are intended to show that the hypothesized therapeutic concept is working in vivo in humans. Late-stage phase II (phase IIb) studies are focused on identifying the appropriate patient populations in which the drug works best and determining appropriate dosing regimens for subsequent large-scale trials.

Phase III studies are conducted to confirm the efficacy and safety of a new drug in a larger patient population (250–1,000 or more subjects) and to detect and evaluate adverse drug effects that may be encountered during subsequent clinical use. For submission of an NDA, the efficacy and safety results of the phase III program usually need to be replicated with the same dosing regimen in two independent, double-blind, randomized, placebo-controlled clinical trials (pivotal trials). Depending on the indication, placebo control might need to be replaced by the current standard of care for ethical reasons.

Phase IV studies, or so-called postmarketing studies, are conducted after drug approval to further refine the use of the drug in different patient populations, different indications, or different formulations.

Although the traditional four phases are helpful in broadly defining a clinical drug development program, the use of these phases in strict chronological order is misleading. Nowadays, drug development is widely accepted as an iterative knowledge-building process with learning phases in which information about the drug's properties and effects are collected and in which the previously established and integrated knowledge and the derived hypotheses are confirmed.

Pharmacovigilance and risk mitigation strategies are growing efforts in postmarketing drug development that are intended to identify new information about side effects and adverse effects associated with medicines and to prevent harm to patients.

7-8 Questions

1. Which of the following statements is correct regarding an antagonist in a system without spare receptors that is stimulated by an agonist?
   - **A.** The effect of an irreversible antagonist can be overcome by increasing the agonist concentration.
   - **B.** The effect of a competitive antagonist is independent of the agonist concentration.
   - **C.** The effect of a noncompetitive antagonist can be overcome by increasing the agonist concentration.
   - **D.** The effect of a competitive antagonist can be overcome by increasing the agonist concentration.

2. Drug A is a full agonist for a specific receptor system; drug B is a competitive antagonist for the same receptor system. If increasing doses of drug B are co-administered with drug A, drug B will
   - **A.** increase the apparent E_{max} of drug A.
   - **B.** reduce the apparent E_{max} of drug A.
   - **C.** increase the apparent EC_{50} of drug A.
   - **D.** reduce the apparent EC_{50} of drug A.

3. Which of the following statements is correct for a receptor system that exhibits a receptor reserve of 90%?
   - **A.** Partial agonists are not able to achieve maximum cellular response.
   - **B.** Only 10% of the available receptors need to be occupied by a full agonist to achieve maximum cellular response.
   - **C.** More than 99% of the receptors need to be occupied by a competitive antagonist to have an effect on the dose–response relationship of a full agonist.
   - **D.** Only 90% in the receptor reserve is available for interaction with competitive antagonists.

4. EC_{50} is a measure of
   - **A.** the intrinsic activity of a drug.
   - **B.** the efficacy of a drug.
   - **C.** the potency of a drug.
   - **D.** the dissociation rate of a drug–receptor complex.

5. Which of the following can act as an antagonist for a full agonist?
   - **A.** Inverse agonist
   - **B.** Partial agonist
   - **C.** Less potent agonist
   - **D.** Noncompetitive agonist

6. An inverse agonist produces what kind of response on its receptor system?
   - **A.** Reduction in the number of spare receptors
   - **B.** Increase in binding affinity for full agonists
   - **C.** Reversal of the effect of irreversible antagonists
   - **D.** Reduction in basal receptor activation

7. Isosorbide dinitrate (ISDN) is used for the treatment of coronary heart disease. Its major effect is vasodilation of coronary arteries. ISDN is known to exhibit functional tolerance. Which of the following will be observed if three doses of ISDN are administered every 8 hours?
   - **A.** The maximum plasma concentration C_{max} for ISDN will be smaller after the third dose than after the first dose.
   - **B.** An ISDN plasma concentration of 10 ng/mL obtained after administration of the third dose results in a higher degree of vasodilation than the same concentration after administration of the first dose.
   - **C.** There is no difference in vasodilation and ISDN plasma concentration between the first and the third doses.
   - **D.** The degree of vasodilation is smaller after the third dose than after the first dose.

8. Which of the following statements is the therapeutically most important distinction between small molecule drugs and biologics such as therapeutic proteins?
   - **A.** Therapeutic proteins are always substantially more expensive than small molecule drugs.
   - **B.** Therapeutics proteins are not defined by structure and purity as are small molecule drugs, but by their production process, which may result in batch-to-batch variability.
   - **C.** Therapeutic proteins are in contrast to small molecule drugs only available as intravenously administered dosage forms.
   - **D.** Therapeutic proteins are always acting as antagonists.

9. An ACE inhibitor has a short elimination half-life of 3 hours and a wide therapeutic range. Why can it be administered once daily and still achieve therapeutic efficacy despite its short elimination half-life?

A. The therapeutic efficacy of ACE inhibitors is independent of the administered dose and resulting drug concentration.
B. After five elimination half-lives (15 hours), more than 90% of the administered drug has been eliminated, and the drug will not be effective any more. Hence, the FDA made a mistake in approving this dosing regimen.
C. Elimination half-life is irrelevant for designing dosing regimens.
D. Because of the wide therapeutic range, the daily dose can be so high that even at the end of the 24-hour dosing interval, drug concentrations are still above the EC_{50} to maintain therapeutic efficacy.

10. Which of the following statements regarding the concept of the therapeutic range is correct?

A. Drug plasma concentrations below the lower limit of the therapeutic range are ineffective in all treated patients.
B. If drug plasma concentrations are maintained within the therapeutic range, the drug's desired therapeutic effect is achieved in all treated patients.
C. The therapeutic range defines a range of drug plasma concentration with high probability of desired clinical efficacy and low probability of unacceptable toxicity.
D. If drug plasma concentrations always remain below the upper limit of the therapeutic range, none of the treated patients will experience drug-related toxicity.

11. Assume a class of drug substances with the same pharmacokinetic characteristics and the same mechanism of action but different EC_{50} values. To achieve the same therapeutic effect, drugs with a higher EC_{50} need to be administered at __________ dose rate than drugs with a lower EC_{50}.

A. a higher
B. one third of the
C. the same
D. a lower

12. In the United States, first-in-humans studies can be initiated after (mark all that apply)

A. research subjects have received financial compensation.
B. the FDA has not objected to an IND filing.
C. subjects have given written informed consent.
D. studies have been approved by an institutional review board.

13. Phase I studies in drug development are usually performed

A. in healthy subjects.
B. in patients with the targeted disease.
C. in special populations such as elderly patients or pediatric patients.
D. in patients who have been cured from the targeted disease.

14. The primary objective of phase III studies is to

A. assess the pharmacokinetics of the drug in healthy individuals.
B. determine the physicochemical stability of the dosage form.
C. determine the pharmacoeconomic benefit of a new drug therapy.
D. determine the efficacy and safety of a new drug therapy.

15. Pharmacovigilance is an approach

A. to increasing drug safety in the postmarketing phase.
B. to preventing theft in the pharmacy.
C. to increasing drug efficacy by switching nonresponders to different therapies.
D. to preventing the use of drugs after their expiration date.

16. Why is selectivity of a drug an important concept to minimize adverse drug reactions?

A. Selectivity determines the fraction of patients who are nonresponders.
B. Selectivity determines in which organ a drug accumulates.
C. Selectivity determines the extent of a drug's interaction with off-target receptors.
D. Selectivity determines how fast a drug is metabolized by hepatic enzymes.

17. Two concurrently administered drugs are metabolized by the same hepatic enzyme system, CYP2D6. What conclusions should the pharmacist draw?

A. There will certainly be a drug–drug interaction because both drugs use the same enzyme system.
B. There is the potential for a drug–drug interaction, but it may not necessarily occur, depending on the doses of the drugs used and their affinities to CYP2D6.
C. There will certainly be no drug–drug interactions because CYP2D6 is polymorphically expressed.
D. There is the potential for a drug–drug interaction, but it will not occur if one drug is given by oral administration and the other drug is given by intravenous administration.

18. The acceptance of a specific benefit-to-risk ratio (mark all that apply)

A. depends on the treated disease.
B. depends on the shelf life of the drug.
C. depends on the treated patient population.
D. depends on the frequency and severity of adverse drug reactions.

7-9 Answers

1. **D.** Competitive antagonism can be overcome by increasing agonist concentrations.

2. **C.** Antagonists increase the apparent EC_{50} of a drug by shifting the effect versus concentration curve to the right.

3. **B.** In a system with spare receptors or receptor reserve, only a fraction of available receptors needs to be stimulated to achieve the maximum pharmacologic response.

4. **C.** The concentration at half maximum effect, EC_{50}, is a measure of drug potency. The more potent a drug is, the smaller is EC_{50}.

5. **B.** A partial agonist can act as an antagonist for a full agonist because it occupies the receptors but has a reduced intrinsic activity.

6. **D.** Inverse agonists decrease the basal activation level of a receptor by stabilizing its inactive form.

7. **D.** Functional tolerance is characterized by a decreasing response to a repeated stimulus.

8. **B.** Therapeutic proteins are produced in genetically modified living organisms and are defined by their production process.

9. **D.** Initial concentrations multiple times higher than the EC_{50} ensure therapeutically efficacious concentrations throughout the dosing interval despite the short half-life.

10. **C.** The therapeutic range is a concentration range with high probability for efficacy and low probability for toxicity.

11. **A.** Drugs with a higher EC_{50} are less potent and need higher drug concentrations and thus a higher dose rate to achieve the same therapeutic effect.

12. **B, C, D.** First-in-human dosing requires an IND filing with the FDA to which it does not object, as well as approval of the study protocol by an institutional review board and written, informed consent by the participating subjects.

13. **A.** Phase I studies establish the safety and tolerability of a new drug in healthy subjects.

14. **D.** Phase III study programs are aimed at determining the efficacy and safety of a new drug therapy.

15. **A.** Pharmacovigilance is a systematic approach to collecting, monitoring, researching, assessing, and evaluating ADR-related information from health care providers and patients.

16. **C.** Selectivity is directly related to the frequency and severity of adverse drug reactions.

17. **B.** The fact that two drugs are metabolized by the same enzyme system indicates only that the potential exists for a drug–drug interaction.

18. **A, C, D.** The benefit-to-risk ratio balances the potential harm and the potential desired therapeutic outcome of a drug therapy.

7-10 Additional Resources

Atkinson AJ, Abernethy DR, Daniels CE, et al. *Principles of Clinical Pharmacology.* 2nd ed. New York, NY: Academic Press; 2006.

Benet LZ, Hoener BA. Changes in plasma protein binding have little clinical relevance. *Clin Pharmacol Ther.* 2002 71(3):115–121.

Brunton L, Hilal-Dandan R, Knollmann B, eds. *Goodman & Gilman's The Pharmacological Basis of Therapeutics.* 13th ed. New York, NY: McGraw-Hill Professional; 2017.

Crommelin DJA, Sindelar RD, Meibohm B, eds. *Pharmaceutical Biotechnology: Fundamentals and Applications.* 4th ed. New York, NY: Springer; 2013.

Meibohm B, Derendorf H. Basic concepts of pharmacokinetic/pharmacodynamic (PK/PD) modelling. *Int J Clin Pharmacol Ther.* 1997;35(10):401–413.

Meibohm B, Evans WE. Clinical pharmacodynamics and pharmacokinetics. In: Helms RA, Quan DJ, Herfindal ET, Gourley DR, eds. *Textbook of Therapeutics: Drug and Disease Management.* 8th ed. Baltimore, MD: Lippincott, Williams & Wilkins; 2006:1–31.

Page C, Curtis M, Walker M, Hoffman B. *Integrated Pharmacology.* 3rd ed. Philadelphia, PA: Mosby Elsevier; 2006.

Rowland M, Tozer TN. *Clinical Pharmacokinetics: Concepts and Applications.* 4th ed. Baltimore, MD: Lippincott, Williams & Wilkins; 2010.

Pharmacognosy and Dietary Supplements

8

C. RYAN YATES AND BILL J. GURLEY

8-1 KEY POINTS

- Dietary supplements are not regulated as rigorously as conventional medications.
- Choice of products with the USP (United States Pharmacopeia) seal ensures that the product contains the contents listed on the label in the amounts indicated and that the product does not contain impurities.
- To have the desired composition, herbal products must be grown under appropriate conditions, must be the appropriate age before harvest, and must contain the appropriate plant part.
- Products may contain inappropriate additives and contaminants, or they may not contain the amounts stated on the label.
- Drug–dietary supplement interactions can occur and result in harm.
- The ingestion of large amounts of vitamins may result in more harm than benefit.
- Persons with hormone-sensitive cancers should not use DHEA (dehydroepiandrosterone).
- Dietary supplements have not been well studied.
- Dietary supplements are difficult to study because the active compounds are not always known.

8-2 STUDY GUIDE CHECKLIST

The following topics may guide your study of this subject area:

- ☐ Consideration of the federal regulations that cover the sale and the manufacture of dietary supplements when counseling patients on their use
- ☐ Human clinical efficacy trials, which investigate the potential utility of dietary supplements in disease
- ☐ Factors that affect the potential for herb–drug interactions

8-3 Introduction

Botanicals have been the archetype for medicines since ancient times and still serve as sources for modern drug discovery. Although their use in contemporary American medicine has all but disappeared, they still underpin the philosophies of traditional Chinese medicine, Ayurvedic medicine (India), and Kampo medicine (Japan). Up until the early 20th century, monographs for botanicals and botanical extracts composed a significant part of the Dispensatory of the United States and the United States Pharmacopeia. However, the modern drug industry supplanted their use, relegating botanicals and botanical extracts to relative obscurity until 1994, when the U.S. Congress passed the Dietary Supplement Health and Education Act (DSHEA). The DSHEA characterized vitamins, minerals, and botanical extracts as dietary supplements.

Today, dietary supplements, formulated as powders, tablets, capsules, liquid tinctures, and other dosage forms, are sold alongside conventional over-the-counter (OTC) medications in retail outlets. Although dietary supplements are not intended to treat, cure, mitigate, or prevent any disease, many consumers view them as substitutes for conventional medications. Since the introduction of the DSHEA regulations in 1994, dietary supplements have gained a significant foothold in the U.S. health care system. As testament to their popularity, almost 50% of U.S. adults regularly consume dietary supplements, spending more than $30 billion annually. Current surveys indicate that 20–30% of prescription drug users take medications concomitantly with herbal supplements, often without notifying their physician or other health care provider. Prospects for herb–drug interactions, therefore, are considerable.

8-4 Effect of DSHEA on Regulation of Dietary Supplements

A dietary supplement, as defined by DSHEA, is "a product (other than tobacco) added to the total diet that contains at least one of the following ingredients: a vitamin, mineral, herb or botanical, amino acid, metabolite, extract, or combination of any ingredient described previously." Many laypersons and health care professionals believe that dietary supplements are not regulated by the U.S. Food and Drug Administration (FDA); however, the FDA does regulate dietary supplements as foods rather than conventional drug products. This approach may seem a bit counterintuitive because many dietary supplements often contain phytochemicals (plant-derived chemicals) that have pharmacologic activity. Unlike conventional medications, dietary supplements do not have to undergo premarket safety and efficacy testing. However, dietary supplement manufacturers must follow good manufacturing practices for food (not drugs), and they must ensure their products are safe.

In addition, product labels must meet the following criteria:

- They should describe the product as a dietary supplement.
- They must not include claims to prevent, treat, diagnose, or cure a specific disease.
- They may state that the product "supports the structure or function of the body" or "general well-being of the body," followed by this wording: "This statement has not been evaluated by the Food and Drug Administration. This product is not intended to diagnose, treat, cure, or prevent any disease."

The FDA inspects dietary supplement manufacturers to ensure that they follow current Good Manufacturing Practices (GMPs) for dietary supplements. In addition, some manufacturers use standards set forth by the United States Pharmacopeia (USP) for dietary supplements to ensure that they are marketing products that meet current GMP standards for content and quality. Proof of efficacy, however, is not required for dietary supplements. Because manufacturers are not regulated as rigorously by the FDA under DSHEA, product quality can vary considerably.

8-5 Crude Drugs, Semipurified Natural Products, and Purified Natural Products

Natural substances have been used to provide treatment and remedies since early humans. *Crude drugs* are substances that are not refined and are used in their natural state. For example, garlic cloves can be ingested to manage hypertension or high cholesterol.

Natural products can be semipurified by extraction procedures to remove unwanted components. An example of a semipurified natural product is echinacea liquid extract.

As a further step, a natural substance can be purified so that only the desired components remain. The pharmaceutical industry may use this process to identify one or more or compounds that have pharmacologic activity. For example, Paclitaxel (Taxol), an important antineoplastic, was first harvested from the Pacific yew tree. However, because yew trees are limited in number, a synthetic version was developed and is now marketed.

8-6 Variability of Occurrence of Pharmacologically Active Substances in Plants

Many currently used pharmaceuticals are based on phytochemicals identified in plants. Although a single phytochemical may be responsible for the pharmacologic activity associated with a plant, most plants have multiple phytochemical constituents. These compounds may work additively or synergistically to elicit the desired response.

Important considerations to ensure appropriate phytochemical composition, dosage form performance, and bioavailability are as follows:

- Growing conditions
  - Rainfall, sun exposure, temperature, soil quality, fertilizer and pesticide use
- Harvesting
  - Appropriate time of year (e.g., saw palmetto berries must be ripe)
  - Appropriate age of plant (e.g., ginseng plant must be 3–10 years old)
  - Appropriate part of plant (e.g., ginkgo leaf)
- Processing of plant materials
  - Powdered plant material versus plant extracts
  - Aqueous extract versus nonaqueous extract
- Dietary supplement dosage form
  - Single-ingredient versus multiple-ingredient product
  - Rare evaluation of disintegration and dissolution profiles of phytochemicals
  - Effect of poor aqueous solubility of phytochemicals on dissolution and bioavailability
  - Conventional dosage form (e.g., tablet, capsule, liquid) versus novel dosage form (e.g., phytosome, microemulsion, nanoparticle)
  - Effect of novel phytochemical dosage forms—marked improvement of bioavailability with concurrent increased toxicity or drug interaction potential
  - Rare bioavailability studies on dietary supplement dosage forms

The final product to the consumer may be a tablet, capsule, liquid gel–capsule, elixir, extract, or, in some cases, part of the dried plant. This variety of dosage forms confounds the comparison of products. The clinical studies discussed in the following sections were conducted using products that contained the expected chemicals at the expected amounts.

8-7 Herbal Products

Dietary herbal supplement sales increased by 7.7% to $7.5 billion in 2016, the second-largest increase in the past decade. The robust growth in herbal supplement sales is indicative of patients' expanding interest in identifying alternative, as well as complementary, approaches to managing their individual health and wellness. This section reviews the top 10 herbal supplements in terms of sales across the mainstream (e.g., grocery and convenience stores, pharmacies) and natural (e.g., supplement and specialty retail outlets, sports nutrition stores) channels.

Black cohosh (*Cimicifuga racemosa* L.)

Class and chemistry

The rhizome of *Cimicifuga racemosa* contains cycloartenol-type triterpene glycosides, including actein, cimicifugoside, cimiracemoside A, and 23-epi-26-deoxyactein, which are thought to be the primary bioactive constituents. Additional ingredients include phenylpropanoids (e.g., hydroxycinnamic acids), alkaloids, N-methylserotonin, starch, fatty acids, resin, and tannins.

Pharmacological actions

Black cohosh has been described as having antiosteoporosis, antiviral, antitumor, antioxidant, and anti-angiogenic activities.

Ethnopharmacological use

Black cohosh may provide relief of menopausal complaints including hot flashes and profuse sweating.

Adverse effects, contraindications, and precautions

- Liver toxicity (hepatitis, jaundice, altered liver enzymes) is possible with the use of black cohosh.
- Skin reactions (urticarial, itching, edema) and gastrointestinal (GI) symptoms (dyspepsia and diarrhea) are possible with the use of black cohosh.
- Patients with a history of liver disease should use black cohosh with caution.
- Preparations should not be used with estrogens in patients who are undergoing treatment for breast cancer or have a history of estrogen-receptor-positive cancer.

Clinical trials

Black cohosh has been evaluated for the treatment of menopausal symptoms with little demonstrated effect. An important caveat is that when the extract quality of black cohosh preparations was verified, black cohosh significantly improved menopausal symptoms.

Cranberry (*Vaccinium macrocarpon*)

Class and chemistry

Cranberries are comprised of water (88%), organic acids (including salicylate), fructose, vitamin C, flavonoids, anthocyanidins, catechins, and triterpenoids. The anthocyanidins and proanthocyanidins, which function as a natural plant defense system, are tannins (stable polyphenols) found only in *Vaccinium* berries.

Pharmacological actions

Cranberry is believed to enhance the urine's ability to prevent uropathogenic bacteria from adhering to urinary tract epithelial cells. The antiadherent activity is attributed to A-type proanthocyanidins, which consist of catechin and epicatechin molecules.

Ethnopharmacological use

Recurrent urinary tract infections.

Adverse effects, contraindications, and precautions

None have been reported.

Clinical trials

The effect of cranberry extract on various urologic conditions has been evaluated in clinical trials:

- The incidence of radiation-induced cystitis and pain and burning were both lower in the cranberry group.
- A Cochrane systematic review concluded that there is some evidence that cranberry juice may decrease the number of symptomatic urinary tract infections (UTIs) over a 12-month period, particularly for women with recurrent UTIs. However, a recent Cochrane systematic review failed to support the use of cranberry products for the prevention of UTIs.

Echinacea (*Echinacea angustifolia, E. pallida,* and *E. purpurea, Eleutherococcus senticosus* [Siberian ginseng], and *Panax quinquefolius* [American ginseng])

Class and chemistry

E. angustifolia contains 3 phenylpropanoids, 15 alkamides, 2 alkaloids, 2 polysaccharides, and 2 essential oils. Aerial parts also include flavonoids.

Pharmacological actions

Echinacea has anti-inflammatory and antibacterial activity. It may assist in wound healing by stabilizing hyaluronic acid via inhibition of hyaluronidase and inhibiting collagen contraction.

Ethnopharmacological use

Prevention and treatment of the common cold have been reported.

Adverse effects, contraindications, and precautions

- Echinacea's adverse effects are, in most cases, rare, mild, and reversible.
- Rash has been reported in children.
- Echinacea is contraindicated in patients with immune-related disorders including tuberculosis, multiple sclerosis, AIDS (acquired immune deficiency syndrome), and HIV (human immunodeficiency virus) infection.
- Pregnant and lactating women and people with allergies and asthma should use echinacea with caution.

- American ginseng and Siberian ginseng interact with the fluorescence polarization immunoassay, causing false elevations in digoxin concentrations, and with the microparticle enzyme immunoassay, causing falsely low digoxin concentrations.

Clinical trials

Echinacea has been evaluated for both prevention and treatment of the common cold. Although no significant difference was seen in cold reduction, an exploratory meta-analysis demonstrated that prophylactic treatment with echinacea products significantly reduced the incidence of colds. There is little evidence to support echinacea's ability to shorten the duration of colds.

An echinacea-based product was as effective as oseltamivir in treating flu-like symptoms in one randomized, clinical trial.

Flax (*Linum usitatissimum*)

Class and chemistry

Flaxseed (or linseed) is used as a cereal and in baking products. *Linum usitatissimum* contains 3 phenylpropanoids, 15 alkamides, 2 alkaloids, 2 polysaccharides, and 2 essential oils. Aerial parts also include flavonoids.

Pharmacological actions

Flaxseed's nutraceutical effects are believed to derive from both the oil and the flaxseed fiber. Flaxseed oil contains high levels (50–60%) of the omega-3 polyunsaturated fatty acid α-linolenic acid. Flaxseed fiber is one of the most concentrated sources of lignans (phenolic resins found in many plants), such as secoisolariciresinol diglucoside.

Ethnopharmacological use

- Bowel stimulation
- Omega-3 supplementation
- Hyperlipidemia
- Atherosclerosis
- GI disturbances (chronic constipation, colon damage by laxative abuse, irritable bowel, diverticulitis, gastritis, enteritis)
- Systemic lupus erythematosus (SLE, or lupus)
- Rheumatoid arthritis
- Application as a poultice for local inflammation

Adverse effects, contraindications, and precautions

None have been reported with the use of recommended amounts.

Clinical trials

Numerous trials have demonstrated the positive effect of flaxseed on a diversity of therapeutic areas including cardiovascular health, breast cancer, prostate cancer, lupus, and arthritis. Examples of the positive effect of flaxseed consumption include the following:

- A significant decrease in low-density lipoprotein cholesterol (LDL-C) and in the rate of bone resorption in postmenopausal women

- A reduction of systolic and diastolic blood pressure, with most benefit derived from the consumption of whole seeds for 12 or more weeks.

Garcinia gummi-gutta (*Garcinia cambogia*)

Class and chemistry

Phytochemical studies of the roots, bark, and fruit of garcinia gummi-gutta have identified xanthones (e.g., carbogiol), benzophenones (e.g., garcinol), organic acids (e.g., hydroxycitric acid [HCA]), and amino acids (e.g., gamma aminobutyric acid).

Pharmacological actions

Garcinia gummi-gutta may exert lipid-lowering, antidiabetic, anti-inflammatory, anticancer, antihelminthic, anticholinesterase, diuretic, and hepatoprotective activity. Garcinia gummi-gutta may have antiobesity activity related to regulation of serotonin levels that lead to satiety and reduced food intake, increased fat oxidation, and decreased de novo lipogenesis (fat production). HCA is a potent inhibitor of adenosine triphosphate–citrate lyase, which catalyzes fatty acid, cholesterol, and triglycerides syntheses.

Ethnopharmacological use

- Weight loss
- Appetite suppressant
- Traditional medicinal uses such as treatment of bowel complaints, intestinal parasites, and rheumatism

Adverse effects, contraindications, and precautions

- Garcinia gummi-gutta is safe in humans if used at recommended doses.
- Because garcinia gummi-gutta enhances serotonin levels, patients should be advised to avoid concomitant use of garcinia gummi-gutta and other medications that affect serotonin levels, such as serotonin selective reuptake inhibitors.

Clinical trials

The majority of trials that have examined products containing garcinia gummi-gutta in weight loss studies have failed to demonstrate a significant effect of garcinia gummi-gutta on weight loss. Interestingly, a randomized, double-blind, placebo-controlled study of a combination product containing *G. mangostana*, rather than *G. cambogia*, showed a significant reduction in weight and serum lipids including LDL-C and triglycerides.

Ginger (*Zingiber officinale*)

Class and chemistry

Phytochemical constituents of *Z. officinale* rhizomes include gingerols, zingiberene, and shogaols. The gingerols, primarily 6-gingerol, are responsible for ginger's pungency.

Pharmacological actions

Ginger exerts antidiabetic, antiobesity, anticancer, anticoagulant, anti-inflammatory, and antioxidant activity. Pharmacologic activity is related to inhibition of the cyclooxygenase (COX) and lipoxygenase (LOX) enzymes. For example, gingerols are nonselective COX inhibitors.

Ethnopharmacological use

- Nausea and vomiting
- Fever
- GI (dyspepsia, irritable bowel syndrome)
- Diarrhea
- Dysmenorrhea
- Arthritis
- Diabetes
- Anticoagulant

Adverse effects, contraindications, and precautions

Ginger is safe in humans if used at recommended doses.

Clinical trials

- In pregnant women, ginger improved nausea symptoms without affecting the number of vomiting episodes.
- In women with dysmenorrhea, ginger significantly reduced pain when administered during the first 3–4 days of the menstrual period.
- Current trial results do not support the use of ginger as an ergogenic or analgesic.

Green Tea (*Camellia sinensis*)

Class and chemistry

Primary chemical constituents include catechins and purine alkaloids including caffeine, theophylline, and theobromine.

Pharmacological actions

Green tea increases plasma antioxidant capacity and decreases serum concentrations of total cholesterol, triglyceride, and atherogenic index.

Ethnopharmacological use

- Reduced risk of cardiovascular disease including reduced lipid levels
- Reduced risk of pancreatic, squamous cell lung, and esophageal cancer
- Prevention of colon cancer
- Decreased recurrence of Stage I and II breast cancer
- Diuresis, dysuria, edema
- Mild diarrhea; digestive aid
- Reduced osteoporosis risk
- Headache, CNS (central nervous system) stimulant
- Weight loss

Adverse effects, contraindications, and precautions

- The major dose-limiting ingredient of green tea extract appears to be caffeine. Thus, most dose-limiting toxicities are caffeine related and include GI (flatulence, nausea, abdominal bloating), neurological (insomnia, restlessness, tremor, headache, pain, paresthesia), and cardiovascular (palpitations, hypertension) adverse effects.
- Human studies demonstrate that 8–16 cups of green tea per day are safe and well tolerated.

- In 2008, the Dietary Supplements Information Expert Committee (DSI EC) of the United States Pharmacopeial Convention systematically reviewed 216 case reports on green tea products, including 34 reports concerning liver damage, in response to concerns over hepatotoxicity related to green tea extract (GTE)–containing weight-loss products. The data suggest that liver-related adverse effects after GTE intake are rare.

Clinical trials

Numerous clinical trials have evaluated the effect of green tea on markers of disease. Findings include that green tea

- significantly lowers systolic blood pressure, total cholesterol, and LDL-C.
- produces modest, but significant, reductions in BMI (body mass index), body weight, and waist circumference.

Horehound (*Marrubium vulgare*)

Class and chemistry

Horehound is a bitter herb that contains bitter principles and tannins. Actives include the diterpene, marrubiin, a bitter lactone that opens to form marrubiinic acid, as well as the flavonoids quercetin, apigenin, and luteolin.

Pharmacological actions

Horehound has been found to produce anti-inflammatory, analgesic, antispasmodic, vasorelaxant, gastroprotective, hepatoprotective, antidiabetic, hypocholesterolemic, antihypertensive, antioxidant, antimicrobial, antifungal, antiasthmatic, expectorant, and neuroprotection actions.

Ethnopharmacological usage

- Expectorant
- Dyspepsia symptoms such as swelling or flatulence, temporary loss of appetite

Adverse effects, contraindications, and precautions

None have been reported.

Clinical trials

M. vulgare aqueous extracts failed to alter metabolic parameters (fasting blood glucose, cholesterol, triglycerides) in a double-blind study in patients with uncontrolled type 2 diabetes.

Ivy Leaf (*Hedera helix*)

Class and chemistry

Phytochemical constituents of *H. helix* include triterpene saponins, flavonoids, polyacetylenes, phenolic compounds (chlorogenic acid), and rutinosides (rutin and nicotiflorin).

Pharmacological actions

Ivy leaf extracts exert bronchospasmolytic, secretolytic, expectorant, and antitussive activity. Note that the saponins, α-hederin and hederacoside C, act to increase β_2-adrenergic receptor density, which accounts for the enhanced response to β_2-adrenergic receptor agonists—both endogenous medications (epinephrine) and those used in inflammatory lung disease.

Ethnopharmacological use

- Adjuvant therapy in inflammatory bronchial diseases (e.g., bronchitis)
- Expectorant, antitussive

Adverse effects, contraindications, and precautions

- GI adverse effects (nausea, vomiting, diarrhea) have been noted.
- Allergic reactions (urticaria, skin rash, dyspnea) have been reported.
- Do not use in children under 2 years of age.
- Use with caution in patients with gastritis or gastric ulcers.
- Concomitant use of ivy leaf and opiate antitussives is not recommended.

Clinical trials

Ethanol extracts of ivy leaf have been purported to be safe and effective in treating inflammatory lung disease such as chronic obstructive pulmonary disease, bronchitis, and asthma.

Turmeric (*Curcuma longa*)

Class and chemistry

Turmeric is a traditional spice and medicine. Diarylheptanoids, collectively termed curcuminoids, represent the most active chemical constituent of turmeric. Curcuminoids including curcumin, demethyoxycurcumin, and bisdemethoxycurcumin account for 1–6% of turmeric by dry weight and impart the spice's characteristic yellow color. The term *curcumin* is used interchangeably with *curcuminoids*.

Pharmacological actions

Curcumin has been identified with several pharmacologic targets including histone acetyltransferase (HAT) p300, histone deacetylase-8 (HDAC8), cannabinoid receptor 1 (CB1), and cystic fibrosis transmembrane conductance regulator (CFTR). However, target engagement and selectivity assays are lacking. Thus, the exact targets are currently unproven. Curcumin possesses numerous pharmacologic properties including antioxidant, anti-inflammatory, hepatoprotective, antimutagenic, anticarcinogenic, antitumor, antibacterial, fungistatic, and wound-healing actions.

Ethnopharmacological use

- A paste or lotion containing turmeric is used for the treatment of dry and flaking skin, skin sores and wounds, external inflammations, and painful arthritis.
- In 1985, the German Commission E approved turmeric for the internal treatment of indigestion.
- The European Medicines Agency's (EMA) draft monograph includes therapeutic indications for turmeric preparations, including powdered rhizome, herbal tea, and 1:10 tincture with 70% alcohol, for dyspepsia.
- Health Canada's turmeric monograph lists approved uses of the dried rhizome or preparations of the rhizome (e.g., herbal tea infusion, 1:1 fluid extract and1:5 tincture) as a carminative to help relieve flatulent dyspepsia and as a digestive aid.

Adverse effects, contraindications, and precautions

- The most common adverse effects are simultaneous abdominal pain and nausea, constipation, vertigo, and itching.
- Other randomized control trials in patients with arthritis reported adverse effects that included mild fever and throat infection, GI symptoms, hair loss, tachycardia, hypertension, and redness of tongue, but the adverse effects profile was similar in placebo and pain medicine (ibuprofen and diclofenac) control groups.
- Turmeric preparations and curcumin are considered safe at doses up to 1,200 mg/day for up to 4 months.

Clinical trials

A recent meta-analysis of seven clinical trials (649 Asian patients) was conducted to assess the lipid-lowering efficacy and safety of turmeric and curcumin in patients at risk of cardiovascular disease. Findings from the trials included the following:

- In patients at significant risk of cardiovascular disease, serum LDL-C and triglycerides were reduced, but there was no change in HDL-C (high-density lipoprotein cholesterol) or total cholesterol.
- Patients with arthritis reported a reduction in pain.
- In patients with ulcerative colitis, the clinical activity index and the endoscopic index were significantly lower at 6 months in the curcumin cohort.

8-8 Nonherbal Products

Probiotics

The GI tract is host to a wide variety of microorganisms that exist in balance and do not cause disease. This balance can be altered by antibiotic therapy, infection, and environmental factors that usually manifest as diarrhea.

Probiotics are live bacteria—including *Lactobacillus rhamnosus strain GG, L. acidophilus, L. reuteri, L. casei, Bifidobacterium lactis, B. bifidum, Streptococcus thermophilus*, and the yeast strain *Saccharomyces boulardii*—that are available as dietary supplements and in yogurt, cheese, and buttermilk.

When ingested, probiotics replicate in the small intestine and maintain or reestablish the balance between the beneficial gut bacteria and the bacteria associated with disease. Probiotics are used to treat infectious diarrhea and antibiotic-associated diarrhea.

Prebiotics

Prebiotics are carbohydrates known as *soluble fiber.* The dietary products help hold water in the colon to promote normal passage of stool, and they also promote the growth of probiotics. Thus, probiotics and prebiotics work together to decrease diarrheal disease.

Omega-3 Fatty Acids and Fish Oil

Linoleic acid, an omega-6 fatty acid, prevents essential fatty acid deficiency. It is chain elongated to arachidonic acid, a 20-carbon fatty acid. Products in this metabolic pathway include prostaglandins and leukotrienes, which are proinflammatory, thrombogenic, and vasoconstrictive.

Linolenic acid is an omega-3 fatty acid that is chain elongated to eicosapentaenoic acid (EPA) and docosahexaenoic acid (DHA). EPA and DHA are precursors to prostaglandins and leukotrienes that are anti-inflammatory, antiarrhythmic, and triglyceride lowering.

The importance of including omega-3 fats in the diet was initially noted in the Inuit population of the Arctic, who ingested large quantities of fatty fish and had a low risk of cardiovascular disease. Current recommendations are that dietary intake of fish be increased to two servings per week to decrease the risk for cardiovascular disease. Short-term increases in dietary omega-3s do little to improve mental acuity in older adults. Thus, long-term, if not lifelong, dietary modification may be needed to achieve this outcome.

Omega-3s can be ingested in the diet from fish, flaxseed, and nuts such as walnuts. Large fish, such as shark, king mackerel, swordfish, or tilefish, should be consumed in moderation and not be consumed at all by pregnant women, women who are planning to conceive, and small children because these fish contain increased amounts of mercury in their flesh. Polychlorinated biphenyls (PCBs) also can be transferred from the environment to fish and, as with mercury, are in higher concentration in the fat and skin of the largest fish. Removal of fat and skin from fatty fish significantly reduces the concentration of PCBs.

Alternatively, omega-3s can be consumed as a fish oil dietary supplement. Supplements containing larger amounts of DHA and EPA are desired.

The concern over potential mercury and pesticide contamination of fish oil supplements has been dismissed because the purification process removes potential toxins, including mercury. In addition, the fish source for many supplements is anchovies and sardines, which are small fish that do not accumulate significant amounts of mercury or PCBs. Cod liver oil is a source of omega-3s; however, concentrations are low, and it contains significant amounts of vitamin A, which can accumulate and result in toxicity.

Adverse effects that have been observed include the following:

- Common side effects include fishy aftertaste and GI symptoms.
- Potential exists for antithrombotic effects; bleeding is a concern, especially with doses that exceed 3 g/day. Use cautiously in patients on anticoagulants.

Glucosamine and Chondroitin

Glucosamine is available as a hydrochloride salt or as a sulfate usually obtained from shrimp, lobster, and crab shells. Persons with shellfish allergy should be informed of the potential for an allergic reaction. Chondroitin is obtained from bovine or shark cartilage. Vegetarians and those with shellfish allergies may opt for a vegetarian glucosamine that is derived from corn and a vegetarian chondroitin that is derived from algae.

An adequate trial of at least 1 month is needed to determine if a benefit will be achieved. Glucosamine and chondroitin have been studied individually and as a combination. The usual outcome measures are decreases in joint pain and stiffness; however, some studies have evaluated joint-space narrowing.

Adverse effects are as follows:

- Side effects are minimal but include GI complaints and headache.
- Because glucosamine facilitates hexosamine pathway flux, it has the potential to interfere with glucose metabolism. However, patients with type 2 diabetes given normal doses of glucosamine and chondroitin for 3 months had no change in their hemoglobin A1C concentrations.

Coenzyme Q10

Like cholesterol, coenzyme Q10 (CoQ10), also known as *ubiquinone,* is a product of the mevalonate pathway. CoQ10 has been used to treat cancer; diabetes; and cardiovascular disease, including congestive heart failure, angina, and hypertension.

A review of studies of congestive heart failure treated with doses of CoQ10 ranging from 50 to 300 mg daily and of angina treated with doses up to 600 mg daily concluded that a benefit existed in both conditions. Other studies have not found benefit, leading to suggestions that dosing was inadequate.

Of note, 3-hydroxy-3-methylglutaryl coenzyme A (HMG-CoA) reductase inhibitors block a step in the mevalonate pathway, resulting in a decrease in cholesterol and ubiquinone concentrations. Two trials evaluating doses of 100 or 200 mg of CoQ10 daily found that statin-related myalgia was not improved. One proposition suggests that long-term statin therapy may deplete CoQ10, and either a larger dose or a longer trial may be needed to see benefit. A serum concentration response relationship has not been established; thus, more study is needed to determine the place of CoQ10 in therapy.

Adverse effects are as follows:

- Side effects are primarily GI related and are usually mild.
- Other side effects include mild insomnia, photosensitivity, and fatigue.

Patients receiving warfarin may experience an increase in PT (prothrombin time) or INR (international normalized ratio); therefore, they should be closely monitored if CoQ10 is administered.

Dehydroepiandrosterone

Dehydroepiandrosterone (DHEA) is an endogenous product of cholesterol metabolism that exists in equilibrium with sulfated DHEA (DHEA-S), and they are precursors to both testosterone and estradiol.

DHEA concentrations begin to decrease in the third decade of life. DHEA as a dietary supplement has been promoted as the "fountain of youth" and has been used as a treatment for depression, arthritis, and cancer and as a performance enhancer.

Adverse effects are as follows:

- Side effects can be problematic and consist of acne, oily skin, voice deepening, hirsutism, menstrual irregularities, gynecomastia, insomnia, and weight gain.
- Because DHEA is a precursor for estradiol and testosterone, patients with hormone-responsive cancers should not take DHEA.

Melatonin

Melatonin is an endogenous hormone diurnally secreted by the pituitary gland. Concentrations increase at night to induce sleep. Exogenous melatonin is derived from bovine pineal gland or may be synthesized.

The most common use for melatonin is for sleep regulation. Minimizing and preventing jet lag is one of the more common uses for melatonin. Persons planning a flight across multiple time zones adjust their time to go to sleep to coincide with their destination and continue supplementation for several days after arrival. Individuals who work different shifts have used melatonin to help adjust to new sleep times.

Studies have shown that sleep latency is improved with melatonin; however, sleep efficiency and length of sleep appear to be unaffected.

Adverse effects are as follows:

- Side effects include drowsiness, disorientation, and nausea.
- Melatonin can decrease sperm counts and motility, so fertility in males can be affected.

8-9 Vitamins and Minerals

A balanced diet leads to better health and prevents many diseases, and because many people do not always eat properly, consumption of vitamin and mineral supplements has become a part of everyday life. Indeed, many health care providers recommend a daily multivitamin to make up for dietary deficiencies. Notably, adequate intake of folic acid during pregnancy prevents neural tube defects. Thus, women of childbearing age should take a multivitamin containing 400 mcg of folic acid, the amount in most multivitamins. Multivitamins do not contain sufficient calcium for either men or women, so a calcium supplement with vitamin D in addition to a standard multivitamin is recommended.

Epidemiological studies suggest an association between the consumption of diets high in vitamin E and a decreased risk of cardiovascular disease. Many dietary supplements, especially those containing beta-carotene, vitamin C, and vitamin E, are promoted as antioxidants. Unfortunately, an idea prevails among consumers that the use of these supplements fills the gaps created by poor diets and that large doses of these antioxidant vitamin supplements protect against cardiovascular disease and cancer.

Antioxidant vitamins provide protection to cells in danger of being damaged by free radicals. Theoretically a benefit, this protection would preserve cellular integrity. However, free radicals do serve a useful purpose in that they can destroy mutant cells that are destined to be cancerous. If there are no free radicals to do this function, the mutant cells can proliferate. Thus, antioxidants may be permissive and allow cancer cells to multiply. Indeed, radiation therapy works by generating free radicals to induce cytotoxicity to the cancerous cells. Therefore, high doses of antioxidants should be avoided in individuals undergoing radiation and certain types of chemotherapy to avoid neutralizing the effects of their cancer therapies.

Vitamin E (tocopherol) and Vitamin A (beta-carotene)

Prevailing trends suggest that the dietary intake of foods high in antioxidant vitamins such as vitamin E (tocopherol) and vitamin A (beta-carotene) may provide some protection from cardiovascular disease. When pharmacologic doses of supplements are taken, however, this protection is lost, and increased cardiovascular morbidity and mortality exist.

One explanation is that the protection seen from dietary intake was not from the individual vitamins but rather from other phytochemicals present in the foods. Eight forms of vitamin E exist in nature; four of these are tocopherols, four are tocotrienols, and some of these exist as stereoisomers. The majority of clinical studies evaluate only alpha-tocopherol. Recent evidence points to the tocotrienols as agents with neuroprotective, anticancer, and cholesterol-lowering properties. Other studies propose that gamma-tocopherol, which is present in the diet in concentrations two to four times greater than the alpha form, is superior in disease prevention. The differences in metabolic effects attributable to these different forms of vitamin E need further study.

Vitamin D

Multiple controlled trials have concluded that vitamin D is important in almost every chronic disease in humans, including infections, cardiovascular disease, type 1 diabetes, arthritis, osteoporosis, and chronic pain syndromes.

Vitamin D deficiency is common. More than 50% of the population has 25(OH)D (25-hydroxyvitamin D) serum levels less than 32 ng/mL. Goal concentrations range from 40 to 70 ng/mL.

Ultraviolet B (UVB) radiation from sunlight photoisomerizes 7-dehydrocholesterol in the skin to form vitamin D_3, or cholecalciferol. Vitamin D_3 is then oxidized in the liver to 25-hydroxy D_3, which is then oxidized in the kidney and other tissues to form 1,25-dihydroxy D_3, the active form of vitamin D. Factors limiting this conversion process include the following:

- ***Dark skin:*** Melanin skin pigment prevents the UVB rays from penetrating the skin.
- ***Distance from the equator:*** Fewer UVB rays penetrate the atmosphere.
- ***Atmospheric pollution:*** Such pollution impedes UVB penetration.
- ***Use of sunscreens to prevent skin cancers:*** SPF (sun protection factor) 8 blocks production by more than 95%.
- ***Increased hours spent indoors:*** Television and video games have limited people's leisure time outdoors.
- ***Obesity:*** Fatty tissue stores vitamin D; thus, in obese individuals, vitamin D may be unavailable for systemic tissue needs.

Vitamin D can be obtained from foods, but few foods contain sufficient amounts. Even foods fortified with vitamin D, such as milk, orange juice, and cereals, contain only about 100 IU (international units) of vitamin D per serving. Although infant formulas are fortified with vitamin D, breast milk contains almost none.

The current Food and Nutrition Board of the Health and Medicine Division of the National Academies of Sciences, Engineering, and Medicine recommends a daily intake of 600 IU (15 mcg) of vitamin D in adults. More recent publications recommend supplements of at least 1,000 IU per day and suggest that even more may be needed. They also recommend that all individuals have at least a yearly measurement of serum levels of 25-hydroxy D_3 to ensure that concentrations are adequate.

8-10 Evaluation of Alternative and Complementary Medication

Natural products do not have to be evaluated for purity, bioavailability, or efficacy. The manufacturer is responsible for ensuring safety. However, the mechanism for ensuring safety has not been well established. Through the recently implemented adverse effects monitoring program, products that are associated with toxicity should be more readily identified. The consumer can be assured that products with the USP, CL (ConsumerLab.com), or NSF (NSF International) seals are pure and contain the labeled amount. Even with the full implementation of the DSHEA, there will not be a requirement to ensure efficacy.

8-11 Herb–Drug Interactions

Current surveys indicate that almost half of the U.S. population takes some form of dietary supplement. In addition, almost 30% of prescription drug users in the United States take botanical supplements concomitantly with conventional medications, often without notifying their physician or other health care provider. Therefore, prospects for herb–drug interactions are considerable.

In vitro studies are very useful for evaluating both purified phytochemicals and multicomponent extracts. Such studies can provide mechanistic information about potential interactions and are relatively simple and inexpensive to perform. Several limitations, however, hamper their utility as predictors of in vivo responses. These limitations include the following:

- Most methods employ solubilizing agents (e.g., dimethyl sulfoxide [DMSO], ethanol, acetonitrile) to facilitate exposure and uptake of poorly water-soluble phytochemicals into cells or microsomes.
- Phytochemical concentrations necessary to modulate enzyme or transporter activity often exceed those achieved in vivo.
- Studies examining purified compounds may not reflect the phytochemical complexity typical of extracts that may contribute to the net inhibitory or inductive effects observed.
- Many phytochemicals undergo extensive intestinal or hepatic metabolism, a condition that may affect their net modulatory effects in vivo.

Herb–drug interaction studies conducted in small animals (e.g., mice, rats, dogs) are less expensive than human clinical studies and can often provide an initial assessment of bioavailability for phytochemicals either in pure form or in the context of a complex extract. Limitations of animal studies are that large, nonphysiological doses are often administered and that because of species variation in metabolism and transport, results are rarely generalizable to humans.

The importance of in vivo human studies for investigating herb–drug interactions came to the forefront in 2000 when a succession of clinical case reports revealed that St. John's wort drastically reduced plasma concentrations of the immunosuppressant cyclosporine, precipitating graft rejection in organ transplant recipients. Several common oversights can influence the outcome and interpretation of human studies:

- Because botanical supplements often exhibit significant brand-to-brand and lot-to-lot variability, commercially available products must be analyzed independently for phytochemical characterization and content.
- Disintegration and dissolution characteristics for specific dosage forms should be conducted before study implementation. Dosage forms failing to properly disintegrate or release their purported *marker* compounds within a reasonable time period will preclude any meaningful results.
- An assessment of phytochemical bioavailability or detection of marker compounds in circulating plasma or urine provides evidence of exposure as well as subject compliance. Although desirable, this prerequisite is often limited by the paucity of validated analytical methods available for measuring unique phytochemicals and their metabolites in biologic fluids.
- Very few studies incorporate positive controls for inhibition (e.g., clarithromycin as cytochrome 450 [CYP] 3A4/ABCB1 inhibitor) or induction (e.g., rifampin as CYP3A4/ABCB1 inducer) as a means of gauging clinical relevance.

Two general categories of herb–drug interactions are recognized—pharmacodynamic and pharmacokinetic:

- Pharmacodynamic herb–drug interactions are situations in which the botanical supplement has a pharmacological effect that is either very similar to or opposite of that of a conventional medication.
- Pharmacokinetic-mediated herb–drug interactions are those in which phytochemicals present in botanical dietary supplements affect the absorption, distribution, metabolism, and excretion of conventional medications.

Although numerous in vitro and animal studies suggest that a wide variety of phytochemicals and botanical dietary supplements can cause pharmacokinetic herb–drug interactions, very few of these findings translate to human clinical results. Two important phytochemical mixtures to keep in mind are St. John's wort and green tea.

Despite the thousands of botanical dietary supplements currently on the U.S. market, very few appear to pose significant risks for clinically relevant herb–drug interactions. This may stem from two key factors. First, only a small portion of the top-selling botanicals have been evaluated in clinical herb–drug interaction studies. The vast majority of new botanical products and multi-ingredient formulations have yet to be examined for their drug interaction potential. Second, many phytochemicals have poor oral bioavailability, and this property likely accounts for their low risk of herb–drug interaction. As mentioned earlier, major contributors underlying inadequate systemic phytochemical exposure are extensive first-pass metabolism and poor solubility in GI fluids. Together, these two issues likely account for the meager efficacy of many botanicals, but they also render commercial botanicals quite safe. Recognizing that poor aqueous solubility impairs the absorption of many phytochemicals, the dietary supplement industry has begun implementing novel phytochemical delivery systems to overcome this deficiency. Novel formulations using technologies such as liposomes, phytosomes, nanoparticles, and microemulsions, as well as the purposeful incorporation of methylenedioxyphenyl-containing phytochemicals (e.g., piperine), have demonstrated marked improvements in phytochemical bioavailability. Although such technologies may improve supplement efficacy, they may also increase the herb–drug interaction potential of many botanicals that have heretofore posed only minimal risks. At present, very few clinical herb–drug interaction studies have evaluated many of these novel formulations.

In summary, botanical dietary supplements can interact with conventional medications. The mechanisms for such interactions are pharmacodynamic, pharmacokinetic, or sometimes both. Many popular botanicals pose little risk for drug interactions; however, most have yet to be evaluated in a clinical setting. Finally, novel dietary supplement dosage forms may increase the herb–drug interaction potential for many botanicals.

8-12 Adulteration and Contamination

Dietary supplements also face challenges with regard to adulteration and contamination. The contamination with heavy metals, microbial pathogens, pesticide residues, and improperly identified plant material and the adulteration with toxic plant extracts, pharmaceutical agents, and other inappropriate additives have generated concern among the medical community and lay public. Although contamination or adulteration with certain less noxious substances or botanicals may not be harmful, other additives have been the cause of serious toxicity. Contamination with heavy metals and various toxic herbs is generally more problematic for imported supplements than for those produced domestically. More disconcerting than unintended product contamination has been the seemingly purposeful adulteration of dietary supplements with conventional drugs. Certain categories of dietary supplements are more apt to be adulterated with undeclared drugs than are other categories. These products include supplements marketed as exercise performance enhancers, which may be adulterated with anabolic steroids or analogues of anabolic steroids; male sexual enhancement products, which may be adulterated with phosphodiesterase 5 antagonists such as sildenafil, tadalafil, vardenafil, or novel analogues of these drugs; and certain weight-loss products that may contain synthetic sympathomimetics like dimethylamylamine, sibutramine, amphetamines, or ephedrine alkaloids. The FDA has removed from the market a variety of dietary supplements containing undeclared prescription medications and anabolic steroids, several of which have produced toxic manifestations in some consumers. Most supplement manufacturers have avoided this problem through rigorous, proactive implementation of GMPs. Others, however, have been less diligent in their approach to product quality. Beginning in 2008, the FDA implemented GMPs for the dietary supplement industry that addressed such issues as proper plant species identification, avoidance of microbial or heavy metal contamination, and preventive steps regarding adulteration with prescription medications. In accordance with GMPs, adulterants continue to be illegal, and testing for certain contaminants is now required. Implementation of these regulations has significantly reduced incidences of adulteration and contamination, but the FDA still removes adulterated dietary supplements from the U.S. market on an almost daily basis.

8-13 Questions

1. Regulation of dietary supplements under the Dietary Supplement Health and Education Act of 1994 requires that products

A. be accurately labeled.
B. provide evidence of product efficacy.
C. contain no more than three excipients.
D. identify all the chemical components.

2. The pharmacological activity associated with herbal medicine

A. is due to a single chemical entity that has been identified.
B. can depend on harvesting conditions.
C. must be measurable in an alcoholic extract.
D. should be present in both the root and the aerial parts of the herb or the plant.

3. Which of the following statements is true for echinacea?

A. *Echinacea pallida, E. angustifolia,* and *E. purpurea* are comparable in effects.
B. *Echinacea* species may be effective in preventing the common cold.
C. Echinacea must be taken with meals to enhance bioavailability.
D. Echinacea products are without adverse effects.

4. The Dietary Supplement and Health Education Act (DSHEA) does *not* allow for which of the following types of claims?

A. Health claims
B. Structure or function claims
C. Nutrient content claims
D. Disease claims

5. Which of the following is the only acceptable route of administration for dietary supplements?

A. Intravenous
B. Intra-arterial
C. Oral
D. Ocular

6. Which of the following has been shown to decrease digoxin serum concentrations?

A. *Panax ginseng*
B. *Linum usitatissimum*
C. *Eleutherococcus senticosus*
D. *Echinacea pallida*

7. Which of the following patients should not be given St. John's wort?

A. A 28-year-old woman who is receiving highly active antiretroviral therapy
B. A 32-year-old woman who is overweight and taking no prescription medications
C. A 45-year-old man who is taking acetaminophen for osteoarthritis
D. A 68-year-old man who receives a weekly massage for sore muscles after tennis

8. A 62-year-old person can use which of the following to lower triglyceride concentration?

A. Fish oil
B. Garlic
C. Ginseng
D. Probiotics

9. Dietary fish intake

A. should include the very large fish that have increased amounts of EPA and DHA.
B. should be increased to decrease the morbidity and mortality associated with cardiovascular disease.
C. benefit can be replaced by large doses of cod liver oil.
D. at least 3 times a week is appropriate in all groups of individuals.

10. Glucosamine and chondroitin combination in the treatment of joint pain associated with rheumatoid disease

A. shows benefit within the first week of therapy.
B. has no potential for allergy because it is not plant based.
C. is more effective in preventing joint-space narrowing.
D. may be effective in treating pain in moderate to severe disease.

11. Individuals who receive HMG-CoA reductase inhibitors for high cholesterol and experience myalgia may be depleted of which of the following?

A. Vitamin A
B. Vitamin K
C. Selenium
D. Ubiquinone

12. Which of the following statements is *not* true regarding green tea?

A. The major dose-limiting ingredient of green tea extract appears to be caffeine.
B. Human studies demonstrate that 8–16 cups of green tea per day are safe and well tolerated.
C. Human data suggest that green tea extract is associated with significant liver injury.
D. Green tea is associated with lower systolic blood pressure, total cholesterol, and LDL-C in humans.

13. Individuals with a hormone-sensitive tumor should *not* receive which of the following agents?

A. DHEA
B. Saw palmetto
C. St. John's wort
D. Vitamin E

14. There are numerous human clinical trials evaluating the potential efficacy of natural products in subjects with various ailments. Which of the following is NOT true regarding evidence to support potential benefit of natural products?

- **A.** There is some evidence that cranberry juice may decrease the number of symptomatic urinary tract infections (UTIs) over a 12-month period, particularly for women with recurrent UTIs.
- **B.** Patients with arthritis who use curcumin report a reduction in pain.
- **C.** Horehound use is associated with improvement in metabolic parameters (e.g., insulin sensitivity) in subjects with type 2 diabetes.
- **D.** In pregnant women, ginger improves nausea symptoms without affecting the number of vomiting episodes.

15. Vitamin D deficiency is related to

- **A.** overexposure to the sun.
- **B.** deactivation of cholecalciferol in the liver.
- **C.** increased skin pigmentation.
- **D.** lack of sunscreen use.

16. Melatonin has been shown to

- **A.** decrease sleep latency.
- **B.** enhance sleep efficiency.
- **C.** increase length of sleep.
- **D.** result in vivid dreams.

17. Cranberry juice (*Vaccinium macrocarpon*) is purported to be beneficial in treating which of the following conditions?

- **A.** Common cold
- **B.** Elevated serum triglycerides
- **C.** Insomnia
- **D.** Urinary tract infections

18. Flax (*Linuum usitatissimum*) may be beneficial in the management of which of the following medical conditions? (Mark all that apply.)

- **A.** Hyperlipidemia
- **B.** Rheumatoid arthritis
- **C.** Irritable bowl
- **D.** Systemic lupus erythematosus

19. Which of the following is a potential drug interaction with patients receiving garcinia gummi-gutta?

- **A.** HMG-CoA reductase inhibitors
- **B.** Selective serotonin reuptake inhibitors
- **C.** Corticosteroids
- **D.** Warfarin

20. Which of the following are administration routes that have been used for turmeric (*Curcuma longa*)? (Mark all that apply.)

- **A.** Buccal
- **B.** Topical
- **C.** Oral
- **D.** Intranasal

8-14 Answers

1. A. Dietary supplements must have an accurate label. Products need not demonstrate efficacy. There is no limit to the number of ingredients, and the chemical components do not have to be identified.

2. B. Harvesting conditions can be critical to ensure a quality herbal product. Often the chemical entities have not been identified, and if they are known, there is no assurance that one particular chemical is responsible for the pharmacologic effects. Some herbal products have the active component in the root, some in the aerial portion, and others in the seed or berry. Because there is no certainty of the active chemical's identity or if it is extractable with alcohol, chemicals do not have to be present in an alcoholic extract.

3. B. Echinacea, in particular *E. purpurea*, is thought to have some activity against the common cold. Studies have not compared effects among the three species that are used. Although adverse effects are minimal, some mild adverse effects can occur. There is no information available on bioavailability with or without food intake.

4. D. The DSHEA specifically prohibits product labeling that refers to the treatment, cure, or diagnosis of "disease."

5. C. Products considered dietary supplements can be administered only orally.

6. **C.** *Eleutherococcus senticosus*, or Siberian ginseng, has been reported to decrease serum digoxin concentrations. Both *E. senticosus* and *Panax quinquefolius* (American ginseng) can interfere with the fluorescence polarization immunoassay and the microparticle enzyme immunoassay. There have not been reports of assay interference with *P. quinquefolius* or *Echinacea pallida*.

7. **A.** St. John's wort has many important drug interactions because it induces CYP450 and P-glycoprotein. St. John's wort decreases concentrations of the antiretrovirals and should not be used with these drugs. Interactions with acetaminophen have not been reported. Getting a massage treatment for sore muscles would not pose a problem in someone receiving St. John's wort.

8. **A.** Fish oil lowers triglyceride concentrations. Garlic has been shown to lower serum cholesterol concentrations but is not specific for triglycerides. Ginseng and probiotics have no effect on triglyceride values.

9. **B.** Increased dietary intake of fish reduces cardiovascular-related morbidity and mortality. Eating large amounts of the very large fish is problematic because they contain more mercury and possibly more PCBs (fatty fish). Pregnant women and young children are recommended to limit their intake of fish that contain more mercury because of heavy metal toxicity. Cod liver oil contains the appropriate fats, but it also contains large amounts of vitamin A that can accumulate and cause toxicity.

10. **D.** Glucosamine-chondroitin shows promise in the relief of joint pain in moderate to severe rheumatoid disease. It must be used for at least 1 month to see benefit. It is not plant based, but it is sourced from shellfish, so potential for allergy exists. Glucosamine alone appeared to be better than the combination in slowing joint-space narrowing in those with more moderate disease.

11. **D.** Ubiquinone is a metabolite of the mevalonate pathway that generates cholesterol. Statins block a step in this pathway that decreases cholesterol concentrations and also decreases ubiquinone (CoQ10) concentrations. Neither selenium nor vitamins A and K has been associated with myalgia related to HMG-CoA reductase inhibitors (statins).

12. **C.** In 2008, the Dietary Supplements Information Expert Committee (DSI EC) of the United States Pharmacopeial Convention systematically reviewed 216 case reports on green tea products, including 34 reports concerning liver damage, in response to concerns over hepatotoxicity related to green tea extract (GTE)–containing weight-loss products. The data suggest that liver-related adverse effects after GTE intake are rare.

13. **A.** DHEA is metabolized to testosterone and estradiol, which stimulate prostate and certain types of breast cancer, respectively. Saw palmetto contains fatty acids and sterols that do not affect hormone concentrations. Vitamin E was not found to decrease the occurrence of cancer. St. John's wort does not affect tumor cells.

14. **C.** Horehound aqueous extracts failed to alter metabolic parameters (fasting blood glucose, cholesterol, triglycerides) in a double-blind study in patients with uncontrolled type 2 diabetes.

15. **C.** Increased skin pigmentation decreases penetration of UVB rays through the skin, so activation of vitamin D is reduced. Insufficient exposure to sunlight and sunscreen use have been associated with vitamin D deficiency. Cholecalciferol is activated (not deactivated) in the liver.

16. **A.** Melatonin appears to decrease sleep latency (the time taken to fall asleep) but has no effect on sleep efficiency or length of sleep. Melatonin does not affect dreaming.

17. **D.** Beneficial effects of cranberry juice (*Vaccinium macrocarpon*) have been reported for the treatment of recurrent urinary tract infections. However, a Cochrane systematic analysis was unable to support this claim.

18. **All apply.** Trials have demonstrated beneficial effect of flax (*Linum usitatissimum*) for a wide variety of conditions, including hyperlipidemia, rheumatoid arthritis, irritable bowl, and systemic lupus erythematosus.

19. **B.** Garcinia gummi-gutta may affect serotonin levels. Therefore, this product should be avoided in patients receiving selective serotonin reuptake inhibitors.

20. **B, C.** Turmeric (*Curcuma longa*) has been administered topically as a paste or lotion as well as orally.

8-15 Additional Resources

Chavez ML, Jordan MA, Chavez PI. Evidence-based drug–herbal interactions. *Life Sciences*. 2006;78(18):2146–2157.

Dasgupta A. Herbal supplements and therapeutic drug monitoring: focus on digoxin immunoassays and interactions with St. John's wort. *Ther Drug Monit*. 2008;30(2):212–217.

Gill HS, Guarner F. Probiotics and human health: a clinical perspective. *Postgrad Med J*. 2004;80(947):516–526.

Halberstein RA. Medicinal plants: historical and cross-cultural usage patterns. *Ann Epidemiol*. 2005;15(9):686–699.

Izzo AA, Carlo GD, Borrelli F, Ernst E. Cardiovascular pharmacotherapy and herbal medicines: the risk of drug interaction. *Int J Cardiol*. 2005;98(1):1–14.

NIH National Center for Complementary and Integrative Health. 2012 National Health Interview Survey. Available at: https://nccih.nih.gov/research/statistics/NHIS/2012.

Shi S, Klotz U. Drug interactions with herbal medicines. *Clin Pharmacokinet*. 2012;51(2):77–104.

Pharmaceutics and Biopharmaceutics

9

HASSAN ALMOAZEN

9-1 KEY POINTS

- A *drug* is defined as a substance used in the diagnosis, treatment, or prevention of a disease or as a component of a medication. Most of the drugs used today are highly potent and require accurately weighed low doses if the drug is to be administered directly for a therapeutic effect.
- Therapeutic efficacy depends on the type of dosage form and route of administration.
- Liquids exhibit certain properties that allow them to flow across surfaces, and they can be studied to determine their viscosity.
- Solid substances can be broadly classified as crystalline solids or amorphous solids.
- A molecular dispersion of a solute in a solvent that results in a homogeneous system is called a true *solution*.
- A *heterogeneous system* can be defined as a chemical system that contains various distinct and mechanically separable parts or phases (e.g., suspension, emulsion).
- A *suspension* is a two-phase coarse dispersion system composed of insoluble solid material dispersed in an oily or aqueous liquid medium.
- An *emulsion* is a thermodynamically unstable heterogeneous system that consists of at least one immiscible liquid that is intimately dispersed in another in the form of droplets.
- A *partition* (*P*) or *distribution coefficient* (*D*) is the ratio of two concentrations of a compound in two immiscible solvents at equilibrium.
- The logarithm of the ratio of the concentrations of the un-ionized solute in the solvents is called *log P* and is represented by the following equation:

$$\log P_{octanol/water} = \log\left[\frac{[solute]_{octanol}}{[solute]_{water}}\right]$$

- The term *bioavailability* indicates the rate and extent that a drug is taken up from a dosage form into the systemic blood circulation and is available to exert its effects.
- A drug product's life is limited. The rate of a reaction, or *degradation rate*, is the velocity by which the reaction occurs. This rate is expressed as dC/dt (the change in concentration, or C, within a given time interval, or dt). The rate of a reaction, dC/dt, is proportional to the concentration to the nth power, where n is the order of the reaction.

9-2 STUDY GUIDE CHECKLIST

The following topics may guide your study of this subject area:

- ☐ The relationship between the pH and the dissociation constant (pK_a) for a weak acid or a weak base drug and the way this relationship affects drug absorption
- ☐ The relationship between solubility and dissolution rate for any drug and the major factors that affect both
- ☐ Rheology and evaluation of selected parameters that are used to describe the rheological behavior of different pharmaceutical systems
- ☐ Surfactants and the factors that affect the formation of micelles
- ☐ Hydrophilic–lipophilic balance and the way it influences the formation of emulsions
- ☐ Dispersed systems and different colloidal systems
- ☐ Excipients and their functions in different dosage forms
- ☐ Drug stability, order of reaction, and shelf life
- ☐ Different routes of administration and corresponding dosage forms

9-3 Introduction

The finished dosage form administered to patients usually contains an active drug entity and excipients. Here, a *drug* is defined as a substance used in the diagnosis, treatment, or prevention of a disease or as a component of a medication.

For a drug to be effectively administered, it is combined with specific excipients that constitute the finished dosage form (e.g., tablets or capsules). Here, an *excipient* is defined as an inert substance that is used to constitute the final dosage form to ensure adequate delivery of the drug. The amount and type of excipient depend on the purpose and type of the dosage form. The field that studies the dosage form is called pharmaceutics. Biopharmaceutics studies the factors that influence the release and absorption of the drug from the dosage form.

Biopharmaceutics enables the design of the dosage form to be based on the physical and chemical properties of the drug substance, the route of drug administration, (oral, topical, injectable, transdermal patch), the desired therapeutic effect (immediate or sustained release), toxicologic properties of the drug, and the safety of the excipients used. Biopharmaceutics also focuses on other factors that can influence drug absorption and metabolism.

9-4 Physical–Chemical Factors that Influence the Drug in a Dosage Form

As the temperature of a substance increases, its heat content, or *enthalpy,* increases proportionally. During such an event, substances can undergo a change of state, or phase change. These transitions from one state of matter to another can occur as a change from a solid to a liquid state (melting) or from a liquid to a gaseous state (vaporization).

Solubility

The solubility of a compound depends on the physical and chemical properties of the solute and the chemical properties of the solvent. Other factors, such as temperature, pressure, and the pH of the solvent, also affect the solubility of solutes.

According to the U.S. Pharmacopeia, the solubility of a drug can be expressed as the number of milliliters of solvent needed to dissolve 1 g of the solute. Table 9-1 describes different types of solubility.

TABLE 9-1. Solubility Terms According to the U.S. Pharmacopeia

Solubility term	Parts of solvent required to dissolve 1 g of solute
Very soluble	Fewer than 1
Freely soluble	1–10
Soluble	10–30
Sparingly soluble	30–100
Slightly soluble	100–1,000
Very slightly soluble	1,000–10,000
Insoluble	More than 10,000

Temperature significantly affects the solubility of solutes. As the temperature increases, the solubility of a solid increases proportionally for an endothermic change of state. However, as the temperature of a system containing a gas in liquid is increased, the solubility decreases because of the change in vapor pressure.

Most therapeutically relevant drugs that are small molecules (less than 500 molecular weight) are generally weak electrolytes (i.e., they are either weak acids or weak bases).

Another important parameter related to solubility is the concept of partition coefficients and log *P*. A *partition* (*P*) or *distribution coefficient* (*D*) is the ratio of concentrations of a compound in the two phases of a mixture of two immiscible solvents at equilibrium. Hence, these coefficients are a measure of differential solubility of the compound between the two solvents. Normally, one of the solvents chosen is water, and the second is hydrophobic, such as octanol (known as an *octanol–water system*).

Both the partition and the distribution coefficients are measures of the hydrophilic ("water loving") or hydrophobic ("water fearing") degree of a chemical substance. Partition coefficients are useful, for example, in estimating distribution of drugs within the body. Hydrophobic drugs with high partition coefficients are preferentially distributed to hydrophobic compartments, such as lipid bilayers of cells and plasma protein, whereas hydrophilic drugs with low partition coefficients preferentially are found in hydrophilic compartments, such as blood serum.

To measure the partition coefficient of ionizable solutes, one adjusts the pH of the aqueous phase so that the predominant form of the compound is nonionized. The logarithm of the ratio of the concentrations of the un-ionized solute in the solvents is called *log P*, which is represented by the following equation:

$$\log P_{octanol/water} = \log\left[\frac{[solute]_{octanol}}{[solute]_{water}}\right]$$

Another method of classification of pharmaceutically relevant compounds is the *biopharmaceutical classification system*, which classifies drugs according to their solubility and permeability through biological membranes. According to this system, drugs are classified into four groups: (1) high solubility: high permeability, (2) low solubility: high permeability, (3) high solubility: low permeability, and (4) low solubility: low permeability.

Surface and interfacial tension

In a liquid state, the cohesive forces between the adjacent molecules are well developed. Molecules in the bulk phase of a liquid are surrounded by other molecules of the same kind (liquid–liquid interface), unlike the molecules at the surface of a liquid, which are not completely surrounded by like molecules (liquid–air interface) (Figure 9-1).

As a result, molecules at or near the surface of a liquid experience a net inward pull or inward intermolecular attraction from molecules in the interior of the liquid, causing the liquid surface to contract spontaneously. Therefore, liquids tend to assume a spherical shape, that is, a volume with the minimum surface area and least free energy.

Any expansion of the surface increases the free energy of the system. Thus, *surface free energy* can be defined by the work required to increase the surface area *A* of the liquid by 1 area unit. This value is expressed as the number of millinewtons (mN) needed to expand a 1 m^2 surface by 1 unit:

$$Work = \gamma \cdot \Delta A$$

where ΔA is the increase in surface area and γ is the surface tension, or surface free energy, in mN/m^2.

Water has a surface tension at 20°C of approximately 72 mN, whereas *n*-octanol has a surface tension of approximately 27 mN. Thus, more work must be expended to expand the surface of water than to expand the surface of *n*-octanol.

At the boundary, or interface (e.g., between two immiscible liquids that are in contact with each other), the corresponding interfacial tension (i.e., free energy, or work required to expand the interfacial

FIGURE 9-1. Molecules in Bulk Liquid State and Liquid Surface State

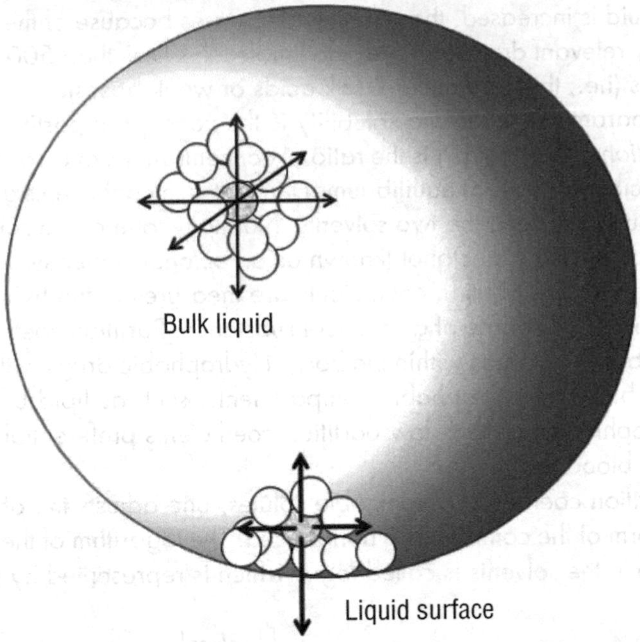

area) reflects the extent of the intermolecular forces of attraction and repulsion at the interface. When the interface is between two liquids, substantial molecular interaction occurs across the two phases. This interaction reduces the imbalance in forces of attraction within each phase.

Flow characteristics

Liquids exhibit certain properties that allow them to flow across a solid surface. These properties can be studied to determine the nature of a particular liquid and its viscosity.

The flow of a liquid across a solid surface can be examined in terms of the velocity, or rate of movement, of the liquid relative to the surface area across which it flows.

The flow can be represented schematically and by assuming the flow of liquid is the movement of numerous parallel layers of liquid between an upper, movable plate and a lower, fixed plate (Figure 9-2).

FIGURE 9-2. Schematic of Liquid Flow

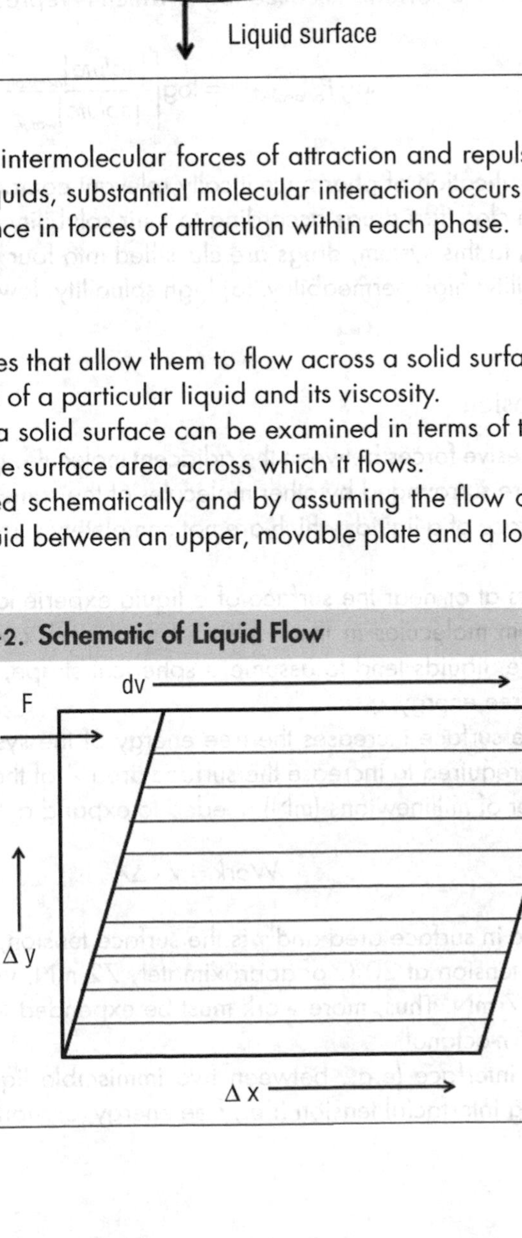

When a constant force (*F*) is applied to the upper plate such that it moves with the constant velocity, each lower plate moves with a velocity directly proportional to its distance from the stationary bottom layer. The velocity (*dv*) of the remaining layers of liquid between the two plates is proportional to their distance from the immovable plate (i.e., $\Delta y/\Delta x$).

The velocity gradient leads to deformation of the liquid with time, or the *rate of shear, dv/dx,* or *D.* Newton defined flow in terms of the ratio of the force *F* applied to a plate of area *A* (shear stress τ) divided by the velocity gradient (*D*) induced by τ:

$$\frac{F}{A} = \eta \circ \frac{dv}{dx}$$

where η is the *coefficient of viscosity,* also known as *viscosity.*

Viscosity is an expression of resistance of fluid flow: the higher the viscosity, the greater the resistance. Liquids that behave according to the preceding equation are known as *Newtonian substances.* Liquids containing dilute dispersions and simple molecules tend to behave in a Newtonian manner.

In contrast, substances that do not follow the preceding equation are known as *non-Newtonian substances.* Substances in this class exhibit shear-dependent or time-dependent viscosities. Solids and heterogeneous liquids (e.g., concentrated colloids, suspensions, emulsions) exhibit non-Newtonian flow. Analyses of non-Newtonian substances using a viscometer yield results that, when plotted, give rise to various consistency curves: plastic, pseudoplastic, or dilatant flows (Figure 9-3).

Suspensions of small, deflocculated particles that have a high solid content can exhibit shear-thickening or dilatant viscosity, whereas solutions of certain polymers often show shear-thinning or pseudoplastic viscosity. In both systems, the apparent viscosity increases or decreases, respectively, with an increase in the rate of shear. This increase or decrease indicates a change of structure (breakdown or ordering) that does not reform immediately when the stress is removed.

Plastic, or Bingham body, behavior is exemplified by flocculated particles in concentrated suspensions that show no apparent response to low-level stress. Flow begins only after a limiting yield stress (yield value) is exceeded.

FIGURE 9-3. Flow Curves of Newtonian and Non-Newtonian Substances

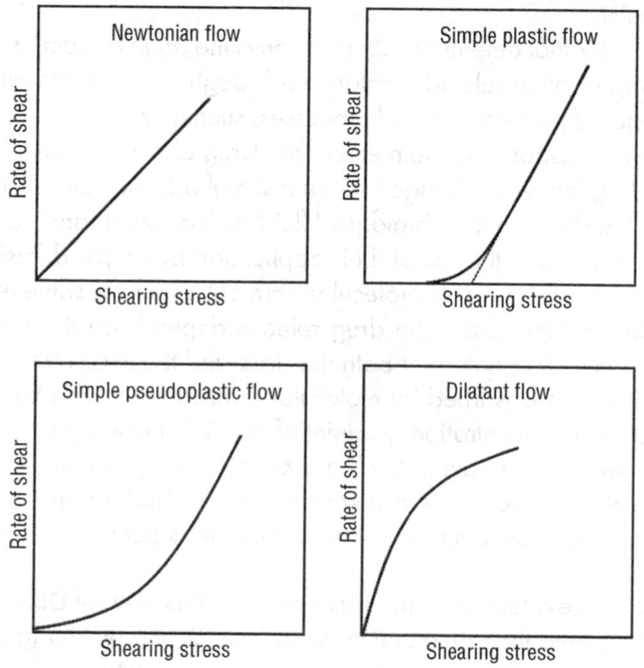

Solids

Certain substances show stronger intermolecular attractions than those seen in liquids and gases. Such substances exist as solids and show a higher order of geometry. Solid substances can be classified broadly as *crystalline* solids or *amorphous* solids.

Crystalline solids, such as ice or sodium chloride, are arranged in fixed geometric patterns or lattices and exhibit definite shape and orderly arrangement of the units. The units involved in the formation of crystals can be atoms, molecules, or ions. Solids, unlike gases, are almost incompressible and show distinct melting points, with the solid-to-liquid transition being very sharp.

Conversely, amorphous solids show a lower degree of order than crystalline solids and have randomly arranged units. They exhibit a wider range of nondistinct melting points and tend to flow when subjected to sufficient pressure over a period of time. They are isotropic (i.e., they display similar properties in all directions).

Polymorphism

Polymorphism is the condition wherein substances can exist in more than one crystalline form.

These polymorphs have different molecular arrangements or crystal lattice structures. Such alternative arrangements of the crystal lattice structure result in different polymorphs exhibiting different properties. For example, the melting point, solubility, dissolution rate, density, and stability can differ considerably among the polymorphic forms of a drug.

Steroids are an example of a drug class with an especially high incidence of polymorphism. Other pharmaceutically relevant compounds that exhibit polymorphism include fatty (triglyceride) excipients (e.g., theobroma oil, cocoa butter).

9-5 Biological Principles of Dosage Forms

For a drug to exert a therapeutic effect, it has to be administered at a specified dose. *Dose* is defined as a specified quantity of a therapeutic agent, such as a drug or medication, prescribed to be taken at one time or at stated intervals.

Another significant factor that determines drug action is the *route of administration,* which is defined as the path by which a drug or other related substance is brought into contact with the body. Once the drug is administered, a number of physicochemical processes, such as diffusion and dissolution, are involved in elucidating the therapeutic response to the medication. Drug absorption may be described as the rate at and extent to which a drug leaves its dosage form and site of administration. The term *bioavailability* indicates the extent to which a drug leaves a biological fluid such as blood and has access to its site of action.

Most drugs are absorbed from the site of their application by simple diffusion. Drug diffusion through a barrier predominantly occurs by simple molecular permeation and to some extent by movement through pores and channels. In the latter case, the drug release depends on the crystallinity and crystal size, degree of swelling, and chemical nature of both the drug and the excipients.

In a case where the drug is absorbed by molecular diffusion, it travels by a *passive transport* mechanism, which is dictated by a concentration gradient of the drug traveling from a region of higher concentration to a region of lower concentration. Such a process is energy independent.

In some cases, the drug molecule is transported across biological membranes by the action of membrane transporters or pumps. Such a process is known as *active transport* and is generally energy dependent.

Passive transport can be explained on the basis of Fick's First Law of Diffusion. This law states that the amount of material (M) flowing through a unit cross section (S) of a barrier in unit time (t), which is known as the flux (J), is proportional to the concentration gradient (dC/dx):

$$J = \frac{dM}{S \circ dt}$$

Because the flux (*J*) is proportional to the concentration gradient (*dC*/*dt*),

$$J = D \circ \frac{dC}{dt}$$

In this equation, *D* is the *diffusion coefficient* (cm^2/sec) and is a physicochemical property of the material (drug); it is not constant and can vary with changes in concentration, temperature, pressure, solvent properties, and chemical nature of the diffusant. Fick's First Law of Diffusion describes the diffusion process under the condition of steady state when the concentration gradient (*dC*/*dx*) does not change with time.

Biopharmaceutics and the design of modern drug delivery systems are based on the concept of diffusion and dissolution. When the drug in its solid form is introduced into the gastrointestinal (GI) tract, the drug begins to pass into a solution state from the intact solid state.

The Noyes–Whitney equation explains the rate of dissolution of many drugs into the surrounding media and is expressed as follows:

$$\frac{dM}{dt} = \frac{D \circ S}{h} \circ (C_s - C)$$

where *M* is the mass of the drug, dissolved in time *t*; *dM*/*dt* is the mass rate of dissolution (mass/time); *D* is the diffusion coefficient of the drug in the solution; *S* is the surface area of the exposed solid; *h* is the thickness of the diffusion layer near the drug surface; C_s is the solubility of the drug; and *C* is the concentration of the drug in the bulk solution at time *t*.

Liquid Systems

Homogeneous systems

A molecular dispersion of a solute in a solvent that results in a homogeneous system is called a *solution*. In such a system, the solvent is the predominant entity. *Saturated solutions* are solutions that, at a given temperature and pressure, contain the maximum amount of solute that can be accommodated by the solvent. If the saturation or if the solubility limit is exceeded, a fraction of the solute can separate from the solution and exist in equilibrium with it.

Solutes can be (1) gases, liquids, or solids and (2) nonelectrolytes or electrolytes. Solutes that do not form ions on dissolution in water are known as *nonelectrolytes*. Some examples of this class of solutes are estradiol, glycerin, urea, and sucrose. The absence of ions in these aqueous solutions prevents the flow of electric current. When the solute forms ions in the solutions, they are called *electrolytes*. Examples of electrolytes include sodium chloride, hydrochloric acid, and atropine sulfate. Their aqueous solutions conduct electric current.

Electrolytes can be classified as strong or weak electrolytes. Strong electrolytes (e.g., sodium chloride, hydrochloric acid) are completely ionized in water at all concentrations, whereas weak electrolytes (e.g., aspirin, atropine) are partially ionized in water.

Heterogeneous systems

A *heterogeneous system* can be defined as a chemical system that contains various distinct and mechanically separable parts or phases (e.g., suspensions, emulsions).

Colloidal dispersions play a significant role in pharmaceutical products. Such dispersions consist of two distinct immiscible entities, the dispersed phase (internal phase) and the dispersion medium (external phase). The particles of the dispersed substance are only suspended in the mixture, unlike a solution, within which they are completely dissolved.

A *colloid* is a type of chemical mixture in which one substance is dispersed evenly throughout another. This state occurs because the particles in a colloid are larger than in a solution and small enough to be dispersed evenly and maintain a homogeneous appearance, but large enough to scatter light and not dissolve (size range 10–500 nm).

Coarse dispersed systems can be classified broadly into two pharmaceutically relevant systems: *suspensions* and *emulsions.*

Suspensions

A *suspension* is a two-phase coarse dispersion system that is composed of insoluble solid material dispersed in an oily or aqueous liquid medium. The particle size of the dispersed solid is usually greater than 0.5 mm.

Insoluble and distasteful drugs can be formulated into a suspension with pleasant taste. Pharmaceutical suspensions can be used for topical, oral, and parenteral routes. However, when suspensions are used parenterally, the particle size of the dispersion has to be considerably lower than that of oral or topical suspensions.

Emulsions

An *emulsion* is a thermodynamically unstable heterogeneous system that consists of at least one immiscible liquid that is intimately dispersed in another in the form of droplets. The droplet diameter is usually between 0.1 μm and 10 μm and is considered a coarse dispersion.

Emulsions are inherently unstable because the droplets of the dispersed liquid tend to coalesce to form large droplets until all of the dispersed droplets have coalesced. This unstable emulsion is stabilized by the addition of a third component to the system, an emulsifying agent. The emulsifying agent prevents coalescence and helps maintain the integrity of the individual droplets.

Emulsions can be of different types depending on the nature of the dispersion medium and the dispersed phase. When the oil phase is dispersed into a continuous aqueous phase, it is an *oil-in-water emulsion,* whereas if the water phase is dispersed in a continuous oil phase, it is a *water-in-oil emulsion.*

Drug stability in solutions and suspensions

A drug in solution or suspension can degrade to form a product or several products. The U.S. Food and Drug Administration restricts the degradation of any drug to no more than 10% of the initial amount over a period of time called shelf life. Shelf life is defined as the time lapsed to maintain 90% of the drug at a specific temperature or pH. Shelf-life calculation depends on the mechanism of the degradation.

Degradation mechanisms

Zero-order mechanism

A drug can degrade according to the following scheme: A→B

The rate of degradation of molecule A is $dA/dt = k$ where dA/dt is the rate of degradation of molecule A and k is degradation rate constant. Integration of a rate equation yields a straight-line equation:

$$A = A_0 - kt$$

where A is the amount of drug remaining at any time, A_0 is initial amount, and k is zero-order rate constant. For zero-order kinetics, a plot of concentration versus time will yield a straight line where the intercept is A_0 and the slope is $-k$. The shelf life for zero-order kinetics is $t_{90} = 0.1A_0/k$ where the unit for zero-order rate constant is concentration time^{-1}.

Suspensions follow zero-order kinetics.

Example: A drug suspension (150 mg/mL) degrades by zero-order kinetics with a reaction rate constant of 0.75 mg/mL*hour. What is the concentration of drug remaining after 1 week (7 days)? Calculate t_{90} (shelf life) for this drug.

$$A = A_0 - kt$$

Concentration of drug remaining after one week $A = 150 - (0.75 \times 168) = 150 - 126 = 24$ mg/mL

$$\text{Shelf life: } t_{90} = \frac{0.1A_0}{k} = \frac{0.1 \times 150}{0.75} = 20 \text{ hours}$$

First-order mechanism

A drug degrades according to the following scheme: $A \rightarrow B$

The rate of degradation of molecule A is $dA/dt - k[A]$ where dA/dt is the rate of degradation of molecule A, $[A]$ is the amount of molecule A remaining at any time, and k is first-order degradation rate constant. Integration of rate yields an exponential function:

$$A = A_0 e^{-kt}$$

where A is the amount of drug remaining at any time, A_0 is initial amount, and k is first-order rate constant. For first-order kinetics, a plot of concentration versus time will yield a curvature. Taking the natural logarithm of concentration versus time will yield a straight-line equation ($\ln A = \ln A_0 - kt$) where the intercept is A_0 and the slope is $-k$. The shelf life for first-order kinetics is $t_{90} = 0.693/k$ where the units for first-order rate constant is time^{-1}.

Example: A drug in solution at a concentration of 5mg/mL follows a first-order reaction with a rate constant of 0.0009 day^{-1}. How much drug will remain after 150 days?

$$\ln A = \ln A_0 - kt$$

Concentration of drug remaining after 150 days:

$$\ln A = \ln 5 - (0.0009 \times 150) = 1.609 - 0.135 = 1.474$$

$$A = 4.36 \text{ mg/mL}$$

9-6 Principles of Drug Delivery via Dosage Forms

Oral Administration

A drug that is absorbed from the stomach or intestine, or both, must first pass through the liver. If the drug is metabolized in the liver or excreted in the bile, some of the active drug will be inactivated before it can reach the general circulation to cause a therapeutic effect; that is, its oral bioavailability is decreased.

Other anatomical, physiological, and pathological factors (e.g., stomach acidity, peristalsis, distribution of drug in the body) can also influence bioavailability. The choice of the route of drug administration or drug product must be based on an understanding of these conditions.

Absorption, regardless of the site, depends on drug solubility. Drugs administered in aqueous (true) solution are more rapidly absorbed than those administered in oily solution, in suspension, or in solid form because they mix more readily with the aqueous phase at the absorptive site. Dissolution is slowed for drugs in solid form, and the rate of dissolution may be the rate-limiting factor in their absorption. Intra-articular injection of triamcinolone solution, for example, is effective for 1–2 days after injection, whereas injection of triamcinolone acetonide suspension is effective for 2 weeks.

Most orally administered products (i.e., tablets, capsules, clear liquids, suspensions) are swallowed too quickly to allow any drug absorption through the mucous membranes in the mouth. In contrast, products that are held under the tongue (sublingual) or between the cheek and gum (buccal) are retained longer at the absorption site and can be absorbed.

The rate and extent of drug absorption at the sublingual and buccal sites are also affected by physiologic factors. Thin mucous membranes in these regions present a low barrier to systemic entry of the drug. Furthermore, high vascularity at these sites quickly flushes away the absorbed drug, thereby maintaining a high-concentration gradient.

With regard to absorption through the stomach, for most drugs administered by the oral route, the drugs must cross the GI epithelium to enter the systemic circulation. Drug penetration across the epithelium occurs by the paracellular route or the transcellular route.

Only low-molecular-weight and highly hydrophilic compounds are absorbed by the paracellular route (i.e., between the epithelial cells, around the cells). The contribution of the paracellular route is relatively small because of the presence of tight junctions between the cells that limit absorption.

Absorption by the transcellular route (i.e., across the epithelial cells) can occur by passive diffusion, carrier-mediated transport, or pinocytosis. *Passive diffusion* is the most common mechanism of absorption. Most drug molecules are absorbed across the GI membrane by passive diffusion. Drugs diffuse across the membrane from a region of high concentration (i.e., gastric fluids) to a region of low concentration (i.e., blood circulation).

The rate of diffusion is proportional to the concentration gradient but also depends on lipid solubility, size, and ionization of the molecule. In some instances, facilitated diffusion occurs if the movement of the drug is in the direction of the concentration gradient (and therefore does not require energy and involves transport proteins).

As the term suggests, *carrier-mediated transport* requires the use of specialized carriers to transport drug molecules across the membrane. It is *active transport* if the movement is against the concentration gradient and requires energy.

Pinocytosis plays a very small role in drug transport. In pinocytosis, molecules or carrier packets are engulfed by a cell. The cell membrane invaginates and encloses the molecule. It then fuses again, forming a vesicle that detaches and moves to the cell interior, where it releases its contents. Liposomes are examples of drugs that enter cells by pinocytosis.

Oral Bioavailability

Oral bioavailability can be defined as the rate and extent of drug absorption from the GI tract. It depends to a great extent on the pH of the gastric contents and the pK_a of the drug. The pH and pK_a relationship regulates the degree of dissolution and ionization of a drug that is administered in solid form. This relationship also controls the extent to which a drug precipitates out of solution.

The pH of the stomach contents is strongly acidic and typically ranges between 1 and 3 for fasted and fed states, respectively. The pH of the small intestine is basic and typically ranges between 7 and 9.

Oral Delivery Systems

Conventional oral delivery products include tablets and capsules, as well as liquids such as clear solutions, suspensions, and emulsions.

A significant majority of products are formulated as tablets. Types of tablets include conventional quick release, effervescent, disintegrating, buccal, sublingual, controlled release, and sustained release. Some drug products are also available in the form of granules and sprinkles, generally for pediatric use.

Liquid drug products

Liquid formulations provide a high degree of flexibility when fine dosage adjustments are needed. In addition, they are convenient for pediatric and geriatric patients, who may have trouble swallowing solids.

Liquids can easily be colored and flavored to make them aesthetically appealing. However, masking the taste of the drug is more difficult. Liquid formulations are more cumbersome to store and transport and are more difficult to dose accurately. In addition, the shelf life of many drugs is shortened in an aqueous medium. The number of available liquid products has been steadily declining over the past few years because of the complexities of manufacturing and the difficulties in packaging, shipping, handling, and storage.

Conventional or immediate-release tablets

Tablets dominate the pharmaceutical market because of their wide acceptance by both patients and physicians, their ease of manufacturing, and the advances and developments in pharmaceutical science that have enabled the formulation of tablets with desired biopharmaceutical profiles.

Tablets come in many different sizes; shapes (round, oblong, triangular, cylindrical, square); and colors. The variety allows patients to distinguish one product from another more easily. Some products are scored, enabling patients to accurately break a tablet into uniform pieces.

Conventional tablets disintegrate in the stomach or intestine into smaller granules. The granules then undergo dissolution or further breakdown into smaller particles. These particles dissolve in the GI tract at a rate that is governed by factors such as the pH of the GI medium, the pK_a of the drug, and particle size. The dissolved drug molecules cross the GI membranes and enter the systemic circulation.

A tablet should be administered with a glass of water to facilitate its disintegration and dissolution. When patients have difficulty swallowing a whole tablet, a conventional tablet is sometimes crushed, broken, or ground to compound an alternative formulation, such as a capsule or a liquid suspension.

Enteric-coated products

Enteric-coated products are designed to minimize exposure of a drug to the acidic pH in the stomach, which could result in its degradation, or to decrease gastric side effects such as ulcers, perforations, and bleeding caused by the local effects of the drug on the gastric mucosa. Enteric-coated aspirin is an example of this type of product.

Sprinkles and granules

Solid formulations also come in the form of sprinkles, granules, and effervescent tablets. These formulations contain excipients similar to those used in tablets and capsules. They are classified differently, however, because of the method of administration.

Sprinkles and granules are aggregated powders. Sprinkles are generally used to administer solid drugs to babies and toddlers who cannot swallow a tablet or capsule. Montelukast (Singulair) is available as a tablet for adults and as sprinkles and chewable tablets for pediatric patients.

Granules also provide a convenient mode of administering drugs in large doses.

Effervescent tablets

Effervescent tablets must be dissolved in water before use. *Effervescence* is the reaction in water between an acid and a base that produces carbon dioxide. Citric acid is the most commonly used acid. Typical bases used are sodium bicarbonate and potassium bicarbonate.

Water-soluble binders are used in effervescent tablets, and the concentration should be just high enough so that the tablet is sufficiently hard to allow handling. Artificial sweeteners are generally used to improve the taste. These formulations are commonly used to administer medications to pediatric patients.

Orally disintegrating tablets

Orally disintegrating tablets (ODTs) allow the ease of swallowing that is afforded by a liquid formulation and provide the convenience of a tablet product. ODTs are not intended to be swallowed. The tablets disintegrate on the tongue instantly, usually within a few seconds, which results in rapid onset of action.

An ideal drug for an ODT formulation is a high-potency drug that is expected to have a quick onset of action. Examples include zolmitriptan (Zomig-ZMT) for migraine and ondansetron (Zofran) for nausea and vomiting. The patient should be advised not to swallow an ODT. Swallowing will likely delay the onset of action and defeat the purpose of taking an ODT. Breaking the ODT into powder or granules for compounding is acceptable because it will not affect the safety and efficacy of the product.

Thin films

Films or strips containing drugs and various biocompatible polymers that are suitable for oral administration have now been developed and marketed. These strips or thin films are small and instantaneously dissolve or "melt" on the tongue.

The thin strips are convenient to use and can be taken without water. They are easy to swallow, which is an advantage for pediatric or geriatric patients. In addition, they dissolve before a child is able to spit out the product.

Capsules

Hard gelatin capsules

In a capsule, one or more drugs and excipients are enclosed within a gelatin shell. The gelatin shell may be hard or soft. As with conventional tablets, most gelatin capsules are designed to be swallowed.

Gelatin capsule shells come in a variety of sizes and colors that improve the aesthetic appeal of the product and mask the unpleasant taste of the drug. Some patients find capsules easier to swallow because of their oblong shape. If the patient is unable to swallow a hard gelatin capsule, it can be opened, and the contents can be mixed with water, juice, pudding, or applesauce.

Capsules are not as dominant in the marketplace as are tablets because they are more complex to manufacture and must be stored in a humidity-controlled environment.

For safety and maintenance of the integrity of a capsule formulation, pharmaceutical companies often use special techniques to make a capsule product tamperproof. Most capsules can be cut with a sharp razor knife or a single-edge blade to empty the contents.

Soft gelatin capsules

The soft gelatin capsule delivery system was invented to allow administration of a small quantity of liquid as a solid formulation. Soft gelatin capsules are typically used for drugs that present solubility-related bioavailability problems if formulated as a tablet or a hard gelatin capsule. The drug is dissolved in an appropriate nonaqueous vehicle, and this solution is then encapsulated (e.g., vitamin E soft caps). Soft gelatin capsules can also be filled with suspensions, pastes, or powders.

Some soft gelatin capsules release the drug more quickly than do compressed tablets or hard gelatin capsules. They may attain a faster absorption because the drug is already in solution.

Controlled-release oral tablets

If an oral dosage form releases drug for 9–12 hours, it is considered to be a controlled-release or, more specifically, a sustained-release product. These products require fewer doses each day and usually produce better patient compliance with the dosing regimen and more constant blood level of the drug.

Advantages of the oral route

Oral ingestion is the most common method of drug administration used around the world for both ambulatory and institutional patients. It is also the safest, most convenient, and most economical route of administration. Oral products are particularly applicable to self-administration by the patient.

The onset of the drug effect can be from 10 to 60 minutes, and the duration of drug release can be from 30 minutes to 24 hours, depending on the dosage form (e.g., aspirin immediate-release tablet compared to controlled-release tablets or capsules).

Oral ingestion is the preferred route of administration of drugs that are not indicated for life-threatening emergency situations for reasons of convenience and dosing regimen compliance. Modified-release products that reduce dosing frequency and provide convenience can have a positive effect on patient adherence and outcomes. Self-administration and increased patient adherence reduce health care costs, a factor that is appealing to third-party payers because of its potential to reduce overall health care costs.

Disadvantages of the oral route

Emesis can result from irritation to the GI mucosa. Some drugs are destroyed by digestive enzymes or low gastric pH. Irregularities in absorption or gastric emptying can occur in the presence of food or other drugs.

Drugs in the GI tract may be metabolized by the enzymes of the mucosa, the intestinal flora, or the liver before they gain access to the general circulation, thereby decreasing the total amount of drug that reaches the site of action.

Onset of response for these drugs is slower (e.g., 15–90 minutes) than for drugs delivered intravenously, where the effect may be almost immediate.

Parenteral Administration

Parenteral (*para* = around; *enteral* = related to the GI tract) literally means around the GI tract. However, in common usage, the term is often considered synonymous with *injectable*. Injectable products are sterile products and may require special handling and administration.

Parenteral injections of drugs have certain distinct advantages over oral administration. In some instances, parenteral administration is essential for the drug to reach its site of action in active form. For example, almost all protein drugs are administered by injection rather than by the oral route because protein drugs are broken down by stomach acid and digestive enzymes.

Parenteral drug delivery is usually more rapid and more predictable than is administration by other routes. It is particularly advantageous in emergency therapy or if a patient is unconscious, uncooperative, or unable to retain anything given by mouth.

Asepsis must be maintained to avoid infection, particularly for an intravascular injection. Wiping the patient's skin with an antibacterial before injection is considered best practice.

Pain may accompany the injection, and if self-medication is a necessary procedure (e.g., insulin, human growth hormone), a patient may have difficulty performing the injection.

The major routes of parenteral administration are intravenous (IV), subcutaneous (under skin), and intramuscular (IM; into muscle). Many other less-used injectable routes are also available for specialized delivery.

- IV administration of true solution drug products delivers 100% of the drug into the systemic circulation.
- Absorption from subcutaneous and IM sites occurs by simple diffusion along the gradient from drug depot at the site of injection into the plasma. The rate is limited by the area of the absorbing capillary membranes and by the solubility of the substance in the interstitial fluid.
- Epidural administration is on or over the dura mater.
- Intra-articular administration is into a joint.
- Intra-arterial administration is into an artery or arteries.
- Intracardiac administration is into the heart.
- Intracavitary administration is into a pathologic cavity, such as occurs in the lung in tuberculosis.
- Intradermal administration is into the dermis, the dermal layer of the skin.
- Intralymphatic administration is into a lymph channel or node.
- Intramuscular administration is into a muscle, such as the muscle fibers of the upper arm or gluteal area.
- Intraosseous administration is directly into the marrow of a bone. The needle is injected right through the bone and into the soft marrow interior.

- Intraperitoneal administration is into the peritoneal cavity.
- Intraspinal administration is into the vertebral column. It refers to both the epidural and the intrathecal routes.
- Intrathecal administration is into the cerebrospinal fluid at any level of the cerebrospinal axis, including injection into the cerebral ventricles. Injection is into the subarachnoid spaces.
- Intracerebroventricular administration is into a ventricle of the brain.
- Intravitreal administration is into the vitreous body of the eye.

Intravenous route

The factors concerned in oral absorption are circumvented by intravenous injection of drugs in aqueous solution. The desired concentration of a drug in blood is obtained with an accuracy and immediacy not possible by any other procedure.

If the dose is administered over a few minutes, it is a *bolus dose* administered through an IV administration set directly into a vein. If administered over hours from a hanging bag, it is an *IV drip* or *infusion*. The effect of short-acting drugs can be maintained by administration as an IV drip (usually with an IV pump to control and help monitor the drip).

The IV route is not without adverse effects. IV injections are administered directly into the venous circulation, and highly vascular organs, such as the heart, lungs, liver, and kidney, are rapidly perfused with the drug. Adverse reactions may occur because high concentrations of drug may be attained rapidly in both plasma and tissues. Often such reactions can be prevented by giving a slow IV bolus injection or controlling an IV drip.

Other drugs with poor aqueous solubility may precipitate from solution and produce adverse reactions, including embolism.

Subcutaneous injections

Injection into a subcutaneous (under skin) site is often used for the administration or patient self-administration of drugs (e.g., some insulin products, human growth hormone). It can be used only for drugs that are not irritating to tissue; otherwise, severe pain, necrosis, and sloughing of tissue may occur.

The rate of absorption following subcutaneous injection of a drug is often sufficiently continuous and slow to provide a sustained input into the systemic circulation over a period of 4–12 hours. The incorporation of a vasoconstrictor agent in a solution of a drug to be injected subcutaneously also retards absorption and prolongs the local effect (e.g., lidocaine with epinephrine injection).

Intradermal injections

Intradermal (ID) injections are administered within the dermis layer of the skin (i.e., the upper layer of the skin just below the epidermis). ID injections are very small volume injections (0.1 mL) and are used to deliver drugs to produce local effects. ID injections may prolong the drug release—sometimes for days.

Examples of uses of ID delivery are injections for skin testing, antigen delivery to evaluate for allergic reactions, and sometimes administration of vaccines (e.g., influenza vaccine).

Intra-articular injections

Intra-articular injection is administration of a drug into a joint. Intra-articular administration of local anesthetics and adjuvants is an alternative method for postoperative analgesia. Patients who have undergone ligament reconstruction and experience moderate to severe postoperative pain can benefit from intra-articular injection of ropivacaine and morphine through a catheter in the knee joint. This approach decreases the need for supplemental IV morphine.

For the first few hours after intrasynovial or intra-articular injection, local discomfort in the joint may occur, but such discomfort is rapidly followed by effective relief of pain and improvement of local function.

Intraspinal injections

Intraspinal delivery is administration of drugs directly into the vertebral column. It includes epidural and intrathecal injections.

Epidural injection

Epidural injections are administered on or over the dura mater, and the drug is delivered to the outside of the dura and not into the cerebrospinal fluid. Thus, the clinical effects are more localized to the spinal cord.

Drugs can be delivered by a single bolus injection or as a continuous infusion. For example, morphine sulfate extended-release liposome injection is a special liposomal dosage formulation injected into the epidural space. This injection is a sterile, preservative-free suspension of multivesicular liposomes containing morphine sulfate present as a suspension in 0.9% sodium chloride solution. On epidural injection, the multivesicular liposomes release morphine systemically into the intrathecal space through the meninges at a slow rate over a prolonged period. When given as a single dose 30 minutes preoperatively, it has produced persistent analgesia for 48 hours postoperatively. The distribution, metabolism, and elimination pattern of liposomal morphine sulfate is similar to that after delivery of other parenteral morphine formulations.

Intrathecal and intracerebroventricular injections

Intrathecal injection is the administration of drugs within the cerebrospinal fluid at any level of the cerebrospinal axis, including injection into the cerebral ventricles.

When lipid-insoluble drugs are needed to treat neurologic disorders, bypassing the blood–brain barrier and delivering drugs directly into the brain are necessary. This bypass can be achieved by intrathecal administration, in which drugs are injected into the cerebrospinal fluid surrounding the spinal cord, or by direct injection of drugs into the brain by intracerebroventricular injection, which is an invasive approach.

Advanced primary or metastatic cancer pain, thoracic and lumbar pain, nerve root injuries, and neuropathic pain are treated with intrathecal injections and infusions of opioids, local anesthetics, clonidine, baclofen, and other drugs used for the treatment of chronic pain, cancer pain, and intractable spasticity.

Intramuscular injections

Drugs in aqueous solution are absorbed quite rapidly after IM injection, depending on the rate of blood flow to the injection site. The IM injection site is usually the deltoid muscle of the upper arm or the vastus lateralis muscle in the anterolateral aspect of the middle or upper thigh (1 or 2 mL). Gluteus muscles are used for a hip injection (usually up to 5 mL).

Very slow, sustained release with constant absorption from the IM site results if the drug is injected in a solution in oil or is suspended in various other repository vehicles rather than as a true aqueous solution. Penicillin suspensions, such as procaine or benzathine penicillin G, are sometimes administered in this manner. Procaine penicillin G blood levels last for several days, whereas benzathine penicillin G may last for a week.

Depot injections release the drug slowly and maintain serum drug concentrations for a longer duration (hours to days). *Depot injections* are long-acting dosage formulations indicated for maintenance treatment rather than for initiation of therapy. Depot formulations are available as oil-based injections (e.g., fluphenazine enanthate, estradiol cypionate); aqueous suspensions (e.g., procaine penicillin G, benzathine penicillin G, methylprednisolone acetate [Depo-Medrol]); and microspheres (e.g., leuprolide acetate [Lupron Depot]).

Rectal Administration

The oral route is the preferred route for the administration of most drugs. Sometimes this route is not practical or feasible, particularly if the patient has nausea, vomiting, or seizures; if the patient is uncooperative; or if oral intake is restricted.

The rectal route can be used to deliver some drugs systemically (e.g., antiemetics). Treatment of certain rectal conditions (itching, swelling, or pain from hemorrhoids or local infections) may also be best achieved by localized drug administration at or near the affected area.

Suppositories

A suppository is a solid delivery system in which the drug is incorporated into a base with or without additional excipients. The base either melts at body temperature (cocoa butter or fat base) or dissolves in the mucous secretions (polyethylene glycol [PEG]), thereby releasing the drug. In many marketed products, surfactants and emulsifiers such as polysorbate 80 and glyceryl monostearate are also used to aid in the dispersion of the drug on release.

Suppositories come in many shapes and sizes, which helps facilitate their insertion and retention in the rectal cavity. Suppositories are generally cylindrical, and one or both of the ends may be tapered. Adult suppositories weigh roughly 2 grams, whereas suppositories for children are about half that weight.

Suppositories are particularly useful for delivering laxatives directly to the site of action to facilitate emptying of the lower bowel, for providing local anti-inflammatory and anesthetic effects, and for delivering a drug to the rectum to produce a systemic effect (e.g., promethazine antiemetic).

The release of the drug and onset of drug action depend on the liquefaction of the suppository base, the dissolution of the active drug in the fluids, and the diffusion of the drug through the mucosal layers. A lipophilic drug is released slowly, whereas a hydrophilic or water-soluble drug is released rapidly from an oleaginous or fatty base. Opposite polarity makes for faster release. Like polarity between the drug and the suppository base makes for slower release. A lipophilic drug shows a moderate rate of release from a water-soluble base. The release rate depends on the aqueous solubility of the drug.

Rectal gels

For treatment of status epilepticus, the rectal route is convenient for the administration of benzodiazepines, because IV access may be difficult to establish.

Diazepam rectal gel is an aqueous solution of diazepam containing the cosolvents propylene glycol and ethyl alcohol. It is marketed in premeasured doses, which increases both the convenience and the accuracy of dosing.

Enemas

Rectal enemas are either aqueous solutions or suspensions of a drug with or without cosolvents such as propylene glycol or ethyl alcohol. The solution or suspension is often buffered using phosphate buffers to adjust the pH and also may contain preservatives and antioxidants.

Viscosity is adjusted using polymers such as cellulose derivatives, carbomers, or gums such as xanthan gum.

Rectal foams

Rectal foams contain inert, pressurized gas propellants such as isobutane and propane.

Foams are better retained than enemas, probably because foams are more viscous than enemas and some foams are sticky. A more uniform coating and better patient acceptance can be achieved with a foam than with an enema.

The drug in a rectal enema or foam can spread over a wider area than a drug in a suppository.

Rectal ointments and creams

Ointments and creams are also used for topical application of drugs to the perianal area as well as for administration of drugs into the rectum, generally with the use of an applicator. Because the contact time between the drug and the mucous membranes is relatively short, no significant systemic absorption occurs.

These formulations are used mainly to deliver steroids, anti-inflammatory agents, and local anesthetics for the treatment of local conditions (e.g., hemorrhoids or anal itching or swelling).

Advantages and disadvantages of rectal administration

As an alternative to the IV route, rectal administration has the advantages of being relatively painless and convenient to use, especially in the pediatric population.

A high concentration of the drug can be achieved in the rectum; hence, this route is useful if local action is desired. For example, for proctitis caused by ulcerative colitis, rectal enemas and suppositories of corticosteroids are standard localized treatment.

Some drugs administered low in the rectum are absorbed into the systemic circulation by the inferior and middle rectal veins without passing through the liver. This form of administration is advantageous for drugs that are subject to first-pass hepatic metabolism. For example, rectal administration of the analgesic methadone results in rapid absorption, long duration of action, and high bioavailability.

Intersubject and intrasubject variability in absorption after rectal administration is probably the most important concern for the health care provider. The absorption of a drug may be delayed or prolonged, or uptake may be almost as rapid as with an IV bolus dose. Diarrhea and disease also affect absorption.

Patient compliance can be a problem because of a reluctance to use rectal formulations.

Certain formulations (PEG-base suppositories) and drugs can cause mucosal irritation in sensitive tissues.

Pulmonary Drug Delivery

The pulmonary route has been used for many years for the delivery of drugs and treatment of diseases. It has been primarily used, however, for drug delivery to the airways and the lungs for local action.

The pulmonary route is widely accepted as the optimal route of administration for first-line drugs to manage asthma and chronic obstructive pulmonary disease and for drugs to treat pulmonary diseases such as chronic bronchitis, respiratory infections, and cystic fibrosis. In such diseases, direct delivery of medication to the lungs and airways represents targeted drug delivery to the site of action. It leads to faster pharmacologic effects and reduced side effects.

The lung has also been studied as a possible route of noninvasive drug administration for the treatment of systemic diseases such as diabetes mellitus (e.g., inhaled insulin). Behind the recent strong interest in the pulmonary delivery of drugs is the development of new inhalation devices that make possible the delivery of larger drug doses to the airways (milligram dosing compared with microgram dosing) and that achieve greater deposition efficiency than did older devices.

Topical Administration

Topical skin administration

Few drugs readily penetrate the intact skin. Absorption of those that do is proportional to the surface area over which they are applied and to their lipid solubility because the epidermis behaves as a lipid barrier.

However, the dermis is freely permeable to many solutes; consequently, systemic absorption of drugs occurs much more readily through abraded, burned, or denuded skin. Inflammation and other conditions that increase cutaneous blood flow also enhance absorption. Toxic effects are sometimes produced by absorption through the skin of highly lipid-soluble substances (e.g., a lipid-soluble insecticide in an organic solvent).

Absorption through the skin can be enhanced by suspending the drug in an oily vehicle and rubbing the resulting preparation into the skin. This method of administration is known as *inunction*.

Because hydrated skin is more permeable than dry skin, the dosage form may be modified or an occlusive dressing may be used to facilitate absorption.

Topical patches

Controlled-release topical patches are recent innovations. For example, a patch containing scopolamine placed behind the ear, where body temperature and blood flow enhance absorption, releases sufficient drug to the systemic circulation to protect the wearer from motion sickness (Transderm SCOP, scopolamine patch).

Patches containing nitroglycerin are used to provide sustained delivery of a drug that is subject to extensive first-pass metabolism after oral administration (Nitro-Dur, Transderm-Nitro). Other examples of transdermal products include the menopausal hormone therapy patch (CombiPatch), which has estrogen and progestin, and the nicotine patch (NicoDerm) to help people quit smoking.

Topical eye administration

Topically applied ophthalmic drugs are used primarily for their local effects.

Systemic absorption that results from drainage through the nasolacrimal canal is usually undesirable. In addition, a drug that is absorbed after such drainage is not subject to first-pass hepatic elimination. Systemic toxicity may occur for this reason when α-adrenergic antagonists are administered as ophthalmic drops.

Local effects usually require absorption of the drug through the cornea. Corneal infection or trauma may thus result in more rapid absorption.

Ophthalmic delivery systems that provide prolonged duration of action (e.g., suspensions, ointments) are useful additions to ophthalmic therapy.

9-7 Principles of Dosage Form Stability and Drug Degradation in Dosage Forms

Dosage form quality is directly linked to product efficacy. Poor-quality drug products are less likely to be effective or safe.

Drug product stability depends on the concentration, time, temperature, pH, and physical or chemical reactivity.

Extensive chemical degradation of the active ingredient can cause substantial loss of active ingredient from the dosage form. Chemical degradation can produce a toxic product that has undesirable side effects. Instability of the drug product can cause decreased bioavailability. As a result, the therapeutic efficacy of the dosage form may be substantially reduced.

According to the law of mass action, the rate of a chemical reaction is proportional to the molar concentration of the reactants each raised to a power equal to the number of molecules of each individual reactant.

The order of a reaction is the way in which the concentration of the drug or reactant in a chemical reaction affects the rate. The rate of a reaction, dC/dt, is proportional to the concentration to the nth power, where n is the order of the reaction.

The rate at which the drug substance or drug product is degraded in the dosage form may follow several kinetic patterns. First-order degradation patterns are the most common, and the rate depends on the concentration of the one drug in solution. A zero-order degradation pattern is the second most common pattern. Here the degradation rate is constant and independent of the drug concentration. Second-order degradation patterns are still less common and depend on the concentration of two chemical species. In reality, when extended-time drug degradation patterns are analyzed, they often contain one mechanism initially and a second or third mechanism as time progresses.

Stability is an essential quality attribute for dosage forms because drug stability information is used to make regulatory decisions on the shelf life of a product. Degraded dosage forms are unacceptable for patient use because they are often less than optimally effective or may even be toxic or antigenic. Therefore, ensuring that a drug product will work effectively means that a time period when the dosage form is likely to work best (shelf life) should be determined, and the information should be made available to the patient and health care professionals.

Everything is subject to decay, and pharmaceuticals are no exception. The rate varies dramatically. For manufactured drug products, the expiration date is determined experimentally when the 95% one-sided lower confidence limit crosses 90% of the labeled amount of active ingredient under specified storage conditions of temperature and relative humidity according to U.S. Food and Drug Administration guidelines. Some radiopharmaceuticals significantly decay within 1 day. Other products may be good for 3 years (e.g., saline solutions, some tablets, and lyophilized products). A 2- to 3-year shelf life for a manufactured drug product is common.

For nonsterile compounded drug products, Chapter <795> of the United States Pharmacopeia (USP) gives guidance for beyond-use dating. When a manufactured drug product is the source of the active ingredient, the beyond-use date is not later than 25% of the time remaining until the product's expiration date or 6 months, whichever is earlier. For formulations containing water, the beyond-use date is not later than 14 days for liquid preparations when stored at cold temperatures between 2°C and 8°C (approximately refrigerator temperature). Chapter <797> of the USP should be consulted for beyond-use dating for compounded sterile products.

In contrast, compounded prescriptions may be acceptable for patient use only for several hours to several months, depending on the physical attributes of the dosage form. For example, a reconstituted antibiotic liquid product may be good for only 2 weeks under storage at refrigerator temperatures, whereas a compounded dermal prescription may be good for only 1 month or less because of the lack of an antimicrobial preservative.

9-8 Materials and Methods Used in Preparation and Use of Drug Forms

When a pharmaceutical product is made, the active ingredients or the drugs are incorporated into acceptable pharmaceutical additives or excipients. The drug with the excipients constitutes a drug delivery system (e.g., tablets, capsules, parenteral solutions, emulsions, suspensions).

In addition to containing the drug, drug delivery systems such as tablets contain excipients that aid processing and manufacture of the drug and effective drug delivery to the patient. Table 9-2 shows some commonly used excipients in tablets.

TABLE 9-2. Commonly Used Excipients in Tablets

Ingredient type	Function	Examples
Diluents	Provide bulk in tablet and accurate dosing of drug	Lactose monohydrate, microcrystalline cellulose (MCC), dextrose, sucrose, dicalcium phosphate, starch
Binders	Bind powders together to aid granulation and compression	Starch, gelatin, polyvinylpyrrolidone (PVP), alginic acid and its derivatives, cellulose derivatives, glucose, sucrose
Lubricants	Prevent adherence of granules and powders to tablet punches and dies; aid smooth ejection of tablets from die cavity	Magnesium stearate, talc, stearic acid, polyethylene glycols (PEGs), sodium or magnesium lauryl sulfate
Disintegrates	Promote disintegration of tablet after administration	MCC, starch, PVP cellulose, modified starches, carboxymethylcellulose, magnesium aluminum silicate
Glidants	Improve flow properties of powders and granules	Colloidal silica (Cab-O-Sil), talc
Polymers	Modulate drug dissolution from tablet	PVP, ethylcellulose, PEG, carboxymethylcellulose, polylactides, polyglycolides
Colors and pigments	Differentiate tablets	FDC Red 40, canthaxanthin, iron oxide, beta carotene

TABLE 9-3. Commonly Used Excipients in Capsules

Ingredient type	Function	Examples
Diluents	Provide bulk in capsule and accurate dosing of drug	Lactose, mannitol, calcium carbonate, magnesium carbonate
Glidants	Improve flow properties during filling of capsules	Silica, starch, talc
Lubricants	Aid ejection of capsule plugs	Magnesium stearate
Surfactants	Wet powder after administration to aid drug dissolution	Sodium lauryl sulfate, sodium docusate
Plasticizers	Aid formation of the soft gelatin capsule	Glycerol, sorbitol, polypropylene glycol
Preservatives	Prevent microbial growth in capsules and prevent degradation of drug	Methylparaben, propylparaben, potassium sorbate, propyl hydroxybenzoate

Capsules can be of two types: hard gelatin and soft gelatin. The hard gelatin capsules have two pieces: a cap and a bottom plug. The drug with the excipients is filled into the two parts. Soft gelatin capsules are manufactured from plasticized gelatin using a rotary die process. They are formed, filled, and sealed in a single step of the manufacturing process. Table 9-3 describes some commonly used excipients in capsules.

Emulsions and suspensions are coarse dispersions and are inherently unstable systems. A number of additives are used to stabilize these systems. Emulsions are made of an oil phase, a water phase, and an emulsifying agent or emulsifier. Suspensions are solid particles of the drug suspended in a liquid medium, and they contain a drug, a liquid medium, and a suspending agent.

True solutions contain miscible solvent that can dissolve the drug in an aqueous or nonaqueous medium. Surfactants are often used to form micellar or colloidal dispersions.

Some of the commonly used excipients in liquid dosage forms are shown in Table 9-4.

TABLE 9-4. Commonly Used Excipients in Liquid Dosage Forms

Ingredient type	Function	Examples
Antimicrobial preservatives	Prevent microbial contamination	Methylparaben, propylparaben, benzalkonium chloride, benzyl alcohol
Antioxidants	Prevent oxidization of active drug	Sodium metabisulfite, butylated hydroxytoluene, butylated hydroxyanisole
Surfactants	Form colloidal (micellar) dispersions	Polysorbate 80, Span 20, poloxamers
Emulsifiers	Stabilize coarse emulsions	Polysorbate 80, Span 20, poloxamers, stearyl alcohol
Suspending agents	Act as thickening agent and stabilize suspension	Carbomer, carrageenan, cellulose, hydroxyethyl cellulose
Chelating agents	Impart stability to formulation	Disodium ethylenediaminetetraacetic acid
Solvents	Aid solubilization of drugs	Ethanol, propylene glycol, t-butyl alcohol, tetraglycol

9-9 Questions

1. A change of state from a liquid to a gas for a compound involves
   - **A.** change in molecular formula of the compound.
   - **B.** overcoming of intermolecular forces of attraction.
   - **C.** a decrease in melting point.
   - **D.** no significant physicochemical effects.

2. Which of the following statements describes the main difference between a solid and a liquid form of a chemical?
   - **A.** Intramolecular forces are virtually nonexistent in solids.
   - **B.** Solids exhibit surface tension, whereas liquids do not.
   - **C.** Solids show very high intermolecular interactions and have more geometric order than liquids.
   - **D.** Intermolecular forces are nonexistent in liquids.

3. Liquids containing dilute dispersions and simple molecules tend to behave in a
   - **A.** Newtonian manner.
   - **B.** non-Newtonian manner.
   - **C.** thixotropic manner.
   - **D.** antithixotropic manner.

4. The rate of *dissolution* of drugs into the surrounding media is expressed by the
   - **A.** Noyes–Whitney equation.
   - **B.** Michaelis–Menten equation.
   - **C.** Stokes equation.
   - **D.** Henderson–Hasselbalch equation.

5. Aspirin (pK_a 3.49) will be most soluble in water at which pH?
   - **A.** 1
   - **B.** 2
   - **C.** 3
   - **D.** 6

6. The droplet diameter of a stable emulsion is usually between which of the following?
   - **A.** 0.1–10 μm
   - **B.** 100–10,000 μm
   - **C.** 0.001–0.01 μm
   - **D.** 0.2 μm–4 μm

7. Which of the following drug species is more likely to cross from the lumen of the gastrointestinal tract into the bloodstream more rapidly?
   - **A.** The salt form of a weak acid drug
   - **B.** The salt form of a weak base drug
   - **C.** The nonionized form of the weak acid drug
   - **D.** A nonelectrolyte drug with a polarity similar to water

8. Most drug species cross biological barriers in the body by which mechanism?
   - **A.** Pinocytosis
   - **B.** Active transport into cells
   - **C.** Facilitated diffusion
   - **D.** Passive diffusion

9. The factor that least affects passage of molecules by passive diffusion is
   - **A.** the concentration gradient between both sides of the semipermeable membrane of the tissue.
   - **B.** the pH difference on each side of the membrane.
   - **C.** the pK_a of the drug molecule.
   - **D.** the body temperature.

10. In general, drugs are best absorbed from the lumen of the gastrointestinal tract into the bloodstream if the dosage form is a
    - **A.** tablet.
    - **B.** capsule.
    - **C.** true solution syrup.
    - **D.** suppository.

11. Noah is a 1-year-old boy in good health except for a bacterial infection and needs an antibiotic. Which of the following is your choice for an antibiotic drug product?
    - **A.** A chewable tablet
    - **B.** A dissolving thin film strip
    - **C.** A liquid suspension
    - **D.** A sprinkle of drug mixed with food

12. The shelf life of a drug product is

A. the expiration date.
B. when 90% of the labeled amount of the active ingredient is still left in the drug product.
C. the time from when the product was manufactured or compounded until the labeled expiration date.
D. the time that the drug degradation ruins the product.

13. Penny, a 45-year-old female, appears in the emergency department of the local hospital experiencing a panic attack after a car wreck in which the other driver experienced some trauma. Your choice for therapy is

A. an intravenous bolus dose of an antianxiety drug.
B. an intravenous infusion of an antianxiety drug.
C. an intramuscular injection of an antianxiety drug.
D. a subcutaneous dose of an antianxiety drug.

14. Elaine is a 23-year-old female who was in a head-on motor vehicle accident and experienced trauma to the head, chest, and abdomen. She was not wearing her seatbelt. She must be administered antibiotics for the infections that will result from the trauma. Her initial antibiotics should be administered as

A. an oral suspension.
B. an intravenous drip.
C. an intramuscular injection.
D. a subcutaneous injection.

15. John is a 53-year-old male with diabetes who is not responding to standard oral antidiabetic medications and must use insulin to control his blood glucose levels. He is expected to self-administer his medications. Which route of administration would you choose for his insulin administration?

A. Intravenous
B. Intramuscular
C. Subcutaneous
D. Oral

16. The intradermal route of administration is best used for

A. antibiotics.
B. antidepressants.
C. allergen testing.
D. nausea and vomiting.

17. The first-pass effect by the liver is most often experienced after

A. oral drug administration.
B. pulmonary drug administration.
C. rectal drug absorption.
D. transdermal drug absorption.

18. Polymorphism is the condition wherein

A. similar substances have the same molecular weight.
B. substances can exist in more than one crystalline form.
C. solids have the same crystal lattice structure.
D. similar solids have similar solubility profiles.

9-10 Answers

1. B. A liquid exhibits short-range order because of the presence of weak forces of attraction, whereas gases show no order. Thus, to convert a liquid to a gas, the weak attractive forces have to be overcome.

2. C. Solids show very high intermolecular interactions and have more geometric order than liquids. Solids do not exhibit surface tension, whereas liquids do so.

3. A. Liquids containing dilute dispersions and simple molecules tend to behave in a Newtonian manner. In contrast, non-Newtonian liquids exhibit shear-dependent or time-dependent viscosities. Thixotropic liquids are thick under normal conditions but become thinner when shaken. In contrast, antithixotropic liquids become thicker when agitated.

4. A. The Noyes–Whitney equation explains the rate of dissolution of drugs into the surrounding media.

5. D. Aspirin is a weakly acidic drug with a pK_a of 3.49 and will exist in its ionized form at relatively basic pH (6).

6. **A.** An *emulsion* is a thermodynamically unstable heterogeneous system that consists of at least one immiscible liquid that is intimately dispersed in another in the form of droplets. The droplet diameter is usually between 0.1 μm and 10 μm and is considered a coarse dispersion.

7. **C.** Charged species of drug molecules do not readily pass through the gastrointestinal barriers. Salts of weak acids or bases may ionize and exist as charged species and retard absorption. Only non-ionized species can pass readily through the barrier.

8. **D.** Most drug species cross biological barriers in the body by the passive diffusion mechanism, a non-energy-dependent process.

9. **D.** Transport of molecules by the passive diffusion process is extensively dependent on the surface area of the absorbing membrane, the pH difference on each side of the membrane, and the pK_a of the drug molecule. Body temperature has little effect on transport of molecules.

10. **C.** Both tablets and capsules undergo disintegration followed by dissolution and then diffusion. However, a true solution does not have to undergo disintegration and dissolution and, hence, is readily absorbed.

11. **D.** A sprinkle of drug mixed with food would be the best choice because it would be easy to administer and more palatable.

12. **C.** The shelf life of a drug product is the time from when the product was manufactured or compounded until the labeled expiration date.

13. **C.** An intramuscular injection of an antianxiety drug is the best choice because it gives rather quick relief but also has some action for several hours.

14. **B.** An intravenous drip will obtain high concentration of the antibiotic quickly and provide the ability to control the dose.

15. **C.** The subcutaneous route is best because the oral route has already failed. Intravenous and intramuscular routes are probably impractical for self-administration.

16. **C.** The intradermal route is the best route for allergen testing because using this route leads to the least exposure of the allergen to the systemic circulation and the effect is localized only to the site of the injection.

17. **A.** The first-pass effect is often experienced after oral drug administration because high concentrations of the drug go directly to the liver once they are absorbed.

18. **B.** Polymorphism is the condition wherein substances can exist in more than one crystalline form. Different polymorphic forms will show different solubilities and crystal lattice structure but have the same molecular weight.

9-11 Additional Resources

Allen LV, Jr, ed. *Remington: The Science and Practice of Pharmacy.* 22nd ed. London, U.K.: Pharmaceutical Press; 2012.

Sinko PJ. *Martin's Physical Pharmacy and Pharmaceutical Sciences.* 5th ed. Baltimore, MD: Lippincott Williams & Wilkins; 2010.

United States Pharmacopeial Convention. Chapter <795>: Pharmaceutical compounding—nonsterile preparations. In: *United States Pharmacopeia 41/National Formulary 36.* Rockville, MD: United States Pharmacopeial Convention; 2017.

United States Pharmacopeial Convention. Chapter <797>: Pharmaceutical compounding—sterile preparations. In: *United States Pharmacopeia 41/National Formulary 36.* Rockville, MD: United States Pharmacopeial Convention; 2017.

U.S. Department of Health and Human Services, Food and Drug Administration, Center for Drug Evaluation and Research, Center for Biologics Evaluation and Research. Guidance for industry: Q1A(R2) stability testing of new drug substances and products. Rockville, MD; U.S. Department of Health and Human Services; 2003.

Clinical Pharmacokinetics

10

S. CASEY LAIZURE

10-1 KEY POINTS

- Steady-state drug concentration is determined by the clearance of the drug.
- Changes in the volume of distribution do not change the steady-state concentration.
- For a drug eliminated by first-order elimination, the ratio of the dose to the steady-state drug concentration remains constant.
- Renal function can be quantitatively estimated from the serum creatinine and used to adjust the dose of renally eliminated drugs.
- Liver function tests measure liver damage, not function, and do not provide a quantitative estimate of liver drug metabolism.
- For high-extraction hepatically eliminated drugs, there will be a large difference between the oral and intravenous dose because of the high first-pass metabolism when the drug is given orally.
- Absolute bioavailability is the difference in the area under the curve (AUC) after oral dosing compared to the AUC after intravenous dosing.
- The most commonly encountered pharmacokinetic drug interactions are the result of changes in renal or hepatic drug elimination, causing a change in the drug's clearance.

10-2 STUDY GUIDE CHECKLIST

The following topics may guide your study of this subject area:

- ☐ Understanding of the basic pharmacokinetic parameters including clearance, volume of distribution, and half-life
- ☐ Estimation of the half-life from two plasma concentrations and determination of the time needed for the concentration to decrease based on *k*
- ☐ Difference between first-order elimination and nonlinear elimination
- ☐ The effect of controlled release ($ka << k$) on drug disposition
- ☐ Renal drug elimination and the estimation of renal function using the Cockcroft–Gault and MDRD (Modification of Diet in Renal Disease) Study equations
- ☐ Estimation of bioavailability
- ☐ Hepatic drug elimination and the venous equilibrium model
- ☐ Drug interactions resulting from hepatic enzyme inhibition and hepatic enzyme induction

10-3 Introduction

Pharmacokinetics is the mathematical modeling of drug concentration versus time used to understand drug disposition and to predict the relationship between drug dose and exposure. Understanding the numerous equations derived from models is an important part of clinical pharmacokinetics. However, performing specific calculations based on pharmacokinetic equations is limited because of the inadequate number of drug concentrations available from patients in clinical practice.

This chapter focuses on how one can apply pharmacokinetics in the clinical setting to achieve therapeutic drug concentrations, interpret drug concentrations in patients, adjust doses, and assess drug interactions. The reader is expected to have an understanding of basic pharmacokinetic equations.

10-4 Basic Pharmacokinetic Parameters

Volume of Distribution

The volume of distribution (V) is the theoretical volume based on the measured drug concentration in the plasma that would occur if the drug were allowed to completely distribute throughout the body without any drug elimination. Knowing the value of V, one can estimate the total amount of drug in the body from the measured drug plasma concentration. For example, if a 75-kg patient is taking digoxin and has a V of 7 L/kg and a digoxin plasma concentration of 0.5 ng/mL, then one can estimate the total amount of digoxin in the body by

$$Amt = Cp \times V$$

where Amt is the amount of drug in the body, Cp is the measured drug plasma concentration, and V is the volume of distribution. For this patient, the Amt is

$$Amt = 0.5\,\text{mcg/L} \times (7.0\,\text{L/kg} \times 75\,\text{kg}) = 262.5\,\text{mcg}$$

Note the plasma concentration is changed from ng/mL to mcg/L so that the units will properly cancel out, giving the final answer in mcg. When performing pharmacokinetic calculations, always include units, which provides a check that the equation is correct and prevents incorrect answers from a mismatch in the units.

Clinically, V is used to determine the amount of drug to administer to a patient to rapidly achieve a specific plasma concentration. In this case, Amt becomes what is most commonly referred to as the loading dose (LD) and can be estimated using the following equation:

$$LD = \frac{(C_T - C_{Obs}) \times V}{F \times S}$$

where LD is a single dose to achieve the desired plasma concentration, C_T is the target plasma concentration one wants to achieve, C_{Obs} is the concentration of drug in the plasma before the loading dose (this will usually be zero), V is the volume of distribution, F is the bioavailability, and S is the fraction of active drug in the salt form (this is usually 1). For most drugs, the loading dose is based on the patient's body weight in mg per kg, which is derived from the V for the specific drug. Thus, this equation is not commonly applied directly in clinical practice, although there are notable exceptions, such as the dosing of theophylline in neonates for prevention of apnea. For example, if one is trying to achieve a theophylline plasma concentration of 8 mcg/mL in an 18-day-old neonate who weighs 3.9 kg, standard mg/kg dose estimates cannot be used. Instead, the loading dose equation must be used to estimate the proper loading dose because the *V* differs between adults and neonates:

$$LD = \frac{8\ \text{mg/L} \times (0.68\ \text{L/kg} \times 3.9\ \text{kg})}{(1 \times 0.8)} = 26.5\ \text{mg}$$

where *LD* is the loading dose to achieve a plasma concentration of 8 mcg/mL; 0.68 L/kg is the *V*; 3.9 kg is the neonate's body weight; *F* is 1 (the dose is given intravenously); and *S* is 0.8 because the drug is given as aminophylline, which is 80% theophylline.

The volume of distribution for drugs ranges from great to very small (e.g., amiodarone with an extremely large *V* of about 66 L/kg and warfarin with a *V* of about 0.14 L/kg). Drugs with a small volume tend to be more hydrophilic, which limits their ability to cross lipophilic cell membranes, while drugs with a large volume tend to be lipophilic compounds that can easily cross cell membranes and distribute to body tissues outside the plasma. Drugs with a *V* less than 0.5 L/kg have very limited distribution outside the plasma (e.g., warfarin and gentamicin), drugs with a *V* around 0.8 to 1 L/kg usually distribute into total body water (vancomycin and theophylline), and drugs with a large *V* widely distribute into other body tissues such as fat (tetrahydrocannabinol) or muscle (digoxin). However, one cannot determine from the *V* alone where a drug distributes—a large *V* by itself indicates only that the drug distributes outside the plasma compartment, but not into which tissue.

Clearance

The vast majority of drugs are eliminated by first-order elimination, which means a constant percentage of drug is eliminated per unit time. The actual elimination rate, the amount per unit of time such as mg/h, changes with changes in a drug's plasma concentration. Where *V* is the parameter that relates the plasma concentration to the total amount of drug in the body, clearance (*Cl*)is the parameter that relates the actual drug elimination rate (velocity) to the plasma concentration. For example, if the plasma concentration of a drug is 2 mcg/mL and the *Cl* is 1 L/minute, then one can determine the velocity (*v*) of drug elimination using the following equation:

$$v = Cp \times Cl$$

where *v* is the velocity of drug elimination, *Cp* is the plasma concentration, and *Cl* is the clearance. Thus, when the plasma concentration is 2 mcg/mL, the rate of drug elimination is calculated as follows:

$$v = 2\ \text{mg/L} \times 1\ \text{L/minute} = 2\ \text{mg/minute}$$

The *Cl* of a drug determines the steady-state plasma concentration that will be achieved in a patient chronically administered a consistent dose of the drug. For example, one can predict the steady-state concentration of lidocaine that will be achieved if one administers a constant intravenous infusion of that drug at 4 mg/minute in a patient with a lidocaine clearance of 1 L/minute using the following equation:

$$C_{ss} = \frac{X_O}{Cl}$$

where C_{ss} is the steady-state plasma concentration that will occur, X_O is the drug dose administered as a constant intravenous infusion, and *Cl* is the clearance. Thus, for this patient

$$C_{ss} = \frac{4\ \text{mg/L}}{1\ \text{L/minute}} = 4\ \text{mcg/mL}$$

and the steady-state plasma concentration achieved when a constant intravenous infusion is given at a rate of 4 mg/minute will be 4 mcg/mL. Steady state occurs when the amount of drug going into the body (X_O) is equivalent to the amount being eliminated from the body (v). In this lidocaine example, X_O is 4 mg/minute, and the v of drug elimination when the concentration reaches 4 mcg/mL is 4 mg/minute. Thus, clearance indicates at what plasma concentration the elimination rate will become equivalent to the dosing rate and steady state achieved. However, in clinical practice, this C_{ss} equation is not useful because the patient's actual drug clearance is not known. Also, the vast majority of drugs are given by chronic oral dosing, not by constant intravenous infusion, and when a plasma concentration is measured, it is most commonly a trough concentration. Furthermore, with oral dosing, one must account for bioavailability (F). Thus, this equation is not used in clinical practice. However, the equation can be rearranged as follows:

$$Cl = \frac{X_O}{C_{ss}}$$

This arrangement provides a clinically useful relationship between the dose and the steady-state plasma concentration. As long as the Cl does not change, the ratio of X_O to C_{ss} cannot change, which leads to the following equation commonly used to adjust dosing based on a measured steady-state drug plasma concentration:

$$\frac{X_{obs}}{C_{ss,obs}} = \frac{X_O}{C_{ss,t}}$$

where X_{obs} is the present dose the patient is receiving that resulted in the steady-state plasma concentration of $C_{ss,obs}$, and X_O is the new dose to achieve the new targeted steady-state plasma concentration $C_{ss,t}$. This relationship remains valid as long as the Cl has not changed in the patient and one assumes that the bioavailability has not changed. Thus, if a patient takes 300 mg of lithium three times per day and has a steady-state trough concentration of 0.55 mEq/L, then the dose required to achieve a lithium steady-state trough concentration of 0.8 mEq/L can be estimated as

$$\frac{900 \text{ mg}}{0.55 \text{ mEq/L}} = \frac{X_O}{0.8 \text{ mEq/L}}$$

$$X_O = \frac{900 \text{ mg} \times 0.8 \text{ mEq/L}}{0.55 \text{ mEq/L}} = 1{,}309 \text{ mg}$$

which, divided into three doses, results in 436 mg and leads to a recommendation of 450 mg of lithium three times per day to achieve a steady-state plasma trough concentration of 0.8 mEq/L.

The vast majority of drugs obey this first-order pharmacokinetics, which means that a plot of the natural log of the plasma concentration versus times results in a straight line and that the clearance remains constant at usual therapeutic doses. However, some hepatically eliminated drugs are subject to nonlinear elimination when dosed in the normal therapeutic range, the most common example being the anticonvulsant drug phenytoin. When a drug is eliminated by enzymes in the liver, the velocity (v) of drug elimination by metabolism is described by the following equation:

$$v = \frac{V_{max} \times C}{K_m + C}$$

where V_{max} is the maximum rate of metabolism by hepatic enzymes possible, C is the plasma concentration of the drug, and K_m is the plasma concentration at the point of one-half of the V_{max}. Most drugs follow first-order (clearance remains constant) pharmacokinetics because the K_m is much greater than the plasma concentration (K_m>>C). As long as this remains true, then $K_m + C$ is approximately equal to K_m and the equation becomes

$$v = \frac{V_{max} \times C}{K_m}$$

For this equation, V_{max} over K_m is a constant that becomes the Cl in first-order pharmacokinetics. However, for phenytoin and a few other drugs and potentially for many hepatically eliminated drugs if taken in overdoses, the plasma concentration approaches the K_m and the equation cannot be simplified. In this case, the clearance of the drug becomes concentration dependent, which means the clearance decreases as the plasma concentration of the drug increases. Thus, if the dose of a first-order elimination drug is doubled, then the steady-state plasma concentration will double, but doubling the dose of a drug that undergoes nonlinear elimination will result in a greater than doubling of the steady-state plasma concentration. The converse is true also—if the dose of a drug with nonlinear elimination is decreased by half, then the new steady-state plasma concentration will decrease by more than half. This unpredictability in the relationship between dose and steady-state plasma concentration makes dosing nonlinearly eliminated drugs more difficult.

Half-Life

The half-life ($t_{1/2}$) of a drug is the time taken for the drug concentration (or the total amount of drug in the body) to decrease by 50%. First-order drug elimination is mathematically identical to radioactive decay where the half-life is a parameter of an asymptotic decay function. It takes five half-lives for a drug to be completely eliminated from the body once dosing is stopped, but technically, 3.125% of the drug will still be left after five half-lives (100%, 50%, 25%, 12.5%, 6.25%, 3.125%). The converse is also true: steady state is considered to be achieved after five half-lives, even though the drug is still 3.125% from the steady-state concentration (0%, 50%, 75%, 87.5%, 93.75%, 96.875%). Knowing these percentage values is important so that you can apply them clinically. If a patient had a digoxin trough concentration determined after being dosed for four half-lives, one would not want to ignore this concentration because it has not reached the threshold of five half-lives that is considered steady state. The concentration is 93.75% complete, which makes this concentration close to the steady-state concentration.

Half-life is commonly equated as the pharmacokinetic parameter determining how fast a drug is eliminated from the body. However, the half-life of a drug is dependent on the V and the Cl of the drug as described by the following equation:

$$t_{1/2} = \frac{0.693 \times V}{Cl}$$

where V is the volume of distribution and Cl is the clearance of the drug. Thus, if the half-life of a drug in a patient changes, it is due to a change in V, Cl, or both. However, in most instances, changes in the drug half-life of a patient or differences in drug half-lives among patients occur because of a change in the Cl or the variability in drug Cl among patients and not because of differences in the V. This change or variability occurs because large changes in V are unusual, whereas large changes in Cl are quite common because of the variability and lability of renal and hepatic drug elimination. Variability in a drug's V among patients is significant, but Cl variability among patients is generally much greater.

Normally, one thinks of the terminal elimination phase of a drug's disposition as defining the elimination rate constant, k, and thus the half-life:

$$-m = k;\ t_{1/2} = \frac{0.693}{k}$$

where m is the slope of line of the semilog plot of the terminal elimination phase and k is the first-order elimination rate constant. This equation presumes that for an orally administered drug, the absorption rate is rapid compared with the elimination rate ($ka >> k$). If this is true, then the drug is completely absorbed before the terminal elimination phase and the slope of the terminal elimination phase is determined by the elimination half-life of the drug. However, if a drug is given in a controlled-release dosage form in which $ka << k$, then the absorption rate becomes rate limiting, the semilog plot of the terminal elimination phase is determined by the absorption rate rather than the elimination rate, and the slope of the terminal elimination phase is dependent on ka instead of k. This is referred to as the *flip-flop* in pharmacokinetics. This flip-flop affects the time to reach steady state and the time to eliminate all of a drug from the body once dosing is stopped. For a controlled-release drug in which $ka << k$, the time to reach steady state is five absorption rate half-lives ($t_{1/2abs}$), and the time to eliminate a drug from the body is also five $t_{1/2abs}$.

A final consideration is the effect of nonlinear drug elimination on the half-life. As discussed previously, the clearance decreases as the drug plasma concentration increases and the clearance increases as the plasma concentration decreases. Thus, because the half-life is inversely affected by the *Cl*, the half-life constantly changes as the drug plasma concentration changes for a drug exhibiting nonlinear elimination such as phenytoin. Though phenytoin is commonly referred to as having a half-life of about 1 day, technically, half-life is not a parameter of a drug that exhibits nonlinear elimination.

10-5 Drug Elimination

The two primary routes of drug elimination are by the kidneys (renal) and by the liver (hepatic). The kidney removes drugs from the body while the liver metabolizes drugs generally into a more water-soluble form that promotes renal elimination. In general, one worries about a patient's renal function when he or she is dosed with a renally eliminated drug and one worries about a patient's liver function when he or she is dosed with a hepatically eliminated drug. However, hepatic elimination results in the formation of a metabolite, which may have therapeutic or toxic activity, that must be considered when a patient has renal disease. Morphine is a typical example of a drug that is rapidly eliminated by hepatic metabolism (glucuronidation) with the removal of the glucuronides (morphine-3-glucuronid, morphine-6-glucruonide) by the kidneys. An expectation that morphine dosing is the same in patients with normal or poor renal function would be incorrect. The morphine-6-glucuronide retains opiate activity and will accumulate in patients with renal failure, potentially leading to respiratory depression. Thus, despite the fact that morphine is rapidly metabolized by the liver, one must still consider renal function when dosing this drug.

Renal Drug Elimination

For drugs primarily eliminated by the kidneys, the dose can be adjusted on the basis of an assessment of the patient's kidney function using the serum creatinine (*SCr*). The Cockcroft–Gault and the Modification of Diet in Renal Disease (MDRD) Study equations are the most commonly used assessments. Both equations provide a quantitative estimate of a patient's renal function. The Cockcroft–Gault equation is the older equation, which was developed to estimate the creatinine clearance from the serum creatinine:

$$CrCl = \frac{(140 - Age)BW}{(72 \times SCr)}$$

where *CrCl* is the creatinine clearance in mL/minute, *Age* is the patient's age in years, *BW* is the body weight in kg, and *SCr* is the serum creatinine in mg/dL. The body weight should be the adjusted body weight:

$$ABW = IBW + 0.4(TBW - IBW)$$

where *ABW* is the adjusted body weight in kg, *IBW* is the ideal body weight, and *TBW* is the patient's actual total body weight. If a patient is overweight, using the *IBW* will underestimate the *CrCl* and using the patient's actual total body weight will overestimate the *CrCl*. The more overweight the patient, the greater is the difference in the *CrCl* estimate when using the different weights (*IBW*, *ABW*, *TBW*). If the patient is female, multiply the estimate by 0.85.

The MDRD Study equation uses the *SCr* as in the Cockcroft–Gault equation, but the equation was developed to estimate the relationship between the *SCr* and the glomerular filtration rate (*GFR*), rather than the *CrCl*:

$$GFR = 175 \times SCr^{-1.154} \times Age^{-0.203}$$

where *GFR* is the glomerular filtration rate in mL/minute/1.73m², *SCr* is the serum creatinine in mg/dL, and *Age* is the patient's age in years. If the patient is female, multiply the estimate by 0.742, and if the patient is African American, multiply the estimate by 1.212. The resulting answer is in units of mL/minute/1.73m². To calculate the patient's actual *GFR* in mL/minute, multiply the estimate by the patient's body surface area divided by 1.73. Both equation estimates are affected by the patient's gender (male versus female) and by the patient's weight (body surface area includes patient's weight). However, weight has a more significant effect on the Cockcroft–Gault equation than on the MDRD Study equation and a bigger gap will appear between these estimates as the patient's weight increases. The MDRD Study equation also has a factor for ethnicity (African American) that is not included in the Cockcroft–Gault equation. Many dosing nomograms that adjust drug dose on the basis of a patient's estimated renal function still use the Cockcroft–Gault equation, but there is discussion about using the MDRD Study equation instead. Hospitals generally report the *GFR* on patient laboratory results estimated from the MDRD Study equation rather than a Cockcroft–Gault equation. Exercise caution when using a *GFR* laboratory result because the units likely will be mL/minute/1.73m² and one will need to convert to the patient's actual *GFR* using the patient's body surface area in order to adjust drug doses.

Hepatic Drug Elimination

Unlike renal function, one cannot derive a quantitative estimate of liver function from a laboratory test. The group of tests often referred to as liver function tests—alanine transaminase (ALT), aspartate transaminase (AST), gamma-glutamyl transpeptidase (GGTP), and alkaline phosphatase (Alk Phos)—cannot be used to estimate drug elimination. These tests measure enzymes produced by cells in the liver that are released into the blood stream when the cells are damaged. Thus, the tests indicate damage to the liver, but they do not correlate quantitatively with the liver's metabolic capacity. Therefore, the elimination of a hepatically eliminated drug is most likely decreased, but the amount is unknown, and there are no dosing nomograms for adjusting drug dose on the basis of any hepatic laboratory parameter analogous to the way the *SCr* is used in the dosing of renally eliminated drugs. Instead, general statements are available, such as "start at a lower dose if patient has abnormal liver function tests" or "avoid the use of the drug in patients with severe hepatic disease."

The role of the liver in drug elimination is also unique because any drug administered orally must pass through the liver before reaching the systemic circulation. All of the drug that is absorbed from the gastrointestinal tract passes through the liver before reaching the systemic circulation and distributing to body tissues. The drug metabolism that occurs upon this first pass of the entire drug dose through the liver is referred to as first-pass metabolism. The model explaining hepatic drug metabolism, including first-pass metabolism, after oral dosing is called the venous equilibrium model. Understanding this model is necessary to properly interpret the pharmacokinetics of hepatically eliminated drugs and the effects of drug interactions and disease states on their disposition. This model has three parameters that determine hepatic drug disposition: the free fraction of drug in the plasma (f_{up}), the maximum clearance of the drug possible by hepatic metabolism referred to as the intrinsic clearance (Cl_{int}), and the liver blood flow (Q). Hepatically eliminated drugs are divided into three classes—low-, intermediate-, and high-extraction drugs. The class is determined by the drug's extraction ratio:

$$ER = \frac{Cl_h}{Q}$$

where ER is the drug's extraction ratio, CL_h is the hepatic clearance of the drug, and Q is the liver blood flow (approximately 1,350 mL/minute in humans). Low-extraction drugs have an ER less than or equal to 0.3, high-extraction drugs have an ER greater than or equal to 0.7, and intermediate-extraction drugs have an ER between 0.3 and 0.7. Thus, propranolol, which has a hepatic clearance of about 1,100 mL/minute, has the following extraction ratio:

$$ER = \frac{1{,}100 \text{ mL/minute}}{1{,}350 \text{ mL/minute}} = 0.81$$

making it a high-extraction drug. Drugs with high-extraction ratios are eliminated as fast as they are presented to the liver, making their elimination flow dependent. Thus, their drug clearance is approximately equal to the liver blood flow:

$$Cl = Q$$

This is in contrast to low-extraction drugs in which the clearance is dependent on f_{up} and Cl_{int}:

$$Cl = f_{up} \times Cl_{int}$$

and the Cl value is much less than the liver blood flow (Q). When a hepatically eliminated drug is given orally, it will undergo first-pass metabolism, which is described as

$$F^* = 1 - ER$$

where F^* is the fraction of the absorbed drug dose that escapes first-pass metabolism. For high-extraction drugs, ER is greater than or equal to 0.7 and a large proportion of the drug is metabolized before reaching the systemic circulation, which is in contrast to low-extraction drugs that will have only a small portion of the drug dose metabolized before reaching the systemic circulation. Thus, for low-extraction drugs, F^* is approximately equal to 1, and for high-extraction drugs

$$F^* = \frac{Q}{f_{up} \times Cl_{int}}$$

when one assumes that $f_{up} \times Cl_{int} >> Q$. These equations, which are based on the venous equilibrium model, cannot be used quantitatively, but they are important in understanding what factors affect the steady-state plasma concentrations of hepatically eliminated drugs and the differences between low- and high-extraction drug disposition. The following equations illustrate the factors that determine the free steady-state (the pharmacologically active drug concentration) and the total steady-state (free concentration plus concentration bound to plasma proteins) drug concentrations.

Low-extraction drug (intravenous or oral)

Determinants of the steady-state total and free plasma concentrations of a hepatically eliminated, low-extraction drug given intravenously or orally are as follows:

$$C_{ss,total} = \frac{Dose}{f_{up} \times Cl_{int}}$$

$$C_{ss,free} = f_{up} \times \frac{Dose}{f_{up} \times Cl_{int}} = \frac{Dose}{Cl_{int}}$$

In the case of a low-extraction drug, there is no first-pass metabolism (no F^*), and the Cl of the drug is equivalent to $f_{up} \times Cl_{int}$.

High-extraction drug (intravenous)

Determinants of the steady-state total and free plasma concentrations of a hepatically eliminated, high-extraction drug given intravenously are as follows:

$$C_{ss,total} = \frac{Dose}{Q}$$

$$C_{ss,free} = f_{up} \times \frac{Dose}{Q} = \frac{f_{up} \times Dose}{Q}$$

For a high-extraction drug, the Cl is equal to Q; when the drug is given intravenously, hepatic first-pass metabolism is bypassed, and thus, there is no F^*.

High extraction drug (oral)

Determinants of the steady-state total and free plasma concentrations of a hepatically eliminated, high-extraction drug given orally are as follows:

$$C_{ss,total} = \frac{F^* \times Dose}{Q} = \frac{\dfrac{Q}{f_{up} \times Cl_{int}} \times Dose}{Q} = \frac{Dose}{f_{up} \times Cl_{int}}$$

$$C_{ss,free} = f_{up} \times \frac{F^* \times Dose}{Q} = \frac{f_{up} \times \dfrac{Q}{f_{up} \times Cl_{int}} \times Dose}{Q} = \frac{Dose}{Cl_{int}}$$

When a high-extraction drug is given orally, the first-pass metabolism is significant. When one substitutes $(Q/f_{up} \times Cl_{int})$ for F^* in the equation, the equations for the steady-state total and free concentrations simplify to the equations identical to a low-extraction drug. Using these equations, one can predict how changes in f_{up}, Cl_{int}, and Q will affect the steady-state total and free concentrations and whether this is likely to alter the therapeutic effect of the drug (see Table 10-1).

Using Table 10-1, one can predict the effect that changes in protein binding (changes the f_{up}), enzyme inhibition and induction (changes the Cl_{int}), and liver blood flow (changes in Q) will have on the steady-state total drug concentration ($C_{ss,total}$) and the pharmacologically active steady-state free drug concentration ($C_{ss,free}$). For example, if propranolol is being administered intravenously to a patient who is started on rifampin, which induces the metabolism of propranolol, then one can predict what will happen to the propranolol $C_{ss,total}$ and $C_{ss,free}$. Propranolol is a high-extraction drug (*ER* is 0.81) being given intravenously in this case. Enzyme induction would be an increase in the Cl_{int} (↑), which (from the table) would result in no change in the $C_{ss,total}$, $C_{ss,free}$, or therapeutic effect. If one refers to the equations, then $Cl = Q$ and neither the steady-state total drug concentration nor the steady-state free drug concentration is affected by changes in Cl_{int} . If the propranolol is being given orally, then according to Table 10-1, the increase in the Cl_{int} alters both the $C_{ss,total}$ and the $C_{ss,free}$, causing both to decrease and most likely decreasing the therapeutic effect. If one refers to the equations for a high-extraction drug given orally, then Cl_{int} is in both the $C_{ss,total}$ and the $C_{ss,free}$ equations and is inversely related to the steady-state concentrations. This route effect caused by the first-pass metabolism of high-extraction drugs also explains why a normal therapeutic intravenous dose of propranolol is about one-tenth of the normal oral dose. Using the table or the equations, one should be

TABLE 10-1. Venous Equilibrium Model

f_{up}	Cl_{int}	Q	$C_{ss,total}$	$C_{ss,free}$	Therapeutic effect
Low extraction (intravenous or oral)					
↑	↔	↔	↓	↔	↔
↓	↔	↔	↑	↔	↔
↔	↑	↔	↓	↓	↓
↔	↓	↔	↑	↑	↑
↔	↔	↑	↔	↔	↔
↔	↔	↓	↔	↔	↔
High extraction (intravenous)					
↓	↔	↔	↔	↑	↑
↓	↔	↔	↔	↓	↓
↔	↑	↔	↔	↔	↔
↔	↓	↔	↔	↔	↔
↔	↔	↑	↓	↓	↓
↔	↔	↓	↑	↑	↑
High extraction (oral)					
↑	↔	↔	↓	↔	↔
↓	↔	↔	↑	↔	↔
↔	↑	↔	↓	↓	↓
↔	↓	↔	↑	↑	↑
↔	↔	↑	↔	↔	↔
↔	↔	↓	↔	↔	↔

↑, increase; ↓, decrease; ↔, no change.

able to predict the change in the $C_{ss,total}$ and $C_{ss,free}$ and the therapeutic effect that will occur for any change in f_{up}, Cl_{int}, or Q for low-extraction and-high extraction hepatically eliminated drugs.

10-6 Bioavailability

The U.S. Food and Drug Administration defines *bioavailability* as "the rate and extent to which the active ingredient or active moiety is absorbed from a drug product and becomes available at the site of action." Because, in practice, drug concentrations are rarely determined at the site of action (e.g., at a receptor site), bioavailability is more commonly defined as "the rate and extent that the active drug is absorbed from a dosage form and becomes available in the systemic circulation." The following factors affect bioavailability:

- Drug product formulation
- Properties of the drug (salt form, crystalline structure, formation of solvates, and solubility)
- Composition of the finished dosage form (presence or absence of excipients and special coatings)
- Manufacturing variables (tablet compression force, processing variables, particle size of drug or excipients, and environmental conditions)
- Rate and site of dissolution in the gastrointestinal tract
- Physiologic determinants

- Contents of the gastrointestinal tract (fluid volume and pH, diet, presence or absence of food, bacterial activity, and presence of other drugs)
- Rate of gastrointestinal tract transit (influenced by disease, physical activity, drugs, emotional status of subject, and composition of the gastrointestinal tract contents)
- Presystemic drug metabolism or degradation (influenced by local blood flow; condition of the gastrointestinal tract membranes; and drug transport, metabolism, or degradation in the gastrointestinal tract or during the first pass of the drug through the liver)

Absolute Bioavailability

Absolute bioavailability is the fraction (or percentage) of a dose administered nonintravenously (or extravascularly) that is systemically available as compared to that available with an intravenous (IV) dose. If given orally, absolute bioavailability (F) is

$$F = \frac{AUC_{po}}{AUC_{IV}} \times \frac{Dose_{IV}}{Dose_{po}}$$

where F is the fraction of the oral dose that is absorbed into the systemic circulation relative to an intravenous administration, AUC_{po} and AUC_{IV} are the area under the curve for oral and intravenous administration, respectively, and $Dose_{IV}$ and $Dose_{po}$ are the doses administered intravenously and orally, respectively. When a drug is given intravenously, the F is always considered to be 1.

Relative Bioavailability

Relative bioavailability refers to a comparison of two or more dosage forms in terms of their relative rate and extent of absorption:

$$F = \frac{AUC_{test}}{AUC_{ref}} \times \frac{Dose_{ref}}{Dose_{test}}$$

where F is the relative bioavailability of the test drug to the reference drug in a dosage form other than intravenous. The equation is identical to the previous equation for absolute bioavailability with the exception that one is not comparing it to the drug administered intravenously. This comparison is often done to compare two different oral formulations of the same drug. Thus, if F is near 1, then the two dosage forms have the same bioavailability. This is not the same as bioequivalence, which includes assessing the rate and the extent of drug absorption.

Bioequivalence

Two dosage forms that do not differ significantly in their rate and extent of absorption are termed *bioequivalent.* In general, bioequivalence evaluations involve comparisons of dosage forms that are pharmaceutical equivalents or pharmaceutical alternatives. Pharmaceutical equivalents are drug products that contain identical amounts of the identical active drug ingredient (i.e., the same salt or ester of the same therapeutic moiety, in identical dosage forms). Pharmaceutical alternatives are drug products that contain the identical therapeutic moiety, or its precursor, but do not necessarily have the same amount or dosage form or the same salt or ester.

Biopharmaceutics Classification System

With minor exceptions, the U.S. Food and Drug Administration requires that bioavailability and bioequivalence of a drug product be demonstrated through in vivo studies. However, the Biopharmaceutics

Classification System (BCS) can be used to justify the waiver of the requirement for in vivo studies for rapidly dissolving drug products containing active moieties or active ingredients that are highly soluble and highly permeable. The BCS classifies drugs on the basis of their solubility, permeability, and in vitro dissolution rate:

- Class 1 has high solubility and high permeability.
- Class 2 has low solubility and high permeability.
- Class 3 has high solubility and low permeability.
- Class 4 has low solubility and low permeability.

10-7 Drug Interactions

Pharmacists are expected to be experts in drug interactions and are commonly asked questions by both patients and health care providers about such interactions. Databases on drug information provide an invaluable source for identifying drug interactions, but pharmacists should have an understanding of the underlying mechanisms and pharmacodynamics of drug interactions. Drug interactions can be divided into four major areas: (1) drug–drug interactions, (2) drug–disease interactions, (3) drug–food interactions, and (4) drug–polymorphism interactions (see Figure 10-1).

Drug–Drug Interactions

Drug–drug interactions are either pharmacokinetic or pharmacodynamic. Pharmacokinetic interactions occur when one drug alters the disposition of another, such as lovastatin and ketoconazole. Ketoconazole is a potent cytochrome P450 (CYP) 3A4 inhibitor that decreases the metabolism of lovastatin, potentially increasing the risk of rhabdomyolysis. Inhibition of drug transporters is another type of

FIGURE 10-1. Drug Interactions

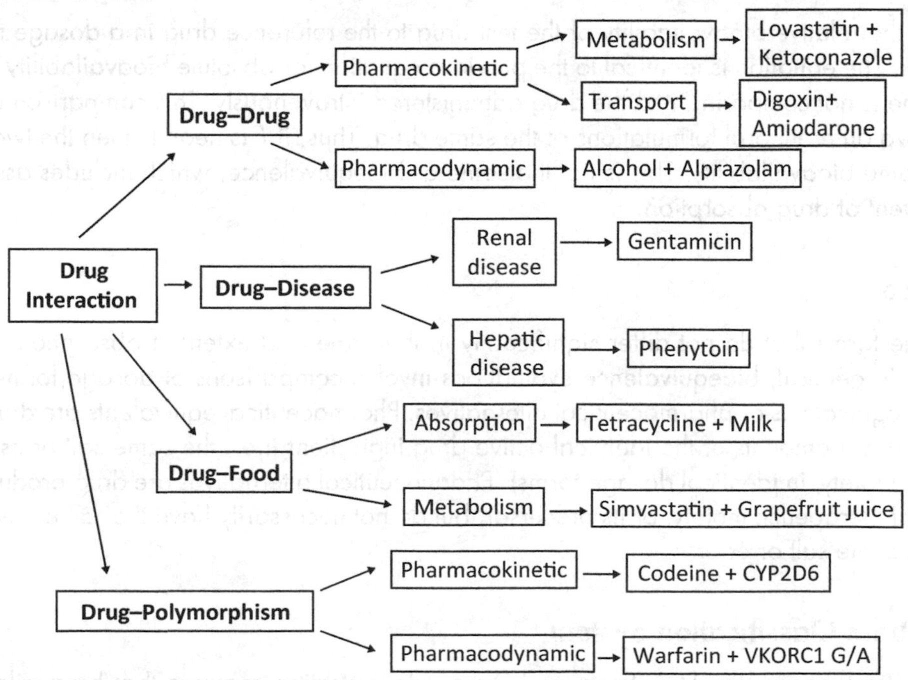

CYP2D6, cytochrome P450 2D6.

pharmacokinetic interaction in which drug transport across a cell membrane is affected by another drug, such as digoxin and amiodarone. Amiodarone is a potent inhibitor to P-glycoprotein, which is an active transporter that pumps substrates in the intestinal cell wall back into the lumen of the gut and reduces absorption. Digoxin is a P-glycoprotein substrate drug whose bioavailability is increased by amiodarone because of inhibition of this drug transporter. Drug–drug pharmacodynamic interactions occur when two drugs have overlapping pharmacological activity, such as alprazolam and alcohol. Alcohol and alprazolam are both central nervous system depressants—when taken together, they synergistically interact, increasing the risk of death from respiratory depression.

Drug–Disease Interactions

Drug–disease interactions are most commonly due to renal or hepatic disease, although there are other less common drug–disease interactions. Gentamicin is completely eliminated by the kidneys, and its elimination directly correlates with a patient's renal function. Hepatically eliminated drugs such as phenytoin will have a reduced elimination in patients with liver disease, increasing the risk of adverse effects.

Drug–Food Interactions

Drug–food interactions are often due to an interaction that reduces absorption, such as the interaction between tetracycline and milk. Milk contains calcium, which combines with tetracycline to form an insoluble salt and reduces the bioavailability and effectiveness of this antibiotic. The intestines contain drug-metabolizing enzymes, such as CYP3A4, which can be inhibited by foods such as grapefruit juice and result in an increase in bioavailability of a CYP3A4 substrate drug such as lovastatin.

Drug–Polymorphism Interactions

Research surrounding drug–polymorphism interactions is intense. Like pharmacokinetic interactions, this class of drug interactions can be divided into pharmacokinetic and pharmacodynamic interactions. Pharmacokinetic interactions affect drug disposition, such as the interaction between codeine and CYP2D6 polymorphisms. Codeine is an opiate analgesic that is a prodrug requiring metabolism by CYP2D6 to morphine to exert its analgesic effect. Patients who are poor metabolizers of CYP2D6 will not convert codeine to morphine and will not have a significant analgesic response when given codeine. The interaction between warfarin and VKORC1 G/A is a pharmacodynamic interaction in which carriers of the "A" allele are more sensitive to the anticoagulant effect of warfarin and therefore require lower doses.

Changes in Drug Clearance

Most clinically significant drug interactions result from a change in the clearance of a drug. For renally eliminated drugs, this change is most commonly a decrease in clearance because of renal disease; for hepatically eliminated drugs, both decreases and increases in clearance are common. Decreases in hepatic metabolism can occur as a result of one drug inhibiting the metabolism of another, a genetic polymorphism associated with decreased enzyme activity, and loss of enzyme because of hepatic disease. Increases in clearance occur because of one drug inducing the metabolism of another by increasing the amount of the hepatic enzyme responsible for the drug's metabolism or because of genetic polymorphisms, resulting in gene duplication of the drug-metabolizing enzyme.

Changes in hepatic clearance are most commonly either a decrease in hepatic drug clearance because of competitive enzyme inhibition or an increase in drug clearance because of enzyme induction. In competitive enzyme inhibition, one drug competes with another drug for the site of hepatic drug metabolism, causing an increase in the K_m:

$$\downarrow v = \frac{V_{max} \times C}{\uparrow K_m + C}$$

The higher the concentration of the interacting drug, the greater the decrease in the elimination of the affected drug. Thus, the maximum reduction in drug clearance will occur when the interacting drug has reached steady state, and the interaction will cease after the interacting drug dosing has been stopped for five half-lives. Enzyme induction does not cause any change in K_m: in the case of enzyme induction, the V_{max} is increased:

$$\uparrow v = \frac{\uparrow V_{max} \times C}{K_m + C}$$

The higher the concentration of the interacting drug, the greater the enzyme induction and the larger the increase in the clearance of the affected drug. However, because enzyme induction requires the production of more enzyme by the liver, maximum effect will not occur until 2 to 4 weeks after the interacting drug reaches steady state. Conversely, after the interacting drug is stopped, hepatic enzyme levels will not return to baseline for 2 to 4 weeks. Thus, the onset and offset of enzyme induction interactions are generally longer than the interactions resulting from competitive inhibition.

Changes in Volume of Distribution

When considering changes in the volume of distribution, one needs to consider both the change relative to the total drug concentration and the pharmacologically active free drug concentration. The following equation defines the volume of distribution at steady state (V_{ss}):

$$V_{ss} = V_P + \frac{f_{up}}{f_{ut}} \times V_T$$

where V_p is the volume of the plasma, V_T is the volume of the tissues, f_{up} is the fraction unbound in the plasma, and f_{ut} is the fraction unbound in tissues. The V_p is small and usually does not contribute significantly to the total volume, simplifying the equation to

$$V_{ss} = \frac{f_{up}}{f_{ut}} \times V_T$$

However, the volume of distribution of the pharmacologically active drug is determined by the free drug concentration, which is the V_{ss} divided by the fraction unbound in the plasma:

$$V_{ss,u} = \frac{V_{ss}}{f_{up}} = \frac{\frac{f_{up}}{f_{ut}} \times V_T}{f_{up}} = \frac{V_T}{f_{ut}}$$

where $V_{ss,u}$ is the unbound volume of distribution at steady state, V_{ss} is the volume of distribution at steady state based on the total drug concentration, f_{up} is the fraction unbound in the plasma, and f_{ut} is the fraction unbound in the tissues. Thus, in a patient, V_T is generally a constant and changes in the active drug concertation will occur only if the f_{ut} changes. There are no clinically documented changes in f_{ut}. Do not interpret this to mean that changes in f_{ut} do not occur because of drug interactions. The problem is that there is no way to measure f_{ut}, unlike the f_{up}, which is simply the free drug concentration in the plasma divided by the total concentration in the plasma. However, clinically, there are no known drug interactions that alter the unbound volume of distribution and require a change in the loading dose of a drug.

10-8 Questions

1. A patient with decreased renal function (serum creatinine 3.2 mg/dL) was given a 1,000 mg dose of vancomycin at 09:30 on 2/12. Vancomycin plasma concentrations measured at 13:20 on 2/12 and 04:30 on 2/13 were 35 and 21.6 mcg/mL, respectively. What is the half-life of vancomycin in this patient?

   A. 8 hours
   B. 14.3 hours
   C. 17.9 hours
   D. 21.7 hours

2. The half-life of gentamicin in a patient is 4.6 hours. A plasma concentration drawn 2 hours after the 30-minute dosing infusion was started is 12.3 mcg/mL. How long with it take for the gentamicin plasma concentration to fall from 12.3 mcg/mL to 1 mcg/mL?

   A. 8.6 hours
   B. 12.7 hours
   C. 16.6 hours
   D. 21.4 hours

3. A drug given by constant intravenous infusion has a half-life of 14 hours. If the drug has been infused for 19 hours, what percentage of the steady-state concentration has been reached?

   A. 38%
   B. 54%
   C. 61%
   D. 75%

4. A patient has been taking 250 mg of valproic acid three times per day for 2 weeks (half-life 16 hours), and a trough concentration drawn is 23 mcg/mL. What dose would come closest to achieving a target steady-state trough concentration of 60 mcg/mL?

   A. 250 mg four times per day
   B. 750 mg three times per day
   C. 500 mg three times per day
   D. 750 mg four times per day

5. A patient has come to the emergency room after overdosing on a medication. His plasma concentration is 38 mcg/mL. The medication has a *k* of 0.175 h^{-1} and a *ka* of 0.052 h^{-1}. How much time is needed for the plasma concentration to decrease to 5 mcg/mL?

   A. 39 hours
   B. 53 hours
   C. 12 hours
   D. 19 hours

6. Phenytoin has a volume of distribution of 0.7/kg. What intravenous loading dose ($S = 0.92$) would be required to achieve a target plasma concentration of 15 mcg/mL in a patient weighing 198 pounds?

   A. 13,508 mg
   B. 854 mg
   C. 923 mg
   D. 1,027 mg

7. A pediatric patient receives an immunosuppressive therapy with oral cyclosporine solution. His concentration-adjusted dosing regimen is 85 mg every 12 hours. Because of a recent change in his insurance coverage, he needs to be switched from the product he is currently using to a generic solution dosage form of cyclosporine that is covered by his insurance. The bioavailability of the dosage form he previously used is 43%; the bioavailability of the generic dosage form is 28%. What is the appropriate dosage regimen for the generic dosage form that will maintain the same systemic exposure obtained from the previously used dosage form?

   A. 25 mg every 12 hours
   B. 55 mg every 12 hours
   C. 184 mg every 12 hours
   D. 130 mg every 12 hours

8. For a phase III study of drug product in clinical drug development, an oral dosing regimen that maintains an average steady-state concentration of 50 ng/mL needs to be established. In single-dose studies, an oral dose of 80 mg resulted in an AUC of 962 ng/mL × h and an elimination half-life of 10.3 hours. What dosing regimen should be used?

   A. 35 mg every 12 hours
   B. 50 mg every 12 hours
   C. 72 mg every 12 hours
   D. 95 mg every 12 hours

9. Beth R. (58 kg, 63 years old) is suffering from symptomatic ventricular arrhythmia. She will be started on an oral multiple-dose regimen with the antiarrhythmic mexiletine. The population average values of mexiletine for clearance and volume of distribution are $Cl = 0.5$ L/h/kg and $V = 6$ L/kg, respectively. Although a therapeutic range of 0.5–2 mg/L has been described, avoiding large peak-to-trough fluctuations is recommended. The available oral dosage forms are 150, 200, and 250 mg capsules with an oral bioavailability of 0.9%. Design an appropriate and practical oral-dosing regimen that keeps the plasma concentrations at an average concentration of approximately 1 mg/L, with a peak-to-trough fluctuation of less than or equal to 100% (between 0.75 and 1.5 mg/L). What dosing regimen should be used?

A. 150 mg every 6 hours
B. 200 mg every 6 hours
C. 200 mg every 8 hours
D. 250 mg every 8 hours

10. When used for drug dosing, the estimated GFR as determined by the MDRD Study equation must be multiplied by which of the following in an overweight or underweight patient?

A. Patient's weight/72 kg × 1.73 m^2
B. Patient's body surface area/patient's weight
C. 1.73m^2/patient's body surface area
D. Patient's body surface area/1.73m^2

11. Dabigatran is a direct thrombin inhibitor used for stroke prevention in patients with non-valvular atrial fibrillation and has a risk of bleeding complications if inappropriately dosed. A patient who has not been previously evaluated is to be started on dabigatran, and the following information is available from today's labs: eGFR 24 mL/minute/1.73 m^2 (reported by lab); BSA 2.30 m^2; estimated *CrCl* by Cockcroft–Gault equation using adjusted body weight is 33 mL/minute. What is the most appropriate recommendation for initial dosing of dabigatran in this patient?

Dabigatran (Pradaxa): Dosing for atrial fibrillation

■ *CrCl* > 30 mL/minute	150 mg po twice daily
■ *CrCl* 15–30 mL/minute	75 mg po twice daily
■ *CrCl* < 15 mL/minute	No recommendation provided

A. Start 75 mg twice daily, and closely monitor for signs of bleeding.
B. Start 150 mg twice daily, and closely monitor for signs of bleeding.
C. Confirm the patient's kidney function is stable before recommending a dosing regimen.
D. Inform the team this drug should not be used because of the patient's poor kidney function.

12. A new drug given to a subject orally (with normal CYP2D6 genotype) has a bioavailability of 12%. When the same subject is given a 10 mg intravenous dose, the calculated AUC is 1,260 ng/mL × h. The drug is completely metabolized by CYP2D6 to an inactive metabolite that is excreted in the urine. What can be concluded from this information?

A. This new drug must be a P-glycoprotein substrate.
B. This new drug is a high-extraction drug that undergoes extensive first-pass metabolism.
C. This new drug is a low-extraction drug with poor oral absorption.
D. Making any conclusions from this information is impossible without knowing the volume of distribution.

13. A patient has been taking oral phenytoin ($F = 0.9$) 300 mg per day for 7 years. During this time, her kidney function has gradually declined from an eGFR of 85 mL/minute to 32 mL/minute and her albumin has declined from 4.5 g/dL to 2.4 g/dL. Phenytoin is highly bound to albumin, so phenytoin binding in the plasma will be lower than normal. How will this patient's steady-state total and free phenytoin concentrations change with the decrease in protein binding?

A. The total and free concentrations will not change.
B. The total and free concentrations will decrease.
C. The total concentration will increase, and the free concentration will decrease.
D. The total concentration will decrease, and the free concentration will be unchanged.

14. Phenytoin is 90% bound to plasma proteins with a therapeutic range based on total drug concentration of 10–20 mcg/mL. Thus, the therapeutic range based on the pharmacologically active drug concentration (the free concentration) is 1–2 mcg/mL ($0.1 \times 10 = 1$; $0.1 \times 20 = 2$). If the plasma protein binding of phenytoin is reduced to 85%, then what is the therapeutic range based on the total phenytoin plasma concentration?

A. 10–20 mcg/mL
B. 12.5–24.6 mcg/mL
C. 6.7–13.3 mcg/mL
D. 8–17 mcg/mL

15. A patient weighing 85 kg is taking metoprolol 100 mg orally twice per day with good control of his blood pressure. Metoprolol is a CYP2D6 substrate with a volume of 4.2 L/kg, a clearance of 15 mL/minute/kg, and a half-life of 3.2 hours. Recently, he was started on paroxetine (a CYP2D6 inhibitor) 20 mg per day. What is the expected effect of paroxetine on metoprolol?

A. Metoprolol free and total concentrations will not change.
B. Metoprolol free and total concentrations will increase.
C. Metoprolol free and total concentrations will decrease.
D. The total concentration will decrease, and the free concentration will remain unchanged.

16. A patient is taking digoxin 0.125 mg per day with a measured steady state of 1.7 ng/mL drawn 5 hours after his last digoxin dose. His heart rate is 81 beats per minute at this time. The desired steady-state concentration is 1.0 ng/mL. What is the most appropriate course of action?

A. Stop dosing, wait for the concentration to fall to 1 ng/mL, and restart dosing at 0.125 mg every other day.
B. Decrease the dose to 0.125 mg every other day.
C. Check the patient's renal function.
D. Redraw the level later in the dosing interval.

17. As part of a patient medication reconciliation, a pharmacist notes that the patient is taking both warfarin and carbamazepine. Because carbamazepine induces the elimination of warfarin, the pharmacist should

A. call the patient's physician and warn the physician that the anticoagulant effect of warfarin is going to decrease.
B. instruct the patient to take an extra warfarin dose and to call his physician.
C. call the patient's physician and suggest the use of an anticonvulsant that does not induce warfarin's metabolism.
D. learn how long the patient has been taking this drug combination and obtain recent international normalized ration (INR) values.

18. Using the Cockcroft–Gault equation, calculate the creatinine clearance of a 67-year-old female with a serum creatinine of 2.8 mg/dL who weighs 187 pounds and is 5 feet 4 inches tall.

A. 21 mL/minute
B. 25 mL/minute
C. 33 mL/minute
D. 18 mL/minute

19. A patient has been taking both warfarin, a hepatically eliminated drug with a *Cl* of 3.5mL/minute, a *V* of 10 L, and a half-life of 37 hours, and rifampin (a potent inducer of warfarin metabolism) for the past 6 months. His dose has been adjusted to keep his INR between 2 and 2.5. His treatment with rifampin is being discontinued. What will happen to the steady-state free and total concentrations of warfarin and to his INR after stopping rifampin?

A. The total concentration will increase, and the free concentration will remain unchanged with no change in his INR.
B. The total concentration and the free concentration will increase, causing an increase in his INR.
C. The total concentration and free concentration will decrease, causing a decrease in his INR.
D. The total concentration will remain unchanged, and the free concentration will increase, causing an increase in his INR.

20. Myocardial infarction has been reported to increase levels of α_1-acid glycoprotein, the major binding protein of lidocaine. What would be the expected effect of the increase in α_1-acid glycoprotein on lidocaine disposition (Cl = 1.0 L/minute, V = 1.1, half-life = 2 hours L/kg) and hepatic elimination?

A. $C_{ss,total}$ will increase, and $C_{ss,free}$ will increase.
B. $C_{ss,total}$ will increase, and $C_{ss,free}$ will be unchanged.
C. $C_{ss,total}$ will be unchanged, and $C_{ss,free}$ will increase.
D. $C_{ss,total}$ will be unchanged, and $C_{ss,free}$ will decrease.

10-9 Answers

1. D. Estimation of *k* from two plasma concentrations is

$$k = \frac{\ln\left(\frac{C_1}{C_2}\right)}{\Delta t}$$

C_1 = 35 mcg/mL
C_2 = 21.6 mcg/mL
Δt = time interval between C_1 and C_2

Time in this case is 24-hour clock time, which is used in all hospitals. Calculate the time interval from 2/12 at 13:20 to 2/13 at 04:30. Calculate the time interval from 13:20 to 24:00 and add 04:30:

$$\begin{array}{r} 23{:}60 \\ \not{24{:}00} \\ -\ \underline{13{:}20} \\ 10{:}40 \\ +\ \underline{04{.}30} \\ 14{:}70 \Rightarrow 15{:}10 \Rightarrow 15.17\text{ h} \end{array}$$

Calculate *k*:

$$k = \frac{\ln\left(\frac{35\text{ mcg/mL}}{21.6\text{ mcg/mL}}\right)}{15.17\text{ h}} = 0.032\text{ h}^{-1}$$

Calculate half-life:

$$t_{1/2} = \frac{0.693}{0.032\text{ h}^{-1}} = 21.7\text{ h}$$

2. C. In this case, calculate the Δt:

$$\Delta t = \frac{\ln\left(\frac{C_1}{C_2}\right)}{k}$$

C_1 = 12.3 mcg/mL
C_2 = 1 mcg/mL
$k = 0.693/4.6$, h = 0.151 h^{-1}

$$\Delta t = \frac{\ln\left(\frac{12.3\text{ mcg/mL}}{1.0\text{ mcg/mL}}\right)}{0.151\text{h}^{-1}} = 16.6\text{ h}$$

3. C. Because the half-life is 14 hours and the drug has been infused for 19 hours, the percentage of steady-state concentration is between 50 and 75%. To calculate the exact percentage of steady state, simply calculate *k* ($k = 0.693/14 = 0.050$) and use the following formula:

$$f_{ss} = 1 - e^{-k \times t}$$

where f_{ss} is the fraction of the steady-state concentration, k is the elimination rate constant, and t is the time since the start of the infusion. Thus,

$$f_{ss} = 1 - e^{-0.050 \times 19} = 0.613 \times 100 = 61\%$$

4. B. Use the ratio between the dose and the steady-state trough concentration.

$$\frac{X_{obs}}{C_{ss,obs}} = \frac{X_O}{C_{ss,t}}$$

$$\frac{750 \text{ mg/day}}{23 \text{ mcg/mL}} = \frac{X_O}{60 \text{ mcg/mL}}$$

$$X_O = \frac{1{,}956.7 \text{ mg/day}}{3}$$
$$= 652 \text{ mg three times per day}$$
$$\sim 750 \text{ mg three times per day}$$

5. A. This is the pharmacokinetic "flip-flop" with the *ka<<k*. Thus, use the *ka* rather than the *k* to calculate the time needed for the concentration to drop from 38 mcg/mL to 5 mcg/mL.

$$\Delta t = \frac{\ln\left(\dfrac{38 \text{ mcg/mL}}{5 \text{ mcg/mL}}\right)}{0.052 \text{ h}^{-1}} = 39 \text{ h}$$

6. D. Use the loading dose equation:

$$LD = \frac{(C_t - C_{obs}) \times V}{F \times S} = \frac{(15 \text{ mg/L} - 0) \times (0.7 \text{ L/kg} \times 90 \text{ kg})}{(1.0 \times 0.92)}$$
$$= 1{,}027 \text{ mg}$$

7. D. First, calculate how much cyclosporine the patient presently receives every 12 hours based on bioavailability of 43%:

$$85 \text{ mg} \times 0.43 = 36.55 \text{ mg every 12 hours}$$

Then calculate the dose needed based on bioavailability of the new dosage form (28%):

$$\frac{36.55 \text{ mg}}{0.28} = 130.5 \text{ mg} \sim 130 \text{ mg every 12 hours}$$

8. B. From the single-dose study, one can calculate *Cl/F*:

$$Cl/F = \frac{Dose}{AUC} = \frac{80 \text{ mg}}{962 \text{ ng/mL} \times \text{h}}$$
$$= \frac{80{,}000 \text{ mcg}}{962 \text{ mcg/L} \times \text{h}} = 83.2 \text{ L/h}$$

Using the oral clearance (*Cl/F*), calculate the dose that will achieve a mean steady-state concentration of 50 ng/mL when given every 12 hours, which is a reasonable time interval given the half-life of about 10 hours:

$$Dose = 50 \text{ ng/mL} \times 83.2 \text{ L/h} = 50 \text{ mcg/L} \times 83.2 \text{ L/h}$$
$$= 4{,}160 \text{ mcg/h} = 4.16 \text{ mg/h} \times 12 \text{ h}$$
$$\sim 50 \text{ mg every 12 hours}$$

For this calculation, assume that the *F* remains constant between the single-dose study and the steady-state dosing estimate.

9. D. The dose needed to achieve a mean steady-state concentration of 1 mg/L is determined by the clearance in this patient, which is 29 L/h (0.5 L/h/kg × 58 kg).

$$Dose = \frac{C_{ss} \times Cl}{F} = \frac{1 \text{ mg/L} \times 29 \text{ L/h}}{0.9} = 32.2 \text{ mg/h}$$

The dosing interval required that will keep the fluctuation between the peak and the trough between 1.5 and 0.75 mg/L is determined by the *k*, which is equal to the *Cl/V*:

$$k = \frac{Cl}{V} = \frac{29 \text{ L}}{(6 \text{ L/kg} \times 58 \text{ kg})} = 0.083 \text{ h}^{-1}$$

Use *k* to determine the time needed for the concentration to drop from 1.5 mg/L to 0.75 mg/L:

$$\Delta t = \frac{\ln\left(\dfrac{1.5 \text{ mg/L}}{0.75 \text{ mg/L}}\right)}{0.083 \text{ h}^{-1}} = 8.35 \text{ h}$$

Thus, the dose is 250 mg (32.2 mg/h × 8 h = 257.6 mg) administered every 8 hours.

10. **D.** To convert from the body surface area (BSA) normalized units of the MDRD Study equation of mL/minute/1.73[2] to mL/minute, calculate the patient's BSA and divide it by 1.73.

11. **C.** The correct answer to the question highlights the importance of knowing more about the patient than just the reported lab value and the danger of making assumptions that may not be accurate. In this case, the estimated renal function by the Cockcroft–Gault equation (33 mL/minute) and the MDRD Study equation (31 mL/minute) both result in a recommendation of 150 mg po twice daily, but because there is no information on whether the patient's renal function is stable, basing a dose on this lab value would be inappropriate. The serum creatinine has a long half-life as renal function declines, and it may continue to rise for several days in patients who have an acute kidney injury. Thus, in this patient, one does not know if the kidney function is still declining.

12. **C.** This is a hepatically eliminated drug, so the first step is to determine its extraction ratio:

$$ER = \frac{Cl_{drug}}{Q} = \frac{\dfrac{Dose}{AUC}}{1{,}350 \text{ mL/minute}}$$

$$= \frac{\dfrac{10{,}000 \text{ mcg}}{1{,}260 \text{ mcg/L} \times \text{h}}}{81 \text{ L/h}} = 0.098$$

Because this is a low-extraction drug (*ER* is less than or equal to 0.3) there is no significant first-pass metabolism that could explain the low bioavailability of 12%. The drug could have reduced absorption if it is a substrate of P-glycoprotein, but there is no information given that would allow that conclusion. However, one does know that the low bioavailability is due to poor absorption.

13. **D.** Phenytoin is a low-extraction hepatically eliminated drug highly bound to albumin. A decline in protein binding results in an increase in the f_{up}. Thus, one can apply the venous equilibrium model equations to determine that the total steady-state concentration of phenytoin will decrease and the free steady-state concentration will remain unchanged.

$$\downarrow C_{ss,total} = \frac{Dose}{\uparrow f_{up} \times Cl_{int}}$$

$$\leftrightarrow C_{ss,free} = \frac{Dose}{Cl_{int}}$$

14. **C.** To determine the total concentration that corresponds to a free concentration range of 1 to 2 mcg/mL, simply divide the free concentration range by the f_{up}:

$$\text{Range} = \frac{1 \text{ mcg/mL}}{0.15} \text{ to } \frac{2 \text{ mcg/mL}}{0.15} = 6.7 \text{ to } 13.3 \text{ mcg/mL}$$

Thus, as the protein binding decreases, the therapeutic range based on the total steady-state drug concentration decreases. Patients with kidney and liver disease have decreased albumin, which could lead to an inappropriate dosage increase resulting in toxicity if one applies a normal therapeutic range of 10 to 20 mcg/mL as the target range.

15. **B.** Because metoprolol is a hepatically eliminated drug, one needs to determine its extraction ratio:

$$ER = \frac{Cl_{drug}}{Q} = \frac{\left(\dfrac{15 \dfrac{\text{mL}}{\text{min}}}{\text{kg}} \times 85 \text{ kg}\right)}{1{,}350 \text{ mL/minute}} = 0.94$$

Thus, this is a high-extraction drug being given orally. The inhibition of CYP2D6 by paroxetine would be a decrease in the Cl_{int}. Thus, applying the venous equilibrium model, one would conclude that the total and the free steady-state concentrations would increase, possibly resulting in an unexpected decrease in blood pressure and heart rate:

$$\uparrow C_{ss,total} = \frac{Dose}{f_{up} \times \downarrow Cl_{int}}$$

$$\uparrow C_{ss,free} = \frac{Dose}{\downarrow Cl_{int}}$$

16. **D.** Digoxin has a significant distribution phase (two-compartment model), but the therapeutic range is based on digoxin trough concentrations. If a level is drawn less than 8 hours after administration of the dose, then the digoxin concentration will be falsely elevated. The patient's heart rate is 81 bpm, which also does not suggest the dose is too high. In this case, redraw an appropriate trough level. Drug-Level Illustration 16-1 below shows the problem.

Drug-Level Illustration 16-1.

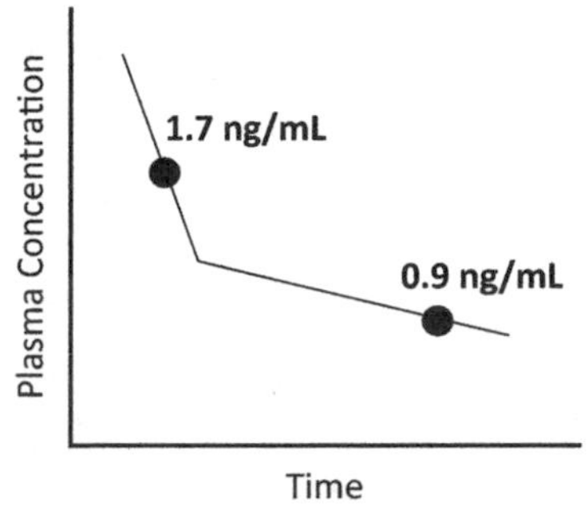

The level of 1.7 ng/mL is not a true trough level and may be significantly higher than the true trough level. To properly interpret drug levels, one must know when the level was drawn in relation to the last dose.

17. **D.** There is a significant drug–drug interaction between warfarin and carbamazepine. Carbamazepine induces the metabolism of warfarin, leading to a decrease in warfarin's effect (decrease in INR) and potentially increasing the risk of blood clot formation. However, if the patient was taking carbamazepine before the initiation of warfarin therapy, then the warfarin dose was stabilized under the condition of enzyme induction. In this case, discontinuation of carbamazepine would be inappropriate because it would lead to an increase in the warfarin level, which could lead to dangerous bleeding. More information is needed to make an appropriate therapeutic decision.

18. **A.** The first step is to calculate the patient's ABW:

$$ABW = IBW + 0.4(TBW - IBW)$$
$$= 54.7\text{ kg} + 0.4(85\text{ kg} - 54.7\text{ kg}) = 66.8\text{ kg}$$

Then use the ABW to calculate the *CrCl*:

$$CrCl = \frac{(140 - 67)66.8\text{ kg}}{(72 \times 2.8\text{ g/dL})} \times 0.85 = 20.6\text{ mL/minute}$$

19. **B.** Warfarin is a low-extraction hepatically eliminated drug. The dose was stabilized while the patient's hepatic enzymes were induced by rifampin. When rifampin is stopped, the Cl_{int} will decrease:

$$\uparrow C_{ss,total} = \frac{Dose}{f_{up} \times \downarrow Cl_{int}}$$

$$\uparrow C_{ss,free} = \frac{Dose}{\downarrow Cl_{int}}$$

Remember that the maximal decrease in enzyme activity will take 2–4 weeks. Therefore, the INR would be expected to increase over the next 2–4 weeks.

20. **D.** Lidocaine is a high-extraction hepatically eliminated drug given by intravenous infusion. The increase in α_1-acid glycoprotein will cause an increase in the protein binding, resulting in a decrease in the f_{up}.

$$\leftrightarrow C_{ss,total} = \frac{Dose}{Q}$$

$$\downarrow C_{ss,free} = \frac{\downarrow f_{up} \times Dose}{Q}$$

Thus, the decrease in f_{up} would be expected to decrease the active free drug concentration, resulting in a decrease in the effects of the lidocaine infusion.

10-10 Additional Resources

Brunton LL, Hilal-Dandan R, Knollmann BC. *Goodman & Gilman's: The Pharmacological Basis of Therapeutics*. 13th ed. New York, NY: McGraw Hill Education; 2018.

Gibaldi M, Perrier B. *Pharmacokinetics*. 2nd ed. New York, NY: Marcel Dekker; 1982.

U.S. Department of Health and Human Services, Food and Drug Administration, Center for Drug Evaluation and Research. Guidance for industry: bioavailability and bioequivalence studies submitted in NDAs or INDs—general considerations. Draft Guidance. March 2014. Available at: https://www.fda.gov/downloads/drugs/guidancecomplianceregulatory information/guidances/ucm389370.pdf.

Clinical Pharmacogenetics and Pharmacogenomics

11

GILLIAN C. BELL

11-1 KEY POINTS

- *Pharmacogenomics* is the study of the multigene influence on drug response, and *pharmacogenetics* is the study of the single-gene influence on drug response.
- The goal of pharmacogenetics and pharmacogenomics is to use genotype and drug phenotype information to optimize drug therapy.
- Variations important to pharmacogenomics can be found in genes encoding drug transporters, drug targets, and disease association.
- Deoxyribonucleic acid (DNA) is a double-stranded molecule that resembles a twisted ladder. The two strands are held together by noncovalent hydrogen bonds between base pairs. In base pairing, adenine pairs with thymine, and cytosine pairs with guanine.
- The central dogma of molecular biology states that the flow of genetic information is from DNA to ribonucleic acid (RNA) to protein. During gene expression, transcription produces RNA from a DNA template. Translation is the process by which RNA produces proteins.
- Functional variations in drug-metabolizing enzymes can influence drug concentrations and therefore are important predictors of drug treatment efficacy and of the risk for toxicity.
- Therapeutic recommendations based on pharmacogenetic results can be found in Clinical Pharmacogenetics Implementation Consortium guidelines. Additionally, there are numerous medications with pharmacogenetic information in the U.S. Food and Drug Administration (FDA) labeling, including several drugs with boxed warnings. A compiled list of medications with pharmacogenetic information can be found in the Table of Pharmacogenomic Biomarkers in Drug Labeling on the FDA Web site.
- Human genome and single nucleotide polymorphism mapping projects have provided researchers with the necessary tools to begin identifying the genes and gene variants that may be predictive of treatment outcome.
- Genomewide and candidate gene association studies are used to identify significant phenotype–genotype associations; they provide the primary step to identifying genetic predictors of drug response.

11-2 STUDY GUIDE CHECKLIST

The following topics may guide your study of this subject area:

- ☐ Key terminology for genetic concepts
- ☐ Basic concepts of genetics, including DNA transcription and translation
- ☐ Differences in the various recombinant DNA technologies used for biomedical research and clinical testing
- ☐ Genetic polymorphisms of metabolic enzymes, drug transporters, and drug targets and their effect on the pharmacokinetics and pharmacodynamics of medications
- ☐ Genetic polymorphisms with disease-associated implications and effect of variation on medication response
- ☐ Resources for using pharmacogenetic information in clinical care

11-3 Introduction to Pharmacogenetics and Pharmacogenomics

The existence of interindividual differences in response to drug therapy is well known. Twin studies have proved that drug pharmacokinetics and pharmacodynamics are indeed highly heritable. The complex interplay of gene–gene interactions and gene–environment interactions is key to disease predisposition as well as to the response to drug therapy. The field of *pharmacogenomics* focuses on how multiple genes determine drug response, whereas *pharmacogenetics* studies a single gene's influence on drug phenotypes. Clinicians now have both a wealth of genomic evidence (Table 11-1) and the necessary resources, including the U.S. Food and Drug Administration (FDA) Table of Pharmacogenomic Biomarkers in Drug Labeling and clinical guidelines, to support routine use in clinical care and to advance the field significantly.

11-4 Key Terminology

- ***Allele:*** An alternative form of a gene or heritable characteristic.
- ***Biomarker:*** A characteristic that is predictive of a biologic, pathogenic, or pharmacologic process or response.
- ***DNA (deoxyribonucleic acid):*** An acid found primarily in the nucleus of the cell that acts as the molecular basis of heredity. DNA consists of purine and pyrimidine bases, phosphate groups, and deoxyribose as the sugar moiety.
- ***Enzyme:*** A protein that catalyzes chemical reactions.
- ***Gene:*** An inherited functional unit occupying a specific locus on a chromosome.
- ***Genomics:*** The comprehensive study of the genome and the factors that influence it.
- ***Genotype:*** The genetic constitution of a cell or individual.
- ***Haplotype:*** A combination of alleles at multiple loci that travel together during recombination.
- ***Heterozygous:*** The presence of more than one allele occupying a specific gene position on homologous chromosomes.
- ***Homozygous:*** The presence of identical alleles at a specific locus on homologous chromosomes.
- ***Indel:*** An insertion or deletion genetic mutation.

TABLE 11-1. Evolution of Pharmacogenetics

Observation	Year
Succinylcholine was observed to produce prolonged neuromuscular blockade after normal doses.	1954
Isoniazid was found to induce neurotoxicity.	1954
Primaquine-induced hemolytic anemia was observed in glucose-6-phosphate dehydrogenase deficiency.	1956
The term *pharmacogenetics* was used for the first time by Friedrich Vogel and was defined as the study of the role of genetics in drug response.	1959
An autosomal recessive inherited deficiency in cytochrome P450 2D6 was linked to the extreme hypotensive effects caused by debrisoquine hydroxylation.	1977
The U.S. Congress commissioned the Human Genome Project.	1988
Human genome sequencing was completed.	2003
Phases I and II of the International HapMap Project were completed. The goal was to identify the most common variations across the human genome.	2007

Evans, Relling, 2004; National Human Genome Research Institute, 2012; Relling, Giacomini, 2006.

- ***Monogenic trait:*** A trait or characteristic determined by a single gene (e.g., hematologic toxicities associated with *TPMT* [thiopurine methyltransferase] gene functional polymorphisms).
- ***Nucleotide:*** Molecules that constitute the structure of RNA and DNA.
- ***Pharmacogenetics:*** The study of a single gene's influence on drug response (i.e., efficacy or toxicity).
- ***Pharmacogenomics:*** The study of how genes across the entire genome interact to influence drug response.
- ***Phenotype:*** The observable characteristic (trait) of an organism or individual.
- ***Polygenic trait:*** A trait or characteristic determined by multiple genes.
- ***Polymorphism:*** Variation in the genetic sequence occurring at a frequency of greater than or equal to 1%. This term is often used interchangeably with *variant allele*.
- ***Protein:*** A macromolecule made up of a sequence of amino acids defined by a gene sequence.
- ***Proteomics:*** The study of the structure and function of the full set of proteins encoded by a genome.
- ***RNA (ribonucleic acid):*** A molecule that is transcribed from DNA and consists of a long chain of nucleotides, each of which includes a nitrogenous base, a ribose sugar, and a phosphate.
- ***Single nucleotide polymorphism:*** A base pair substitution occurring in every three hundred bases, on average.

11-5 Genetic Concepts

The basic principles and capabilities related to heredity are contained within the structure of the DNA molecule. The nucleotide is the basic unit of DNA. A nucleotide consists of a sugar (deoxyribose) connected to a phosphate group and to one of four possible nitrogenous bases: adenine (A), guanine (G), cytosine (C), or thymine (T).

In a DNA strand, many nucleotides are joined together, with the sugars and phosphates alternating in a linear chain, forming the backbone of the molecule. The bases of each nucleotide project from the backbone.

DNA is a double-stranded molecule. The DNA molecule consists of two strands of opposite polarity (antiparallel) held together by complementary base pairing. In double-stranded DNA, A always pairs with T, and G always pairs with C (Figure 11-1).

Unlike the covalent bonds throughout the rest of the molecule, complementary base pairs are held together by the relatively weak attraction of noncovalent hydrogen bonds. This feature is critical to how DNA transfers information. The low energy of hydrogen bonds permits the two strands to come apart and serve as templates for transfer of the encoded information.

The information stored in DNA goes through an RNA intermediate in the process of making protein. This flow of information, from DNA to RNA to protein, is called the *central dogma of molecular biology.* The two key cellular processes involved are transcription and translation:

- *Transcription* describes those activities related to gene expression, in which the DNA serves as a template to produce an RNA transcript.
- In *translation,* the sequence of the RNA transcript is read as a triplet code to direct production of a protein.

The human genome contains approximately 3 billion base pairs of DNA, with genes making up only a small fraction of the total. A *gene* is a DNA segment containing the sequences that physically code for a gene product (coding sequences) plus the surrounding sequences required for transcription. The elements of a typical gene include a promoter, a start codon, multiple exons with intervening introns, and a stop codon. Genes vary widely in size and complexity; there are several classes of genes.

The most common types of genetic variation are single nucleotide polymorphisms (SNPs), which account for about 90% of genetic variations among individuals. Other variations include insertion–deletion mutations

FIGURE 11-1. **Structure of the DNA Molecule**

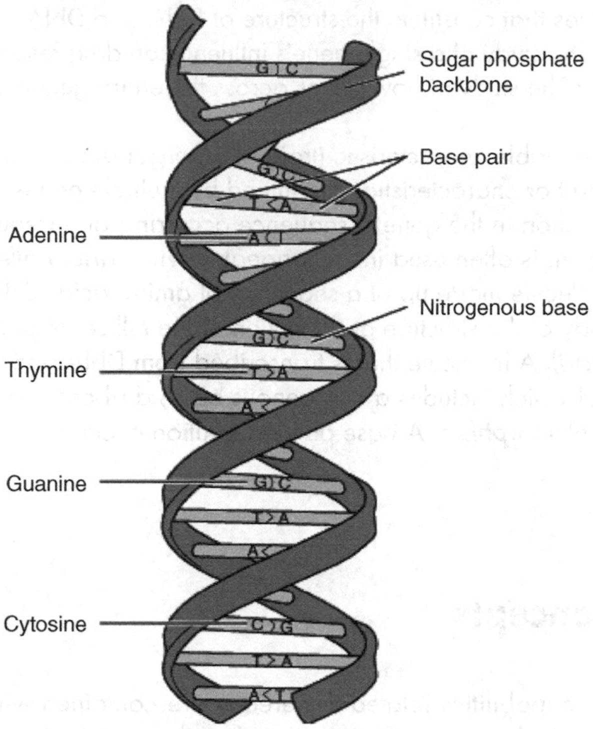

National Human Genome Research Institute (https://www.genome.gov/Pages/Hyperion/DIR/VIP/Glossary/Illustration/dna.cfm?key=deoxyribonucleic%20acid%20%28DNA%29).

(indels) and copy number variations, which can result in gene segments or whole genes being duplicated or deleted. The frequency at which polymorphisms occur differs among individuals from different ethnic, racial, or geographic origins.

11-6 Recombinant DNA Technology

The ability to manipulate nucleic acids in vitro has revolutionized all fields of biomedical research. Since the 1960s, science has taken advantage of the naturally occurring inner workings of cells and genomes to develop increasingly sophisticated technologies for biomedical research and clinical testing. Most laboratory methodologies rely at their core on the intrinsic biochemical principles of nucleic acids and proteins.

Polymerase Chain Reaction

Since the technique of polymerase chain reaction (PCR) first became available in the 1980s, it has become an integral component of the majority of molecular technologies. PCR provides an elegantly simple method to make large quantities of DNA that can be used for further analysis in a large number of applications.

PCR requires a small sample of the double-stranded DNA to be amplified, as well as two oligonucleotides to serve as primers. The requirements of the primers are that they are homologous to sequences flanking the region of interest and that their polarity directs bidirectional DNA synthesis across the region of interest (Figure 11-2). Additional reagents required are DNA nucleotides (deoxynucleotide triphosphates, or dNTPs) and thermostable DNA polymerase in an appropriately buffered cationic solution.

FIGURE 11-2. Polymerase Chain Reaction[a]

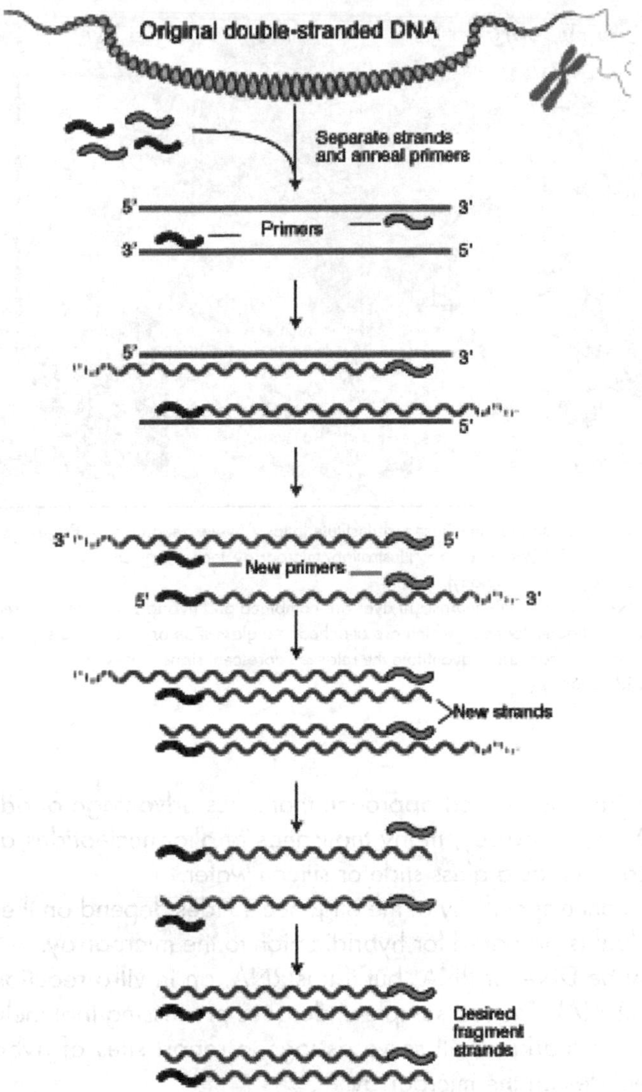

National Human Genome Research Institute (https://www.genome.gov/Pages/Hyperion/DIR/VIP/Glossary/Illustration/PCR.cfm?key=polymerase%20chain%20reaction%20%28PCR%29).

a. In PCR, multiple rounds of DNA denaturation, annealing of primers, and extension (new DNA synthesis from each primer) are carried out to make many copies of the DNA sequence between the two primers.

In a reaction consisting of 20–30 cycles, millions of copies of the sequence spanning the primers are produced. PCR products thus produced can be analyzed in numerous ways. In DNA sequencing, the exact order of bases in a segment of DNA is determined. Typical components of a sequencing reaction include DNA polymerase and standard DNA nucleotides, as well as limited quantities of specially modified dideoxynucleotides (ddNTPs), the DNA to be sequenced (template), and a single primer complementary to the template and adjacent to the region to be sequenced.

Like PCR, sequencing is a cyclic reaction, but new DNA synthesis occurs in only one direction—off the end of the sole primer. Over the course of multiple rounds of primer annealing and unidirectional synthesis, an array of different lengths is produced, with each new chain having a base-specific fluorescent tag at its 3′ terminus. Analysis of fluorescence as a function of length allows determination of the DNA sequence of the template.

FIGURE 11-3. Microarray Technology[a]

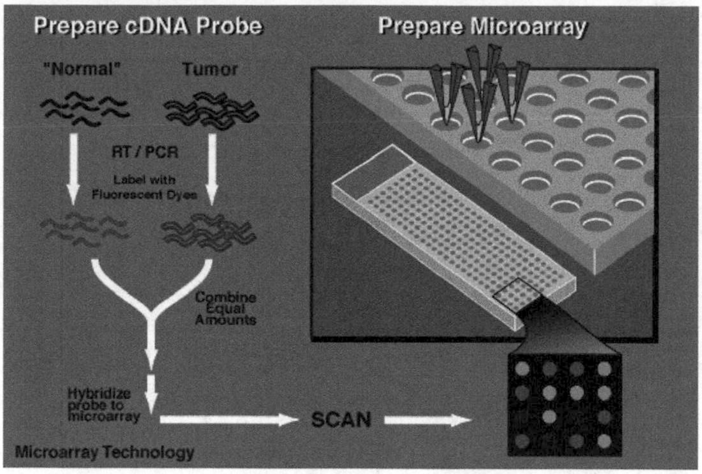

National Human Genome Research Institute (https://www.genome.gov/Pages/Hyperion/DIR/VIP/Glossary/Illustration/microarray_technology.cfm?key=microarray%20technology).

a. DNAs labeled with fluorescent dyes are combined and hybridized to an ordered array of oligonucleotides, which are attached to a glass slide or other solid support. The array is scanned to quantitate the relative fluorescent signals at each site of hybridization.

Microarrays

Microarrays are a hybridization-based approach that takes advantage of advances in microtechnology and bioinformatics. On a microarray, many thousands of oligonucleotides are attached as an ordered array to a small surface, such as a glass slide or silicon wafer.

The number and sequence specificity of the oligonucleotides depend on the specific application. A test sample from an individual is prepared for hybridization to the microarray.

The test sample may be DNA or RNA, but if it is RNA, an in vitro reaction is used to convert it to its complementary DNA (cDNA). The test sample undergoes processing that includes covalent labeling with fluorescent markers; these markers will serve as tags to report sites of hybridization between the test sample and oligonucleotides on the microarray.

Often, two samples (e.g., patient and normal control) are tagged with two different fluorescent markers. The two samples are then combined and hybridized to the microarray. A scanner quantitates the amount of fluorescence at each spot on the array, and complex computer analyses compare relative levels of the two fluorescent markers (Figure 11-3).

Any number of questions can be addressed using microarrays. For example, patterns of gene expression can be characterized through analyses of messenger RNA (mRNA) expressed in specific populations of cells. Alternatively, DNA arrays can be used to determine the genotype or gene sequence at thousands of positions in the genome of an individual. The advent of microarrays has vastly increased the scale of data that can be obtained from molecular analyses of nucleic acids.

11-7 Genetic Basis for Alterations in Drug Response

The goal of pharmacogenetics is to use an individual's genetic profile to optimize drug therapy. This optimization can be achieved by minimizing the likelihood of toxicity while maximizing efficacy by choosing the most effective drug or dose of drug. Genetic variations important to pharmacogenetics can be found in genes encoding drug-metabolizing enzymes, drug transporters, drug targets, and disease-associated enzymes.

Polymorphisms in Genes Involving Drug Metabolism

Genetic variants in genes encoding drug-metabolizing enzymes play a major role in determining drug concentrations and, therefore, dictate drug efficacy and toxicity. Several polymorphic genes are important to drug metabolism (Table 11-2). Enzyme pharmacogenetics has been studied in great detail for many phase I enzymes, including cytochrome P450 isoenzymes, esterases, and dehydrogenases, as well as conjugating phase II enzymes. A few examples are discussed in this section.

Polymorphic Phase I Enzymes

Glucose-6-phosphate dehydrogenase (G6PD) deficiency results in the oxidation of a sulfhydryl group of hemoglobin, causing hemolysis when oxidative drugs are administered. G6PD deficiency is a sex-linked recessive trait with more than 30 known functional polymorphisms affecting individuals of different ethnic backgrounds at differing proportions. Men of African or Mediterranean descent have a high frequency of G6PD deficiency.

The cytochrome P450 (CYP) isoenzyme family consists of more than 50 proteins that metabolize a vast array of drugs. Functional polymorphisms have been discovered in a number of CYP enzymes. In many cases, individuals who possess a variable drug phenotype can be classified as poor, intermediate, rapid, or ultrarapid metabolizers (Table 11-3). Individuals classified as ultrarapid metabolizers can have as many as 13 copies of a functional CYP protein.

CYP2D6 has the largest number of variations of all the CYP enzymes with more than 100 known alleles, and as much as 25% of all medications are metabolized by CYP2D6. Poor metabolizers possess two or more nonfunctional alleles, while ultrarapid metabolizers possess multiple copies of functional alleles. CYP2D6 poor metabolizers are at an increased risk of toxicity during therapy with many antidepressant and antipsychotic drugs because of the decreased metabolism of active metabolites. Conversely, CYP2D6 poor metabolizers are at risk of decreased analgesic response to codeine and tramadol therapy.

CYP2C19 is primarily responsible for inactivating proton pump inhibitors such as omeprazole. Polymorphisms resulting in decreased metabolism of proton pump inhibitors by CYP2C19 can cause increased drug concentrations and, consequently, increased gastric pH, thus leading to an increased cure rate in peptic ulcer treatment. CYP2C19 is responsible for the bioactivation of clopidogrel to the active thiol metabolite in a two-step process. Poor metabolizers of CYP2C19 can have reduced platelet inhibition and can be at an increased risk for adverse cardiovascular events. CYP2C19 ultrarapid metabolizers may have decreased efficacy with the selective serotonin reuptake inhibitors (SSRIs) citalopram and escitalopram, tertiary amine tricyclic antidepressants, and voriconazole because of increased metabolism of active metabolites.

CYP2C9 is responsible for the metabolism of warfarin. Low activity results in decreased warfarin clearance and subsequent increased risk of bleeding. Phenytoin and nonsteroidal anti-inflammatory drugs are also major substrates of CYP2C9; variations resulting in decreased metabolism can result in patients at risk for adverse effects with these agents.

Polymorphic Phase II Enzymes

N-acetyl transferase (NAT) is responsible for the acetylation of arylamine carcinogens and heterocyclic amines. Individuals with slow acetylation activity can experience toxicity, such as hydralazine- and procainamide-induced lupus-like syndrome and sulfonamide hypersensitivity.

UDP-glucuronosyltransferase 1 family, peptide A1 (UGT1A1) isoenzyme is a member of the UGT1A1 superfamily of phase II drug-metabolizing enzymes. It is responsible for the catalysis of the glucuronidation reaction of xenobiotics. In colon cancer, irinotecan is a common treatment option for metastatic disease

TABLE 11-2. Examples of Polymorphic Drug-Metabolizing Enzymes Affecting Drug Response

Enzyme	Medication	Therapeutic implication
CYP2B6	Efavirenz	Possible increased plasma concentrations and decreased clearance of efavirenz in patients with HIV infection compared with patients with normal metabolizer status
CYP2C19	Clopidogrel	Reduced platelet inhibition and increased risk for adverse cardiovascular events in IMs and PMs
	Voriconazole	Decreased likelihood of achieving therapeutic concentrations in UMs with standard dosing
	SSRIs (citalopram, escitalopram)	Possible decreased efficacy in UMs and increased adverse effects in PMs
	Tricyclic antidepressants	Possible decreased efficacy in UMs and increased adverse effects in PMs
	Proton pump inhibitors	Possible decreased efficacy in UMs and improved *Helicobacter pylori* cure rates (along with antibiotics) with decreased CYP2C19 metabolism
CYP2C9	Phenytoin	Increased risk for adverse effects in IMs and PMs
	Warfarin	Decreased metabolism in IMs and PMs; lower initial dosing may be warranted in those with concomitant variations in VKORC1
	NSAIDs	Increased risk for adverse effects in PMs
CYP2D6	Opioid analgesics (codeine, tramadol)	Possible lack of efficacy because of decreased formation of more active metabolites in PMs; possible risk of adverse effects in UMs
	Ondansetron, tropisetron	Decreased likelihood of achieving therapeutic concentrations in UMs with standard dosing
	SSRIs (paroxetine, fluvoxamine)	Possible decreased efficacy in UMs and increased adverse effects in PMs
	Tricyclic antidepressants	Possible decreased efficacy in UMs and increased adverse effects in PMs
	Tamoxifen	Decreased active metabolite (endoxifen) concentrations in IMs and PMs and increased risk of disease recurrence when using it as adjuvant treatment in early breast cancer
	Antipsychotics (aripiprazole, risperidone, brexpiprazole)	Increased risk of adverse effects in PMs with standard dosing
	Atomoxetine	Increased risk of adverse effects in PMs with standard dosing
CYP3A5	Tacrolimus	Lower-dose adjusted trough concentrations in IMs and NMs
DPYD	Capecitabine, fluorouracil, tegafur	Reduced or absent DPYD activity can result in severe toxicity (neutropenia, nausea, vomiting, severe diarrhea, stomatitis, mucositis, hand–foot syndrome)
TPMT	Thiopurines (azathioprine, mercaptopurine, thioguanine)	Increased concentrations of active metabolites and risk of myelosuppression in IMs and PMs; risk of life-threatening myelosuppression in PMs with standard dosing
UGT1A1	Atazanavir	High likelihood of bilirubin-related discontinuation in PMs
	Irinotecan	Increased risk of neutropenia in PMs

PharmGKB (https://www.pharmgkb.org); Clinical Pharmacogenetics Implementation Consortium (https://cpicpgx.org.)
DPYD, dihydropyrimidine dehydrogenase; IM, intermediate metabolizer; NM, normal metabolizer; NSAID, nonsteroidal anti-inflammatory drug; PM, poor metabolizer; SSRI, selective serotonin reuptake inhibitor; UM, ultrarapid metabolizer.

TABLE 11-3. Effect of Phenotype on Metabolism of Medications

Metabolizer	Activity	Effect
Ultrarapid and rapid metabolizer (UM and RM)	Higher-than-normal enzymatic activity	■ Increased metabolism of active drugs that are inactivated by enzyme ■ Generation of active drug metabolites to a greater extent
Normal metabolizer (NM)	Full function enzymatic activity	■ Expected metabolism of drugs inactivated by enzyme ■ Expected generation of active drug metabolites
Intermediate metabolizer (IM)	Decreased enzymatic activity (between normal and poor)	■ Decreased metabolism of active drugs that are inactivated by enzyme compared to normal metabolizers ■ Generation of active drug metabolites to a lesser extent than normal metabolizers
Poor metabolizer (PM)	Little to no enzymatic activity	■ Greatly decreased metabolism of active drugs that are inactivated by enzyme compared to normal metabolizers ■ Generation of active drug metabolites to much less extent than normal metabolizers

as well as other types of solid tumors. Patients who have a protein-deactivating polymorphism in *UGT1A1* can experience severe toxicities, including myelosuppression and diarrhea.

Thiopurine methyltransferase (*TPMT*) encodes a protein responsible for the deactivation of thiopurine drugs (i.e., mercaptopurine, thioguanine, azathioprine). Polymorphisms in *TPMT* that cause a loss of protein function can result in the accumulation of high levels of the cytotoxic thioguanine nucleotide (TGN) metabolites when normal thiopurine drug doses are given (Figure 11-4). Patients with excessively high levels of TGNs are at considerable risk for severe adverse effects such as life-threatening myelosuppression and secondary cancers.

Polymorphisms in Genes Encoding Drug Transporters

Genetic variations in drug transporters can affect the distribution of drugs, which can alter the concentration at the site of action. A few selected examples are discussed in this section.

P-glycoprotein is a well characterized member of the ATP (adenosine triphosphate)-binding cassette (ABC) transporter family; it is encoded by the *ABCB1* gene (also known as the *MDR1* gene), which is known to be highly polymorphic. Numerous studies have demonstrated associations between genetic variations in *ABCB1* and the efficacy or toxicity of medications, including digoxin, simvastatin, ondansetron, and methotrexate.

The solute carrier organic anion transporter family member 1B1 (*SLCO1B1*) gene encodes a membrane-bound organic anion transporter protein (OATP1B1) involved in active transport of endogenous and exogenous substances. It is responsible for the uptake of 3-hydroxy-3-methylglutaryl coenzyme A (HMG-CoA) reductase inhibitors (statins) into the liver. Variations in the *SLCO1B1* gene, resulting in decreased activity of the OATP1B1 transporter, have been associated with increased systemic exposure of simvastatin and increased risk of myopathy.

Polymorphisms in Genes Encoding Drug Targets

Genetic variations in drug targets can alter response and affect efficacy. A few selected examples are shown in Table 11-4 and discussed in this section.

The μ-opioid receptor gene (*OPRM1*) encodes the μ-opioid receptor, which is the primary binding site for endogenous opioid peptides and opioid analgesics. Numerous studies have examined the relationship of variations of *OPRM1* to opioid dose requirements and pain scores. Several studies reported higher

FIGURE 11-4. TPMT Polymorphism Predicts Thiopurine Drug Levels[a]

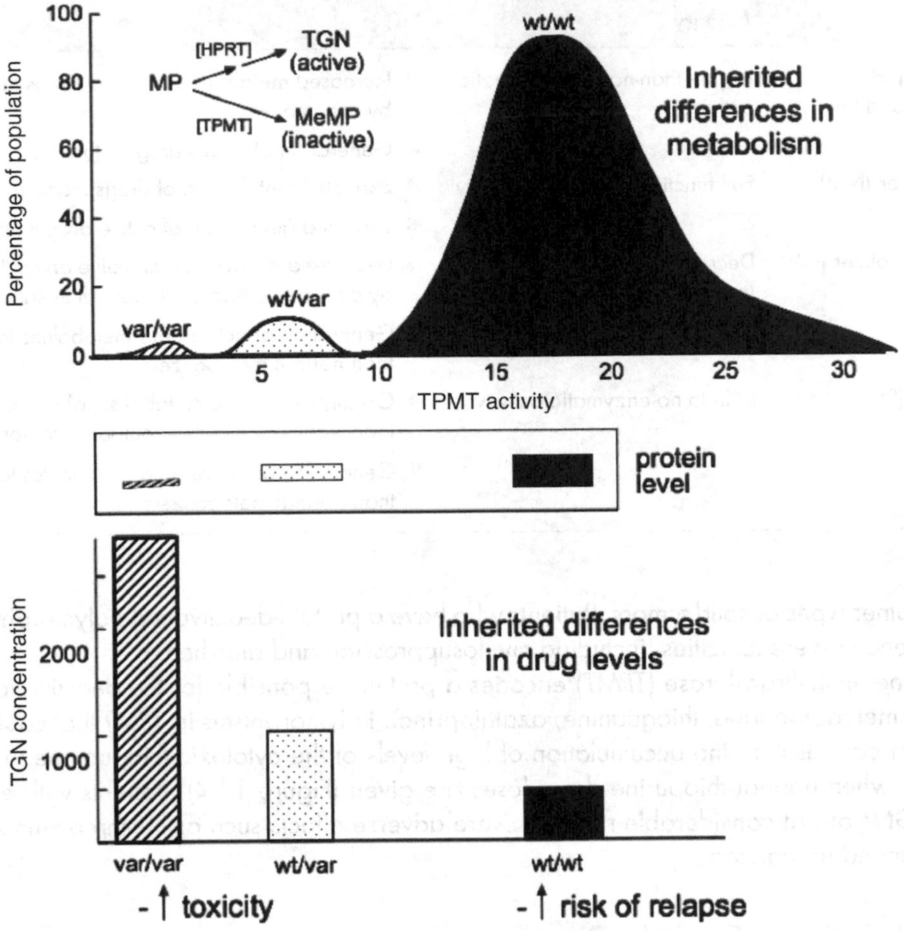

Jones et al., 2007.
HPRT, hypoxanthine phosphoribosyl transferase; MeMP, methylmercaptopurine; MP, mercaptopurine; TGN, thioguanine nucleotide; TPMT, thiopurine methyltransferase; var, variant or dysfunctional alleles; wt, wild-type or normal alleles.
a. MP can be deactivated by TPMT or converted to the active thioguanine nucleotide metabolites catalyzed by HPRT. Polymorphisms in TPMT result in a trimodal population frequency distribution in TPMT protein activity. TPMT protein activity is directly correlated with the level of TPMT protein expressed and is inversely correlated with the cytotoxic TGN metabolite levels.

consumption of intravenous opioids (morphine, fentanyl) postoperatively in patients with one or two copies of the variant allele but other studies have reported no difference.

Vitamin K epoxide reductase complex subunit 1 (*VKORC1*) is the warfarin target gene and is important to the post-translational carboxylation of vitamin K–dependent clotting factors. Polymorphisms in *VKORC1* have been found to account for about 30% of the variation in the required dose. Initial dosing recommendations based on *VKORC1* variations, in addition to CYP2C9, which is involved in the metabolism of warfarin, can be found in the drug label or package insert. A more comprehensive dosing algorithm is also available at http://www.warfarindosing.org.

Targeted Therapy for Somatic Variations in Tumors

For some types of cancers, there are variations in normal signaling pathways that can be targeted by medications designed to interfere with these aberrant pathways.

TABLE 11-4. Examples of Polymorphisms in Drug Target and Disease-Associated Genes

Gene (gene symbol) or protein	Drug class (drug examples)	Response influenced
β_2-adrenergic receptor (ADRB2)	β_2-agonist (albuterol, terbutaline)	Bronchodilation
Arachidonate 5-lipoxygenase (ALOX5)	Leukotriene modifiers (montelukast)	FEV_1 improvement
Ion channels (HERG, KvLQT1, MinK, MiRP1)	Antibiotics (erythromycin, clarithromycin); cholinergic agents (cisapride); antiarrhythmics (quinidine)	Risk of torsades de pointes
Serotonin transporter (5-HTT)	Selective serotonin reuptake inhibitors (e.g., fluoxetine)	Antidepression response
Human leukocyte antigen (HLA-B)	Abacavir, carbamazepine, phenytoin	Hypersensitivity reactions
Factor V Leiden, prothrombin	Estrogen-containing oral contraceptives	Increased risk of deep vein thrombosis and pulmonary embolism
Alpha-adducin (ADD1)	Diuretics (hydrochlorothiazide)	Reduction of blood pressure, risk of heart attack and stroke
Angiotensin-converting enzyme (ACE)	ACE inhibitors (enalapril)	Left ventricular mass reduction, hypotension, renoprotection
β_1-adrenergic receptor (ADRB1)	β-blockers (metoprolol)	Reduction in blood pressure
Dopamine receptors (D3)	Neuroleptics	Adverse effects (i.e., tardive dyskinesia, acute akathisia)
5-hydroxytryptamine (serotonin) receptors	Clozapine	Schizophrenia response

Evans, Relling, 2004; Relling, Giacomini, 2006.
FEV_1, forced expiratory volume in 1 second.

Epidermal growth factor receptor (EGFR) is a tyrosine kinase receptor that plays a key role in regulating cell proliferation. EGFR is overexpressed in some cancers such as non–small cell lung cancer. Tumors with activating mutations that result in EGFR overexpression respond better to the EGFR inhibitor gefitinib than do tumors without overexpression.

v-erb-b2 avian erythroblastic leukemia viral oncogene homolog 2 (HER-2/neu or ERBB2) is a member of the EGFR family of tyrosine kinase receptors. Breast tumors that overexpress HER-2/neu are more likely to recur and, therefore, afford a worse prognosis. Trastuzumab is a monoclonal antibody that targets the HER-2/neu receptor, ultimately halting cell proliferation. It is indicated in the treatment of breast tumors that overexpress HER-2/neu. Studies have shown that patients with metastatic breast cancers that overexpress HER-2/neu respond significantly better to trastuzumab in combination with a taxane (i.e., paclitaxel) than do patients who are treated with a taxane alone.

O-6-methylguanine-DNA methyltransferase (MGMT) is important to DNA repair associated with endogenous and exogenous genomic insults. The MGMT promoter status has been associated with response to alkylating agents (i.e., temozolomide, carmustine) in glioma patients. Patients with a methylated MGMT promoter are more likely to respond to alkylating chemotherapeutics.

Genes with Disease-Associated Polymorphisms

Genes that affect the disease itself or the risk of adverse effects when drugs are given are considered disease-associated genes. Polymorphisms occurring in disease-associated genes can influence the drug-associated efficacy and toxicity. A few selected examples are shown in Table 11-4 and discussed in this section.

Abacavir is an antiviral used in the treatment of HIV/AIDS (human immunodeficiency virus/acquired immune deficiency syndrome) that can lead to life-threatening toxicities that have been associated with genetic variations. Studies suggest that patients who are treated with abacavir and have a specific human leukocyte antigen allele (*HLA-B*5701*) are at risk for developing *abacavir hypersensitivity syndrome*. The *HLA-B*5701* genetic test has been shown to reduce the incidence of this adverse outcome and provide more optimal treatment for patients affected by HIV/AIDS.

Variations in the coagulation factors prothrombin and factor V Leiden are associated with a higher risk of developing a deep vein thrombosis (DVT) and pulmonary embolism (PE). The use of estrogen-containing oral contraceptives is also associated with an increased risk of these thromboembolic disorders, and when they are used by individuals with these variations, the risk increases further.

11-8 Guidance for Use of Pharmacogenetics in Clinical Care

There are more than 140 medications with pharmacogenetic information in the FDA Table of Pharmacogenomic Biomarkers in Drug Labeling. Although a large number of these are genetic biomarkers for targeted therapy in oncology, there are many other drugs with pharmacogenetic information associated with metabolism and hypersensitivity. This information can be found in various sections, including boxed warnings for several drugs. Abacavir and carbamazepine have boxed warnings recommending testing to help prevent hypersensitivity reactions. The boxed warning for codeine reports that respiratory depression and death have occurred in children who received codeine following tonsillectomy or adenoidectomy and had evidence of being ultrarapid metabolizers of codeine. Labeling for the antiplatelet drug clopidogrel warns that patients who are poor metabolizers of CYP2C19 may experience diminished effectiveness of clopidogrel compared with patients with normal function and that one ought to consider a different drug for these patients. Additional drugs with pharmacogenetic information in FDA labeling can be found in the FDA table of pharmacogenomics biomarkers in drug labeling.

Guidelines are now available to help clinicians translate pharmacogenetic results into actionable therapeutic recommendations. The Clinical Pharmacogenetics Implementation Consortium is an international group of more than 200 experts in the field of pharmacogenetics and laboratory medicine who help create peer-reviewed, evidence-based, detailed gene–drug clinical practice guidelines outlining how to use pharmacogenetic information to optimize prescribing. These guidelines can be found at https://cpicpgx.org. Additionally, the Pharmacogenetics Knowledge Base (PharmGKB) is a Web-based comprehensive resource of curated knowledge about genetic variation affecting drug response (https://www.pharmgkb.org).

11-9 Genomic and Proteomic Principles of Disease and Drug Development

Genomic and proteomic studies provide an important resource for current efforts in disease understanding, systems biology, and drug discovery. Research has progressed tremendously through technical achievements that have allowed the high-throughput quantitative analysis of DNA sequence, transcribed RNA, and expressed protein in tissues of interest. Microarrays, two-dimensional gels, and mass spectrometry are vital technologies that provide innovative approaches to identification of drug targets, thus providing a gateway to drug discovery. Association studies have become a key mechanism for linking genomic and proteomic signatures to disease. The principle behind association studies is that if one is given a sample size for a patient group with enough power to detect a significant correlation between the disease and the phenotype of interest, then genes or proteins that are predictive of the phenotype can be identified.

Genomics

Advances in genomics have stimulated the drug regulatory process such that recommendations are frequently made to incorporate genomic studies in clinical study design. The mapping of the whole genome nucleotide sequence (the Human Genome Project) along with common variations (the International HapMap Project) has provided research scientists with the opportunity to perform genomewide association studies (GWASs) to validate drug-associated phenotypes discovered in the clinic.

GWASs are important for the identification of novel drug targets that may predict the phenotype of interest (treatment efficacy versus toxicity). Indeed, such identification does not always lead to a direct relationship between the disease and the associated biological marker, but it does provide grounds for validation through preclinical functional studies and ultimately in independent study populations. The hope for GWASs is that genotypes important to drug response will be determined and used as biomarkers to identify individuals who will respond to specific drugs and to tailor drug doses to optimize treatment outcome.

Clinical studies can be designed to test new drugs in the subset of patients who are more likely to respond to or who have a lower risk of adverse effects from a drug. These studies will provide the opportunity to define drug treatment parameters in the subset of patients who will have the greatest benefit from the drug.

Overall, genomics has redefined how clinical scientists approach drug discovery. The significant amount of available biomolecular information that has evolved over the past decade provides a very rich and a very challenging foundation on which to build.

Emerging Technology

In addition to genomic technologies discussed earlier, other "-omics" are being used to elucidate the differences in drug response, including whole genomic sequencing, epigenomics, and proteomics. Proteomics aims to provide a comprehensive understanding of a set of proteins (proteome) expressed in a cell or tissue at a given point in time. It promises to provide a better understanding of disease and the effective therapies.

Proteomics can be applied in a variety of clinical research environments, with an aim of determining the protein profile of a cell, tissue, or bodily fluid. This information can ultimately be used to compare and contrast profiles of healthy and diseased biomaterials to identify protein differences in the search for novel drug targets.

One goal for proteomic studies is to develop assays that can screen drug candidates by using a comparative analysis approach of reference protein profiles from normal profiles versus diseased profiles.

Proteomics offers the necessary complement to genomic-based studies in drug development by providing a means for identifying and validating novel targets and for understanding the biological consequences of the newly discovered biomarkers, when compared with using either approach alone.

11-10 Questions

1. Pharmacogenomics is the study of

A. how the environment affects drug response.
B. how genes and the environment interact.
C. the effect of a single gene on the response to drug therapy.
D. how multiple genes influence the response to drug therapy.

2. The central dogma of molecular biology describes

A. strand polarity in nucleic acids.
B. the order of chromosomes in the karyotype.
C. the flow of information from genes to proteins.
D. the correspondence between codons in mRNA and anticodons in tRNA.

3. Which of the following methodologies could be used to analyze the amount of mRNA expressed from many genes?

   A. PCR amplification of genomic DNA
   B. DNA sequencing
   C. RNA processing
   D. Microarray analysis

4. The most common genetic variations in humans are

   A. insertion–deletion mutations.
   B. nonsynonymous mutations.
   C. SNPs.
   D. missense mutations.

5. Which of the following statements is true regarding the International HapMap Project?

   A. It was a project initiated with the goal of sequencing the human genome.
   B. Its ultimate goal was to identify the most common human variations in the genome.
   C. It was initiated to study the influence of environmental factors on drug response.
   D. Its goal was to perform genotype-to-phenotype association studies to identify genetic predictors of cancer risk.

6. Genes that affect a disease or the risk of drug-induced adverse effects are considered

   A. drug targets.
   B. disease-associated genes.
   C. drug metabolizers.
   D. drug enhancers.

7. The observable characteristic of an organism is a

   A. genotype.
   B. phenotype.
   C. protein.
   D. haplotype.

8. The large-scale study of the structure and function of proteins is

   A. genomics.
   B. bioinformatics.
   C. proteomics.
   D. biostatistics.

9. A genetic variation that occurs at a frequency of greater than or equal to 1% is considered a

   A. polymorphism.
   B. genotype.
   C. tagSNP.
   D. monogenic trait.

10. Which of the following drugs has a boxed warning including pharmacogenetic information?

    A. Carbamazepine
    B. Aripiprazole
    C. Oxycodone
    D. Warfarin

11. MGMT promoter status is predictive of which of the following clinical responses to drug therapy?

    A. Improved tumor response in hormone-expressing breast tumors
    B. Improved response in non–small cell lung cancer when gefitinib is given
    C. Response to alkylating agents in patients with brain tumors
    D. Response to warfarin therapy in patients with variants in VKORC1

12. Which of the following statements is correct about HER-2/neu expression?

    A. HER-2/neu expression is predictive of the response to warfarin therapy.
    B. Low expression predicts an increased risk for brain tumors.
    C. Low expression in patients with non–small cell lung cancer is a positive prognostic factor.
    D. Overexpression predicts a better response to trastuzumab therapy.

13. Which of the following genetic variations is important to the risk of hypersensitivity reactions after abacavir therapy?

    A. *MGMT*
    B. *HLA-B*5701*
    C. *CYP2C19*
    D. *TPMT*

14. Thiopurine methyltransferase is important to the deactivation of which of the following drugs?

A. Azathioprine
B. Methotrexate
C. Warfarin
D. Irinotecan

15. Which of the following genes is important to the risk of neutropenia with irinotecan therapy?

A. *PACSIN2*
B. *TPMT*
C. *UGT1A1*
D. *EGFR*

16. Omeprazole is primarily inactivated by which cytochrome P450 enzyme?

A. CYP2C19
B. CYP2D6
C. CYP2C9
D. CYP2D6*4

17. The study of how a single gene influences drug response defines the field of

A. proteomics.
B. bioinformatics.
C. pharmacogenomics.
D. pharmacogenetics.

18. Which of the following genes is important to drug-induced bronchodilation in asthmatics?

A. *HLA*
B. *EGFR*
C. *CRHR1*
D. *ADRB2*

19. Individuals who have deactivating mutations in *CYP2D6* and are determined to be poor metabolizers will likely have which of the following type of drug response?

A. Toxicity associated with codeine treatment
B. Toxicity associated with antipsychotic therapy
C. Increased bleeding risk after warfarin therapy
D. Increased response to proton pump inhibitors

20. In the mid-1950s, which of the following genes was found to be important to the risk of hemolysis after primaquine exposure?

A. *G6PD*
B. *TPMT*
C. *CYP2D6*
D. *NAT2*

21. Which of the following drugs has a boxed warning that includes pharmacogenetic information?

A. Carbamazepine
B. Aripiprazole
C. Oxycodone
D. Albuterol

11-11 Answers

1. **D.** The field of pharmacogenomics focuses on how multiple genes determine drug response, whereas pharmacogenetics studies a single gene's influence on drug phenotypes.

2. **C.** The central dogma states that the flow of genetic information is from DNA to RNA to protein. Genes are composed of DNA, which is transcribed to RNA before being translated to protein.

3. **D.** Microarrays can quantitatively analyze patterns of gene expression by measuring levels of hybridization across an array. Although not covered here, modified PCR approaches are capable of quantitating RNA; however, genomic DNA would not be useful for this purpose.

4. **C.** The most common types of DNA variation are single nucleotide polymorphisms. SNPs account for about 90% of genetic variation between individuals.

5. **B.** The ultimate goal of the International HapMap Project was to identify the most common human variations in the genome. This project has provided researchers with the necessary tools to perform candidate gene and genomewide association studies to validate findings discovered in the clinic.

6. **B.** Disease-associated genes can influence a disease or the risk for other phenotypes such as drug-induced adverse effects.

7. **B.** A phenotype is an observable (or measurable) characteristic, such as blood pressure or the activity level of a particular protein.

8. **C.** *Proteomics* is defined as the large-scale study of the structure and function of proteins.

9. **A.** A *polymorphism* is a variation in the genetic sequence occurring at a frequency of greater than or equal to 1%.

10. **A.** Carbamazepine has a boxed warning regarding the risk of serious dermatologic reactions and *HLA-B*1502* allele.

11. **C.** MGMT promoter status is predictive of the response to alkylating agents in patients who have brain tumors.

12. **D.** HER-2/neu overexpression predicts a better response to trastuzumab therapy.

13. **B.** *HLA-B*5701* is a genetic variant that is associated with the risk for hypersensitivity reactions after abacavir therapy.

14. **A.** TPMT is responsible for the deactivation of thiopurine drugs (azathioprine, mercaptopurine, thioguanine).

15. **C.** *UGT1A1* variants are associated with the risk for neutropenia with irinotecan therapy.

16. **A.** The cytochrome P450 enzyme CYP2C19 is primarily responsible for the inactivation of omeprazole. Deactivating polymorphisms can cause decreased metabolism of proton pump inhibitors, resulting in an increased drug concentration and, consequently, an increased gastric pH and ulcer cure rate.

17. **D.** Pharmacogenetics studies a single gene's influence on drug phenotypes.

18. **D.** β_2-adrenergic receptors (encoded by *ADRB2*) are targets for β_2-agonists used in the treatment of asthma.

19. **B.** Deactivating mutations in *CYP2D6* can result in a "poor metabolizer" phenotype and can result in toxicity when antipsychotic drugs are given.

20. **A.** *G6PD* was found to be important to the risk of hemolysis after primaquine exposure.

21. **A.** Carbamazepine, abacavir, clopidogrel, and codeine all have FDA labeling with boxed warnings containing pharmacogenetic information.

11-12 Additional Resources

Caudle KE, Dunnenberger HM, Freimuth RR, et al. Standardizing terms for clinical pharmacogenetic test results: consensus terms from the Clinical Pharmacogenetics Implementation Consortium (CPIC). *Genet Med.* 2017;19(2):215–223.

Cavallari LH, Lam YWF. Pharmacogenetics. In: Dipiro JT, Talbert RL, Yee GC, et al., eds. *Pharmacotherapy: A Pathophysiologic Approach.* 10th ed. New York, NY: McGraw Hill; 2017:e5.

Clinical Pharmacogenetics Implementation Consortium. Guidelines [gene–drug pairs]. Available at: https://cpicpgx.org/guidelines/. Accessed December 8, 2017.

Evans WE, McLeod HL. Pharmacogenomics: drug disposition, drug targets, and side effects. *N Engl J Med.* 2003;348(6):538–549.

Evans WE, Relling MV. Moving towards individualized medicine with pharmacogenomics. *Nature.* 2004;429(6990):464–468.

International HapMap Project. 2012. National Human Genome Research Institute Web site. 2012. https://www.genome.gov/10001688/international-hapmap-project. Accessed March 29, 2018.

Jones TS, Yang W, Evans WE, Relling MV. Using HapMap tools in pharmacogenomic discovery: the thiopurine methyltransferase polymorphism. *Clin Pharmacol Ther.* 2007;81(5):729–734.

Nielsen LM, Olesen AE, Branford R, et al. Association between human pain-related genotypes and variability in opioid analgesia: an updated review. *Pain Pract.* 2015 Jul;15(6):580–594.

PharmGKB Web site. https://www.pharmgkb.org. Accessed December 8, 2017.

Relling MV, Evans WE. Pharmacogenomics in the clinic. *Nature.* 2015;526(7573):343–350.

Relling MV, Giacomini KM. Pharmacogenetics. In: Brunton LL, Lazo JS, Parker KL, eds. *Goodman and Gilman's The Pharmacological Basis of Therapeutics.* 11th ed. New York, NY: McGraw-Hill; 2006: 93–115.

Table of Pharmacogenetic Biomarkers in Drug Labeling. July 2017. U.S. Food and Drug Administration Web site. https://www.fda.gov/downloads/Drugs/ScienceResearch/UCM578588.pdf. Accessed December 8, 2017.

Extemporaneous Compounding and Parenteral and Enteral Products

12

JAMES W. TORR

12-1 KEY POINTS

- Traditional pharmacy compounding involves the triad relationship between the prescriber, patient, and pharmacist.
- Pharmacy compounding is regulated differently than pharmaceutical manufacturing.
- State boards of pharmacy generally regulate pharmacy compounding.
- The U.S. Food and Drug Administration (FDA) regulates pharmaceutical manufacturers and 503B outsourcing facilities.
- The United States Pharmacopeial Convention provides compounders with standards and guidance for the preparation of both sterile and nonsterile compounded formulations.
- The United States Pharmacopeia (USP) identifies three classes of nonsterile preparations: simple, moderate, and complex.
- The USP identifies three microbial risk levels of compounded sterile preparations (CSPs), which are determined according to the corresponding probability of microbial contamination. The three risk levels are low, medium, and high.
- In the absence of stability information applicable to a specific drug and preparation, the USP provides guidance on establishing appropriate beyond-use dates (BUDs).
- A thorough knowledge of and proficiency in pharmacy calculations is required for the extemporaneous compounding of prescriptions.
- Care must be taken to not lose components during the preparation process. Doing so can alter the concentration of active pharmaceutical ingredient(s) in the finished preparation.
- All weighing and measuring must be accurate (avoiding errors of ± 5%).
- Particle size reduction and geometric dilution are essential compounding methods to ensure uniform preparations.

12-2 STUDY GUIDE CHECKLIST

The following topics may guide your study of this subject area:

- [ ] Compare and contrast the characteristics of an extemporaneously compounded preparation with those of a manufactured product.
- [ ] Apply regulatory and professional guidelines pertaining to pharmacy compounding.
- [ ] Apply calculations and procedures required for compounding various dosage forms.
- [ ] Describe the following terms and their application to compounding: geometric dilution, trituration, levigation, and eutectic mixture.
- [ ] Differentiate between the three categories of nonsterile preparations.
- [ ] Differentiate between the microbial risk levels of CSPs.
- [ ] Apply BUD guidelines to compounded preparations that lack stability data.
- [ ] Describe USP Chapter <797> standards for personnel training.

12-3 Pharmacy Compounding

Compounding is defined as the mixing or combining of ingredients to prepare a pharmaceutical preparation customized to meet a patient's needs. The United States Pharmacopeial Convention further defines *compounding* as "the preparation, mixing, assembling, packaging, and labeling of a drug, drug-delivery device, or device in accordance with a licensed practitioner's prescription or medication under an initiative based on the practitioner–patient–pharmacist relationship in the course of professional practice." Additionally, compounding includes the following:

- Preparation of drugs or devices in anticipation of prescription drug orders based on routine, regularly observed prescribing patterns
- Reconstitution or manipulation of commercial products that may require the addition of one or more ingredients because of a licensed practitioner's prescription drug order
- Preparation of drugs or devices for the purposes of, or as incident to, research, teaching, or chemical analysis

In general, pharmacy compounding may be categorized as either sterile or nonsterile. Pharmacists extemporaneously compound medications to provide patients and prescribers options for treatment and therapy in addition to those available commercially. Individualized, custom-prepared medications are needed for several reasons, including but not limited to: (1) the therapeutic agent is unavailable (i.e., discontinued or back ordered by the manufacturer); (2) the preferred dosage form is not available; and (3) the commercial product(s) may contain an offending component such as dyes, preservatives, fillers, and binders. In addition, from time to time, commercially manufactured products are unavailable. Several segments of the population are not sufficiently served by pharmaceutical manufacturers, including pediatric, geriatric, and veterinary patients, as well as patients with rare or complicated diseases. Prescribers and pharmacists working closely with patients may improve quality of life by providing compounded medications that meet their unique needs. Table 12-1 summarizes the differences between compounded preparations and manufactured products.

12-4 Regulations and Guidelines for Compounding

The U.S. Food and Drug Administration (FDA) describes compounding as "a practice in which a licensed pharmacist, a licensed physician, or, in the case of an outsourcing facility, a person under the supervision of a licensed pharmacist, combines, mixes, or alters ingredients of a drug to create medication tailored to

TABLE 12-1. Compounding versus Manufacturing

Compounded preparations	Manufactured products
Regulated by a state board of pharmacy	Regulated by the U.S. Food and Drug Administration (FDA)
Extemporaneously prepared pursuant to a prescription or medication order	Manufactured in FDA-approved facilities in accordance with current good manufacturing practices
Prepared for specific patient in conjunction with the prescriber	Not prepared for specific patient
Labeled with beyond-use dates (BUDs)	Labeled with expiration dates
Not advertised (or limited advertising)	Often advertised and promoted
Not prepared in advance except in the case of documented usage or demand	Prepared in advance and subject to FDA–approved labeling
Not given National Drug Code (NDC) numbers	Given NDC numbers

the needs of an individual patient." Generally, the FDA delegates regulatory responsibility of traditional pharmacy compounding to state boards of pharmacy. Therefore, regulations related to pharmacy compounding will vary by state.

In November 2013, the Drug Quality and Security Act (DQSA) was enacted. The federal law consists, in part, of Sections 503A and 503B. Section 503B addresses outsourcing facilities where sterile dosage forms are compounded in the absence of the traditional compounding three-party team of the prescriber, the patient, and the pharmacist. These facilities compound larger quantities of such dosage forms, register voluntarily with the FDA, must be compliant with good manufacturing processes (GMPs), and are subject to inspection by the FDA. Section 503A addresses traditional pharmacy compounding where the three-party team exists. It clarifies FDA involvement in compounding and recognizes that state boards of pharmacy are responsible for regulatory oversight.

The United States Pharmacopeia (USP) sets quality standards for improving public health. The USP has several chapters intended to enhance the practice of pharmacy compounding. Specific general chapters of importance include USP Chapter <795>, *Pharmaceutical Compounding—Nonsterile Preparations*, and Chapter <797>, *Pharmaceutical Compounding—Sterile Preparations*. USP general Chapter <800>, *Handling Hazardous Drugs in Healthcare Settings*, was published in 2016 and is currently scheduled to be enforceable in 2019. The USP expects that pharmacists engaged in compounding will do so in accordance with state and federal compounding laws as well as FDA regulations and guidelines. Additionally, the American Society of Health-System Pharmacists (ASHP) publishes guidelines such as those for compounding sterile preparations and for the handling of hazardous drugs. Because specific pharmacy compounding regulations vary by state, this chapter focuses on general best practices, such as those outlined by the USP and ASHP.

12-5 Compounded Nonsterile Preparations

Compounded nonsterile preparations are intended for oral, topical, transdermal, or rectal administration. This administration includes, but is not limited to, the following dosage forms: topical and oral solutions, suspensions, and emulsions; solid oral dosage forms (tablets, capsules, and lozenges); suppositories; and topical and oral powders. USP Chapter <795> is intended to assist compounders in preparing nonsterile preparations that are of acceptable strength, quality, and purity.

Categories of Nonsterile Preparations

USP Chapter <795> identifies three general categories of compounded nonsterile preparations. These categories are classified according to their complexity, desired site of action (local or systemic), and risk of harm to compounding personnel or patients:

- ***Simple:*** Preparations that follow an official compendial monograph or peer-reviewed literature
- ***Moderate:***
  - Preparations that require special procedures or calculations
  - Preparations that lack stability data
- ***Complex:*** Preparations that require specialized processes, environment, or equipment to achieve desired outcomes (i.e., systemic effect, specialized drug delivery)

Beyond-Use Dates for Nonsterile Preparations

The *beyond-use date* (BUD) is the date after which a compounded preparation is not to be used. Pharmacists assign BUDs to compounded preparations to guide patients in the proper duration of use and storage of the preparation. BUDs are assigned from the date of preparation. The goal is to provide a BUD that

TABLE 12-2. Maximum Beyond-Use Dates of Nonsterile Compounded Preparations[a]

Beyond-use date	14 days	30 days	6 months
Storage condition	Cold temperature (2–8°C, 36–46°F)	Room temperature (20–25°C, 68–77°F)	Room temperature (20–25°C, 68–77°F)
Preparation type	Oral preparations containing water	Liquid and semisolid topical preparations, dermal-mucosal preparations containing water	Preparations containing no water

United States Pharmacopeia, Chapter <795>.

a. The BUD cannot be greater than the expiration date of any component used to compound the preparation. Inclusion of an antimicrobial agent should be considered, if appropriate. Dispense in a container that reduces exposure to light and moisture.

will allow the patient enough time to fully use the amount of preparation dispensed but not enough time to allow the preparation to degrade, lose potency, or be stored for future use.

In the absence of references on the stability of the specific dosage form compounded or sufficient experience with it, the section "General Guidelines for Assigning Beyond-Use Dates" in USP Chapter <795> is followed. Table 12-2 summarizes beyond-use dating for compounded nonsterile preparations.

12-6 Compounded Sterile Preparations

USP Chapter <797> provides procedures and requirements for compounding sterile preparations, and its contents are intended to apply to health care institutions, pharmacies, physician practice facilities, and other facilities in which sterile compounds are prepared, stored, and dispensed. The chapter covers the following topics:

- Preparations compounded according to the manufacturer's labeled instructions and other manipulations when manufacturing of sterile products expose the original contents to potential contamination
- Preparations containing nonsterile ingredients or using nonsterile components and devices that must be sterilized before administration
- Biologics, diagnostics, drugs, nutrients, and radiopharmaceuticals that possess either of the above two characteristics, including, but not limited to, baths and soaks for live organs and tissues, implants, inhalations, injections, powders for injection, irrigations, metered sprays, and ophthalmic and otic preparations

Sterile compounding, as compared to nonsterile compounding, involves several extra requirements:

- Testing for sterility of compounded preparations
- Using cleaner facilities than are required for nonsterile compounding
- Training and testing personnel in the specific principles and practices of aseptic manipulations
- Evaluating and strictly maintaining air quality

Personnel should maintain basic knowledge of sterilization and solution stability principles and practices. USP Chapter <797> is divided into the following sections:

- Responsibilities of all compounding personnel
- The basis for the classification of compounded sterile preparations (CSPs) into low-, medium-, and high-risk levels, with examples of quality assurance practices in each of the risk levels
- Verification of compounding accuracy and sterilization
- Personnel training and evaluation in aseptic manipulation skills, including representative sterile microbial culture medium transfer and fill challenges

- Environmental quality and control during the processing of sterile preparations
- Equipment used in the preparation of sterile compounding
- Verification of automated compounding devices for parenteral nutrition compounding
- Finished preparation release checks and tests
- Storage and beyond-use dating
- Maintenance of product quality and control after preparations leave the compounding facility, including education and training of personnel
- Packing, handling, storage, and transport of sterile compounding
- Patient or caregiver training
- Patient monitoring and adverse effects reporting
- Quality assurance programs for sterile compounding

Microbial Contamination Risk Levels

USP Chapter <797> assigns risk levels of low, medium, or high according to the corresponding probability of contaminating a preparation with microbial contamination (microbial organisms, spores, and endotoxins) and chemical and physical contamination (foreign chemicals and physical matter). Table 12-3 summarizes beyond-use dating for CSPs.

Low-risk level

Low-risk preparations are compounded with aseptic manipulations entirely within International Organization for Standardization (ISO) Class 5 or better air quality using only sterile ingredients, products, components, and devices.

The compounding involves only transferring, measuring, and mixing manipulations with three or fewer sterile products and two or fewer entries into a single sterile product. Manipulations are limited to aseptically opening ampules, penetrating rubber stoppers on vials with sterile needles, and transferring sterile liquids in sterile syringes to sterile administration devices and packages of other sterile products.

In the absence of passing a sterility test and before administration, a low-risk preparation cannot be stored for a period exceeding the following times: 48 hours at controlled room temperature, 14 days at controlled cold temperature, and 45 days in solid frozen state at –20°C or colder.

Medium-risk level

Multiple individual or small doses of sterile products are combined or pooled to compound a medium-risk preparation that will be administered either to multiple patients or to one patient on multiple occasions.

The compounding process includes complex aseptic manipulations other than the single-volume transfer. It requires an unusually long duration, such as that required to complete dissolution or homogeneous mixing. An example of a medium-risk CSP is a total parenteral nutrition (TPN) intravenous admixture.

TABLE 12-3. CSP Risk Levels and BUDs

	CSP storage		
CSP risk level	**Room temperature**	**Refrigerated**	**Frozen**
Low risk	48 hours	14 days	45 days
Medium risk	30 hours	9 days	45 days
High risk	24 hours	3 days	45 days

United States Pharmacopeia, Chapter <797>.

In the absence of passing a sterility test and before administration, a medium-risk preparation cannot be stored for a period exceeding the following times: 30 hours at controlled room temperature, 9 days at controlled cold temperature, and 45 days in solid frozen state at –20°C or colder.

High-risk level

High-risk conditions apply to the manipulation of manufactured products, especially when their content is exposed to potential contamination, when nonsterile ingredients and components are being used, or when a device is used that should be sterilized before use.

These conditions also apply to sterile ingredients, components, devices, and mixtures that are exposed to air quality inferior to ISO Class 5. This provision includes the storage of opened or partially used packages of manufactured sterile products that lack antimicrobial preservatives in environments inferior to ISO Class 5.

In the absence of passing a sterility test and before administration, a high-risk preparation may not be stored for a period exceeding the following times: 24 hours at controlled room temperature, 3 days at controlled cold temperature, and 45 days in solid frozen state at –20°C or colder.

Stability and Sterility Testing and Dating

Stability is defined as the extent to which a product retains, within specified limits and throughout its period of storage and use (i.e., its shelf life), the same properties and characteristics that it possessed at the time of its manufacture. Five types of generally recognized stability are shown in Table 12-4.

Factors affecting product stability

Stability is affected by both environmental factors and dosage form factors. Environmental factors include exposure to adverse temperatures, light, humidity, oxygen, and carbon dioxide. Dosage form factors include particle size (especially in emulsions and suspensions); pH; solvent system composition (i.e., percentage of "free" water and overall polarity); compatibility of anions and cations; solution ionic strength; primary container; specific chemical additives; and molecular binding and diffusion of drugs and excipients.

Sterility testing

The USP requires testing to ensure that all high-risk sterile preparations for administration by injection into the vascular and central nervous systems are sterile before they are dispensed or administered if (1) they are prepared in groups of more than 25 identical individual single-dose packages (e.g., ampules, bags,

TABLE 12-4. Types of Stability

Type of stability	Conditions maintained throughout the shelf life of the drug product
Chemical	Each active ingredient retains its chemical integrity and labeled potency within the specified limits.
Physical	The original physical properties, including appearance, palatability, uniformity, dissolution, and suspendability, are retained.
Microbiological	Sterility or resistance to microbial growth is retained in accordance with the specified requirements. Antimicrobial agents that are present retain effectiveness within the specified limits.
Therapeutic	The therapeutic effect remains unchanged.
Toxicological	No significant increase in toxicity occurs.

United States Pharmacopeia, Chapter <1191>.

syringes, vials); (2) they are prepared in multidose vials for administration to multiple patients; or (3) they are exposed longer than 12 hours at 2–8°C and longer than 6 hours at warmer than 8°C before they are sterilized.

The membrane filtration method is the method of choice if feasible (e.g., components are compatible with the membrane). The method of direct inoculation of the culture medium is used if the membrane filtration method is not feasible.

Bacterial endotoxin (pyrogen) testing is required of all high-risk sterile preparations for administration by injection into the vascular and central nervous systems.

Storage and beyond-use dating

BUDs for compounded sterile preparations are usually assigned on the basis of professional experience. Assigning these dates requires careful interpretation of appropriate information sources for the same or similar formulations. In rare cases, dates are assigned on the basis of preparation-specific chemical assay results; in such cases, the Arrhenius equation is used to determine expiration dates.

Clean-Room Requirements

Requirements of facilities (clean rooms) for compounding sterile preparations are described in USP Chapter <797>. Facilities should be designed to incorporate primary engineering controls (PECs) and secondary engineering controls (SECs) to provide a suitable environment for the compounding of CSPs. PECs include horizontal and vertical laminar airflow workbenches (LAFWs) that use high-efficiency particulate air (HEPA) filters. These LAFWs are the cornerstone of aseptic processing. SECs include the buffer room and anteroom, which generally provide segregated areas for placement of the PEC.

Clean rooms should have a *buffer room* for measuring, weighing, mixing, and performing other manipulations for preparation of CSPs. The buffer area should have LAFWs to provide an adequate critical-site environment, barrier isolator systems to minimize the extent of personnel contact, and clean rooms separate from the external environment. In every LAFW, unidirectional HEPA filters should provide an ISO Class 5 environment.

In addition to a buffer room, the *anteroom* provides a controlled area for personnel to prepare for entering the buffer room. Personal protective equipment (PPE), such as hair covers, face masks, shoe covers, and isolation gowns, is stored and donned in the anteroom. Sterile gloves, which are the last piece of PPE to be donned, may be donned in the anteroom or buffer room.

Table 12-5 describes the ISO classification of the acceptable number of particles of 0.5 μm or larger per cubic meter of air (current ISO) and per cubic foot that may be present in clean rooms designed for

TABLE 12-5. ISO Clean-Room Classifications

Class name		Particle size	
ISO class	U.S. Federal Standard 209E	ISO, m^3	U.S. Federal Standard 209E, ft^3
3	Class 1	35.2	1
4	Class 10	352	10
5	Class 100	3,520	100
6	Class 1,000	35,200	1,000
7	Class 10,000	352,000	10,000
8	Class 100,000	3,520,000	100,000

United States Pharmacopeia, Chapter <797>.

CSPs. For example, 3,520 particles of 0.5 µm per cubic meter or more (ISO Class 5) is equivalent to 100 particles per cubic foot (Class 100) (1 m^3 = 34.314 ft^3).

In addition to the acceptable number of particles in air, the USP specifies the requirements for air filters, such as the HEPA filter, which is unidirectional and produces the cleanest air free from airborne particulates.

12-7 Personnel Training and Competency for CSP Preparation

USP Chapter <797> notes that before preparing CSPs, compounding personnel must complete training and documentation of training. Concepts of training include skills of gowning and garbing; aseptic technique; provision of appropriate environmental conditions; and procedures for cleaning and disinfecting. The training, provided by expert personnel or other professional resources, should include didactic training with written competence and observed skill assessments. Gowning, garbing, and hand hygiene skills and competency are verified through administration of gloved fingertip sampling. A media-fill test is administered for assurance of aseptic technique. Evaluation of competency should occur initially and periodically on the basis of the risk level of CSPs prepared. Table 12-6 summarizes the minimum evaluation schedule for compounding personnel.

12-8 General Compounding Procedures and Techniques

Mixing

- *Geometric dilution* is the preferred method for mixing components to achieve a uniform and homogenous preparation.
- *Comminution*, defined as particle size reduction to achieve uniform particle size, is generally the first step when compounding with solid components. Comminution is accomplished manually by trituration, levigation, or pulverization by intervention and mechanically by grinders and various types of mills through the manual processes of trituration and levigation or through mechanical processes.
- *Trituration* is used to reduce the particle size of powders to make a greater surface area available.
- *Levigation* is the process of mixing or triturating a powder with a liquid in which it is insoluble to reduce particle size and to aid in incorporating the powder into a liquid or semisolid base.
- *Eutectic mixtures* may be achieved by combining solid ingredients that liquefy when mixed together. Examples include camphor, menthol, methyl salicylate, and thymol.

TABLE 12-6. Competency Evaluation Schedule for Personnel Responsible for Preparing CSPs

	CSP risk level		
Test	Low risk	Medium risk	High risk
Glove fingertip test	At least annually (every 12 months)	At least annually (every 12 months)	At least semiannually (every 6 months)
Media-fill test	At least annually (every 12 months)	At least annually (every 12 months)	At least semiannually (every 6 months)

United States Pharmacopeia, Chapter <797>.

Weighing and Measuring

- Care should be taken during compounding to minimize product loss.
- The sensitivity of the pharmacy balance must be determined, and the minimum weighable quantity must be known for that particular balance.
- When weighing and measuring, the percent error should not exceed ± 5% of the theoretical quantity or volume.
- For finished preparations, the percent error should generally not exceed ± 10% of the theoretical quantity or volume. An exception would be for an official compendial monograph with a specified acceptable range.

Compounded Dosage Forms

On the basis of their physical appearance, extemporaneous preparations may be divided into solids, semisolids, and liquids.

Solid preparations

Solids typically include capsules, powders, lozenges, and suppositories. In preparing these dosage forms, the pharmacist must reduce solid ingredients to the smallest reasonable particle size and ensure that all ingredients are blended together to achieve a homogeneous mixture.

When compounding, the pharmacist should monitor humidity to avoid hydrolysis, dosage form adhesion to containers, and softening of capsule shells. Before packaging and dispensing of a preparation, each dosage form should be evaluated to verify accuracy and consistency.

Capsules

Capsules are the most widely used solid dosage form in pharmaceutical compounding. The powder content (drug plus filler) is usually enclosed in a hard gelatin body that is sealed off by a hard gelatin cap.

This dosage form is intended to be swallowed by the patient. If the patient cannot swallow the capsule, the capsule can be opened and the contents mixed with food or drink according to the pharmacist's instructions.

Lactose is the main excipient (filler) used to prepare capsules. The pharmacist mixes the drug (mixed geometrically with lactose) before filling each capsule by hand. Colors can be added to capsules to ensure proper mixing. Capsule filling machines are available to assist the compounder when preparing capsules.

Capsule size is assigned according to the following rule:

Capsule size	0	1	2	3	4	5
Fill weight in grams	0.390	0.325	0.260	0.195	0.130	0.065

Example:

Rx:

Estriol	200 mg
Estrone	25 mg
Estradiol	25 mg
Lactose	qs

Procedures:

1. Calculate the quantity of each ingredient required for the prescription.
2. Accurately weigh each ingredient.
3. Using geometric dilution, mix the estrogen powders.

4. Depending on the size of the capsule, fill each capsule completely with each ingredient, and determine the total weight.
5. Set up a ratio between the weight that fills the capsule completely with each ingredient separately and with the one filled with lactose only. This ratio will enable a compounder to determine the weight of lactose that is equal to each ingredient in the capsule.
6. Determine the amount of lactose needed to prepare the prescription by subtracting the total weight of lactose that fills all the capsules from the equivalent weight of lactose to each drug in the content.
7. Mix drug content with lactose needed geometrically.
8. Fill the capsules by hand or use the Jaansun machine.
9. Package and label the preparation.

Suppositories

Suppositories are solid dosage forms used to administer medicine through the rectum, vagina, or urethra. After insertion, they soften or melt by body temperature.

Several bases are used with suppositories: oil-soluble bases such as cocoa butter; hydrogenated vegetable oils derived from triglycerides such as Fattibase, Wecobee, and Witepsol; and water-soluble bases such as polyethylene glycol (PEG) 300, 400, 1450, 3350, 6000, and 8000.

Example:

Rx:

Progesterone	50 mg
PEG 8000	50%
PEG 1450	30%
PEG 300	20%

Procedures:

1. Calculate the quantity of each active ingredient required for the prescription.
2. Prepare the required base by melting each PEG to 50–60°C.
3. After determining how much base mixture is needed to fill one suppository, pour the base into a beaker and mark the level.
4. Remove some of the base, and add the drug.
5. Add base to the marked level.
6. Pour the mixture into the mold, and refrigerate.
7. Package and label the preparation.

Semisolid preparations

Semisolid dosage forms include creams (emulsions), topical gels, lotions (suspensions), ointments, and pastes. When compounding any of these dosage forms, the pharmacist should prepare an excess amount of the total formulation to allow the prescribed quantity to be accurately dispensed.

The pharmacist is also advised to pay attention to the following: not using ingredients that are caustic or irritating and thoroughly comminuting solids that are abrasive to the mucous membranes, selecting a base that allows active ingredients to provide the intended local or systemic therapeutic effect, and reducing solid ingredients to the smallest reasonable particle size before mixing with the semisolid base. Active ingredients and excipients (inactive ingredients) should be incorporated by geometric dilution to achieve an acceptable uniformity of the dispersion. Spreading a thin film of a finished semisolid formulation on a flat transparent surface (e.g., clear glass ointment slab) may be performed to visually inspect for uniformity.

Ointments and creams

Ointments and creams are semisolid topical preparations. Ointments are made of oleaginous bases such as petrolatum, absorption bases such as petrolatum with lanolin, or water-soluble bases such as PEG ointments. Creams are oil-in-water or water-in-oil emulsions.

Ointments and creams contain waxes and other fatty materials. Ointments have no water, whereas creams contain water up to 50% or more. Surfactants are added to creams to emulsify the oil or water. The most often used surfactants are Tween 80, Span 80, and sodium lauryl sulfate.

Ointments and creams are prepared by heating the waxes on a hot plate and mixing with other ingredients on an ointment slab or in a casserole.

Gels

Gels are classified as two-phase systems: (1) a polymer that forms a three-dimensional network of particles or solvated macromolecules of the dispersed phase, and (2) an aqueous or an alcoholic solvent. Polymers used to prepare gels are bentonite, gelatin, tragacanth, alginic acid, carboxymethylcellulose sodium, colloidal silicon dioxide, methylcellulose, polyvinyl alcohol, carbomer, and poloxamer (Pluronic).

Example:

Rx:

Ketoprofen	10 g
Lecithin-isopropyl palmitate	22 mL
Pluronic F-127 30% gel qs	100 mL

Procedures:

1. Calculate the quantity of each ingredient required for the prescription.
2. Accurately weigh or measure each ingredient.
3. Add the ketoprofen to the lecithin-isopropyl palmitate solution, and mix well.
4. Add sufficient Pluronic F-127 gel to volume, and mix well.
5. Package and label the preparation.

Liquid preparations

Liquid dosage forms include emulsions, solutions, and suspensions. When compounding these dosage forms, the pharmacist has to prepare a 2–3% excess amount of the total formulation to allow for accurate dispensing of the prescribed amount.

Solutions and suspensions

Solutions are liquid preparations containing one or more drug substances dispersed in a suitable solvent or a mixture of miscible solvents. *Suspensions* are liquid preparations containing one or more drug substances dispersed in a solvent such as water; however, the drug is insoluble in the solvent.

Oral solutions contain solubilization agents (surfactants) to improve the solubility of the drug in water or, in the case of suspensions, wetting agents (surfactants) to improve the dispersing ability of the solid drug in the aqueous phase. These surfactants have hydrophilic and hydrophobic groups. The most common surfactant is Tween 80.

Buffers are used to adjust the pH of the medium to improve solubility or stability of the solution. Buffers used are hydrochloric acid, citric acid, acetic acid, and sodium phosphate.

Viscosity-increasing agents are used in suspensions to reduce the sedimentation rate of solid particles. These agents are polymers such as hydroxymethyl or propyl cellulose.

Sweetening agents such as sucrose, aspartame, sorbitol, and cherry syrup are used to add flavor to solutions and suspensions.

Aqueous suspensions are prepared by levigating the powder mixture to a smooth paste with an appropriate wetting agent. This paste is converted to a free-flowing fluid by adding adequate vehicle. Successive portions of the vehicle are used to wash the mortar or other vessel and to transfer the suspension quantitatively to a calibrated dispensing bottle or graduate. The preparation may be homogenized to ensure a uniform final dispersion, and solid ingredients should be reduced to the smallest reasonable particle size.

Solutions should contain no visible undissolved matter when dispensed. Emulsions and suspensions are labeled "Shake well before using."

Parenteral preparations

Parenteral preparations include standard injections (i.e., intravenous, intramuscular, intradermal, subcutaneous, intrathecal, epidural); parenteral admixtures; and parenteral nutrition.

The following ingredients are used to prepare parenteral formulations:

- A solvent such as water is the primary solvent. Co-solvents, such as ethyl alcohol, glycerin, polyethylene glycol (PEG), and propylene glycol, are secondary solvents.
- Buffers are used to adjust the pH of the solution for solubility and stability reasons (e.g., phosphate, citrate, acetate).
- Preservatives are used to prevent bacterial growth in the preparations (benzalkonium chloride 0.01%, benzyl alcohol 1–2%, thimerosal 0.01%).
- Antioxidants are used to enhance stability (ascorbic acid 0.01–0.5%, sodium bisulfate 0.1–1%, sodium metabisulfite 0.1–1%).
- Surfactants are used to increase the solubility of the drug (Tween 80 0.1–0.5%, Span 80 0.05–0.25%).
- Complexation and chelating agents such as EDTA (ethylenediaminetetraacetic acid) 0.01–0.075% are used to improve stability.

Example:

Rx:

Doxorubicin hydrochloride 2 mg/mL	80 mL
Vincristine sulfate 1 mg/mL	4 mL
0.9% sodium chloride injection	qs 100 mL

Procedures:

1. Calculate the quantity of each ingredient required for the prescription.
2. Reconstitute the doxorubicin hydrochloride, if necessary, according to the manufacturer's directions.
3. Carefully measure the required volumes of the reconstituted doxorubicin hydrochloride solution and the vincristine sulfate injection.
4. Add the measured volumes of doxorubicin hydrochloride and vincristine sulfate injections to a sterile container.
5. Add 16 mL of 0.9% sodium chloride injection to the container, and mix well.
6. Withdraw the solution into a sterile syringe, and fill the required reservoir or administration device container.
7. Expel any excess air, and seal the reservoir or container.
8. Package and label the preparation.

Note: All procedures should be carried out in a clean-air environment.

12-9 Dosage Form Preparation Calculations

Capsule Calculations

The following example demonstrates the dosage form calculation for capsules.

Rx:

Diphenhydramine hydrochloride	25 mg
Acetaminophen	325 mg
Lactose	qs

Make 30 capsules size 1:

1. Determine the amount of each drug and of lactose that fully fills a size 1 capsule:

Diphenhydramine hydrochloride	400 mg
Acetaminophen	425 mg
Lactose	475 mg

2. Calculate the diluent displacement weights for the two drugs:

$$\text{Weight of drug in filled capsule/weight of lactose in filled capsule} =$$
$$\text{Weight of drug per capsule/lactose displacement } (x)$$

Diphenhydramine:

400 mg/475 mg = 25 mg/x
x = 29.69 mg of lactose are displaced by 25 mg of diphenhydramine per capsule
For 30 capsules: 29.69 mg × 30 = 0.89 g lactose

Acetaminophen:

425 mg/475 mg = 325 mg/x
x = 363.24 mg of lactose are displaced by 325 mg of acetaminophen per capsule
For 30 capsules: 363.24 mg × 30 = 10.90 g lactose

3. Total amount of lactose needed to prepare this prescription:
Amount of lactose needed per capsule (qs) = 475 mg – (29.69 mg + 363.24 mg) = 82.07 mg
Amount of lactose needed for 30 capsules = 82.07 mg × 30 = 2.46 g

Ointment Calculations

The following example shows the dosage form calculation for an ointment.

Rx:

Sulfur	2 g
Salicylic acid	2 g
Calamine	5 g
Urea	2 g
Hydrophilic petrolatum qs	100 g

1. Weigh total amounts of sulfur, salicylic acid, calamine, and urea.
2. Triturate (reduce particle size) each powder in a porcelain mortar, and mix geometrically.
3. Add small amounts of mineral oil, and levigate with the solid mixture until a paste has formed. Determine the weight of mineral oil used.
4. Amount of hydrophilic petrolatum needed qs to 100 g:

$$x = 100\text{ g (total weight ointment)} - 11\text{ g (solid mixture)}$$
$$- \text{ weight of mineral oil used to levigate the solid mixture}$$

Suppository Calculations

Suppository calculations can be made using the density factor or using a PEG base.

Using the density factor

$$\text{Density factor} = \frac{B}{A - C - B}$$

where *A* is the average weight of a blank suppository, *B* is the weight of medication per suppository, and *C* is the average weight of a medicated suppository.

Rx:

Acetaminophen	300 mg
Cocoa butter	qs

Make 12 suppositories:

Note: The average weight of the cocoa butter blank is 2 g, and the average weight of a medicated suppository is 2.3 g.

1. The density factor for acetaminophen is 0.5.
2. The weight of base that was replaced by drug is 0.3/0.5 = 0.6 g base.
3. The weight of base to prepare one suppository is 2 – 0.6 = 1.4 g.
4. The weight of base to prepare 12 suppositories is 1.4 g × 12 = 16.8 g.
5. The weight of acetaminophen for 12 suppositories is 0.3 × 12 = 3.6 g.
6. Weigh 16.8 g of cocoa butter and heat in a beaker to 38°C until it becomes a liquid, and then mix with 3.6 g of acetaminophen.
7. Pour molten suppositories into a metal mold, and wait until it is congealed.

Using a PEG base

Rx:

Acetaminophen	50 mg
Base qs	2.4 g

Make 12 suppositories:

Base:

PEG 400	30%
PEG 1450	30%
PEG 8000	40%

1. Total weight of acetaminophen needed is 50 mg × 12 = 600 mg.
2. Total weight of 12 suppositories is 2.4 g × 12 = 28.8 g.
3. Weight of PEG base needed is 28.8 g – 0.6 g (acetaminophen) = 28.2 g.
4. Weight of PEG 400 needed is 28.2 g × 0.3 = 8.46 g.
5. Weight of PEG 1450 needed is 28.2 g × 0.3 = 8.46 g.
6. Weight of PEG 8000 needed is 28.2 g × 0.4 = 11.28 g.
7. Heat the PEG bases to 55°C and mix, and then add 0.6 g of acetaminophen to the mixture and mix well.
8. Pour the mixture into the mold, and wait until it is congealed.

Oral Solution Calculations

The following example illustrates the dosage form calculation for an oral solution.

Rx:

Dimenhydrinate	250 mg
Glycerin	qs
Ora-Plus	50 mL
Ora-Sweet qs	100 mL

Sig. 12.5mg/5mL oral solution

1. Dissolve 250 mg of dimenhydrinate in the smallest quantity of glycerin in a beaker.
2. Add 50 mL of Ora-Plus to the drug–glycerin mixture, and mix well.

3. Transfer the mixture to a 100 mL graduated cylinder, and qs to 100 mL with Ora-Sweet. Each teaspoon contains 12.5 mg of dimenhydrinate.

Oral Suspension Calculations

The dosage form for an oral solution can be calculated as shown in the following example.

Rx:

Progesterone, micronized	4 g
Glycerin	5 mL
Methylcellulose 1% solution	50 mL
Flavored syrup qs	100 mL

1. Levigate the progesterone with glycerin (levigating agent) in a glass mortar.
2. Add 50 mL of methylcellulose 1% solution (suspending agent) to the mortar, and mix thoroughly.
3. Transfer the mixture to a graduated cylinder, and qs with flavored syrup to 100 mL.

12-10 Questions

1. What agency generally regulates traditional pharmacy compounding?

A. FDA
B. USP
C. PCAB
D. State boards of pharmacy

2. Which USP general chapter provides guidance for nonsterile compounding?

A. <797>
B. <1075>
C. <795>
D. <800>

3. Which USP general chapter provides guidance for sterile compounding?

A. <1075>
B. <797>
C. <795>
D. <800>

4. According to the USP, how would nonsterile preparations that follow an official compendial monograph or peer-reviewed literature be categorized?

A. Simple
B. Moderate
C. Complex
D. Low risk

5. Which of the following actions by a compounding pharmacist would be outside the scope of traditional pharmacy compounding and require FDA enforcement action?

A. Compounding of drugs in anticipation of prescription drug orders based on routine, regularly observed prescribing patterns
B. Compounding of drug preparations as a result of the prescriber–patient–pharmacist relationship triad
C. Compounding of drugs for third parties who resell to individual patients or offering of compounded drug products at wholesale to other state-licensed persons or commercial entities for resale
D. Compounding of drug preparations for the purpose of, or as incident to, research, teaching, or chemical analysis

6. Which federal legislation enacted in November 2013 amended the Food, Drug, and Cosmetic Act to make a distinction between traditional pharmacy compounding regulated by a state board of pharmacy and a compounding outsourcing facility regulated by the FDA?

A. Drug Quality and Security Act
B. Food and Drug Administration Modernization Act
C. Pharmacy Compounding Compliance Act
D. American Medicinal Drug Use Clarification Act

7. Compared to a manufactured product, a compounded preparation has which of the following characteristics?

A. Made according to current GMP
B. Subject to an approved NDA
C. Is patient specific in conjunction with the prescriber
D. Has an NDC number

8. Which of the following techniques is commonly used to prepare even dispersion of ingredients and homogenous compounded preparations?

A. Comminution
B. Geometric dilution
C. Levigation
D. Trituration

9. Consider a compounding formula of 30 g of diltiazem 0.3% ointment. What is the maximum acceptable weight range for dispensing the preparation?

A. 29–31 g
B. 27–33 g
C. 24–36 g
D. 21–39 g

10. According to USP Chapter <795>, for which of the following preparations would a beyond-use date of 6 months at room temperature be most appropriate?

A. Water-containing oral preparations
B. Water-containing, topical semisolid formulations
C. Water-containing, topical liquid formulations
D. Non-water-containing (nonaqueous) solid formulations

11. According to USP Chapter <797>, what is the maximum BUD for a medium-risk-level CSP stored under refrigeration?

A. 45 days
B. 14 days
C. 9 days
D. 3 days

12. Which of the following types of preparations are considered parenteral preparations? (Mark all that apply.)

A. Intrathecal
B. Intradermal
C. Epidural
D. Topical

13. What is a function of surfactants in suspension preparations?

A. Wetting agent
B. Improve solubility
C. Improve stability
D. Improve palatability

14. Which of the following statements describes a difference between ointments and gels?

A. Ointments have water.
B. Gels are aqueous, two-phase systems.
C. Gels contain petrolatum.
D. Ointments are aqueous, two-phase systems.

15. In the compounding of suppositories, the density factor represents the ratio

A. between the weight of the drug and the weight of the base replaced by the drug.
B. between the weight of the drug and the weight of the base.
C. between the weight of the drug and the weight of the medicated suppository.
D. between the weight of the drug and the weight of a blank suppository.

16. According to USP Chapter <797>, what CSP risk level should be designated to CSPs prepared with nonsterile components?

A. High risk
B. Medium risk
C. Low risk
D. No risk

17. The maximum number of particles of 0.5 µm allowed in 1 m^3 under ISO Class 5 conditions is

A. 35,200 particles.
B. 3,520 particles.
C. 352,000 particles.
D. 3,520,000 particles.

18. According to the USP, which of the following preparations requires the bacterial endotoxin test?

A. Every low-risk preparation
B. Every medium-risk preparation
C. Every high-risk preparation
D. Every CSP

19. According to USP Chapter <797>, what minimum ISO classification is required for HEPA-filtered air within a laminar airflow workbench?

A. ISO Class 6
B. ISO Class 5
C. ISO Class 8
D. ISO Class 4

20. According to USP Chapter <797>, after initial passage of the glove fingertip competency evaluation, what is the minimum frequency for reevaluation of compounding personnel responsible for preparing high-risk-level CSPs?

A. At least monthly
B. At least quarterly
C. At least semiannually
D. At least annually

12-11 Answers

1. **D.** The regulation of pharmacy compounding is generally regulated by individual state boards of pharmacy. This is true for pharmacies operating as traditional pharmacies (i.e., compounding is performed for specific patients, pursuant to a valid prescription). Pharmacies operating outside of this scope may be subject to FDA jurisdiction.

2. **C.** USP Chapter <795> describes the major requirements for nonsterile compounding to which every pharmacist should adhere.

3. **B.** USP Chapter <797> describes the major requirements for sterile compounding to which every pharmacist should adhere.

4. **A.** USP Chapter <795> categorizes nonsterile compounding into three categories: simple, moderate, and complex. Nonsterile preparations that follow an official compendial monograph or peer-reviewed literature would be categorized as simple.

5. **C.** The FDA states that compounding drugs for third-party resale to individual patients or at wholesale to other state-licensed persons or commercial entities is not within the traditional scope of pharmacy compounding. For example, the prescriber–patient–pharmacist relationship is not established.

6. **A.** The Drug Quality and Security Act was enacted in November 2013. The Pharmacy Compounding Compliance Act does not exist, and the other federal acts were enacted before November 2013.

7. **C.** Extemporaneous pharmacy compounding requires the three-party team of physician, patient, and pharmacist in which the physician writes a prescription requiring the pharmacist to compound a preparation for a specific patient. All the other characteristics are for pharmaceutical manufactured products.

8. **B.** Geometric dilution is a mixing process used for even dispersion of ingredients and for promoting of a homogenous preparation. Comminution is a method for particle size reduction. Trituration and levigation are methods of comminution.

9. **B.** When determining the percent error for a preparation, the maximum acceptable error is generally ± 10%. 30 g × 0.9 = 27 g, and 30 g × 1.1 = 33 g.

10. **D.** Usually, solid formulations are more stable than other types of formulations. According to USP Chapter <795>, in the absence of stability data, nonaqueous preparations may be given a 6-month BUD.

11. **C.** In the absence of stability data, USP Chapter <797> defines the maximum BUDs for low-, medium-, and high-risk level CSPs. A medium-risk-level CSP may be stored under refrigeration for 9 days.

12. **A, B, C.** Parenteral preparations involve intrathecal, intradermal, and epidural delivery. Compounded topical preparations are considered nonsterile dosage forms.

13. **A.** The surfactant tends to lower the surface tension between solid surfaces and liquids, thus improving the wetting ability.

14. **B.** Gels are highly aqueous two-phase systems, whereas ointments consist of oleaginous (fatty) bases such as petrolatum.

15. **A.** The density factor is used to determine the amount of suppository base replaced by the presence of the drug.

16. **A.** USP Chapter <797> designates CSPs prepared using nonsterile components and nonsterile equipment and processes as high-risk level.

17. **B.** ISO Class 5 allows 3,520 particles per cubic meter.

18. **C.** The bacterial endotoxin test is required of all high-risk preparations because of the fear of contamination.

19. **B.** HEPA filters should provide ISO Class 5 air within the LAFW.

20. **C.** USP Chapter <797> states that compounding personnel responsible for preparing high-risk-level CSPs shall undergo competency evaluation at least semiannually (i.e., every 6 months).

12-12 Additional Resources

Allen LV Jr. *The Art, Science, and Technology of Pharmaceutical Compounding.* 5th ed. Washington, DC: American Pharmacists Association; 2016.

American Society of Health-System Pharmacists. ASHP Guidelines on Compounding Sterile Preparations. *AM J Health-Syst Pharm.* 2014;71(2):145–166. Available at: https://www.ashp.org/-/media/assets/policy-guidelines/docs/guidelines/compounding-sterile-preparations.ashx. Accessed November 28, 2017.

American Society of Health-System Pharmacists. ASHP Guidelines on Handling Hazardous Drugs. *AM J Health-Syst Pharm.* 2006;63:1172–1193. https://www.ashp.org/-/media/assets/policy-guidelines/docs/guidelines/handling-hazardous-drugs.ashx. Accessed November 28, 2017.

Compounding and the FDA: questions and answers. U.S. Department of Health and Human Services, Food and Drug Administration Web site. https://www.fda.gov/Drugs/GuidanceComplianceRegulatoryInformation/PharmacyCompounding/ucm339764.htm. Accessed November 28, 2017.

United States Pharmacopeia. Chapter 795: Pharmaceutical compounding—nonsterile preparations. In: *United States Pharmacopeia and National Formulary* (USP 41-NF 36). Rockville, MD: United States Pharmacopeia; 2018.

United States Pharmacopeia. Chapter 797: Pharmaceutical compounding—sterile preparations. In: *United States Pharmacopeia and National Formulary* (USP 41-NF 36). Rockville, MD: United States Pharmacopeia; 2018.

United States Pharmacopeia. Chapter 1191: Stability considerations in dispensing practice. In: *United States Pharmacopeia and National Formulary* (USP 41-NF 36). Rockville, MD: United States Pharmacopeia; 2018.

United States Pharmacopeial Convention. *United States Pharmacopeia 41/National Formulary 36.* Rockville, MD: United States Pharmacopeial Convention; 2017.

U.S. Food and Drug Administration. *Guidance for FDA Staff and Industry: Compliance Policy Guides Manual, Sec. 460.200 Pharmacy Compounding.* Rockville, MD: U.S. Department of Health and Human Services, Food and Drug Administration, Office of Regulatory Affairs, Center for Drug Evaluation and Research; 2002.

U.S. Food and Drug Administration. Section 503A of the Federal Food, Drug, and Cosmetic Act. U.S. Department of Health and Human Services, Food and Drug Administration, Office of Regulatory Affairs, Center for Drug Evaluation and Research, Rockville, MD; 2002. Available at: https://www.fda.gov/Drugs/GuidanceComplianceRegulatoryInformation/PharmacyCompounding/ucm376733.htm. Accessed November 28, 2017.

Fundamentals of Pharmacy Practice

13

GLEN E. FARR

13-1 KEY POINTS

- The Pharmacists' Patient Care Process is applicable to any practice setting where pharmacists provide patient care. It includes collecting, assessing, planning, implementing, monitoring, and evaluating the delivery of patient care.
- Characteristics of tertiary, secondary, and primary literature resources differ and are sources of evidence-based drug information.
- Accurate, up-to-date, and unbiased drug information from various sources, particularly the Internet, should be determined by assessment of the reliability of the source before its use.
- The U.S. Food and Drug Administration (FDA) has programs on medication safety, which include a system to manage medication risk through risk evaluation and mitigation strategies (REMSs) and the issuance of boxed warnings in drug package inserts.
- Three price measures are typically used for the payment system for prescription drugs in the retail pharmacy market: average manufacturer price, average wholesale price, and wholesale acquisition cost.
- The Institute for Safe Medication Practices has resources and notices to help health care practitioners prevent errors and ensure that medications are used safely.
- Adverse drug effects and medication errors should be reported to the FDA MedWatch Web site; after clinical review, these adverse drug effects and medication errors become part of the FDA Adverse Event Reporting System.
- All medications that are out-of-date or no longer needed should be safely disposed of as described by the Drug Enforcement Administration.
- Because three of four patients do not adhere to medication instructions, pharmacists should counsel patients on ways to remember to take a prescribed medication and to fill a prescription. In addition, pharmacists should counsel patients to avoid both taking more or less than the recommended dosage and substituting an over-the-counter medication or dietary supplement for the prescribed medication.
- Pharmacist impairment from substance abuse, alcoholism, or behavioral disorders leads to poor performance, which jeopardizes patient care and increases risk of patient harm. Impaired pharmacists can seek help from a pharmacist recovery network.
- Pharmacists function as managers of the pharmacy team members, general operations, and the medication use system. In this managerial role, having communication and problem-solving skills will allow pharmacists to maximize productivity and foster a positive workplace.

13-2 STUDY GUIDE CHECKLIST

The following topics may guide your study of this subject area:

- ☐ Familiarity with the delivery of patient care as described in the *Pharmacists' Patient Care Process*
- ☐ The characteristics of literature sources for drug information and the hierarchy of evidence
- ☐ Factors to consider when responding to drug information requests from health care providers or patients
- ☐ Awareness of "sound alike, look alike" drugs and confusing abbreviations
- ☐ Medications that have REMSs or boxed warnings
- ☐ The way to report an adverse drug effect or a medication error to the FDA's MedWatch
- ☐ Procedure for the disposal of out-of-date or unused drugs versus controlled substances
- ☐ Factors leading to medication nonadherence and counseling points to minimize its negative consequences
- ☐ Assistance for impaired pharmacists through a pharmacist recovery network
- ☐ General drug supply chain and the flow of drug costs
- ☐ Principles of management in a pharmacy practice
- ☐ Successful strategies for effective communication with patients, health care professionals, coworkers, and supervisors

13-3 Overview

Pharmacy practice encompasses a plethora of different knowledge, skills, and attitudes. There are numerous fundamentals necessary for good pharmacy practice. Many of these principles will be addressed in subsequent chapters of this text. However, some of the more general fundamentals are discussed in this chapter.

Recognizing the need for a consistent process in the delivery of patient care across the profession, in 2014 the Joint Commission of Pharmacy Practitioners released the Pharmacists' Patient Care Process. The process is applicable to any practice setting where pharmacists provide patient care and any patient care service provided by pharmacists. Using principles of evidence-based practice, pharmacists practicing patient-centered care should perform the following processes: collect, assess, plan, implement, monitor, and evaluate. To optimize pharmacist-provided patient care, pharmacists should incorporate these five fundamental elements into practice (Figure 13-1).

Collect necessary subjective and objective information about patients to understand their relevant medical and medication history and clinical status. Pharmacists can use multiple sources, including existing patient records, the patient, and other health care providers. This process includes collecting the following:

- A current medication list and medication use history for prescription and nonprescription (over-the-counter [OTC]) medications, herbals, and other dietary supplements
- Relevant health data, which may include medical history, health and wellness information, biometric test results, and physical assessment findings
- Patient lifestyle habits, preferences and beliefs, health and functional goals, and socioeconomic factors that affect access to medications

Assess the information collected and analyze the clinical effects of patients' therapy in the context of their overall health goals to identify and prioritize problems and achieve optimal care. This process includes assessing all medication for appropriateness, effectiveness, safety, and patient adherence. When appropriate, a pharmacist should determine immunization status, the need for preventive care, and other health care services.

FIGURE 13-1. Model of the Pharmacists' Patient Care Process

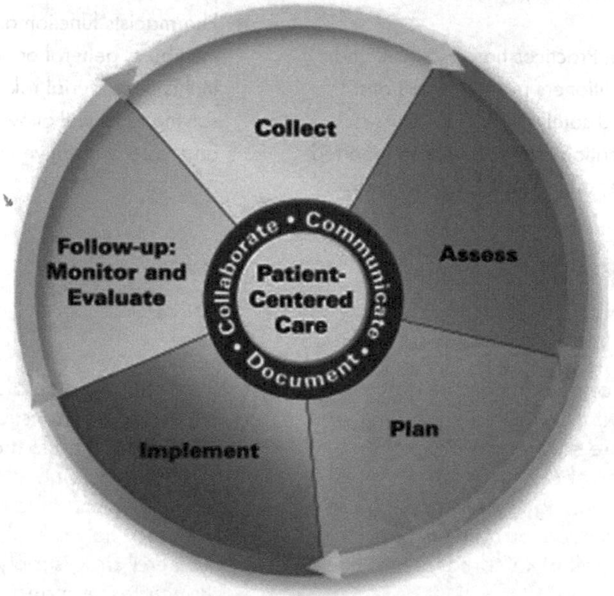

Joint Commission of Pharmacy Practitioners, 2014.

In collaboration with other health care professionals and with the patient or caregiver, develop a care **plan** that is evidence based and cost-effective. It should address medication-related problems and optimize medication therapy. The plan should engage the patient and set goals of therapy for achieving clinical outcomes in the context of the patient's overall health care goals and access to care. The plan should support care continuity, including follow-up and transitions of care as appropriate.

Implement the care plan in collaboration with other health care providers and the patient or caregiver. This process should address medication and health-related problems and engage in preventive care strategies, including vaccine administration. Implementation includes initiation, modification, discontinuation, or administration of medication therapy as authorized or referral or transition of the patient to another health care professional.

Monitor and **evaluate** the effectiveness of the care plan and modify the plan in collaboration with other health care providers and the patient or caregiver as needed. This critical process includes the continuous monitoring and evaluation of clinical endpoints that contribute to the patient's overall health and outcomes of care, including progress toward or the achievement of goals of therapy.

13-4 Fundamentals of Drug Information

Drug information is printed, electronic, or verbal information pertaining to prescription and nonprescription medications and dietary supplements. The term *medication information* is also used and pertains to the use of information to influence medication therapy outcomes. Providing drug information to health care providers and the patient is at the core of all types of pharmacy practice. Drug information can be a simple verbal response to a patient's question, or it can be an involved, researched monograph presented to a hospital's pharmacy and therapeutics committee to aid in the decision of whether or not a drug is added to the formulary.

Biomedical and pharmaceutical literature is generally categorized as primary, secondary, and tertiary sources. Primary sources are original research publications and are usually published in peer-reviewed journals such as *American Journal of Health-System Pharmacy, Annals of Pharmacotherapy, Journal of the American Medical Association, Journal of the American Pharmacists Association, New England Journal of Medicine,* and *Pharmacotherapy.* Secondary literature consists of interpretations and reviews of primary sources and abstracting/indexing services. Examples include review articles; meta-analyses; and systematic reviews, practice guidelines, and indexing programs such as PubMed, Scopus, Embase, CINAHL, Cochrane Library, and Web of Science. Tertiary literature distills a collection of primary and secondary sources to create textbooks, encyclopedic articles, guidebooks, handbooks, and electronic information databases (e.g., UpToDate, Micromedex, *AHFS Drug Information* Online). The resources provide an overview of key research findings, practice guidelines, and an introduction to the principles and practices for a discipline or topic.

Biomedical literature is further classified by clinical levels of evidence that are based on the quality of the design, validity, and applicability to patient care and provide a grade (or strength) of recommendation (Table 13-1). For some topics, few high-level studies are available for a clinical question. The level of evidence descends in the following order:

- Meta-analysis: A systematic review that uses quantitative methods to summarize the results
- Systematic review: A systematic search, appraisal, and summary of all of the literature for a specific topic
- Randomized controlled trials (RCTs): A study of a randomized group of specified patients in an experimental group and a control group with specific variables and outcomes of interest
- Cohort study: Identification of two groups (cohorts) of patients, one that received a treatment and one that did not, and studies of these cohorts going forward for the outcome

TABLE 13-1. Example of Clinical Levels of Evidence Hierarchy

Level	Description
I	Evidence obtained from a systematic review or meta-analysis of all relevant randomized controlled trials (RCTs) or evidence-based clinical practice guidelines based on systematic reviews of RCTs or three or more RCTs of good quality that have similar results
II	Evidence obtained from at least one well-designed RCT (e.g., large multisite RCT)
III	Evidence obtained from well-designed controlled trials without randomization
IV	Evidence obtained from well-designed case-control or cohort studies
V	Evidence obtained from systematic reviews of descriptive and qualitative studies (meta-synthesis)
VI	Evidence obtained from a single descriptive or qualitative study
VII	Evidence obtained from the opinion of authorities or from the reports of expert committees

- Case-control study: Identification of patients who have the outcome of interest (cases) and control patients without the same outcome and studies of the outcome of an exposure or treatment of interest
- Background information and expert opinion: Handbooks, textbooks, electronic information databases, and editorials and commentaries that provide a foundation and a summary of generalized information about a treatment and condition
- Animal research and laboratory studies: Research studies that are at the bottom of clinical evidence but generate critical scientific ideas and foundational knowledge, which ultimately may lead to therapies, diagnostic tools, and an understanding of disease pathogenesis and treatment mechanisms of action

Major compendia contain drug monographs and are commonly used by pharmacists in a variety of practice settings. Many major compendia of drug information, such as *AHFS Drug Information* (http://www.ahfsdruginformation.com), Micromedex (http://truvenhealth.com/products/micromedex), Lexicomp (http://www.wolterskluwercdi.com/lexicomp-online/), UpToDate (http://www.uptodate.com/home), and *Drug Facts and Comparisons,* provide many different aspects of drug information, including information on pediatrics and neonates, intravenous incompatibilities, toxicology, and patient education materials. Some compendia include documented off-label (non–U.S. Food and Drug Administration [FDA] approved) indications. The *Physicians' Desk Reference,* however, contains only FDA-approved medication uses.

The FDA's *Orange Book: Approved Drug Products with Therapeutic Equivalence Evaluations* (or *Orange Book*) can be accessed on the FDA Web site (https://www.fda.gov). (*Note:* http://www.fda.com is not the official FDA Web site.) This reference provides bioequivalence data on chemical entities. The FDA's *Lists of Licensed Biological Products with Reference Product Exclusivity and Biosimilarity or Interchangeability Evaluations* (or *Purple Book*) lists biological products, including any biosimilar and interchangeable biological products, licensed by the FDA. "Biosimilars" is defined by the FDA as biologic agents developed to be "highly similar" to approved drugs with expired patent protection. The term is used to describe officially approved subsequent versions of innovator biopharmaceutical or biological products made by a different sponsor following patent and exclusivity expiry on the innovator product.

The PDR Network's *Red Book* contains information regarding availability and pricing for prescription and OTC medications, as well as information regarding dosage form, size, strength, and routes of administration. This reference also includes the product's National Drug Code numbers and average wholesale price (AWP). Lists of sugar-free, lactose-free, and alcohol-free preparations also can be found in the *Red Book* (https://truvenhealth.com/products/micromedex/product-suites/clinical-knowledge/red-book).

Information from government agencies can be identified through the Web sites of the FDA, the Drug Enforcement Administration (DEA) (https://www.dea.gov), and the Centers for Disease Control and Prevention (CDC) (https://www.cdc.gov). These Web sites also include clinical information and information about new drug approvals, drugs of abuse, and FDA-required information on the drug product label. A product package insert can be obtained from the Web site of the pharmaceutical company or the official provider of FDA label information (https://dailymed.nlm.nih.gov/).

The National Institutes of Health (NIH) operates PubMed (https://www.ncbi.nlm.nih.gov/pubmed), which comprises more than 26 million citations for biomedical literature from MEDLINE, life science journals, and online books. Citations may include links to full-text content from PubMed Central and publisher Web sites.

The Web site of the American Pharmacists Association (http://www.pharmacist.com) provides drug news updates and drug information, and the Web site of the American Society of Health-System Pharmacists (https://www.ashp.org) provides timely information on drug shortages and other drug information. The FDA has a mobile device app to speed public access to information about drug shortages, such as current drug shortages, resolved shortages, and discontinuations of drug products.

Several proprietary sources provide general reviews and reports that are searchable and provide an excellent resource for many questions pharmacists receive from patients and practitioners. For example, Pharmacist's Letter (http://pharmacistsletter.com) and Prescriber's Letter (http://prescribersletter.com) offer print and online access to practical information, including patient information materials for subscribers. The Natural Medicines Comprehensive Database (http://naturaldatabase.therapeuticresearch.com) provides well-researched and useful information on dietary supplements. Web sites for news on the pharmaceutical industry, drug development, and links to several drug information sites include Internet Drug News.com (http://www.coreynahman.com) and FirstWord Pharma (https://www.firstwordpharma.com), which provide information from the pharmaceutical industry.

Medscape (http://www.medscape.com) is a general drug information database that may be freely accessed through the Internet and mobile devices. The drug information contained in this reference is considered broad in scope and depth and relies on authoritative sources of drug information.

Clinical decision support systems (CDSSs) are used to support decision making in a variety of clinical settings. These systems are computer-based programs designed to provide information support for health professionals making clinical decisions typically at the point of care and to provide drug information, and are integrated in pharmacy computer systems. These systems have emerged as an important part of any clinical information system, particularly for computerized physician order entry (CPOE) systems that allow the direct entry of orders and instructions for the treatment of patients. The orders are communicated through a computer network to the appropriate hospital department responsible for fulfilling an order, which includes pharmacy, radiology, or laboratory. Used properly, CPOE decreases delays in order completion, reduces errors related to handwriting or transcriptions, allows order entry at the point of care or off site, provides error checking for duplicate or incorrect doses or tests, and simplifies inventory and posting of charges. Similar CDSSs are used in many community pharmacy computer programs to support monitoring for appropriate doses, drug interactions, and safety warnings.

Wikipedia (http://www.wikipedia.org) is a free Internet resource that is edited by its worldwide users. It may be a useful source for providing information supplementary to other more reliable sources, but its recognized shortcomings include errors in information, lack of referenced documentation, and omissions of information. Pharmacists should be cautious of user-edited sites and blogs as definitive sources of drug information and advise patients of the shortcomings of information contained in Wikipedia.

13-5 Pharmaceutical Supply Chain and Costs

As pharmaceuticals move from manufacturers to consumers, a complex set of market transactions involving prices, discounts, and rebates occurs along the supply chain (Figure 13-2). Although the drugs themselves move in a relatively straightforward path from manufacturers to wholesalers to retail pharmacies or nonretail providers (such as hospitals and clinics) to final consumers, the flow of costs and payments is more complicated.

FIGURE 13-2. Example of the Drug Supply Chain from Manufacturer to Consumer

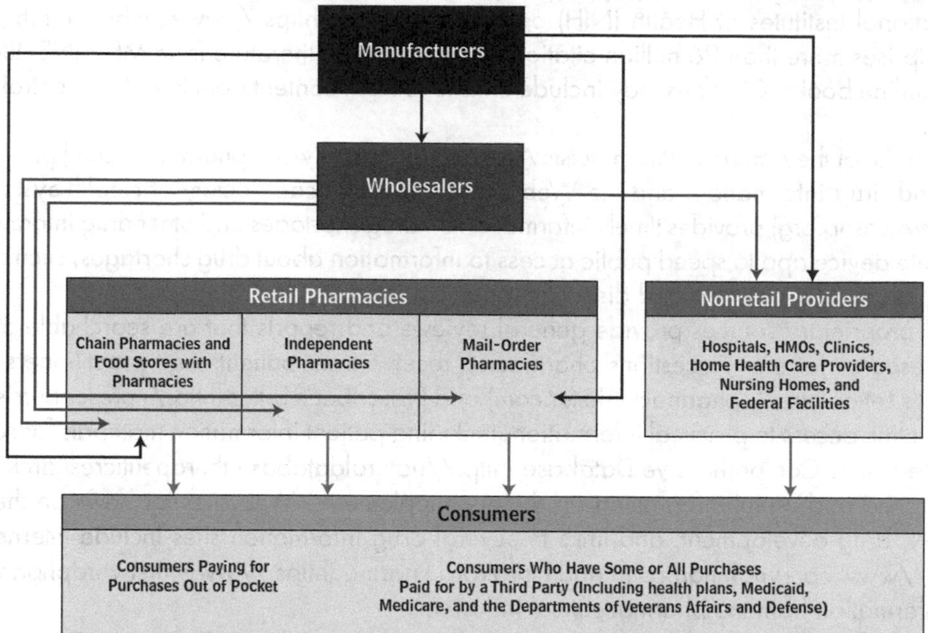

Congressional Budget Office, 2007.
HMO, health maintenance organization.

In 2007, the Congressional Budget Office examined the process by which payments are determined and provided estimates of the relative prices that retail pharmacies and nonretail providers pay for prescription drugs. Several factors determine the price that consumers and health plans ultimately pay for prescription drugs, and interactions often become complicated and confusing (Figure 13-3).

The price that a purchaser pays depends on both the degree of competition in a marketplace and the purchaser's bargaining power. In the pharmaceutical marketplace, competition depends on whether a brand-name drug has patent protection or whether brand-name and generic versions of the drug are available. In addition, even brand-name drugs under patent protection can face competition from other brand-name drugs that are considered to be therapeutic substitutes. A purchaser's bargaining power depends on both the volume purchased and the purchaser's ability to choose which drug to purchase from a set of competing drugs.

A chain pharmacy or a community pharmacy that is a member of a buying group usually dispenses prescriptions as written by the prescriber for brand-name drugs under patent protection. Although a chain pharmacy or a buying group may buy a large volume of brand-name drugs under patent protection, it generally cannot significantly negotiate prices as effectively as a health plan that can choose to cover only one or two brand-name drugs from a set of drugs considered to be therapeutic substitutes. A health plan can negotiate lower prices from manufacturers in the form of rebates by buying large volumes of the brand-name drugs of the plan's choice. For generic drugs, the chain pharmacy or buying group has greater negotiating leverage compared to a health plan. Chain pharmacies and buying groups can choose which of several generic drugs to stock, and by purchasing large volumes of those drugs, they can negotiate lower prices from manufacturers. In contrast, a health plan does not choose which generic drugs to dispense. Instead, the health plan's beneficiaries go to their pharmacies to fill prescriptions, and the pharmacies dispense the generic drugs that they have chosen to stock. Manufacturers have no incentive to negotiate price terms with a health plan for generic drugs even if the health plan buys a large volume.

FIGURE 13-3. Example of the Flow of Funds for Brand-Name Drugs Purchased at a Retail Pharmacy and Managed by a Pharmacy Benefit Manager

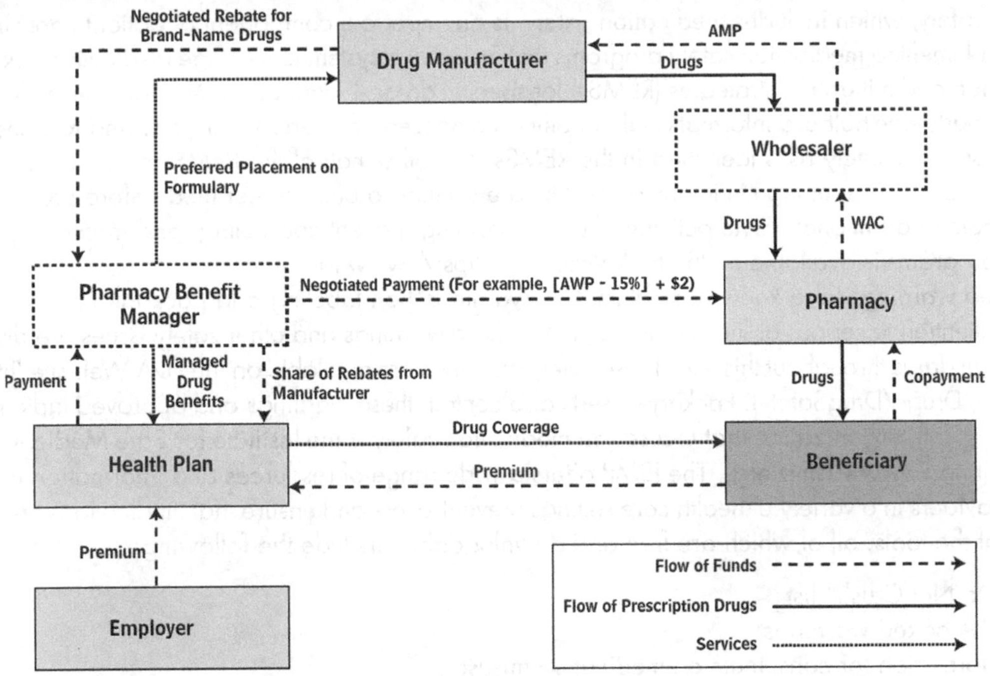

Congressional Budget Office, 2007.
AMP, average manufacturer price; AWP, average wholesale price; WAC, wholesale acquisition cost.

Three price measures are important in understanding the payment system for prescription drugs in the retail pharmacy market:

1. Average manufacturer price (AMP)
2. Average wholesale price (AWP)
3. Wholesale acquisition cost (WAC)

The AMP is an average of actual transaction prices. In contrast, the AWP and WAC are list prices, like a "sticker price" in the automobile industry. The AMP is the average price paid by wholesalers to manufacturers or by retail pharmacies that buy directly from manufacturers for drugs distributed through those pharmacies. It reflects all rebates paid by manufacturers to wholesalers and retail pharmacies. It does not include rebates paid by manufacturers to pharmacy benefit managers, Medicaid, or other third-party payers. Manufacturers are required to report the AMP to the Department of Health and Human Services Centers for Medicare and Medicaid Services, which uses it to calculate the rebates that manufacturers are required to pay state Medicaid programs for sales to Medicaid beneficiaries. For manufacturers, such rebates are a cost of participating in the Medicaid market.

The WAC represents manufacturers' published catalog, or list, price for sales of a drug (brand name or generic) to wholesalers. However, in practice, the WAC is not the price paid by wholesalers. To the extent that the WAC is meaningful in conveying information about actual transaction costs, the utility is limited to single-source drugs (that is, brand-name drugs still under patent protection). For those drugs, the WAC often approximates the prices that retail pharmacies pay to wholesalers. The AWP is a published list price for a drug sold by wholesalers to retail pharmacies and nonretail providers. However, in practice, the AWP is not the price paid by retail pharmacies and nonretail providers but, instead, is often used as a basis for payment to retail pharmacies by, for example, the Medicaid program, pharmacy benefit managers, and health plans. Those organizations often pay pharmacies a price discounted from the AWP.

13-6 Medication Safety

Patient safety, which includes medication safety, is an important component of patient care. In 2010, the FDA implemented medication safety programs that included a system to manage medication risk through risk evaluation and mitigation strategies (REMSs) for specific drugs. Numerous REMSs are currently in place. Of these, nearly one-half are informational in nature, composed of letters, Web sites, and fact sheets describing the specific safety risks identified in the REMSs. The other half of the REMSs also include "elements to assure safe use," requiring clinicians or health care settings to become certified before prescribing and to participate in additional REMS activities, such as training, patient counseling, and monitoring. A listing of REMS programs is available on the FDA Web site (https://www.fda.gov).

Boxed warnings (also known as "black box warnings") on labeling and package inserts are designed to call attention to serious or life-threatening risks. These warnings and other safety issues are discussed with individual drugs throughout this text. These safety warnings are available on the FDA Web site (https://www.fda.gov/Drugs/DrugSafety). Package inserts also contain these warnings and approved indications.

A nonprofit organization that focuses on medication safety is the Institute for Safe Medication Practices (ISMP) (http://www.ismp.org). The ISMP offers a wide range of resources and information to help health care providers in a variety of health care settings prevent errors and ensure that medications are used safely. Some of the tools, all of which are free and downloadable, include the following:

- "Do Not Crush" list
- FDA boxed warnings
- Information for consumers on medication misuse
- Error-prone abbreviations list
- FDA patient safety news, videos, and alerts
- High-alert medications consumer leaflets
- Reports on medication errors and the root cause analysis workbook
- SALAD (sound-alike, look-alike drugs) listing, including "Tall Man" lettering

There are more than 10,000 generic drug names and 40,000 trademarked brand names in use in the United States—but still only 26 letters in the alphabet! Examples of SALAD drugs leading to injury cited by the FDA:

- An 8-year-old child died after receiving methadone instead of methylphenidate.
- A 19-year-old man showed signs of potentially fatal complications after he was given clozapine instead of olanzapine.
- A 50-year-old woman was hospitalized after taking Flomax, instead of Volmax.

Some drug products are branded with a sales-leading product's name, but contain different active ingredients. For example, Dulcolax enteric-coated tablets and suppositories contain bisacodyl, a stimulant laxative. Other Dulcolax products include Dulcolax Stool Softener (docusate sodium), Dulcolax Milk of Magnesia (magnesium hydroxide), and Dulcolax Balance (polyethylene glycol 3350). Product names that previously contained unique active ingredients include Pepto Bismol, Maalox Total Stomach Relief, and Kaopectate; these products now all have bismuth subsalicylate as the active ingredient.

13-7 Adverse Drug Effect and Medication Errors Reporting

Patients should report adverse drug effects or medication errors to both the prescriber and the pharmacist. If the reaction or error is serious or unusual in the clinical judgment of the prescriber or the pharmacist, it should be reported to the FDA via the MedWatch Web site (https://www.fda.gov/Safety/MedWatch/HowToReport).

The FDA Adverse Event Reporting System (FAERS) is a database (https://www.fda.gov/Drugs/GuidanceComplianceRegulatoryInformation/Surveillance/AdverseDrugEffects/) that contains information on adverse events and medication error reports submitted to the FDA. The database is designed to support the FDA's postmarketing safety surveillance program for drug and therapeutic biological products

Reporting of adverse events and medication errors by health care providers and consumers is voluntary in the United States. The FDA receives some adverse event and medication error reports directly from health care providers and consumers (such as patients, family members, and lawyers). However, health care providers and consumers may also report adverse events and medication errors to a product's manufacturer. If a manufacturer receives an adverse event report, it is required to send the report to the FDA. The reports received directly by the FDA and those from manufacturers are entered into FAERS after clinical review and are made available to the public.

The FDA uses FAERS to identify new safety concerns that might be related to a marketed product, evaluate a manufacturer's compliance to reporting regulations, and respond to outside requests for information. The reports in FAERS are evaluated by clinical reviewers in the Center for Drug Evaluation and Research and the Center for Biologics Evaluation and Research to monitor the safety of products after they are approved by the FDA. If a potential safety concern is identified in FAERS, further evaluation is performed. Further evaluation might include conducting studies using other large databases, such as those available in the FDA's Sentinel Initiative (https://www.fda.gov/safety/fdassentinelinitiative/ucm2007250.htm). Based on an evaluation of the potential safety concern, the FDA may take regulatory action(s) to improve product safety and protect the public health, such as updating a product's labeling and package insert information, restricting the use of the drug, communicating new safety information to the public, or, in rare cases, removing a product from the market.

There are limitations to the interpretation and application of FAERS data. There is no certainty that the reported event (adverse event or medication error) was actually due to the product. The FDA does not require that a causal relationship between a product and an event be proven, and reports do not always contain enough detail to properly evaluate an event. Further, the FDA does not receive reports for every adverse event or medication error that occurs with a product. Many factors can influence whether or not an event will be reported, such as the time a product has been marketed and publicity about an event. Therefore, FAERS data cannot be used to calculate the incidence of an adverse event or medication error in the U.S. population.

13-8 Destruction of Drugs

Drugs that are out-of-date or no longer needed should be disposed of safely. Almost all medications can be safely disposed of by using medication take-back programs or DEA-authorized collectors. DEA-authorized collectors safely and securely collect and dispose of pharmaceutical controlled substances and other prescription drugs. Authorized collection sites may be retail pharmacies, hospital or clinic pharmacies, and law enforcement locations. Some pharmacies may also offer mail-back envelopes and drop boxes to facilitate consumers' safely disposing of their unused medications.

If a take-back, mail-back, or drop-box program is not available, most unused or expired medications can be disposed of in household trash. First, mix the medications (do not crush tablets or capsules) with an unpalatable substance such as dirt, cat litter, or used coffee grounds. Then place the mixture in a container such as a sealable plastic bag, and discard the container in household trash. Before discarding an empty bottle or other empty medication packaging, scratch out all personal information on the prescription label to make it unreadable.

Medications that contain controlled substances are especially harmful if taken accidentally by someone other than the patient. Thus, these medications should not be discarded in the trash because this method may still provide an opportunity for a child or pet to accidentally take the medication. If a DEA-authorized collector or drug take-back program is not available, the FDA recommends that these medications be disposed of by flushing them down the toilet. For safety reasons to fish, wildlife, and drinking water, the FDA recommends that only these few, select medications be disposed of in wastewater.

13-9 Medication Nonadherence or Misuse

Nearly three of four consumers admit they do not always take their prescribed medications as directed. Forms of nonadherent behavior include forgetting to take a prescribed medication, not filling a prescription, taking less than the recommended dosage, or substituting an OTC medication or dietary supplement. In some studies, almost one-third of all initial drug prescriptions were not filled within 9 months, with nonadherence highest for expensive drugs and chronic preventive therapies.

Medication nonadherence can have negative consequences for the patient, the prescriber, the pharmacist, and health care researchers all seeking to establish the value of the medication for a patient or target population. Medication adherence presents a particularly complex issue for the elderly patient. For these patients, medication issues and abuses may also result in accidents, such as a fall that causes a hip fracture. In addition, elderly patients could forget that they have already taken the prescribed amount of medication and unwittingly overdose.

Many factors are involved in patient nonadherence, including factors related to the disease, medication side effects, duration of drug therapy, frequency and complexity of treatment, dosage form, and cost. For example, patients are less likely to continue their medication regimen over long periods and are less likely to be adherent when the daily doses increase from 1 tablet to 4 tablets. To help prevent this problem of nonadherence in a multidosage regimen, medications to be taken once a day should be prescribed for ingestion in the morning or at bedtime, those prescribed twice a day can be scheduled to be given in the morning and bedtime, and those prescribed three times a day can be taken after each meal. Schedules calling for medication to be taken four or more times a day create an unnatural division of the day for most people, increasing the possibility of nonadherence. Studies reported that 40–60% of patients could not correctly report their physicians' expectations of them 10–80 minutes after they were provided the information. One study reported that more than 60% of the patients interviewed immediately after their medical visit had misunderstood the directions regarding prescribed medications.

Health care providers generally overestimate adherence rates. Asking patients themselves is a more valid procedure, but it has many difficulties. Patients may not be truthful to avoid displeasing their health care providers, or they may simply not know their rate of adherence. Patients not only under-report poor adherence but also over-report good adherence.

Gender, personality, and cultural factors also may influence adherence rates. Women are generally better than men at adhering to their medication regimens, particularly for drugs that treat behavioral health conditions, such as antidepressant medication. Cultural traditions are important factors in determining who is and who is not likely to adhere to medication regimens.

To help improve adherence, patients should be encouraged to indicate to their physicians and pharmacist verbally or in writing that they understand the choice of medication and its requirements. Patients are more likely to adhere to medication regimens when they are convinced that the medication they are taking is clearly linked to future health and wellness and when they are made an active participant in the decision-making process regarding the medication. Patient interpretation of instructions also varies widely. For example, instructions for a diuretic that is ordered "as needed for water retention" may be interpreted to mean that the drug would be used to cause water retention.

Patient nonadherence to medication has many facets. The seriousness of the illness, the cost of treatment, and treatment side effects can all affect adherence. The patient's age, mental status, and memory capacity are also important factors. The complexity of the recommendation, the duration of the regimen, the type of medical advice, the clarity of the written instructions based on the person's health literacy, and the amount of instruction provided are examples of these factors.

13-10 Impaired Pharmacists or Coworkers

Substance abuse, which includes abuse of alcohol, medications, and illicit substances, leading to impairment is an issue that affects every profession. The consequences to the pharmacy profession are numerous, leading to drug diversion and poor performance by the impaired pharmacist who jeopardizes safe and effective patient care.

Most states, through the state pharmacists association or the state board of pharmacy, have established a pharmacist-assistance program, often called the pharmacist recovery network (PRN). A PRN is a confidential program providing assistance in the recognition and treatment of substance abuse of affected pharmacists. Most PRN treatment programs function with a multidisciplinary staff trained in substance abuse and often include formerly impaired recovering pharmacists.

Each state pharmacy board has its own procedures for dealing with a pharmacist suspected of substance abuse. Once the pharmacist has demonstrated a commitment to recovery and a substance-free lifestyle, reinstatement by the state pharmacy board to practice pharmacy can begin. Generally, the state pharmacy board will require the pharmacist to complete a rehabilitation program, maintain regular contact with an assigned counselor, submit to random drug testing, and participate in support group meetings on a regular basis.

Pharmacists should recognize that resources are available for treatment of either themselves or an affected coworker who is at risk. In many cases, those individuals have placed their professional careers and the public's safety in jeopardy. Information about the various pharmacy recovery programs is available from state pharmacy boards or state-specific pharmacy associations.

Many pharmacists with substance abuse problems initially think that their training will somehow cure their substance abuse. They may perceive themselves functioning normally in their daily pharmacy practice; however, these individuals may exhibit behavioral characteristics that can alert others to the problem. Examples of signs and symptoms of a potentially impaired pharmacist are listed in Box 13-1.

13-11 Basic Principles of Management

Whether planned or not, most pharmacists will become managers in title or actions. Management is the art of maximizing productivity by using and developing people's talents, while providing them self-enrichment and opportunities for growth. Classical management descriptions involve several functional elements (Box 13-2) and the skills of leadership, decision making, and communication.

The most effective managers are those who understand the context in which their organization exists, the organization's culture, and industry- and organization-specific knowledge to get things

BOX 13-1. Indicators of a Potentially Impaired Pharmacist or Coworker

- Personality changes or mood swings
- Frequent absences from work
- Volunteering to check in controlled substances or inventory-controlled substances
- Long or frequent disappearances from the work area or showing up in the work area during unscheduled times
- Increase in medication errors
- Changes in physical appearance (e.g., weight loss/gain or poor hygiene)
- Signs of forgetfulness, irritability, and tardiness
- Decrease in work performance
- Excessive ordering of certain drugs
- Overreaction to criticism
- Increased complaints from patients

BOX 13-2. Classical Elements of Management

- ***Planning:*** Look ahead with the active participation of the entire organization with consideration of available resources and flexibility of personnel.
- ***Organizing:*** Maintain a well-organized operation with sufficient resources and staff so work runs smoothly with a clear division of functions and tasks.
- ***Commanding:*** Communicate clear working instructions so everybody knows what is required of them.
- ***Coordinating:*** Harmonize staff activities and behaviors to stimulate motivation, positive behavior, and discipline within the group.
- ***Controlling:*** Verify that the functions of the organization are going according to plan by adhering to the following four steps:
  1. Establish performance standards based on organizational objectives.
  2. Measure and report on actual performance.
  3. Compare results with performance and standards.
  4. Take corrective or preventive measures as needed.

done. By understanding their environment, managers are able to understand organizational decisions and pharmacy-related changes, anticipate emerging needs, and help employees make sense of new directions.

Effective managers surround themselves with talented people and develop these individuals into high-performing team members who can translate vision into reality. Managing human resources involves establishing goals and performance standards and providing feedback. Employees look to managers to establish clear expectations and outcome measures. Communication is a critical skill to good management as well as overall patient care. Several strategies can be used to successfully communicate with team members (Box 13-3). Communicating with supervisors to achieve the best possible results by considering aspects of *managing up* is also important (Box 13-4). Another primary role for a manager is problem solving; to optimally solve problems and issues that arise, a manager must be adept at many aspects of problem solving (Box 13-5).

BOX 13-3. Elements of Communication

- What you say may not be what the receiver hears.
- Sender and receiver have different levels of interest in a subject.
- Receiver may not be interested in the message.
- Communication is influenced by factors such as body language, facial expressions, and location of the exchange (e.g., office, hallway, parking lot, social event).
- A message's format and presentation can enhance or deter message transmission.
- People differ in how they prefer to receive information such as by text, e-mail, written letter, person-to-person, or group message.
- People often need to receive a message in multiple ways and times.
- Having the receiver repeat the message may help determine if the message is understood.

BOX 13-4. Strategies for the Managing Up Process

- Clarify roles and expectations.
- Recognize a supervisor's work and communication styles.
- Provide a supervisor with complete information.
- Be dependable and trustworthy.
- Assist a supervisor in better managing his or her time.
- Be positive and appreciative.
- Disagree with tact and respect.

BOX 13-5. Strategies for Problem Solving

- Define the problem.
- Analyze the problem.
- Develop possible solutions to the problem.
- Analyze proposed solutions.
- Select the best solution given the environment, resources, and parties involved.
- Plan the next course of action (how a solution will be implemented).
- Involve others in the process.

13-12 Summary

Pharmacists are an integral part of the patient care process. Pharmacists should be collecting, assessing, planning, implementing, monitoring, and evaluating the delivery of patient care in any patient setting. Part of the patient care process is providing evidence-based drug information from reliable sources and ensuring adherence to medication instructions. Impairment is an issue that affects every profession and can lead to patient harm. Pharmacists should be aware of PRNs. Pharmacists are managers with or without a managerial title and should strive to communicate effectively, use sound and effective management principles, and surround themselves with talented, motivated people.

13-13 Questions

1. Which actions are described in the Pharmacists' Patient Care Process as outlined by the Joint Commission of Pharmacy Practitioners in the delivery of patient care across the profession of pharmacy? (Mark all that apply.)

A. Assessing
B. Planning
C. Implementing
D. Judging

2. Which elements apply to the pharmacist's collection of necessary subjective and objective information about patients to understand their relevant medical and medication history and clinical status? (Mark all that apply.)

A. Current prescription medications and medication use history, including OTC medications, herbals, and other dietary supplements
B. Medical history, health and wellness information, biometric test results, and physical assessment findings
C. Marital status and birth order, if they have siblings
D. Patient lifestyle habits, preferences and beliefs, health and functional goals, and socioeconomic factors that affect access to medications

3. Which of the following references would be the best source to identify drug information regarding whether a medication is lactose free?

A. *AHFS Drug Information*
B. FDA *Orange Book*
C. *Red Book*
D. *Martindale: The Complete Drug Reference*

4. Which of the following drug information resources would provide information on biosimilars?

A. *AHFS Drug Information*
B. FDA *Orange Book*
C. FDA *Purple Book*
D. CDC Web site

5. Which element of medication use does the FDA's REMSs program target for reduction?

A. Cost
B. Risk
C. Nonadherence
D. Error

6. For which of the following aspects of appropriate medication use does the Institute for Safe Medication Practices provide tools? (Mark all that apply.)

   A. Cost of medication
   B. Error-prone abbreviations list
   C. High-alert medications
   D. "Do Not Crush" list

7. Which of the following is true about the FAERS database? (Mark all that apply.)

   A. It is a database designed to support the FDA's post-marketing safety surveillance program.
   B. Reporting of adverse events and medication errors by pharmacists is required by the FDA.
   C. If a manufacturer receives an adverse event report, it is required to send the report to the FDA.
   D. Reports in FAERS have been evaluated by clinical reviewers in the FDA's Center for Drug Evaluation and Research and the Center for Biologics Evaluation and Research.

8. What are the proper methods to dispose of medications? (Mark all that apply.)

   A. Pharmacies that are approved as DEA-authorized collectors may accept out-of-date drugs or drugs no longer needed by patients.
   B. Controlled substances should be flushed down a toilet because they are not acceptable for drug take-back programs.
   C. Only licensed pharmacies may be approved as a medication take-back site.
   D. If a take-back program is not available, noncontrolled medications can be mixed with an unpalatable substance and placed in the trash.

9. What is the approximate percentage of patients who do not take their prescription medications as directed?

   A. 25%
   B. 50%
   C. 75%
   D. 100%

10. Which of the following describes aspects of adherence to medications? (Mark all that apply.)

   A. Patients are more likely to adhere to once-a-day or twice-a-day dosing than four-times-a-day dosing.
   B. Prescribers generally overestimate adherence rates of their patients.
   C. Men are generally better at adhering to their medication regimen than women.
   D. Elderly patients are at a greater risk from nonadherence to medications.

11. A pharmacist recovery network, a confidential program providing assistance in the recognition and treatment of impaired pharmacists, is generally under the auspices of which of the following?

   A. The American Pharmacists Association
   B. The American Society of Health-System Pharmacists
   C. A state board of pharmacy or a state pharmacy association
   D. A criminal court

12. Which of the following concepts comprise managing up communications? (Mark all that apply.)

   A. Provide your supervisor only the basic facts regarding the issue in question to save time.
   B. Know your supervisor's work and communication styles.
   C. Express appreciation for positive operational suggestions made by your supervisor.
   D. Disagree with your supervisor with tact and respect.

13. Which of the following price measures reflects all rebates paid by manufacturers to wholesalers and retail pharmacies, but does not include rebates paid by manufacturers to pharmacy benefit managers, Medicaid, or other third-party payers?

   A. Average manufacturer price
   B. Wholesale acquisition cost
   C. Average wholesale price
   D. List price

13-14 Answers

1. **A, B, C.** Judging is not one of the elements of the Pharmacists' Patient Care Process, which includes collecting, assessing, planning, implementing, monitoring, and evaluating a consistent process in the delivery of patient care across the profession.
2. **A, B, D.** A pharmacist does not need to know patients' marital status and birth order to understand their relevant health care, medication history, and clinical status.
3. **C.** Of the choices provided, the *Red Book* would be the best source to identify information regarding whether a medication is lactose free.
4. **C.** The FDA *Purple Book* contains information on biosimilars; chemical bioequivalence is found in the FDA *Orange Book*.
5. **B.** The risk evaluation and mitigation strategies are targeted toward mitigating medication risks.
6. **B, C, D.** Cost of a medication is not found on the ISMP Web site.
7. **A, C, D.** Reporting adverse events and medication errors by pharmacists is voluntary.
8. **A, D.** Controlled substances are acceptable for take-back programs. In addition to pharmacists who are approved, law enforcement sites can serve as a take-back site.
9. **C.** Nearly three of four patients are nonadherent.
10. **A, B, D.** Women are generally more compliant than men.
11. **C.** A state board of pharmacy or a state pharmacy association generally oversees a PRN.
12. **B, C, D.** Your supervisor should be provided complete information to resolve an issue.
13. **A.** The average manufacturer price (AMP) is the average price paid by wholesalers to manufacturers or by retail pharmacies that buy directly from manufacturers for drugs distributed through such pharmacies. It reflects all rebates paid by manufacturers to wholesalers and retail pharmacies, but does not include rebates paid by manufacturers to pharmacy benefit managers, Medicaid, or other third-party payers.

13-15 Additional Resources

Congressional Budget Office. *Prescription Drug Pricing in the Private Sector.* Washington, DC: Congress of the United States; 2007. Available at https://www.cbo.gov/sites/default/files/110th-congress-2007-2008/reports/01-03-prescription drug.pdf. Accessed May 17, 2017.

Joint Commission of Pharmacy Practitioners. Pharmacists' patient care process. 2014. Available at: https://jcpp.net/wp-content/uploads/2016/03/PatientCareProcess-with-supporting-organizations.pdf.

McEvoy GK, ed. *AHFS Drug Information 2014.* Bethesda, MD: American Society of Health-System Pharmacists; 2014.

PDR Network. *Physician's Desk Reference.* 68th ed. Montvale, NJ: PDR Network; 2014.

PDR Network. *Red Book.* Montvale, NJ: Thomson Healthcare/Thomson PDR; 2010.

U.S. Food and Drug Administration. *Orange Book: Approved Drug Products with Therapeutic Equivalence Evaluations.* 34th ed. Silver Spring, MD: U.S. Food and Drug Administration; 2014.

U.S. Food and Drug Administration. *Purple Book: Lists of Licensed Biological Products with Reference Product Exclusivity and Biosimilarity or Interchangeability Evaluations.* Silver Spring, MD: U.S. Food and Drug Administration; 2015.

Wolters Kluwer Health. *Drug Facts and Comparisons 2017.* Philadelphia, PA: Lippincott Williams and Wilkins; 2016.

SOCIAL, BEHAVIORAL, AND ADMINISTRATIVE PHARMACY SCIENCES

area
3

EDITORS: *ANDREA S. FRANKS (14), PETER A. CHYKA (15–21), AND BRADLEY A. BOUCHER (22–24)*

Health Care Delivery Systems 14

KENNETH C. HOHMEIER

14-1 KEY POINTS

- The origin of the modern U.S. health care system can be traced back to the early and mid-20th century.
- Over the past 30 years, there has been a shift from an illness model of disease treatment to a wellness model of chronic disease prevention.
- Pharmacists can practice in a variety of settings but most are located in a community pharmacy or a hospital practice.
- There are four means of health care financing: out of pocket, individual private insurance, employer-sponsored private insurance, and government.
- The distribution of national health care expenditures by source of payment for 2016 was as follows: private insurance, 34%; Medicare payment, 20%; Medicaid payment, 17%; out-of-pocket payment, 11%; and other, 18%.
- Employer-sponsored insurance generally uses principles of managed care to control costs; as a result, most plans can be considered either a health maintenance organization (HMO) or a preferred provider organization (PPO).
- An HMO is a managed care insurance plan where the payer is accountable for both the cost and the quality of care within a closed system.
- A PPO, which is mainly concerned about reducing the cost of care, creates a larger but still restrictive network of physicians who agree to a contracted rate before care delivery.
- An evolution of the HMO and PPO, accountable care organizations (ACOs) are models of managed care that tie payment to cost control and quality of care, theoretically keeping health care providers more accountable for resource use and quality of care.
- If a health care insurer does not manage prescription benefits for its beneficiaries, a pharmacy benefits manager will separately administer the benefits, including formulary development, customer service, and pharmacy contracting.
- Americans can access health care via a variety of systems including for-profit and not-for-profit health care systems, U.S. Department of Veterans Affairs, Indian Health Service, religion-affiliated health care systems, and public health care systems.
- Trends and innovation in health care include growth in retail clinics, expansion of telemedicine and technology, and advances in personalized medicine.

14-2 STUDY GUIDE CHECKLIST

The following topics may guide your study of this subject area:

- ☐ Describe settings where pharmacists may practice within the U.S. health care system.
- ☐ List the various ways in which health care is financed in the United States and which populations are served by each type of financing.
- ☐ Describe the organization of health care delivery systems at the national, state, and local levels.
- ☐ Compare the varying structures of health care delivery systems including managed care organizations, accountable care organizations, and health departments.
- ☐ Differentiate between various types of managed care delivery (e.g., ACO, PPO, HMO).
- ☐ Explain underlying social, political, and economic factors that influence the delivery of health care in the United States.
- ☐ Describe the efforts taken to shift the United States health care system from an illness model of disease treatment to a wellness model of chronic disease prevention.
- ☐ Compare and contrast the U.S. health care system with that of other developed nations.

14-3 Introduction to the U.S. Health Care System

During the 20th century, hospitals and health care systems became the central institutions providing medical care in the United States. In the 1950s, 1960s, and 1970s, the health care focus was on access; from the 1980s to the present, the focus has been on health care cost and quality. Over time, U.S. health care delivery has shifted from a physician-centric model to one of a diverse set of health care professionals working collaboratively and within their own specialty to provide patient care. The role of pharmacists within the U.S. health care system has evolved as well. Whereas pharmacists primarily were found in community pharmacies and hospitals at the beginning of the 20th century, today pharmacists can also be found in specialty pharmacies, medical offices and ambulatory care sites, long-term care, infusion locations, insurance companies, and industry-related sites (manufacturers and researchers). However, the majority of pharmacists practice in either hospitals or community pharmacies. According to the American Hospital Association, 5,564 acute care hospitals currently exist in the United States. There are about 62,000 community pharmacies according to the National Community Pharmacists Association (NCPA).

Financing

Health care financing is central to all other aspects of the U.S. health care system. There are four means for U.S. health care financing: out of pocket, individual private insurance, employer-sponsored private insurance, and government (public). The U.S. health care system was founded on individuals paying out of pocket for their health care expenses. The start of the 20th century saw the introduction of third-party payers—outside entities that pay for health care costs for an individual. The first of these third parties was the individual private insurance. Similar to automobile or life insurance, this insurance for an individual and his or her family is fully funded by the individual patient. This form of third-party payer represents only a small fraction of health care financing. In contrast, employer-sponsored private insurance is the standard means for health care financing for Americans under the age of 65 years. It is similar to individual private insurance but is largely subsidized (financially supported) by an individual's employer. There are dozens of different private insurance companies, and they vary in terms of premiums (the amount of money paid monthly by the insured for the plan), deductibles (specified amounts of money that the insured must pay before an insurance company will pay a claim), out-of-pocket maximums (the maximum amount the insured will pay in a given year after which the insurance pays 100%), and co-payments (the payment made by a beneficiary to the health care provider or organization in addition to that made by the insurer).

Government-funded (or public-funded) health care represents the largest payer of health care in the United States. Government health plans use taxes to fund health care purchases on behalf of the covered individual, whereas private insurance companies use the funds provided by an individual or employer. In contrast to private insurance, there are only a handful of government health care plans (although under each plan, there may be dozens of privately contracted companies that administer the benefit).

Medicare

On July 30, 1965, President Lyndon B. Johnson signed the Social Security Amendments of 1965 into law. This legislation created Medicare and Medicaid, which today provide benefits to more than 43 million Americans. Persons 65 years of age or older, persons under 65 years of age with certain disabilities, and persons with end-stage renal disease requiring either dialysis or kidney transplant are eligible for health insurance coverage through Medicare.

Medicare has four major subdivisions: Part A, Part B, Part C, and Part D. Medicare A and B pay for medical claims. Part C pays for medical and prescription claims. Part D is for prescription claims only.

Medicare Part A

Medicare Part A, commonly called *hospital insurance,* helps cover the costs of inpatient hospital care, skilled nursing facility care, hospice, and home health care. For most people who choose to buy Part A, Part B is required, and premiums must be paid for both.

Medicare Part B

Medicare Part B, commonly called *medical insurance,* helps cover the costs of doctors' services, outpatient care, and some preventive services. Preventive services include diabetes screenings; bone density screenings; colorectal cancer screenings; and flu, hepatitis B, and pneumococcal vaccinations. It may also be used to pay for durable medical equipment (e.g., blood sugar test strips, nebulizers).

Medicare Part C

Medicare Part C, commonly called *Medicare Advantage Plan,* is a program that is operated by private insurance companies on behalf of Medicare. Coverage includes Medicare Parts A and B plus other coverage, which usually includes prescription drug costs.

Medicare Part D

Medicare Part D, or *prescription drug coverage,* was added to Medicare when Congress passed the Medicare Prescription Drug, Improvement, and Modernization Act (MMA) in 2003. Part D was launched in January 2006. Similar to Medicare Part C, Part D is operated by private insurance companies on behalf of Medicare. The MMA defines the drugs that are covered and excluded under Part D. However, all plans are not required to cover all drugs; each plan is allowed to develop its own formulary. The Centers for Medicare and Medicaid Services, or CMS (https://www.cms.hhs.gov), provides regulatory guidance and oversight of the provision of health care benefits to eligible individuals. CMS also reviews formularies to determine if benefit design discriminates against certain beneficiaries and to ensure that drugs are included under each medication class. Enrollment in Part D is optional for beneficiaries enrolled in Part A or B.

Individuals enrolled in Part D may also qualify for medication therapy management services (MTMS) under the MMA. Individuals must meet three criteria for MTMS eligibility:

- Have multiple chronic diseases
- Take multiple drugs
- Be likely to incur expenses that exceed a level specified by the secretary of the U.S. Department of Health and Human Services

Pharmacists and pharmacy interns are the only health care providers specifically identified in the MMA to provide MTMS. According to the American Pharmacists Association (APhA), MTMS may include managing and monitoring drug therapy, consulting with patients and families on proper medication use, conducting disease prevention and wellness screenings, and overseeing medication use.

Medicaid

Medicaid began in the mid-1960s and has become the health care delivery method for poor people and people uninsurable by the commercial market (employer or individual). Jointly funded by the federal and state governments, Medicaid, together with Medicare, is considered an entitlement program. In addition to those classified as poor, other groups of patients eligible for Medicaid include the following:

- Children
- People with chronic disabilities
- People suffering from HIV/AIDS (human immunodeficiency virus/acquired immune deficiency syndrome)

If a patient qualifies for the respective program, health care services should be provided. Health care is a local issue that reflects mainly the patient's accessibility to and the affordability of hospitals, clinics, and health care practitioners.

Funding

Funding for state, city, and county health programs and services is generated through a mix of federal, state, and local taxes as well as grant dollars frequently matched by the state, county, or city health department or commission. These entities provide myriad health care services, including state Medicaid services; emergency medical services; childhood clinic exams; breast and cervical cancer screenings; water quality, pollution, and environmental control; and restaurant inspections. In addition, the respective state health commissions or departments serve as a licensing agency for health care professionals (e.g., physicians, pharmacists, nurses, dentists).

Health Care Trends and Numbers

Currently, the illness model for patient care receives the majority of health care expenditures. The wellness model for preventing disease and promoting health receives only 3% of health care spending and covers procedures such as blood pressure checks, cancer screenings, immunizations, and blood tests.

Some important health care numbers include the following:

- The national health care expenditure for the United States for 2015 was $9,990 per person, which is more than twice the average of the industrialized world.
- The United States ranks only 26th in life expectancy in the industrialized world.
- U.S. health care expenditure in 2015 was $3.2 trillion.
- U.S. total health care spending as a percentage of gross domestic product for 2015 was 17.8%.

In the United States, several health care systems combine to provide care directly or indirectly to the majority of citizens. Those systems include, but are not limited to, the following:

- U.S. Department of Veterans Affairs
- For-profit and not-for-profit health systems
- Indian Health Service (IHS)
- Religion-affiliated health care systems
- Public health care systems

In 2016, the distribution of national health care expenditures by source of payment was as follows: private insurance, 34%; Medicare payment, 20%; Medicaid payment, 17%; out-of-pocket payment, 11%; and other, 18%.

Controlling Health Care Costs

Over the past 30 years, health care cost reduction has been a major issue in the United States. With the rise of third-party payers (private insurers and government), individuals were no longer exposed to the costs associated with health care expenditures, and normal market forces, which typically reduce costs in other industries, were unable to control costs in health care. This phenomenon of rising costs and the need for cost controls directly led to the development of the concept of *managed care*.

Managed care is an evolutionary concept reflecting a different approach to provision of and reimbursement for health care services. It focuses on appropriate use of health care resources. The two main configurations of managed care are health maintenance organizations (HMOs) and preferred provider organizations (PPOs). The accountable care organization (ACO) is the newest form of cost control and ties payment to performance (quality of care).

- HMOs coordinate the provision and financing (insurance) of comprehensive care (provided by a panel of employed physicians or a network of physicians) to a defined population. They are more restrictive than a PPO in terms of where a patient may go to receive care and which provider can provide that care. An example of an HMO is Kaiser Permanente.
- PPOs are networks of health care providers, similar to an HMO. However, these providers are not employees of the PPO—rather, these physicians and hospitals contract with the PPO to have access to a group of insured individuals. PPOs are less restrictive and allow an insured member to see any number of physicians, hospitals, and other health care providers within the network.

- ACOs are health care organizations that tie payment to cost control and quality of care provided. Quality of care is quantified through the use of quality measures that are predetermined metrics defined by Medicare that evaluate domains including patient satisfaction, patient safety, and preventive health care. The primary payer for ACOs is Medicare, but private insurance companies may also participate in ACO models. Most ACOs are experimental, and their characteristics, implementation, and numbers are expected to remain fluid for the next decade.

Social, Political, and Economic Factors of the U.S. Health Care System

Social factors

In today's health care environment, Uwe Reinhardt, a health care economist from Princeton University, has indicated that Americans expect three things:

- They want the latest health technology, procedures, and medications.
- They want them immediately.
- They want someone else to pay for these things.

Health care reform

Prompted in large part by the growing numbers of uninsured individuals, stakeholders at the federal level began advocating for comprehensive health care reform. Although universal health care (aka single-payer health care), a system by which all Americans would be covered with health insurance and no patient would be denied care for his or her inability to pay, was initially considered as the central solution for health care reform, the idea of universal coverage was abandoned because of its unlikely passage by Congress. Instead, the use of an individual mandate (requiring, under financial penalty, U.S. citizens to purchase some form of health insurance) was chosen as the foundation for increasing insurance coverage in the United States. This individual mandate, in combination with government subsidies, expansion of the Medicaid program, and creation of insurance exchanges (marketplaces for individuals to buy insurance), formed the Affordable Care Act (ACA). It was passed as law in March 2010.

By 2013, public opinion of the law as a whole was mostly negative, particularly regarding the individual mandate. Polls taken during the same time frame also indicated that the public expected to pay more for health care because of the ACA. This shift in public opinion, combined with increasing premiums for ACA plans, reopened the debate on health care reform. Currently, a multitude of solutions are being discussed on the federal level, ranging from single-payer health care to free market solutions that include plans for catastrophic health care insurance.

Health care innovations and future delivery models

Although elements of uncertainty exist in today's economy, the following trends and innovative business models in health care warrant attention:

- ***Growth in retail clinics:*** These clinics often are based in pharmacies; are staffed by a nurse practitioner; and achieve increased accessibility and decreased cost per visit for uncomplicated conditions such as ear infections, bronchitis, and conjunctivitis.
- ***Expansion of telemedicine and technology:*** The business model for these services focuses on convenient care for patients—frequently at home. Examples are the use of Internet access, medical devices, advanced telephony, and video conferences.
- ***Advances in personalized medicine:*** In personalized medicine, patients are grouped according to specific diseases and their responses to drugs or treatments. The 2003 sequencing of the human genome now allows genetic tests to deliver predictably effective therapy. An example is the use of genetic information from a simple cheek swab to determine warfarin dosing. Such advances could save $1.1 billion annually in health care costs.

14-4 Organization of Health Care Delivery

Health care delivery in the United States is undergoing significant change. Over the past two to three decades, the model of independent physician practices and small organizations of medical offices and hospitals has been replaced with large health care systems. This horizontal integration occurs when similar entities (such as multiple medical practices) combine into a single organization. Additionally, vertical integration is occurring concurrently whereby entities representing different levels of care delivery combine into a single organization (e.g., hospitals, medical offices, pharmacy). Similarly, a rapid expansion of chain pharmacies occurred in the 1990s and 2000s when a large number of independent pharmacies sold their businesses to large chain pharmacy corporations (horizontal integration). Both in medicine and pharmacy, large and integrated organizations now dominate most regions of the country.

General Health Care Delivery Systems

As described earlier, traditional health care in the United States was physician centric—centered around independent physician practices or solo practitioners in small groups. Physicians would refer a patient to local hospitals if the patient was in need of inpatient care. This arrangement made hospitals dependent on physician referrals; hospitals had difficulty maintaining a steady stream of income to ensure their financial viability, especially if a physician began referring to a competing hospital in the same region. Conversely, physician specialists were highly dependent on referrals from hospital physicians. Because of these and other issues, different types of health system structures emerged throughout the 20th century.

Vertically integrated systems

In a vertically integrated health care system, one large organization takes responsibility for the delivery of care across all levels of care (hence the term *vertical*), including primary care providers, specialists, hospitals, urgent care clinics, pharmacies, and home health agencies. There are substantial improvements to care efficiency, quality, and cost with this model because a single organization acts as employer and administrator for the entire system. However, for both health care providers and patients, this type of health care system can be restrictive. Physicians may view quality-of-care measures and formulary restrictions as barriers to providing care. Patients may believe that the requirement to seek care only within hospitals, medical offices, and pharmacies that belong to the organization limits the choice of care, especially when another hospital or pharmacy not associated with the system is closer to the patient's home or job. Vertically integrated systems are financed under the HMO managed care model.

Semi-integrated models

Scenarios also exist in which hospitals, physicians, specialists, and other members of a typical integrated health care delivery system are not employed by the same organization, yet they still coordinate their services to reduce costs and optimize care. These semi-integrated models may include several independent entities who contract with an HMO plan to deliver care. Although the goal of these organizations is the same as that of a vertically integrated system, managing to reduce costs or improve quality typically is more difficult because the various entities are not part of the same organization. In this model, physicians will typically join independent physician associations to contract with HMOs as part of the network, but they still may see patients who are outside of the HMO, unlike physicians in the vertically integrated system.

Nonintegrated models

Both semi-integrated and vertically integrated systems add significant restrictions on patient choice, which is especially evident when patients switch employers or when employers switch their private insurance plan. In either of these scenarios, patients may find that the physician, pharmacy, or hospital that they have been using for years is no longer in the HMO network and therefore will no longer be covered by the insurance plan. For this reason, PPOs were developed to allow broader access to a multitude of physicians who are members of the organization. Unlike previously described care models, PPOs do not provide the same focus on care efficiency, quality, or cost-control mechanisms. However, PPOs do provide broader access to physicians and other health care providers—increasing the likelihood that patients may keep their health care providers even when switching employers or when employers change insurance providers.

Miscellaneous Health Care Delivery Systems

Health departments

Hospitals, medical offices, and community pharmacies are traditional sites where care is provided for individuals. However, when looking at the health of an entire population, a different organization is necessary. Health departments serve the role of providing localized services to keep residents healthy and informed. Their functions are varied, depending on the needs of the community. Examples of services offered include vaccinations, welfare program administration (such as the Women, Infants, and Children program), and inspection of public facilities (such as swimming pools). Health departments also monitor and report infectious disease data and report numbers and trends to other local, state, and federal organizations to minimize disease outbreak.

Veterans Health Administration

The Veterans Health Administration (VHA) is responsible for providing health care for U.S. military veterans. It is a component of the U.S. Department of Veterans Affairs (VA). Such care is provided at VA medical centers, outpatient clinics, and nursing homes.

Indian Health Service

The Indian Health Service (IHS) is responsible for providing health care and public health services to federally recognized Native American tribes and Alaska natives. Currently, IHS operates in 36 states in the United States. It includes 59 health centers, 26 hospitals, and 32 health stations.

14-5 Pharmacy Benefit Managers

Pharmacy benefit managers (PBMs) may be used to decrease costs associated with prescription drugs, ensure appropriate use of medications, and improve overall quality of care. PBMs may be contracted by managed care organizations, employers, or private insurers and are responsible for more than 90% of all retail prescription drug purchases. PBMs often use mail-out services for prescription delivery to decrease operation costs and increase revenue. In addition, they rely heavily on a drug formulary.

Formularies

A *drug formulary* is a list of medications that are available for patient drug therapy. It is maintained in organized health care settings, such as hospitals. Alternatively, as defined by the Academy of Managed Care Pharmacy, a formulary is "a continually updated list of medications and related products supported by current evidence-based medicine, judgment of physicians, pharmacists, and other experts in the diagnosis and treatment of disease and preservation of health." Formularies are the driving force for a successful PBM. Formulary decisions are made on the basis of scientific evidence and economic considerations to provide optimal and cost-effective drug therapy. Typically, a pharmacy and therapeutics committee comprising pharmacists, physicians, and other health care professionals should be responsible for managing the formulary system.

Levels of PBM Services

PBM services fall into three levels:

- Basic services include claims processing only.
- Intermediate services also are responsible for formulary management.
- Advanced services include disease state management for chronic conditions such as diabetes, hypertension, and hyperlipidemia.

PBMs may provide only one of these services or they may provide all three. PBMs will generally charge co-insurance payments to patients and are similar to other prescription drug plans that offer a tiered system for generic, brand-preferred, and brand-nonpreferred drugs. Over the past few years, PBMs have made an effort to promote the use of generic drugs as a means of lowering health care costs. Generic drugs now make up 64% of all prescriptions dispensed in the United States, and this trend is expected to grow.

14-6 Questions

1. In reference to the change to business-like management of health care, freestanding hospitals becoming multihospital systems is an example of

A. changes in the types of ownership.
B. horizontal integration.
C. vertical integration.
D. parallel integration.

2. What are the two main forms of managed care?

A. HMOs and PPOs
B. HMOs and ACOs
C. PPOs and ACOs
D. MTMS and ACOs

3. Integrated health care delivery systems may include which of the following? (Mark all that apply.)

A. Pharmacy
B. Hospital
C. Home services
D. Outpatient offices

4. What source of payment is the largest contributor to U.S. health care expenditures?

A. Private insurance
B. Medicare
C. Medicaid
D. Out of pocket

5. Which of the following Medicare plans includes coverage for both prescription drugs and medical care?

A. Part A
B. Part B
C. Part C
D. Part D

6. What government agency is responsible for the health care benefits of the majority of Americans age 65 years or older and is funded by the federal government only?

A. Medicare
B. Medicaid
C. Social Security
D. MTMS

7. What form of Medicare is solely for prescription drug coverage?

A. Part A
B. Part B
C. Part C
D. Part D

8. What is one criterion that an individual must meet to be eligible for MTMS enrollment through Medicare?

A. Takes multiple medications
B. Has only one disease state
C. Is older than age 55 years
D. Was enrolled in Medicare for at least 2 years

9. What source of health care is funded by federal and state governments and is the main form of coverage for people uninsured by the commercial market?

A. Medicare
B. Medicaid
C. MTMS
D. Social Security

10. What is the main source of funding for government-sponsored health care programs?

A. Taxes
B. Donations
C. Free for all in need
D. Federal reserve

11. Which of the following is a health care organization that ties Medicare payment to the quality of care provided?

A. ACO
B. HMO
C. PPO
D. IHS

12. Which of the following is an example of managed care? (Mark all that apply.)

A. An insurer contracting with a group of independent physicians to provide care specified by a set of quality measures
B. A patient paying out-of-pocket for a recent hospitalization at a local community hospital
C. A group of independent physicians forming an organization that agrees to provide its services at a discount to contracted insurance plans
D. A vertically integrated health system that employs its physicians, pharmacists, nurses, and other health care workers to coordinate efficient, quality, and cost-effective care

13. Which of the following statements about PBMs is true?

A. PBMs increase overall health care costs.
B. A Pharmacy and Therapeutics Committee is not used by PBMs.
C. PBMs never use a drug formulary.
D. Mail-out services are often used by PBMs.

14. PBM services may include (mark all that apply)

A. claims processing.
B. formulary management.
C. disease state management.
D. new drug development and approval.

15. What piece of legislation created Medicare Part D?

A. Medicare Prescription Drug, Improvement, and Modernization Act of 2003
B. Social Security Amendments of 1965
C. Occupational Safety and Health Administration Act of 1970
D. Food, Drug, and Cosmetic Act of 1938

14-7 Answers

1. **B.** *Horizontal integration* describes the buying of similar business entities by the same owner or group of owners.

2. **A.** HMOs and PPOs are the two main managed care categories, whereas MTMS is an example of pharmaceutical services.

3. **All apply.** Integrated health care systems align multiple levels of health care delivery settings under a single organization.

4. **A.** Private insurance companies carry the majority of financial burden with regard to health care expenditures.

5. **C.** Also known as Medicare Advantage Plans, Medicare Part C includes both drug and medical coverage.

6. **A.** Medicare provides health care benefits for Americans age 65 years and older. The government funds this form of health care.

7. **D.** Medicare Part D provides prescription drug coverage to Medicare recipients.

8. **A.** Patients must be enrolled in Medicare, suffer from multiple chronic disease states, use multiple Part D medications, and incur high annual drug costs.

9. **B.** Medicaid provides health care to those who cannot afford it.

10. **A.** Taxes are the main source of revenue for government-sponsored health care.

11. A. The ACO is a novel, experimental Medicare-funded health care organization model.

12. A, C, D. Each answer except B is correct because there is some intentional action to reduce cost and improve quality of care. Answer B is incorrect because in this scenario the payer (the patient) cannot hold the hospital accountable to providing either higher-quality or more cost-effective care.

13. D. Mail-out services are commonly used to reduce overall drug costs.

14. A, B, C. PBMs are generally not involved in research and development.

15. A. The Medicare Prescription Drug, Improvement, and Modernization Act of 2003 created Part D.

14-8 Additional Resources

Centers for Medicare and Medicaid Services. *Medicare and You*. 2018. Baltimore, MD: U.S. Department of Health and Human Services. Available at: https://www.medicare.gov/medicare-and-you/medicare-and-you.html.

Centers for Medicare and Medicaid Services. *National Health Expenditure Data 2015*. 2015. Baltimore, MD: U.S. Department of Health and Human Services. Available at: https://www.cms.gov/research-statistics-data-and-systems/statistics-trends-and-reports/nationalhealthexpenddata/nhe-fact-sheet.html.

Formulary management. November 2009. Academy of Managed Care Pharmacy, Alexandria, VA. Available at: http://www.amcp.org/WorkArea/DownloadAsset.aspx?id=9298.

Kaiser Family Foundation. *Timeline: History of Health Reform in the U.S.* March 25, 2011. Washington, DC: Kaiser Family Foundation. Available at: https://kaiserfamilyfoundation.files.wordpress.com/2011/03/5-02-13-history-of-health-reform.pdf.

Population-Based Care and Pharmacoepidemiology

15

A. SHAUN ROWE

15-1 KEY POINTS

- Epidemiology is a public health science that studies the risks for disease, distribution of disease, and effects of disease on a human population.
- Pharmacoepidemiology applies the tenets of epidemiology to evaluate medication use in a large population.
- Incidence is the occurrence of new cases of disease in a population at risk during a time period.
- Prevalence is the occurrence of disease cases (new or old) in a population at risk during a time period.
- Mortality rate is a special type of incidence rate that measures the occurrence of death in a population. It can be age adjusted so that mortality rates between different populations can be compared.
- A case report or case series is a descriptive report consisting of single or multiple reports of a new or unusual condition.
- A case-control study is a retrospective study evaluating the risks for a specific condition by comparing a group of patients with the disease to a group without the disease.
- A cohort compares the occurrence of a specific condition in a group that was exposed to a risk factor to a group that was not exposed to a risk factor.
- By applying measures of incidence and of prevalence to data from the U.S. Food and Drug Administration, Centers for Disease Control and Prevention, or other publicly available and proprietary sources, one can estimate the beneficial and harmful effects of medications on large populations.
- Continual monitoring of unwanted effects related to medications is conducted through active and passive surveillance.
- Passive surveillance involves health care providers voluntarily reporting unwanted medication effects to a central database.
- Among other causes, passive surveillance reports can be incomplete because of the time taken to report the cases, fear of malpractice, and the belief that someone else has already reported the information.
- Active surveillance involves the planned systematic collection of information concerning specific conditions, such as adverse effects, disease states, and medication adherence.
- Compared to passive surveillance systems, active surveillance systems provide a more accurate representation of a specific condition; however, active surveillance systems may include only patients from a small number of institutions.

15-2 STUDY GUIDE CHECKLIST

The following topics may guide your study of this subject area:

- ☐ Describe the measures of disease occurrence in large populations.
- ☐ Contrast the advantages and disadvantages of epidemiological study designs in the estimation of beneficial and harmful medication effects in large populations.
- ☐ Demonstrate how to report a medication adverse effect or vaccine adverse effect to the U.S. Food and Drug Administration.
- ☐ Contrast the advantages and disadvantages of passive and active surveillance.
- ☐ Identify key sources of information for the estimation of beneficial or harmful effects of medication use in large populations.

15-3 Overview

Pharmacoepidemiology is the study of the relationship between drug use and its outcomes (beneficial and adverse) in a large number of people. It is often used for postmarketing surveillance to continually monitor drug safety. As compared to randomized controlled trials (RCTs), pharmacoepidemiological studies can evaluate the use of medications in a larger and broader population, which allows for the identification of rare adverse drug effects and shifts in efficacy observed in rigorously conducted RCTs.

Whereas RCTs are best at establishing a causal relationship between drug use and outcomes and are the basis for approval for use by the U.S. Food and Drug Administration (FDA), RCTs may not adequately address the risk of adverse drug effects (ADEs) or may overestimate the true treatment effect. This is due in part to the relatively small number of patients enrolled in RCTs, the short study duration of RCTs, and the strict inclusion and exclusion criteria of RCTs. After a medication is approved for use by the FDA, continual monitoring of use in the general population allows for the generation of new information that may change the balance of the medication's risks and benefits. Using the new information, the FDA can restrict the drug's distribution, or it may request the manufacturer to withdraw the drug from the market. For example, rofecoxib (Vioxx), a nonsteroidal anti-inflammatory drug, was approved on May 20, 1999, and gained wide acceptance for treating chronic pain such as arthritis. However, on September 30, 2004, Merck voluntarily withdrew Vioxx from the market because of concerns about increased risk of heart attack and stroke associated with long-term, high-dosage use based on data from clinical trials.

Unlike RCTs, pharmacoepidemiology systematically evaluates new information generated after medications enter the market. As they relate to the study of medication safety, pharmacoepidemiological studies offer several advantages over RCTs. RCTs are not a feasible study design for the systematic evaluation of adverse medication effects because giving a harmful medication to a patient just to evaluate the societal burden of medication adverse effects would be unethical. Moreover, RCTs are cost-prohibitive for the study of rare ADEs. For example, if one person out of 1 million people who are given a drug develops stroke, and at least five people must develop stroke for a statistically significant finding for the support of the relationship between drug use and stroke development, an RCT would require the recruitment of at least 5 million subjects. Hence, the study would not be financially feasible. Furthermore, there would not be enough people from which to recruit study subjects. In contrast, a pharmacoepidemiological study could make use of real-world data generated from natural practice settings. This capability would allow for an ethical and financially feasible evaluation of the relationship between medication use and stroke development.

This chapter covers the epidemiological tools used to estimate the effects of medications in large populations, the most common epidemiological studies, and the methods for continual monitoring of drug safety and efficacy.

15-4 Principles of Epidemiology and Analytic Tools

Epidemiology is the study of how disease is distributed in populations and what factors influence the disease distribution. Disease has been classically described on the basis of the epidemiologic triad. According to the triad, disease is the product of an interaction of the host, the agent, and the environment. For such an interaction to occur, the host (the human) possesses certain characteristics that make him or her predisposed to or protected against a variety of different diseases. These protective or harmful characteristics are primarily genetic in origin or are the result of past exposures and vaccination history, whereas the disease-causing agents are biologic, physical, or chemical factors. Environmental conditions affecting the relationship between the host and the agent are multifactorial, but climatic and cultural conditions, such as health economics and health care access, are particularly important.

To evaluate the beneficial and harmful effects of a medication in a large population, one must measure the risks of disease occurrence and deaths from the disease. Incidence and prevalence quantify the rate of disease occurrence, whereas mortality rates quantify the rate of death. These measures are the most common measures used in pharmacoepidemiological studies.

Incidence Rates

Two types of incidence measures exist, depending on whether the measure takes into account the time during which each member of the population is at risk. Incidence proportion does not take into account the different times in which a given population is at risk. It is computed as the number of new cases within a specified period divided by the number of the population initially at risk. For example, if a population of 10,000 disease-free persons at the beginning of the observation generates 200 new cases of the disease over 2 years, the incidence proportion is 20 cases per 1,000 persons.

In contrast, incidence rate controls for the different times during which each population member is at risk. The need to control for the different time at risk exists because the population may lose old members or add new members during the 2-year observation period. *Incidence rate* is defined as the number of new cases per person-time at risk. If one assumes the population stays constant over the 2 years in the preceding example, the incidence rate would be 10 cases per 1,000 person-years, because there are 200 new cases per 20,000 person-years (10,000 persons × 2 years). When 5,000 people stay for 1 year only, then the incidence rate is 200 new cases divided by 15,000 person-years ([2 × 5,000] + [1 × 5,000] = 15,000) or 15 cases per 1,000 person-years. Thus, incidence rate is more appropriate when the time during which each individual is at risk differs among the population. However, it does not take into account that the risk of developing a new disease could also be different depending on specific points in time. For example, the incidence rate of 10 per 1,000 person-years can be 20 cases for 1,000 persons for the first year and zero cases per 1,000 persons for the second year.

Prevalence Rates

Prevalence is a measurement of the number of all individuals affected by a certain disease (existing as well as new cases) within a particular period. If a survey identified 20 new cases of prostate cancer in addition to 580 existing cases of prostate cancer in a community of 100,000 people in 2008, then the prevalence rate is 6 per 1,000 people in 2008 while the incidence is estimated at 0.2 per 1,000 people. Prevalence can be viewed as a snapshot of the population at a point in time at which all the members of the population are screened for the disease. Prevalence considers all the individuals with disease at the time of screening as cases. It does not pay attention to when the disease developed. In other words, whether the disease developed yesterday, last month, last year, or even 10 years ago does not matter in computing prevalence rates. However, prevalence rates can change either when new cases develop or when old cases are resolved because some individuals are cured or have died by the time of screening.

Prevalence rates do not control for disease duration. Chronic diseases last longer; thus, more chronic cases will accumulate over time than will acute cases. Hence, when incidence rates are comparable between chronic and acute diseases, the chronic diseases will have higher prevalence rates than will the acute ones. Prevalence is useful for chronic diseases such as HIV (human immunodeficiency virus) and diabetes, whereas incidence is useful for acute diseases such as infection-related conditions.

Mortality Rates

Mortality measures the risk of dying. *Mortality rate* is typically defined as the number of deaths in a given year, scaled to the size of that population. Mortality rate is often reported as the number of deaths per 1,000 individuals per year. For example, a mortality rate of 8 would mean 8 deaths in a given year per 1,000 individuals or 80 deaths in a given year in 10,000 individuals.

Annual mortality rate for all causes is calculated by dividing the total number of deaths from all causes in a year by the population size as of July 1 (i.e., midyear population). The population size at midyear is generally used to control for changing population over time. The equation is expressed as follows:

$$\text{Annual mortality rate for all causes} = \frac{\text{Number of deaths from all causes in 1 year}}{\text{Number of persons in population at midyear}}$$

The mortality rate for a certain age group or for one ethnic group rather than for the entire population is often of interest and can be calculated for that group. The mortality rate for a specific group is called a *specific mortality rate,* such as the age-specific mortality rate. Likewise, when a restriction is placed on a specific disease, it is called a *disease-specific* or *cause-specific mortality rate*. For example, the diabetes-specific mortality rate is computed by dividing the number of patients who have died from diabetic complications by the number of persons in the population at midyear.

Crude mortality rates do not address that mortality rates can differ depending on characteristics of a population under investigation. Virtually all populations are heterogeneous; they are different in terms of age, sex, and other sociodemographics. Age is a major determinant of mortality, and thus, populations would have different mortality rates depending on their age distributions. There are two ways to control for different age distributions:

- ***Compute age-specific mortality rates:*** Here, the population under investigation is divided into several age categories and then age-specific mortality rates are computed for each age category.
- ***Compute age-adjusted mortality rates:*** To compute an overall age-adjusted rate for a given population under investigation, first compute age-specific rates for each age category of the population. Next, compute the number of expected deaths in each age category of a standard population by multiplying the age-specific rate of the population under investigation and the number of people in the respective age category of the standard population. The age-adjusted mortality rate for the population under investigation is the ratio of the sum of expected deaths over all age categories of the standard population and the size of the standard population. Age-adjusted mortality rates are used to compare mortality rates between different populations.

15-5 Common Epidemiological Study Designs

Case Series

Case series may refer to the study of a single patient (*case report*) or a small group of patients (*case series*) who are experiencing a disease. This type of study is purely descriptive and cannot be used to make inferences about the general population of patients with that disease. Studies of this type may lead to the formation of a new hypothesis. On the basis of the information obtained, analytic studies such as case control studies or cohort studies could be designed to investigate a possible link between the disease and its risk factors.

Case Control Studies

Case control studies compare rates of exposure to risk factors for a specific condition between subjects who have that condition (the *cases*) and subjects who do not have the condition (the *controls*). As part of a case control study, the cases and controls should have very specific definitions. For example, the time period for the condition to develop, diagnostic criteria for the condition, population of interest, and other potential contributing factors should all be identified and described. Once cases are identified, controls

TABLE 15-1. A Case Control Study Design

Risk factor	Cases	Controls
Exposed	*a*	*b*
Unexposed	*c*	*d*

from a similar population with a similar chance of developing the condition are chosen. Each selected subject is then evaluated through time to assess the status of exposure to risk factors. Data can be sorted into a 2×2 table (Table 15-1), and an odds ratio (OR) can be calculated to measure the association between the exposure factor and the outcome.

Each cell of Table 15-1 represents the number of exposed cases (a), exposed controls (b), unexposed cases (c), and unexposed controls (d). The ratio of a/c is the odds of exposure in the cases, whereas the ratio of b/d is the odds of exposure in the controls. The OR is the ratio of the two odds (i.e., the odds of exposure in the cases to the odds of exposure in the controls) and is expressed as follows:

$$OR = \frac{(a/c)}{(b/d)}$$

The OR measures the association between the exposure to a disease risk factor and the disease outcome. An OR significantly greater than 1 indicates that those with the disease are more likely to have been exposed to the risk factor than those without the disease. An OR of 1 indicates no association between the risk factor and the disease outcome. An OR less than 1 indicates that those with the disease are less likely to have been exposed to the risk factor than those without the disease. The data in Table 15-2 provide an example of a case control study involving the use of acid-suppressive drugs and the risk of gastric cancer among people registered in Quebec's health insurance plan in Canada.

The OR is

$$OR = \frac{a/b}{c/d} = \frac{ad}{bc} = \frac{679 \times 8{,}728}{4{,}263 \times 919} = 1.51$$

This OR illustrates that gastric cancer patients were more likely to have used acid-suppressive drugs.

Case control studies are usually faster and more cost effective than cohort studies. They are particularly useful for the study of a rare disease because they guarantee a sufficient number of cases with the disease. However, they are prone to bias. The main challenge is to identify the appropriate control group. The identification of controls is typically done by drawing a random sample from the original population at risk. Alternatively, controls can be selected by matching to cases in terms of risk factors that can cause the disease.

TABLE 15-2. Gastric Cancer and Use of Acid-Suppressive Drugs

Acid-suppressive drugs	Cases	Controls
Used	679 (*a*)	4,263 (*b*)
Not used	919 (*c*)	8,728 (*d*)
Total	1,598	12,991

Tamim et al., 2008.

Cohort Studies

Cohort studies compare the risk of developing a disease between those who are exposed to a risk factor and those who are not exposed. A *cohort* is a group of people who share a common characteristic within a defined period. Thus, those who are exposed to a drug in a defined period form an exposure cohort, whereas those who are not exposed form a nonexposure cohort. The subjects should be at risk of getting a certain disease but be free of disease at the beginning of the cohort study. Thus, the selection of a cohort is independent of the occurrence of the condition of interest.

Each cohort is followed prospectively through time to assess the status of disease development. For example, smokers and nonsmokers can be followed through time to assess the development of lung cancer. The relationship between exposure to smoking and risk of lung cancer can be quantified using relative risk (RR) or absolute risk reduction (ARR). The RR is a ratio of the risk of getting lung cancer in those who are exposed to smoking versus those who are not exposed. In contrast, the ARR would be the absolute difference in the risk of getting lung cancer in those not exposed to smoking and those who are exposed (i.e., ARR = $P_{unexposed} - P_{exposed}$).

$$RR = \frac{P_{exposed}}{P_{unexposed}}$$

A cohort study typically generates a 2 × 2 table (Table 15-3). From Table 15-3, the risk of disease in the exposed group ($P_{exposed}$) is $a/(a + b)$, whereas the risk of disease in the unexposed group ($P_{unexposed}$) is $c/(c + d)$. An RR greater than 1 shows association between exposure and disease outcome and can be interpreted as showing that those with exposure are more likely to develop the disease than those without exposure. An RR less than 1 means that the exposure is protective, because it is associated with a lower risk of developing the disease. A relative risk of 1 means no association exists between the exposure and the risk of developing the disease. However, because the ARR is the difference between the risk in the unexposed and exposed groups, zero indicates there is no association between the exposure and the risk of developing the disease. If the ARR is less than zero, then the exposure would indicate an increased risk (i.e., the reduction is negative; therefore, the risk is increased), but if the ARR is greater than zero, then the exposure is associated with an absolute decrease in disease. For simplicity, in the situation where the ARR is negative, the negative sign is generally ignored and the statistic is referred to as the absolute risk increase (ARI). The ARR can also be used to calculate another useful statistic—the number needed to treat (NNT). The NNT is the number of patients who need to be treated during a time period to prevent the development of one outcome. It can be useful when relaying the clinical significance of an intervention or observation. As with the ARR, if the NNT is negative, then the negative sign is generally ignored and the statistic is referred to as the number needed to harm (NNH).

For example, data from the Tennessee Medicaid program obtained between January 1, 1987, and December 31, 1998, were used to identify a cohort of new nonsteroidal anti-inflammatory drug (NSAID) users (n = 181,441) excluding aspirin and an equal number of nonusers, matched for age, sex, and date the NSAID use began. During a 275,565 person-year of follow-up for NSAID users, 3,313 cases of serious coronary heart disease occurred, or 12.02 per 1,000 person-years, while during a 257,069 person-year of follow-up for nonusers, 3,049 cases of serious coronary heart disease occurred, or 11.77 per 1,000 person-years. Thus, the relative risk is 1.02 (12.02/11.77), indicating almost no association

TABLE 15-3. A Cohort Study Design

Risk factor	Disease positive	Disease negative	Total
Exposed	*a*	*b*	$(a + b)$
Not exposed	*c*	*d*	$(c + d)$

between NSAIDs and coronary heart disease, whereas the ARI and NNH are 0.00025 and 4,000, respectively. As with the RR, the ARI and NNH indicate that there is almost no association between NSAIDs and coronary heart disease.

Cohort studies are typically prospective. However, retrospective cohort studies can be designed if historical records of exposure and disease outcomes are available. They are designed when the rate of exposure to a risk factor is rare. Cohort studies offer many advantages over case control studies. The RR is a more powerful association measure than the OR of case control studies; case control studies cannot be used to estimate risk of disease, because subjects are selected on the basis of the status of disease outcome. Time-specific characteristics can be established in prospective studies, and one can more easily control for confounders. The disadvantages of cohort studies are that they are costlier and are subject to a greater chance of losing subjects during the long follow-up period.

15-6 Continual Monitoring of Large Populations

Surveillance systems aim to continually monitor unwanted effects and other safety-related outcomes for safe use of drugs in large populations. Overall, there are two types of surveillance: passive and active. Passive surveillance relies on voluntary reports of adverse drug effects (ADEs) and does not involve any organized efforts to collect complete data on ADEs and outcomes.

Passive Surveillance

Passive surveillance involves health care providers' voluntary reporting of unwanted medication effects. Such reports are submitted voluntarily or by contract by pharmaceutical companies, consumer organizations, or regulatory authorities. The systematic evaluation of the voluntary reports can lead to the detection of safety signals associated with the extensive use of the drug in a large population. In many instances, the systematic evaluation of these reports can identify the occurrence of rare adverse effects that were not identified at the time of the medication's approval and identify risk factors for such adverse effects.

However, spontaneous reports are often incomplete. The reason for incomplete reports is multifactorial. Time since the drug entered the market, the regulatory surveillance activity, the media attention, and the drug market are all potential reasons for such incomplete reports.

Spontaneous reporting by health care providers can be intensified when a need arises to obtain more complete data. For example, when new drugs are first launched, drug companies should encourage voluntary reports of any potential ADEs for the cautious use of new products. Intensified spontaneous reporting in the early phase of postmarketing surveillance can lead to the early detection of new safety signals. Although intensified self-reporting may improve reporting rates, it is not completely free of the limitations of passive surveillance, such as selective reporting and incomplete information.

An example of a voluntary surveillance system is the FDA's MedWatch program (https://www.fda.gov/Safety/MedWatch/default.htm). The MedWatch program enables health care professionals and the public to voluntarily report safety problems associated with medical products, such as drugs and medical devices. All data contained on the MedWatch form will go into the FDA Adverse Event Reporting System (FAERS). FAERS (https://www.fda.gov/Drugs/GuidanceComplianceRegulatoryInformation/Surveillance/AdverseDrugEffects/default.htm) is a computerized information database that supports the FDA's postmarketing surveillance efforts. The FDA uses MedWatch to rapidly communicate new safety information to the medical community for improved patient care.

Active Surveillance

Active surveillance aims to obtain the most complete data possible on drug safety problems. It uses a meticulously planned process to capture comprehensive data on drug safety problems. It also implements an organized system to capture all events of drug safety problems. Two prominent examples of active surveillances are sentinel sites and registries.

Sentinel sites are a limited number of selected reporting sites, from which the information collected may be extended to the general population. Sentinel surveillance systems are useful because a rich source of data collected from the sentinel sites enables more accurate estimation of a risk than is available from broader passive surveillance programs.

Medical records from sentinel sites can be reviewed for complete and accurate data on adverse effects. Patients and physicians can also be interviewed for comprehensive data on risk factors associated with adverse effects. The sentinel surveillance system thus offers the advantage of being able to generate data for specific patient subgroups that would not be available in a passive spontaneous reporting system. Sentinel surveillance systems are most efficient for those drugs used mainly in institutional settings such as hospitals, nursing homes, and hemodialysis centers. These institutions treat specific types of patients and thus serve as a rich data source for certain types of drugs. Sentinel sites, however, are not free of weaknesses. Major weaknesses are selection bias, small numbers of patients, and increased costs of implementation.

An example of a sentinel surveillance system can be found in the National Poison Data System (NPDS), formerly the Toxic Exposure Surveillance System (TESS). Since 1983, NPDS has collected data on calls to U.S. poison control centers regarding poisonings principally from health care providers and members of the public and law enforcement. The American Association of Poison Control Centers (AAPCC) maintains the surveillance program (http://www.aapcc.org/data-system/). Information from AAPCC members is continually uploaded to the NPDS, providing a near real-time evaluation of poison call conditions nationwide. In addition to describing exposures to potentially toxic substances, the NPDS can be used to detect emerging public health concerns, such as potential exposures to harmful biological substances. When these public health concerns are detected by the NPDS, the CDC (Centers for Disease Control and Prevention) notifies state health departments about the potential need for intervention.

Registries aim to maintain a database of individuals with the same characteristic or characteristics. The database establishes a list of people who share the same characteristics and tracks them for additional information. Two types of registries exist, depending on whether the shared characteristic is a disease or a specific exposure.

A *disease registry* (e.g., a cancer registry) attempts to make a list of all the patients with the disease. It can be used to estimate prevalence, incidence, and mortality rates for the specific disease population. It also can be used for case control studies, in which case exposure information is further collected by administering survey questionnaires to the patients, and the cases and controls are compared. An example of the disease registry is the Surveillance, Epidemiology, and End Results (SEER) Program of the National Cancer Institute in the United States (https://seer.cancer.gov/). The SEER Program began collecting data on cancer cases in 1973. Currently, the SEER Program allows the estimation of incidence, survival, and prevalence from cancer data on specific geographic areas representing 26% of the U.S. population.

In contrast, an *exposure registry* (e.g., a drug registry) first identifies a cohort exposed to a certain risk factor, such as a prescription drug, and then follows up on the cohort to collect data on occurrences of adverse effects. Single-exposure cohorts enable the measurement of incidence rates, whereas the comparison with a nonexposed cohort provides RR estimates. An important example of an exposure registry is a requirement created by the 2007 Food and Drug Administration Amendments Act. As part of this law, the FDA was given authority to require a risk evaluation and mitigation strategy (REMS) (https://www.accessdata.fda.gov/scripts/cder/rems/index.cfm) from drug manufacturers. REMSs are designed by the manufacturers to ensure the benefits of a medication outweigh the potentially harmful effects. An REMS may require a plan of elements to assure safe use (ETASU). As part of the ETASU plan, health care professionals must follow specified procedures before prescribing or dispensing a medication, and patients must be monitored and enrolled in a registry. Among other uses, the information in this registry helps describe usage patterns of medications, adverse drug effects, and understanding of monitoring requirements. More information about specific medications in the REMS program is available on the FDA Web site (https://www.accessdata.fda.gov/scripts/cder/rems/index.cfm).

Thus, pharmacoepidemiology is often used in postmarketing surveillance of approved drug products to estimate beneficial and unwanted medication effects in the general population. Current FDA postmarketing surveillance systems are passive, relying on voluntary reports of adverse effects related to use of prescription medications. However, the implementation of active surveillance systems is being discussed. Although building an active surveillance system is complex, progress in computerized medicine will pave the way for the development of effective active surveillance systems.

15-7 Population Health and Pharmacy

Population health is outcomes focused and related to public health. Several pharmacist activities and practice models have a significant effect on the outcomes associated with population health. As one of the most accessible health care professionals, and through activities such as health screenings, immunizations, medication therapy management, clinical research, smoking cessation, family planning, and emergency preparedness, pharmacists play an active role in the improvement of health outcomes in high-risk populations. Though these activities are outside of the traditional fee-for-product pay structure, national pharmacy organizations are advocating for insurance pay structures that include compensation of pharmacists for such activities. Despite the lack of compensation for many of these activities, there is a growing body of evidence that pharmacist-led population health initiatives improve health outcomes.

15-8 Questions

1. Randomized clinical trials cannot adequately address the risk of adverse drug effects at drug approval for which of the following reasons? (Mark all that apply.)

A. Small number of patients
B. Short study duration
C. Strict inclusion criteria
D. Randomization

2. Randomized clinical trials can be inferior to epidemiological studies in drug safety research. Which of the following statements *incorrectly* describes the disadvantages of RCTs in the study of drug safety?

A. RCTs are ethically challenging because subjects are given a drug that may cause harm.
B. RCTs are more expensive to perform than epidemiological studies.
C. RCTs may not be able to recruit enough subjects to find the statistical significance in rarely occurring drug safety problems.
D. RCTs randomize subjects to different comparison groups.

3. Which one of the following statements *incorrectly* describes epidemiology?

A. Epidemiological tools have proved effective in establishing major causes of diseases such as cholera and lung cancer.
B. Epidemiological findings can be refuted by randomized controlled trials.
C. Epidemiology uses data generated through real-world practice environments.
D. Epidemiology uses randomization to compare two groups.

4. Which of the following statements correctly defines epidemiology?

A. Epidemiology is the study of how disease is distributed in populations and what factors influence the disease distribution.
B. Epidemiology is the study of how disease is distributed in sentinel sites and what factors influence the disease development.
C. Epidemiology is the study of what factors cause a specific disease in populations.
D. Epidemiology is the study of causal relationships between diseases and their risk factors in populations.

5. Which of the following is *not* part of the epidemiologic triad?

A. Host
B. Environment
C. Agent
D. Vector

6. Which of the following measures the *risk* that a certain disease newly develops in a given population within a specified period?

A. Incidence
B. Prevalence
C. Mortality
D. Morbidity

7. When do epidemiologists prefer incidence rates to incidence proportions?

A. When the population at risk varies with time
B. When the amount of observation time between people is the same
C. When new cases outnumber existing cases
D. When existing cases outnumber new cases

8. Which of the following statements is *not* a reason that mortality rates are often standardized by age?

A. Mortality rates vary by age.
B. Different populations have different age distributions.
C. Epidemiologists are interested in comparing mortality between different populations.
D. Populations are aging.

9. Which of the following statements is *not* true about case control studies?

A. Case control studies are done when exposure is rare.
B. The odds ratio is reported at the end of the study.
C. Case control studies are done when a disease is rare.
D. Case control studies are retrospective.

10. Which of the following statements correctly describes cohort studies?

A. They are often retrospective.
B. They are conducted to evaluate rare risk factors.
C. They are done when disease is rare.
D. All cohort studies are prospective.

11. Which of the following is a characteristic of a passive surveillance system?

A. Voluntary reporting
B. Sentinel sites
C. Requirement by the federal government
D. Registries

12. As compared to active surveillance systems, which of the following is an advantage of passive surveillance systems?

A. Complete data collection
B. Voluntary reporting by many health care professionals
C. Planned process
D. Automatic collection of data

13. Which of the following is a characteristic of an active surveillance system?

A. It includes only sentinel site reporting.
B. It is a meticulously planned process.
C. It includes only disease or exposure registries.
D. Ii is required by the federal government for all medications.

14. As compared to passive surveillance systems, which of the following is an advantage of active surveillance systems?

A. Voluntary reporting by many health care professionals
B. Low amount of selection bias
C. Complete information in the database
D. Low cost of implementation

15. A prevalence study conducted from January 1 to December 31, 2017, on a population of 125,000 identified 500 cases of a disease. The incidence rate of this disease is 2 per 1,000. What percentage of the cases was newly diagnosed in 2017?

A. 5%
B. 50%
C. 2%
D. Answer cannot be calculated from this data set.

16. A city contains 100,000 people (52,000 males and 48,000 females), and 2,000 people die per year (1,100 males and 900 females). What is the crude mortality rate?

A. 21.2 per 1,000
B. 20 per 1,000
C. 18.8 per 1,000
D. 18.8 per 10,000

17. A cohort study can be used for which of the following factors? (Mark all that apply.)

A. Smoking
B. Physical activity
C. Obesity
D. Congenital anomalies

18. Within a 5-year period, 10,000 residents of a community of 100,000 people were diagnosed with diabetes. What is the incidence rate of diabetes among the members of this community during the 5-year period?

A. 7 per 1,000
B. 142.86 per 1,000
C. 100 per 1,000
D. None of the above

19. Of 100 people who had a disease, 10 had been exposed to a risk factor. Of 100 matched controls, 2 had been exposed to a risk factor. Which of the following is true?

A. The relative risk is 5.
B. The odds ratio is 5.
C. The relative risk is 0.2.
D. The odds ratio is 0.2.

20. In 1945, 1,000 women worked in a factory painting radium dials on watches. A study compared the incidence of bone cancer in these women, up to 1975, with the incidence of bone cancer in 1,000 women who worked as telephone operators in 1945. Twenty of the radium dial painters and 4 of the telephone operators developed bone cancer between 1945 and 1975. This study is an example of

A. a cohort study.
B. an experimental study.
C. a cross-sectional study.
D. a case control study.

15-9 Answers

1. **A, B, C.** RCTs cannot adequately address the risk of ADEs because of their small number of patients, short study duration, and strict inclusion and exclusion criteria. Randomization does not influence the ability of an RCT to detect adverse drug effects.

2. **D.** RCTs are superior to epidemiological studies because they use randomization, which makes different groups comparable at baseline. Giving a patient a medication known to cause harm just to measure the occurrence of adverse drug effects is unethical. As compared to epidemiological studies, RCTs are expensive. Because the occurrence of adverse drug effects may be rare, RCTs are impracticable and financially infeasible and thus inferior to epidemiological study designs for the detection of adverse drug effects.

3. **D.** RCTs, not epidemiology, use randomization. In general, epidemiological studies are well designed to evaluate rare diseases, diseases that develop over long periods of time, or rare risks of disease. RCTs are considered the highest level of evidence; thus, in many instances, an RCT will overturn the results of an epidemiological study. Data used to conduct epidemiological studies are generated from real-world practice environments.

4. **A.** Epidemiology is the study of how disease is distributed in populations and what factors influence the disease distribution. Sentinel sites are an important component of active surveillance, but they are only a component of pharmacoepidemiology. Though risk factors for disease are important, there are three components of disease: the host, the agent, and the environment. Epidemiological studies are not designed to identify causal relationships.

5. **D.** The epidemiologic triad consists of the host, the agent, and the environment.

6. **A.** Incidence measures the risk of developing a new disease. Prevalence is a measure of both new and old cases of disease in a population at risk. Mortality is defined as death; whereas, mortality rate is a special type of incidence. Morbidity is the negative effects of a disease, but it is not a rate.

7. **A.** Incidence rate controls for the different periods during which each population member is at risk. The need to control for the different period at risk exists because the population may lose old members or add new members during the observation period. Although evaluation of the differences in prevalence and incidence by evaluating new cases and existing cases is important, that evaluation is not pertinent to the question.

8. **D.** The standardization is needed because different populations have different age distributions, not because they are aging. Because age is a significant factor in the mortality rate and different populations have different age distributions, standardization of mortality rates is necessary to allow for the comparison of different populations.

9. **A.** Cohort studies are used to study rare exposures. By definition, case control studies use the odds ratio, are used for rare diseases, and are retrospective (answers B, C, and D are incorrect).

10. **B.** Cohort studies are conducted when the risk factors are rare. They can be retrospective or prospective.

11. **A.** Passive surveillance systems are defined by voluntary spontaneous reporting. Sentinel sites, federal requirements, and registries are all characteristics of active surveillance systems.

12. **B.** A significant advantage of passive surveillance systems is the large number of health care professionals reporting into the database. This increases the number of patients in the database and allows for the detection of rare effects that may otherwise go undetected. Unfortunately, because of the voluntary nature of the reporting, many times the data are incomplete. Passive surveillance systems do not include a planned collection system, nor do they currently use automatic data collection.

13. **B.** Active surveillance systems involve meticulously planned processes. Disease registries, exposure registries, and sentinel sites are all part of active surveillance systems. Active surveillance through the REMS program is only required by the FDA when the risks of medication use may outweigh the benefits or new safety information is discovered on an existing medication.

14. **C.** Because of the planned process and required data collection elements, the information contained in active surveillance systems is complete as compared to that in passive systems. Unfortunately, because of the relatively small numbers of health care professionals who are reporting into the system and because of the nonvoluntary reporting nature of the system, there is significant selection bias. In addition, active surveillance systems are very costly to maintain.

15. **B.** Of 125,000 people, there were a total of 500 cases. An incidence rate of 2 per 1,000 means 250 new cases per 125,000 people. Thus, 50% are new cases.

16. **B.** Crude mortality is 2,000 people divided by 100,000 people. Thus, 20 people die per 1,000.

17. **A, B, C.** Smoking, physical activity, and obesity are all key risk factors for disease. Congenital anomalies are disease outcomes, not risk factors.

18. **C.** A Community of 100,000 has 10,000 new cases of diabetes during a 5-year period. Thus, $(10{,}000/100{,}000) \times 1{,}000 = 100$ per 1,000.

19. **B.** The case control study results in an odds ratio of $(10/100)/(2/100) = 5$.

20. **A.** Cohort studies compare the risk of developing a disease between those who are exposed to a risk factor and those who are not exposed. Subjects were not assigned to a treatment, and patients were followed through time for the development of bone cancer. Patients were identified by their exposure to radium by painting watch dials and compared to people who were not exposed to radium but had a risk of developing bone cancer.

15-10 Additional Resources

Centers for Disease Control and Prevention. *Principles of Epidemiology in Public Health Practice: An Introduction to Applied Epidemiology and Biostatistics*. 3rd ed. Atlanta, GA: U.S. Department of Health and Human Services, Centers for Disease Control and Prevention; 2012. Available at: https://www.cdc.gov/ophss/csels/dsepd/ss1978/index.html.

FDA Basics Webinar: a brief overview of risk evaluation and mitigation strategies (REMS). 2017. U.S. Food and Drug Administration Web site. https://www.fda.gov/AboutFDA/Transparency/Basics/ucm325201.htm.

National Cancer Institute. Surveillance, epidemiology, and end results program. Division of Cancer Control and Population Sciences, National Cancer Institute, Bethesda, MD; 2010. Available at: https://www.seer.cancer.gov/.

Postmarketing surveillance programs. June 2017. U.S. Food and Drug Administration Web site. https://www.fda.gov/Drugs/GuidanceComplianceRegulatoryInformation/Surveillance/ucm090385.htm.

Public Health Agency of Canada. Sentinel sites. April 2015. Government of Canada Web site. https://www.canada.ca/en/public-health/services/surveillance/foodnet-canada/sentinel-sites.html.

Tamim H, Duranceau A, Chen L-Q, et al. Association between use of acid-suppressive drugs and risk of gastric cancer: a nested case-control study. *Drug Saf.* 2008;31(8):675–684.

Economic and Humanistic Outcomes of Health Care Delivery

16

JUSTIN GATWOOD

16-1 KEY POINTS

- The world has limited resources, and the study of economics looks at how individuals and organizations engage in the production, distribution, and consumption of goods and services in an environment of limited resources.
- Mankiw's Principles of Economics outline 10 concepts that describe overarching elements of how people make decisions and interact with each other.
- Health care decision makers need to have some way of knowing that they are receiving the most value for their dollar, and pharmacoeconomic approaches help in making those decisions.
- Several assumptions of general economic markets do not necessarily apply to the health care environment, and one must take these differences into account when conducting a pharmacoeconomic analysis.
- The typical patient pays only a portion of the cost of prescription medications, either through a co-pay or co-insurance, and the typical hospital pays a discounted rate for medications and receives further discounts in the form of rebates from the manufacturer or supplier, which are based on the amount of medication purchased.
- A less expensive medication may not be the best choice if it is not as effective as a more expensive medication or if treatment of the side effects or adverse events associated with the medication is costlier than would be the case had a more expensive medication been used.
- A health utility measure can be either disease specific or generic. These humanistic outcome measures allow the patient to specify how much better he or she is feeling or is able to perform activities of daily living when taking a specific medication.
- When conducting pharmacoeconomic studies, researchers must establish the perspective for the study because it determines which costs will be included in the analysis. The typical perspectives are those of the society, the patient, and the payer. The most common perspective used is the payer's perspective.
- The most typical pharmacoeconomic assessments include cost-burden of illness, cost-benefit, cost-utility, cost-effectiveness, and cost-minimization analysis.
- The basic framework for cost-effectiveness analyses is $(\text{Cost}_{\text{Drug A}} - \text{Cost}_{\text{Drug B}})/(\text{Effectiveness}_{\text{Drug A}} - \text{Effectiveness}_{\text{Drug B}})$.

16-2 STUDY GUIDE CHECKLIST

The following topics may guide your study of this subject matter:

- ☐ Understand the extent to which Mankiw's 10 Principles of Economics apply to health care, health economics, and pharmacoeconomics.
- ☐ Define the key macroeconomic principles as they apply to the U.S. health care system.
- ☐ Recognize how microeconomic theory can explain health economics and where market failures exist.
- ☐ Identify types of patient-reported outcomes and their role in determining the effect of various therapies.
- ☐ Understand the elements used to calculate a quality-adjusted life year based on utility tied to a specific health outcome.
- ☐ Understand the elements of the various types of cost-effectiveness analyses as well as the implications of their findings.
- ☐ Define the types and sources of costs, benefits, and probabilities needed to populate a pharmacoeconomic model.

16-3 Microeconomic and Macroeconomic Principles

The world has limited resources, and interpreting how individuals and firms behave within these limitations forms the basis for economic theory. In general, these behaviors are understood in aggregate (macroeconomic) and individual (microeconomic) perspectives. Several economic theories, models, and principles have been created to help identify and predict what will happen in various economic situations, including health-related decisions. Understanding the microeconomic and macroeconomic principles applied to health care can help people better interpret how resources are distributed throughout the system.

Underlying basic economic theory is a series of principles that are useful in understanding the way the economy at large should perform given changes that occur. Mankiw's 10 Principles of Economics outline three categories of assumptions that guide how people make decisions (Box 16-1). The first four principles relate to how people make decisions, the next three relate to how the economy works as a whole, and the last three relate to how people interact. However, one must understand that while Mankiw's principles as well as other well-accepted concepts of economic theory are useful to interpret most decisions, they may not be applicable to all health-related scenarios. For instance, the decision being made by a patient may not be rational because he or she is not always entitled to full information or is unable to fully assess the treatment being offered. Additionally, prices are often set by insurers—who control access to most resources—rather than being dictated by a free market (see Chapter 13 for the flow of funds of the drug supply chain). Also, the cost of giving up health may be quality of life or life

BOX 16-1. Mankiw's Principles of Economics

1. "People face trade-offs."
   To get one thing, you have to give up something else. Making decisions requires trading off one goal against another.
2. "The cost of something is what you give up to get it."
   Decision makers have to consider both the obvious and the implicit costs of their actions.
3. "Rational people think at the margin."
   A rational decision maker takes action if and only if the marginal benefit of the action exceeds the marginal cost.
4. "People respond to incentives."
   Behavior changes when costs or benefits change.
5. "Trade can make everyone better off."
   Trade allows each person to specialize in the activities he or she does best. By trading with others, people can buy a greater variety of goods or services.
6. "Markets are usually a good way to organize economic activity."
   Households and firms that interact in market economies act as if they are guided by an "invisible hand" that leads the market to allocate resources efficiently. The opposite of this is economic activity that is organized by a central planner within the government.
7. "Governments can sometimes improve market outcomes."
   When a market fails to allocate resources efficiently, the government can change the outcome through public policy. Examples are regulations against monopolies and pollution.
8. "A country's standard of living depends on its ability to produce goods and services."
   Countries whose workers produce a large quantity of goods and services per unit of time enjoy a high standard of living. Similarly, as a nation's productivity grows, so does its average income.
9. "Prices rise when the government prints too much money."
   When a government creates large quantities of the nation's money, the value of the money falls. As a result, prices increase, requiring more of the same money to buy goods and services.
10. "Society faces a short-run trade-off between inflation and unemployment."
    Reducing inflation often causes a temporary rise in unemployment. This trade-off is crucial for understanding the short-run effects of changes in taxes, government spending, and monetary policy.

Mankiw, 2007.

itself, either of which is difficult to quantify in dollars. As a result, health care markets, unlike most in the economy, may not be efficient.

Perhaps the most well-known economic theory is supply and demand. At a basic level, the supply and demand model indicates how prices will change given a change in supply and demand for goods or services. As demand increases, supply increases to meet this greater demand, resulting in a larger quantity of a good being sold and at a higher price. The supply-demand curve depicts this relationship (Figure 16-1). In most instances, this relationship is relatively straightforward to visualize, and one can interpret how consumers and businesses would behave in relation to a physical good. However, in the context of health care, the good being sought is health while the service being supplied is health care, both of which can be challenging to quantify. In this case, the supply-demand curve illustrates how, at a given price, one would demand a certain *amount* of health that would be supplied by a certain level of *health care*.

Macroeconomics Affecting Health Care

Macroeconomic studies aggregate output, employment, and the general price level, which provides insight to the performance of the overall economy. These analyses also can focus on specific sectors or functions of the economy, such as labor markets, inflation, and international trade. The U.S. health care system is massive; in 2015, it accounted for more than $3 trillion of spending per year, or roughly 18% of the country's gross domestic product (GDP). The GDP is a measure of the amount of goods or services produced within a country over a period of time and it is an important indicator of an economy's health.

Considering its size, the U.S. health care system plays a considerable role in the exchange of goods and services within the country. As a result, the government has a vested interest in how the system is run, and regulations and policies are regularly put in place in an effort to improve how it functions. Well-known forms of government intervention include programs such as Medicare (care for the elderly), enacted in 1965; Medicaid (care for the poor), enacted in 1965; and the Patient Protection and Affordable Care Act (ACA), enacted in 2010, which sought to provide health insurance for those who did not qualify for, were not offered, or could not afford other forms of health insurance coverage. Although these programs were implemented to improve access to care for millions of Americans, they can have adverse effects on the economy. Government intervention to health care markets may "crowd out" private business investment in health care, meaning these businesses have less of an incentive to invest in health services. Because government programs fetch the lowest prices in the market, more government intervention may lower GDP where otherwise increased private firm activity may have led to higher growth rates related to health

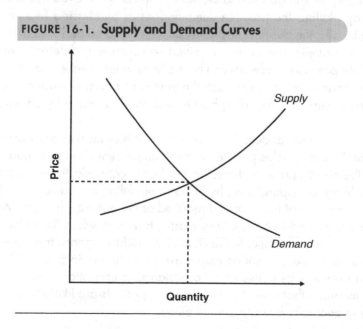

FIGURE 16-1. Supply and Demand Curves

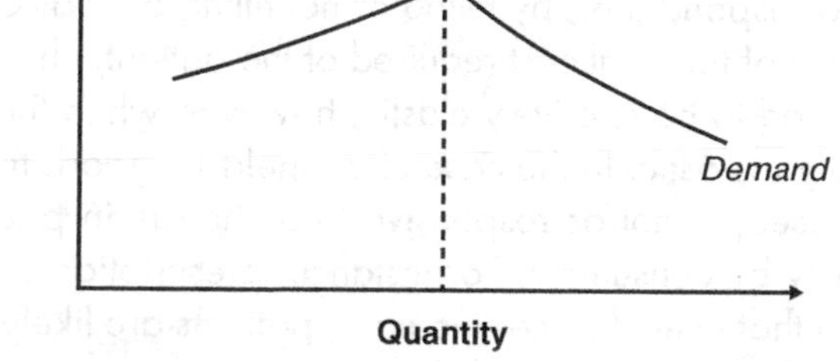

services. Because the U.S. health care sector is a mix of government and private business programs, the balance of these entities is a delicate interaction.

Government intervention in health care also can be seen in the form of recommendations made by public entities, such as the Centers for Disease Control and Prevention (CDC). The CDC collects and reviews evidence on matters relevant to public health, primarily within the United States. At a societal level, these recommendations can affect how certain diseases, both communicable and noncommunicable conditions, are controlled by giving direction to state and local health departments as well as health systems and individual providers. For instance, the CDC provides regular guidance on vaccination schedules for infants, children, and adults. In seeking to limit the spread of infectious disease, the CDC is actually creating what economists refer to as a positive externality. An externality exists when an individual unintentionally benefits or is harmed by another individual consuming a good or service. In the case of vaccinations, the more people vaccinated, the less likely a disease will spread throughout a community, even among those who chose not to be vaccinated. Although this example demonstrates positive effects of an externality, negative ones, such as air pollution, also exist.

Although the role of government in health care has expanded in recent years, private employers are still the single largest payer for health insurance in the United States. The rising and significant cost of health benefits for employees has caused many businesses to shift more of these costs onto their employees. As costs increase for businesses, both in connection with and independent of health care costs, this increase can negatively affect how employers are able to support jobs, as pointed out by Mankiw. In fact, potential negative effects on jobs was a major concern surrounding the ACA, but research on this program has thus far indicated no significant effect.

Microeconomics of Health Care

Whereas macroeconomic theory addresses concepts across the economy, microeconomics studies the individual decision makers, such as consumers, resource owners, and businesses. At this level, one can examine the way health is interpreted as a good, the way consumers may decide between health and other goods or services, and the extent to which health systems can supply health care as a service.

The concept of "health" as a good is an ambiguous one because it is more challenging to quantify than other tangible goods. However, the pursuit and consumption of it can still be interpreted like other goods when considering the concept of budget constraints. Even the demand for health cannot escape the fact that the health care system has limited resources. Consequently, choices must be made when deciding between consuming certain goods and services on the basis of available resources. This relationship can be visualized by plotting the possible combinations of purchasing two goods given a set income (Figure 16-2). Graphically, the budget constraint can then be combined with an indifference curve, which represents the amount of utility (i.e., value) received by consuming different levels of goods or services. Together this helps interpret how trade-offs can be made between consuming health or health care services and other goods or services. When aggregated across consumers, a sense of the market demand curve, or the level of goods or services, including health, that are demanded by consumers at a given price, is achieved.

Within each market, understanding how consumers in that market are likely to respond to changes in price is important. Elasticity helps people interpret the percent change in quantity demanded for each percent change in the good's price. In the context of health care, elasticity could be represented in terms of how patients are likely to respond (i.e., by filling or not filling a medication) when their co-payment or co-insurance (i.e., the portion of the total cost required of the patient) changes. When elasticity is greater than 1, the good is considered to be relatively elastic; however, when this value is less than 1, the good is considered to be relatively inelastic. In the case of an inelastic good, this means that consumer behavior (i.e., the amount purchased) is not as responsive to a change in price. Often this is due to a good being considered a necessity by consumers. For instance, prescription drugs have been observed to be relatively inelastic, meaning that even if prices increase, patients are likely to demand them or the amount demanded is likely to decrease by only a small amount.

FIGURE 16-2. Budget Constraint and Decision Interactions

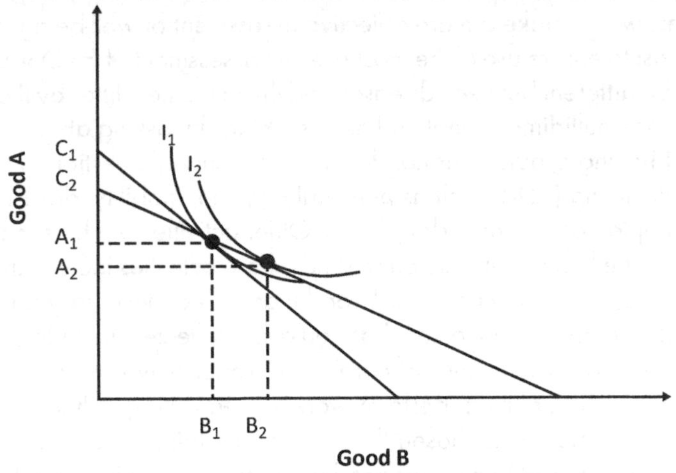

Budget constraints display the quantity of goods (A and B) that can be purchased given a particular level of income. C_1 and C_2 represent budget constraint curves. Value is maximized by selecting the bucket of goods where the indifference curve (I), which represents levels of utility, intersects the budget constraint line. Optimal scenarios are represented by the dots on the I curve.

As mentioned previously, health care and health as goods do not necessarily behave like other products and services as outlined by accepted economic theory. As a result, situations often arise where the assumptions of perfect competition are not satisfied. This can lead to monopolies or similar market structures where significant barriers to entry exist that limit free market competition. In health care, monopolies are perhaps best exemplified by both the pharmaceutical and the hospital industries. In both examples, significant costs are tied to entering each market: the development, manufacturing, and marketing of a drug may exceed $2 billion, while construction of a hospital requires significant investment in infrastructure, human capital (people) for operation, and demonstrated demand in a given area. As a result, people often view pharmaceutical companies as having a monopoly over a certain drug class if they are first to market because the manufacturer, rather than the market, is able to set the price, at least within a threshold that will be acceptable to payers. Similarly, a hospital can be viewed as a monopoly, at least in the geographical sense, if it is the only provider of certain health care services in a particular area. However, in both cases, measures are generally taken to control the extent to which either type of firm has complete control over setting prices in order to protect consumer (i.e., patient) interests.

16-4 Humanistic Outcomes and Their Application to Improve the Allocation of Limited Health Care Resources

Although therapeutic efficacy is an important measure of a drug, other considerations must be made when evaluating how well a treatment works. When building and interpreting pharmacoeconomic models, one must consider such humanistic outcomes of a health intervention. Multiple measures of humanistic outcomes exist, and their application to the medical decision-making process has important implications.

Humanistic Outcomes

By considering humanistic outcomes, one accounts for the effect of a treatment on other aspects of a patient's life in conjunction with the therapeutic effect or discrete health outcome. Perhaps the most widely used humanistic outcome is health-related quality of life (HRQoL). This concept considers how a patient's perceived well-being is affected by a condition or disease over time. Generally, HRQoL is assessed by surveys or questionnaires, which make a more objective assessment of well-being. Both generic and disease-specific instruments exist to ensure use of the most specific assessment of HRQoL possible because the effect on quality of life may be different between diseases and the outcomes differ by the treatment chosen. Generally, these instruments are multidimensional and assess HRQoL by asking about physical, social, emotional, or cognitive effects of having a particular condition. Often, survey questions will focus on how a disease affects activities of daily living (ADL), such as personal hygiene, mobility, dressing oneself, and other common behaviors that people perform on a daily basis. Other activities, such as managing money, preparing meals, and maintaining the home, can also be studied. These activities include those that are performed on a regular basis but perhaps not as often as ADLs and that are not necessary for fundamental functioning.

Other examples of humanistic outcomes that could be collected include patient satisfaction (with a treatment, services provided, or outcomes of care) and productivity (i.e., effect of treatment outcomes, a condition on work loss, or the ability to perform work-related duties). Although often included in HRQoL calculations, side effects related to a chosen therapy can certainly affect daily living by affecting physical, emotional, and cognitive well-being. Intermediate outcomes, such as medication adherence, patient knowledge, and willingness to pay, can be important to consider because they affect decision making and, therefore, can lead to different levels of well-being based on the choice made by the patient. Collectively, the information provided by a patient regarding his or her health condition and functional status is a patient-reported outcome (PRO). PROs represent an important source of information related to health status because they provide insight without interpretation by a health care provider. These measures may be collected as part of a regular clinic visit or in a clinical drug trial.

By capturing HRQoL, either in generic or condition-specific forms, one can gain a sense of the value, or utility, that patients derive from various treatment options and their resulting health states (e.g., ill, well, dead). Utility allows for the determination of patients' preferences between the results of available treatment options as they relate to particular conditions and their effects on HRQoL. These preferences can then serve as weighing factors when the interpretation of HRQoL is transformed into numeric form for analysis. This process allows assignment of more weight to preferred health states, such as better health, and less weight to nonpreferred health states, such as the disease worsening or death. Once the patients' preferences for certain health states are understood, one can calculate quality-adjusted life years (QALYs), which numerically represent the effects of a particular treatment or intervention on the quality and quantity of life lived. The calculation of QALYs is discussed in the next section.

Measuring Outcomes

Unlike discrete clinical measures, such as blood pressure, cholesterol, and blood glucose, that provide a numerical monitoring parameter of a disease, measurement of humanistic outcomes is more subjective and, potentially, complicated. The basic idea is to transform what the patient perceives about his or her well-being into a numeric form that is both a reliable and comparable measure. To accomplish this, multiple survey instruments have been developed, both generic and disease specific, to create a more objective interpretation of quality of life.

Two widely used generic, standardized HRQoL scales are the 36-Item Short Form Health Survey (SF-36) and the EQ-5D. The SF-36 was developed in the United States by the Rand Corporation and measures eight domains of health status: vitality, physical functioning, pain, general health perceptions, physical role functioning, emotional role functioning, social role functioning, and mental health. Other forms of the survey exist if only a select number of domains are needed for analysis. Each domain is scaled on a score from 0 to 100, and every question carries equal weight in importance. A higher score indicates less disability (i.e., a better health status). The EQ-5D was developed by the EuroQol Group and is more commonly used outside of the United States; it has been translated into more than 150 languages and takes into account differences in utilities tied to health status observed across countries. The five domains of the EQ-5D are mobility, self-care, usual activities, pain and discomfort, and anxiety and depression. Results of each domain are combined to produce a value that indicates a precise health state. The instrument also asks patients to report an overall estimate of their HRQoL from 0 to 100 using a visual analog scale. Both the EQ-5D and the SF-36 can be used to create QALYs that then can be used in pharmacoeconomic modeling.

Disease-specific HRQoL instruments also exist and may be used if researchers or health care providers want an estimate of well-being tied to a particular condition. Prominent examples include the Minnesota Living with Heart Failure Questionnaire and the EORTC QLQ-C30, which assesses quality of life for patients with cancer. These scales can be particularly useful in capturing patient well-being when factors related to a condition are known to have particularly significant effects on daily functioning.

A step-wise process is used to calculate HRQoL and transfer it into a measure that can be used in pharmacoeconomic analyses. The first step involves determining utility, which ranges from 0 to 1. For some conditions or outcomes, utility already may be known and people can use those values instead of determining them directly. For example, the EQ-5D and Health Utilities Index (HUI) have prescored utility values for certain health states. A utility score also can be derived in several ways to match the situation. Examples of measures of utility include standard gamble, time trade-off, and visual analog scale. Using standard gamble, one compares the certainty of remaining in a certain health state, taking a "gamble" of being in a better health state (e.g., full health or cured of disease), or risking death. This is calculated by varying the probability of experiencing death until the respondent is indifferent to any changes. Using time trade-off, one determines the amount of time a patient would prefer given two alternative outcomes. The comparisons are generally provided as living in a particular poorer health state for the rest of life or living with full health for a shorter amount of time. Similar to standard gamble, the amount spent in full health is varied until the individual is indifferent to the options provided. The final measure, visual analog scale, is the simplest way to measure utility. To calculate utility in this way, a range of possible health is represented on a scale from 0 (worst possible health) to 100 (best imaginable health) and then individuals are asked to indicate an estimated value of where on the scale they believe a particular health state ranks.

Once utility is determined, one can then calculate QALYs for the particular outcome. The basic premise is that 1 QALY represents a year of life lived in perfect health. Because certain health states affect HRQoL, the perceived quality of life lived given a particular condition or outcome needs to be considered. To do so, the number of years in a health state is multiplied by the utility value associated with that health state. For example, if taking a particular medication allows a person to live 10 additional years, but at only 70% of the patient's optimal level, the number of QALYs would be $10 \times 0.7 = 7$. In other words, although the person may live 10 additional years, the medication gives him or her the equivalent of only 7 years of perfect life during those 10 years.

Calculating the QALYs in the context of medications is also important because the side-effect profiles of two medications may be quite different. If both medications will add 10 years of life, but Drug A has a health utility of 0.5 and Drug B has a health utility of 0.9, then Drug B would result in an increase of 4 additional healthy years of life over Drug A. This allows one to determine the incremental number of QALYs between the two options, which in this example is 4. Using that value, and then using the costs of each treatment, one can determine the incremental cost-effectiveness ratio (ICER) between the two drugs. Continuing this example, if Drug A costs $500 per year and Drug B costs $1,000 per year, then the ICER is the incremental cost ($1,000 – $500 = $500) divided by the incremental QALYS (4 years). The result of this comparison would be $125 per QALY gained.

16-5 Pharmacoeconomic Analysis and Its Application to Improve the Allocation of Limited Health Care Resources

Pharmacoeconomic analysis assists the health care community in making decisions by bringing together clinical, humanistic, and economic aspects of patient care. The basic approach to conducting these analyses is to determine and then interpret the ratio of costs to benefits of a particular treatment. That ratio can be used to determine what therapy is most appropriate based on the perspective of the analysis. Another purpose of pharmacoeconomic analyses is to provide decision makers with objective information to make a decision about which medications to include on their formulary.

Pharmacoeconomic Concepts

The most common techniques used for pharmacoeconomic assessment are cost-burden of illness, cost-minimization, cost-effectiveness, cost-utility, and cost–benefit analysis. In general, these latter three analyses can be summarized by the following equation to compare two drugs, where "Effectiveness" denotes "Benefit," "Effectiveness," or "Utility":

$$\text{Ratio} = (\text{Cost}_{\text{Drug A}} - \text{Cost}_{\text{Drug B}})/(\text{Effectiveness}_{\text{Drug A}} - \text{Effectiveness}_{\text{Drug B}})$$

Cost-burden of illness identifies and measures the costs of the illness but not the treatment outcomes, so it is merely a summation of the direct and, potentially, indirect costs tied to a particular disease or condition. Similarly, cost-minimization analysis assumes that two treatments are equally effective and seeks to determine which therapy will result in the lowest cost of care. However, cost-minimization studies are rarely conducted because the effectiveness and the risks rarely are exactly equal.

The typical type of pharmacoeconomic analysis used for decision making is the cost-effectiveness study. Cost-effectiveness studies are important for decision makers because no immediate evidence exists that the less expensive medication should be preferred or that the more expensive medication is always the wrong choice. A less expensive medication may not be the best choice if it is not as effective as a more expensive medication or if treatment of the side effects or adverse effects associated with the medication is costlier than if a more expensive medication had been used. A medication with a less expensive purchase price may not be the best choice if more of the medication is required to reach the same level of effectiveness as a lesser quantity of a more expensive medication. Cost–benefit analysis measures the costs of treating an illness, along with monetary equivalents for the treatment's outcomes. Cost-effectiveness analysis measures the costs of treating an illness but uses clinical measures for the treatment outcomes.

Increasingly, decision makers are using cost-utility studies to decide which medications should be on the formulary (i.e., the list of approved drugs for a hospital, health system, or health plan). A cost-utility study attempts to include more humanistic benefits of a particular medication to help in the decision-making process. Cost-utility measures the costs of treating an illness but uses preference equivalents for the treatment outcomes, which are often given in health utility measures to calculate QALYs. These measures allow the patient to specify how much better he or she is feeling or is able to do activities of daily living when taking a specific medication. Humanistic outcomes, such as those described in the previous section of this chapter, can be used to determine and measure QALYs and then to determine ICERs. As described, these health utility measures can be age or disease specific, or they can be a generic health measure.

An important consideration when conducting a pharmacoeconomic study is determining the perspective of the analysis. Perspective refers to the viewpoint of the study, which centers around a particular stakeholder. Generally, a stakeholder can be the patient, provider (e.g., physician, pharmacist or pharmacy), health system, payer (e.g., insurance company, government), or, at its widest scope, society as a whole. Perspective matters both in how the results will be interpreted and used and in what inputs are included in the analysis. For instance, if a study is conducted from the payer's perspective, the likely focus would be on direct costs to the payer and not indirect costs, such as those tied to patient time or lost wages, or other matters that do not directly affect the payer. In contrast, a study from the patient's or societal perspective often would be interested in such indirect costs because they would be important to patients and society in general—a perspective that seeks to interpret all possible factors.

The primary way to determine which perspective to use is to ask who will be paying the costs that will be included as inputs in the analysis. For example, in a study looking at the cost-effectiveness of two medications, the prescription costs will differ if the study is from the payer's perspective versus society's perspective. In a study from the perspective of a payer (e.g., a health plan), the cost of the prescription drug will be only the cost that the health plan pays, because the health plan is responsible for only that portion. However, a study from society's perspective will include the cost portion paid by the health plan and the portion paid by the patient, as well as any portion paid by anyone else in society. Furthermore, a study from the patient's perspective would include only the patient's portion of the prescription cost.

Pharmacoeconomic Modeling

Often, the basic analytical structure of a pharmacoeconomic analysis is a decision-tree model, which seeks to compare two or more treatment options in terms of some form of cost-effectiveness. Figure 16-3 shows the basic structure of a decision-tree model that compares two treatments and their respective outcomes.

The first step in this process is to determine the perspective from which to run the model. The next step is to decide the treatments or procedures to include in the comparison. For most pharmacoeconomic analyses, this involves comparing two or more drugs to each other, but it could also include comparing surgical procedures, behavioral interventions, or even doing nothing at all. Importantly, these options should focus on fairly comparable treatments that are both available and likely to be considered.

Once the comparisons and perspective are determined, the model is populated by determining several critical elements: outcomes or benefits, costs, and probabilities. A wide range of options exist to define the outcomes or benefits of a certain treatment or procedure. These options may include curing disease, reducing symptoms, improving disease management, enhancing physical functioning, or improving quality of life. Most often this information is sourced from published literature on the benefits of certain treatments, but patient-reported outcomes could be used or data could be collected prospectively if primary sources of clinical measures or medical outcomes are wanted.

As previously mentioned, the chosen perspective will assist in determining the types of costs that should be included. The vast majority of analyses will use direct costs that measure the goods and services associated with a particular treatment or procedure, but those can differ on the basis of the perspective. This is especially true in the U.S. health care system where costs can vary widely for the same treatment or procedure depending on who is paying. Both public and proprietary sources of information may be needed to determine the proper cost for a study. The other major category of costs to consider are indirect costs. Factors such as patient time, leisure, productivity loss owing to illness, or, similarly, absenteeism

FIGURE 16-3. Decision Tree

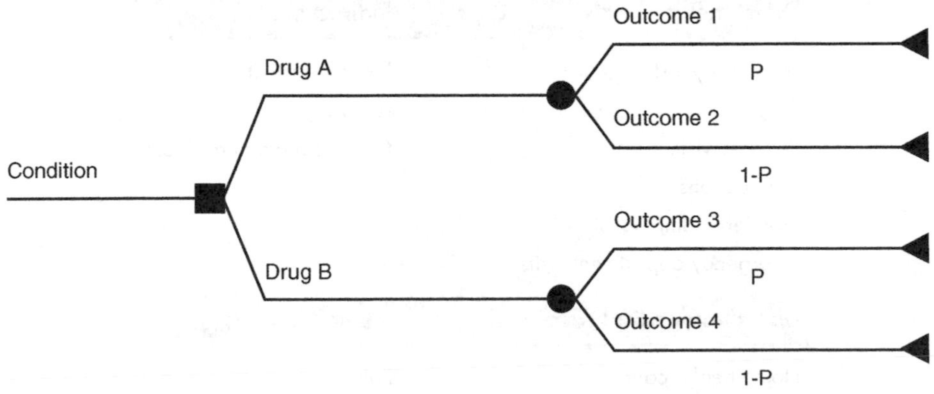

The basic structure of a decision-tree analysis compares one or more treatment options that lead to two or more known outcomes. First, a discrete treatment choice (square) is defined for a condition. These treatments then lead to a set of potential outcomes (circles). The probability of these outcomes is represented by P and sum to 1 among all potential outcomes. At the end of the model, each outcome is associated with a particular payoff (triangle), such as costs or quality-adjusted life years.

may be considered to be indirect costs tied to certain treatments or procedures, but opinions vary widely on what is truly an indirect cost. Regardless, these costs are important to consider in certain perspectives because they are factors often contemplated when making medical decisions. Table 16-1 lists examples of common direct and indirect costs used in pharmacoeconomic models.

Next, the analysis must determine the odds, or probabilities, of certain outcomes in order to reflect what is likely to happen in the real world. Commonly used probabilities include the odds of a treatment curing a disease, the rate at which side effects may happen, the chances of a particular outcome, or even the likelihood that a drug will be taken. Using probabilities that reflect real world evidence is important because the goal is to build a model as close to reality as possible. As a result, probability data from peer-reviewed literature, clinical trials, or directly observed patient behavior are often used.

Three final elements are important to consider as part of a pharmacoeconomic analysis. The first is the time horizon of the study, or the length of time over which one wants to understand the ratio of costs to benefits. Again, this decision has much to do with the chosen perspective, but it is dependent also on the treatments to be studied and their related outcomes. For drugs that manage chronic disease, a time frame of 30 years or longer is not uncommon, but for acute illness, such as seasonal influenza, the focus may be on a single year. For certain surgical procedures, such as coronary artery bypass grafting, the time horizon may be as little as 30 days. For longer time horizons, researchers frequently vary probabilities included in the model because the odds of certain outcomes are likely to change over time.

The second consideration is discounting the values used, which adjusts inputs that are being evaluated over a period longer than one year. In discounting, the present value of inputs or outcomes (i.e., current dollars) is used to reflect people's preference to receive health benefits today rather than years in the future. This approach is often accomplished by using accepted inflation rates or the more precise medical component of the consumer price index to discount medical costs.

The final consideration is the extent to which variability affects the results of the analysis. Because many assumptions are made in economic modeling, such as outcomes and probabilities, determining how a range of these values changes the interpretation of results so that a variety of potential results can be reported is common. To accomplish this, researchers perform sensitivity analyses after conducting the initial analysis with acceptable ranges of the inputs. This approach can be done by varying inputs one at a time or by varying the values of two or more inputs at the same time.

TABLE 16-1. Examples of Common Costs Used in Pharmacoeconomic Analyses

Direct medical costs	**Indirect costs**
Laboratory tests	Lost productivity
Surgery	Lost wages
Provider visits	Costs of premature death
Medications	
Inpatient admissions	
Emergency department visits	
Direct nonmedical costs	**Intangible costs**
Home health care	Pain
Transportation	Suffering
Food	Lost leisure time
Family care	Inconvenience

16-6 Questions

1. Which of the following statements are true regarding economics in general? (Mark all that apply.)

A. We live in a world of limitless resources.
B. Economics is largely broken up into macroeconomics and microeconomics.
C. Macroeconomics studies aggregate output, employment, and the general price level.
D. Microeconomics studies the individual decision makers such as consumers, resource owners, and business firms.

2. Which of the following statements are true regarding economic theory? (Mark all that apply.)

A. The most well-known economic theory is the theory of supply and demand.
B. The supply and demand model provides a visualization of how prices will change given a change in supply and demand for a given commodity.
C. As demand increases, supply increases to meet this increased demand, resulting in a larger quantity being sold and at a higher price.
D. A well-known economic theory is Maslow's Hierarchy of Needs.

3. Which of the following statements is part of Mankiw's 10 Principles of Economics? (Mark all that apply.)

A. People face trade-offs.
B. People respond to incentives.
C. Prices tend to fall when the government prints too much money.
D. Society faces a short-run trade-off between inflation and unemployment.

4. Which of the following statements are true regarding economics and pharmacoeconomics? (Mark all that apply.)

A. One purpose of pharmacoeconomic analyses is to provide decision makers with objective information from which to make a decision.
B. Economics is focused on the economy in general.
C. The main purpose of pharmacoeconomic analyses is to provide information that will help improve patient care, patient health, and patient health outcomes.
D. Pharmacoeconomics is focused on the efficiencies of various inputs and outputs specific to nonprescription products within the health care economy.

5. Which of the following statements are true related to cost-effectiveness analysis? (Mark all that apply.)

A. A cost–benefit analysis measures the costs of treating an illness, along with monetary equivalents for the treatment's outcomes.
B. Cost-effectiveness measures the costs of treating an illness but uses preference equivalents for the treatment outcomes.
C. Cost–benefit ratio = $\text{Cost}_{\text{Drug A}} - \text{Cost}_{\text{Drug B}} / \text{Benefit}_{\text{Drug A}} - \text{Benefit}_{\text{Drug B}}$
D. Cost-effectiveness ratio = $\text{Cost}_{\text{Drug A}} - \text{Cost}_{\text{Drug B}} / \text{Effectiveness}_{\text{Drug A}} - \text{Effectiveness}_{\text{Drug B}}$

6. Which of the following statements are true in reference to health utility? (Mark all that apply.)

A. Cost-utility studies often use health utility measures to calculate QALYs.
B. Health utility measures are always disease specific.
C. The SF-36 and EQ-5D are the most common generic health measures.
D. The SF-36 is a multipurpose health survey that has only 36 questions.

7. Which of the following statements are true about pharmacoeconomic analysis? (Mark all that apply.)

A. The most typical perspectives for pharmacoeconomic studies are those of the society, the patient, and the payer.
B. The primary way to determine which perspective to use is to determine who will be paying the costs that will be included as the inputs in the analysis.
C. The most commonly used perspective is the patient perspective.
D. A pharmacoeconomic study from the patient's perspective would include only the portion of the prescription cost paid for by the patient.

8. Which of the following statements are true about economic markets? (Mark all that apply.)

A. The economic market assumes that the buyer pays the full cost of the commodity; however, in the pharmaceutical market, the payer rarely pays the full price.
B. The economic market assumes that prices will be kept low because of competition, supply, and demand; however, these forces have very little effect on pharmaceutical pricing.
C. The economic market assumes ease of entry for companies desiring to begin producing a commodity; however, the cost of starting a major pharmaceutical company is so high that it limits the number of companies able to enter the pharmaceutical market.
D. The pharmaceutical and health care markets are free from government regulations.

9. Which of the following statements are true regarding medication access? (Mark all that apply.)

A. Pharmacoeconomic data are used by health care companies, government agencies, and other entities to pay for or manage prescriptions.
B. Each therapeutic class of medications typically has multiple available products. Multiple brand-name products as well as multiple generic medications may be available.
C. Because of the cost of purchasing and keeping medications on hand in the hospital, decisions must be made about which medications to purchase and stock.
D. Health insurance companies use pharmacoeconomic data to keep patients from getting the medications that they really need.

10. Which of the following statements are true regarding cost-minimization analysis? (Mark all that apply.)

A. A cost-minimization study assumes that the effectiveness and the risks associated with two medications are equal.
B. Cost-minimization studies are rarely conducted because the effectiveness and the risks rarely are exactly equal.
C. The most common type of pharmacoeconomic analysis used for decision making is the cost-minimization study.
D. In a cost-minimization study, the medication with the lower cost is preferred.

11. Which of the following statements are true regarding cost-effectiveness analysis? (Mark all that apply.)

A. Cost-effectiveness studies are important for decision makers because both the cost and the benefits are stated in monetary terms.
B. A less expensive medication may not be the best choice if its side effects are costlier to treat than those of a more expensive medication.
C. A medication with a less expensive purchase price may not be the best choice if it requires using more of the medication to reach the same level of effectiveness as a lesser quantity of a more expensive medication.
D. The typical type of pharmacoeconomic analysis used for decision making is the cost-effectiveness study.

12. Which of the following equations is correct? (Mark all that apply.)

A. Cost–benefit ratio $= \text{Cost}_{\text{Drug A}} - \text{Cost}_{\text{Drug B}} / \text{Benefit}_{\text{Drug A}} - \text{Benefit}_{\text{Drug B}}$
B. Cost-effectiveness ratio $= \text{Cost}_{\text{Drug A}} - \text{Cost}_{\text{Drug B}} / \text{Effectiveness}_{\text{Drug A}} - \text{Effectiveness}_{\text{Drug B}}$
C. Cost-utility ratio $= \text{Cost}_{\text{Drug A}} - \text{Cost}_{\text{Drug B}} / \text{Utility}_{\text{Drug A}} - \text{Utility}_{\text{Drug B}}$
D. Cost-minimization ratio $= \text{Cost}_{\text{Drug A}} - \text{Cost}_{\text{Drug B}} / \text{Cost}_{\text{Drug B}} - \text{Cost}_{\text{Drug A}}$

13. Which of the following is best described as an unintended positive or negative effect on one individual resulting from the behavior(s) of others?

A. Externality
B. Indirect cost
C. Cost-utility
D. Standard gamble

14. Which of the following is best described as preference weights that help decision makers understand value of or desirability for particular health states?

A. Patient-reported outcome
B. Quality-adjusted life-year
C. Utility
D. Time trade-off

15. Which of the following best describes why values are commonly discounted as part of a multiyear cost-effectiveness model?

A. Patients receive lower costs of care by receiving services now rather than in the future.
B. Improved health is worth more in the future than the present.
C. The discount reflects the expected lower costs of care in the future.
D. Health benefits are preferred in the present versus the future.

16. Which of the following best describes why sensitivity analyses are conducted as part of a pharmacoeconomic model?

A. Sensitivity analyses help double check the work for errors.
B. This type of analysis allows the assessment to be changed from a cost–benefit study to a cost-effectiveness study.
C. Sensitivity analyses account for assumptions made by varying the values applied to inputs used throughout the model.
D. This analysis changes the primary perspective from that of the patient to that of the payer.

17. Which of the following is an example of how utility values commonly are determined? (Mark all that apply.)

A. Reference established values from the Health Utilities Index.
B. Derive values from the amount of time patients would exchange for time lived in perfect health.
C. Compare the amount of risk a patient would accept when comparing one or more outcomes.
D. Ask patients to describe their health in terms of a letter grade.

18. Which of the following best describes the value of collecting patient-reported outcomes as a measure of health status?

A. Patient-reported outcomes are an exact measure of health status.
B. Patient-reported outcomes provide an interpretation of health status without provider input.
C. These measures directly calculate QALYs.
D. Quantitative patient-reported outcome values more consistently describe health status than clinical measures of disease.

19. Which of the following describes the comparison of costs per QALY gained?

A. Incremental cost-effectiveness ratio
B. Cost–benefit analysis
C. Health utility
D. Sensitivity analysis

20. Which of the following best describes the concept of crowding out in terms of health care markets?

A. The physical removal of a firm from operating in a certain market
B. A situation where too much government involvement limits private market investment in health care
C. Increased interest in certain health care markets resulting in too many firms competing for a limited number of patients
D. The reduction of disease incidence as a result of high rates of medication use or vaccination

16-7 Answers

1. B, C, D. Resources are not limitless, and this is a basic underlying economic concept.

2. A, B, C. Maslow's Hierarchy of Needs theory is a psychological theory, not an economic theory.

3. A, B, D. The opposite tends to be true: prices generally rise when too much money is in circulation.

4. A, B, C. Pharmacoeconomics is not specific to nonprescription products. Most pharmacoeconomic studies are performed on prescription products because they are the most costly.

5. A, C, D. A cost-utility analysis uses preference equivalents, not a cost-effectiveness analysis.

6. **A, C, D.** Health utility measures are not always disease specific. They can also be age specific as well as be a generic health measure. Hence, they are useful in all ages and disease states.

7. **A, B, D.** In general, the most common perspective used is the payer perspective, not the patient perspective.

8. **A, B, C.** The pharmaceutical and health care markets are actually heavily regulated. The pharmaceutical market is regulated by the U.S. Food and Drug Administration and the Federal Trade Commission. The health care markets are also heavily regulated by various state and federal government agencies.

9. **A, B, C.** Although some patients may feel this way, pharmacoeconomic data are in fact used to help health insurance companies determine how to provide access to the largest number of beneficial medications given their limited budgets. However, given the limited resources available, providing coverage for any and all medications is impossible.

10. **A, B, D.** The most common type of analysis used is actually the cost-effectiveness study. Cost-minimization is used, but because it simply measures differences in costs, it does not consider other elements important to making a decision.

11. **B, C, D.** The cost–benefit analysis provides both cost and benefits in monetary terms, whereas cost-effectiveness is more likely to use a concrete outcome as a benefit.

12. **A, B, C.** The equation for cost minimization is simply $Cost_{Drug\ A} - Cost_{Drug\ B}$.

13. **A.** An externality exists when one person's behavior has an unintended good or bad effect on someone else. An indirect cost measures factors such as time or other items that may be affected by an approach but are not necessarily the primary foci. Cost utility is a ratio of the costs of a certain approach relative to its perceived usefulness. Standard gamble is a popular approach to measuring health utility.

14. **C.** Utility describes the relative value that an individual perceives to gain from achieving certain levels of health. Patient-reported outcomes is an overarching term for results of interventions that are not interpreted by a provider yet still measure the effect of a therapy. A QALY is how one measures the quality of a year lived based on a particular treatment's likely outcomes. Time trade-off is a popular way to determine health utility.

15. **D.** Generally, people prefer to be healthier today rather than in the future, so discounting shows the health benefits in today's dollars. Lower costs for care are not guaranteed just because treatment was received in the short term rather than the long term, and expected costs are not likely to be lower in the future.

16. **C.** Sensitivity analysis allows for varying the inputs used, which helps account for the assumptions made across the variables that were used. Sensitivity analysis is not constructed to uncover errors made in the primary analysis; if errors are made in the primary analysis, then they will affect every analysis conducted in the model. Generally, only one type of model is run even though this could be changed if needed. Similarly, the perspective is set from the onset of the study, and conducting a sensitivity analysis would not change it.

17. **A, B, C.** Although patients usually are asked to rate their health status, generally this is done using a scale from 0 to 100.

18. **B.** Understanding health status independent of provider interpretation is an important way to determine how a patient is doing. PROs reflect health status but not in a precise, quantitative way like other clinical measures. The values derived from PROs are used to calculate QALYs, but this cannot be done directly without other considerations. Although these values are useful and provide important measures of health status, they are not necessarily a more consistent measure of health status than established, validated clinical measures.

19. **A.** Constructing an incremental cost-effectiveness ratio allows one to determine the cost of each QALY when comparing treatment options. A cost–benefit analysis is an overarching type of model within which one might create an incremental cost-effectiveness ratio. Health utility is a measure used to determine QALYs, and sensitivity analysis may be used when conducting a cost-effectiveness analysis as a way to see how varying the inputs leads to different interpretations of results.

20. **B.** Although government intervention can often be efficient, in some cases too much involvement can reduce how many private firms get involved with health care. Crowding out is a concept that describes what happens to the overall market and not necessarily the physical removal of a firm from that market. Answer C is incorrect because one would likely see the opposite happen, and Answer D describes an externality.

16-8 Additional Resources

EuroQoL. EQ-5D Instruments. EuroQoL Web site. https://euroqol.org/eq-5d-instruments.

Furlong WJ, Feeny DH, Torrance GW, Barr RD. The Health Utilities Index (HUI) system for assessing health-related quality of life in clinical studies. *Ann Med.* 2001;33(5):375–384.

Health insurance status. Henry J. Kaiser Family Foundation Web site. https://www.kff.org/state-category/health-coverage-uninsured/health-insurance-status.

Kaiser Family Foundation and Health Research and Educational Trust. *2017 Employer Health Benefits Survey.* Menlo Park, CA: Henry J. Kaiser Family Foundation; 2017. Available at: https://www.kff.org/health-costs/report/2017-employer-health-benefits-survey.

Lobo BL. Pharmacoeconomic considerations. *Am J Health-Syst Pharm.* 2003;60(suppl 7):S11–S14.

Mankiw NG. *Principles of Economics.* 4th ed. Mason, OH: Thomson South-Western; 2007.

Odedina FT, Sullivan J, Nash R, Clemmons CD. Use of pharmacoeconomic data in making hospital formulary decisions. *Am J Health-Syst Pharm.* 2002;59(15):1441–1444.

Prieto L, Sacristán JA. Problems and solutions in calculating quality-adjusted life years (QALYs). *Health Qual Life Outcomes.* 2003;1:80.

Salvatore D, Diulio EA, Bartley WA. *Schaum's Easy Outline of Principles of Economics.* New York, NY: McGraw-Hill; 2003.

Ware JE. SF-36 health survey update. *Spine.* 2000;25(24):3130–3139. Available at: https://journals.lww.com/spinejournal/Citation/2000/12150/SF_36_Health_Survey_Update.8.aspx.

17 Pharmacy Practice Management

KIMBERLY C. MASON

17-1 KEY POINTS

- Pharmacy practice management requires significant effort in various forms of planning to assure high-quality, efficient operations.
- Given the proportion of health care expenses made up by pharmaceuticals, having a dedicated pharmacy leader overseeing this resource is imperative. Pharmacy staff members are critically important to the clinical and financial success of any health care organization. Pharmacy leaders must work diligently to attract and hire talented individuals who can work effectively as a team toward a common goal.
- Goals should be set on the basis of an organization's vision and reviewed for continued relevance at regular intervals. The goals and underlying objectives make up the strategic plan.
- A common exercise in the development of any strategic plan is completion of an analysis that identifies the organization's strengths, weaknesses, opportunities, and threats—a SWOT analysis.
- Specific programs under consideration should be analyzed and summarized in a business plan to assess the feasibility and wisdom of continued pursuit.
- Marketing tools can be used to bring attention to and build relationships, both short and long term, for programs that encompass goods or services.
- Pharmacy leaders also have oversight of pharmaceutical contracting, inventory control, and drug security. The four main factors that drive drug expense are utilization, price, mix, and innovation. As biologics and high-cost therapies come to the market, the need for precision in budget projection rises.
- A budget is a detailed plan of how resources will be acquired and used in a certain time period. Many sources of data go into budget projections for both revenue and expenses.
- Although these inputs are needed to forecast the operational budget, other information must be evaluated to consider capital budget needs (building, equipment, other assets).
- Communicating the budget targets to the team with the ability to influence whether or not they are met is crucial.
- Communication is an important aspect of leadership.
- In the rare instance that a pharmacist or other health care provider makes a mistake, open lines of communication within the team not only help team members learn of the error quickly but also help them develop preventive strategies.

17-2 STUDY GUIDE CHECKLIST

The following topics may guide your study of this subject area:

- ☐ Understand the key areas of business and the clinical and quality responsibilities of pharmacy leaders.
- ☐ Describe the steps involved to recruit, interview, and hire pharmacy team members.
- ☐ Distinguish the various types of planning and the way each relates to strategic planning.
- ☐ Demonstrate knowledge of the primary elements of marketing and the way each is used.
- ☐ Describe the mechanisms to contract for better pricing of pharmaceuticals.
- ☐ Understand the determinants for accurately projecting a budget to control drug expenses.
- ☐ Demonstrate an understanding of relevant regulatory standards and their application to pharmacy practice.
- ☐ Describe the importance of medication reconciliation and other components of transitional care to reimbursement rates and quality care.

17-3 Management Principles

In all aspects of pharmacy practice, leaders are called on to plan and direct activities to achieve optimal patient care as well as financial performance (Box 17-1). Health care sectors may vary from inpatient care to outpatient care and retail settings, but the common need among all is a coordinated approach. Pharmacy leaders must observe and analyze current and future trends with their unique clinical and business perspectives. They bring to health care systems their experience leading evidence-based clinical and formulary initiatives while controlling drug expenses to maximize patient benefit. Pharmacy leaders have in-depth knowledge of the pharmaceutical supply chain, physicians' prescribing practices, medication-use policies, clinical therapeutics, technology, and medication management systems to successfully support patient care.

With respect to information technology, pharmacy leaders must plan the purchasing, implementation, and maintenance of numerous information systems to support patient care. A commitment to long-term investment in electronic health records, computerized prescriber order entry and electronic prescribing, clinical decision support databases, barcoded medication administration, medication surveillance, smart infusion pumps, automated medication reconciliation, and other clinical applications is necessary. The complexity of these systems requires qualified and appropriately trained pharmacy team members to safely develop and test the systems before putting them into practice.

In addition to guaranteeing continuous cycles of improvement in pharmacy operations, pharmacy leaders must also ensure that clinical outcomes continually improve. Reimbursements are tied more and more to high-quality outcomes; therefore, pharmacies must support value-based purchasing, hospital readmission reduction programs, and medication-related customer satisfaction. An additional area of focus is the core measures published by the Centers for Medicare and Medicaid Services that delineate key quality measures by which the government determines levels of reimbursement for health care providers. Leaders must ensure that highly skilled pharmacists are on staff to communicate with physicians and patients to achieve the highest levels of quality. Continuing education and competency assessment are essential to ensure a minimum standard of practice across pharmacy professionals.

Pharmacy leaders work with pharmacists and physicians to develop medication utilization and formulary initiatives that ensure cost-effective therapy, reduce drug-related problems, and optimize therapeutic outcomes. These activities are usually presented and approved at a multidisciplinary, organizational committee, often called the pharmacy and therapeutics committee.

In both hospitals and community pharmacies, the terms *pharmacy manager* and *pharmacist in charge* are sometimes used interchangeably, but there are differences. Whereas a department manager may have ultimate responsibility for all personnel and their activities in the pharmacy area, the pharmacist in charge (PIC) has the full legal responsibility for the entire operation of the pharmacy in a manner that complies with all applicable state and federal laws and regulations. These roles can be served by two individuals or combined and served by one individual. All states require a pharmacist who is licensed

BOX 17-1. Health System Pharmacy Executive Responsibilities

- Designing, managing, measuring, and improving the medication management system
- Providing strategic planning
- Ensuring quality outcomes through performance improvement activities
- Optimizing the use of technology and information systems
- Leading drug utilization efforts
- Managing financial operations, human resources, and the pharmaceutical supply chain
- Ensuring compliance with regulatory and accreditation requirements
- Providing institutional representation and leadership
- Fulfilling the organization's research and educational missions

in the respective state to sign the application for the pharmacy's permit and to serve as PIC at only one community or institutional pharmacy at the same time. The specific responsibilities for the PIC vary from one state to another, and each state's board of pharmacy publishes these requirements.

17-4 Personnel Management

Managing people in the work setting is both rewarding and challenging. As individuals, each team member has a unique set of skills to contribute to the work of the team overall. Sometimes the most difficult part of management may be motivating the various team members, in ways that are meaningful to each one, to deliver their specific contribution in a collaborative manner that achieves a timely and accurate result. To determine the appropriate management tactics, one must first establish an approach and plan.

Management is more of an art than a science, and therefore, many approaches are used. The more commonly applied approach is one of a positive-thinking style of management whereby leaders coach and inspire their teams toward success. First, leaders must determine the appropriate type, number, and qualifications of staff required to achieve the organization's mission, satisfy regulatory and accreditation requirements, meet patient care needs, and advance pharmacy practice. The mix of skills, such as the number of pharmacists versus technicians on staff as determined by a state's law or regulation, is an important consideration. Programs that advance the use of pharmacy technicians allow pharmacists to spend more time in drug therapy management activities where they can more efficiently affect clinical and financial outcomes. Pharmacy leaders can also develop programs to more fully use the talents and work effort of pharmacy residents and students within the organization. All these individuals rely on pharmacy leaders for their recruitment, training and orientation, mentoring, performance review, and career development.

Maintaining, and even increasing, productivity in the workplace is important. Employees who recognize and share in the desire for productivity will flourish. However, employees who are not performing their duties face progressive discipline, up to termination. Finding and hiring individuals whose values are well aligned with the organization's mission is key for success. Turnover of staff members reduces productivity; therefore, significant effort should be made to retain staff. One of the many strategies for staff retention is recognition and awards. Methods of employee recognition include designating an employee of the month, writing thank-you notes and commendations, acknowledging staff members at department meetings, supporting attendance at professional meetings, and giving small awards such as gift certificates for coffee or a movie.

If a human resources department is available to pharmacy managers, it can be a great asset in regard to procedures for recruiting, interviewing, and hiring employees. The initial applicant screening and application processing can be done by the human resources staff, sparing the time of the pharmacy manager. The screening should compare the applicant's experience to the job description. Job descriptions should include several elements: position, title, duties, required or preferred skills, supervisory oversight and responsibilities, qualifications, education, required work experience, hours, schedule, salary, and benefits. The candidate's application, resume, or CV (curriculum vitae) should be reviewed, noting potential questions to clarify during the interview such as gaps in employment dates, length of employment, reasons for leaving past positions, salary expectations, and outside interests.

The interview team should ideally consist of the position's immediate supervisor and perhaps the leader to whom the supervisor reports. Sometimes, group interviews by administrative or senior staff can provide valuable insights and broader input regarding the individual's potential success and longevity with the organization. The interview itself should begin with some conversational time to put the applicant at ease and then proceed to gathering information from the applicant. The interviewer should seek to ask questions that shed light on the applicant's strengths, motivation, job satisfaction, and work experience.

All interviewers must understand the legal implications of certain interview questions. Potentially discriminatory areas of questioning should be carefully considered or avoided, such as age, arrest record, credit rating, handicaps, marital or family status, military record, nationality of names, religion, or national origin. Also, avoid questions that can have quick, categorical answers such as yes or no, and instead use open-ended questions so the applicant talks more about himself or herself. Clarifying questions can be helpful to ensure a clear understanding of the applicant's answers.

The applicant should then be given information on the position, including the job description and the positive and negative aspects of the position for transparency. The applicant should be allowed sufficient opportunity and time to ask questions. A tour of the work area is also a customary component of an interview. As the interview ends, a discussion of possible start dates should be reviewed, particularly if the interview has gone well. Expressing appreciation to the applicant for coming to interview is a pleasant way to end the discussion. A check of the applicant's references can be done either before or after the actual interview and should be completed no matter how strong the applicant may seem. Other items requiring verification are state board of pharmacy records, academic records, and criminal background searches when permitted by law or by the applicant.

Pharmacy managers primarily want to hire an employee who is supportive and trustworthy. Pharmacy managers should continually recruit talented individuals, even if there are currently no open positions. This approach builds the pool of applicants for future positions and keeps the manager apprised of the supply of resources, both quantitatively and qualitatively. Another way to grow an applicant pool is to advertise, typically when a specific position is available. Of course, an open position should first be shared with current staff members in case they are interested or know of an interested party. The salary for the position should reflect equity and fairness with respect to the salaries of current staff.

Additional responsibilities of pharmacy leaders include ensuring personnel safety such as infection prevention and hazardous waste management, incident reporting, and medical and emergency preparedness. Adequate facilities must be allocated to receive, store, and prepare medications in order to maintain product integrity and personnel safety.

17-5 Planning

As with any organization or business, detailed planning is crucial to success. In terms of successful business performance, planning and executing that plan is essential to meet the productivity and other performance targets set out for the business. The day-to-day and year-to-year performance of the business relies on meeting the key customer and other requirements as set out in the business plan. However, to be able to modify the business in the midst of changing external factors, having a continually evaluated strategic plan is important.

Planning represents purposeful efforts to maximize future success (Box 17-2). Planning is a key managerial function that actually supports the other three functions—leading, controlling, and organizing. Pharmacy organizations require multiple types of planning such as financial planning, business planning, organiza-

BOX 17-2. Steps in the Planning Process

1. Define the planning process with a singular purpose or desired result (mission and vision).
2. Assess the current situation.
3. Establish goals.
4. Identify strategies to reach those goals.
5. Create objectives that support progress toward those goals.
6. Define the timeline and responsibilities for each objective.
7. Write and communicate the plan.
8. Monitor progress toward goals and objectives.

tional planning, operational planning, strategic planning, and resource planning. Each type has a different purpose and may be used by pharmacy managers to varying degrees. Outside consultants are often engaged to assist small- to mid-sized organizations with their planning efforts, while large companies often have dedicated planning departments. Planning can range from use of simple and straightforward concepts to extensive analysis of data with complicated algorithms, decision-making models, and forecasting. All types of planning include assessing the purpose, situation, and goals while developing action plans to accomplish those goals.

Strategic planning is the process of selecting goals, determining programs and policies necessary to achieve the goals, and establishing methods to implement those programs. It ensures that the correct steps are being taken, both now and for the future. Strategic planning enables the optimal deployment of organizational resources within current and future constraints to increase the likelihood of the organization's survival and future success. It helps determine what business the organization ought to be in and the long-term goals that will be needed. An important part of strategic planning is determining the time period within which the goals should be met. Although strategic planning is for the long term, the future is unknown, and therefore, predicting when the plan will lose its relevance is difficult. Strategic plans may be relevant for 2 to 20 years, but they are often refreshed every 2 to 4 years.

To distinguish business planning from strategic planning (Table 17-1), one must understand that strategic planning is about achieving broad, long-term success while business planning is more focused on a specific program and its feasibility. Business planning occurs within the context of the organizational strategic plan, which is the overarching guidance for day-to-day activities.

Given the rapid pace of change in health care, strategic planning is often too reactive. Proactive planning helps organizations control their environments rather than allowing external influences to dictate direction. Some plans may take significant periods of time to complete, but not simplifying the goals to make them more readily attainable is important. Motivating personnel and creating momentum are important parts of strategic planning. Employees want to know and share the story of their company.

Strategic goals are based on the organization's vision for the future, and as such, all team members need to be aligned with that vision. Vision is what the organization wants to be at some future point. A vision statement can be multidimensional and complex, but it must be concise. It is used at both the beginning and the end stages of the strategic planning process. Once the vision is set, planning begins in order to reach that endpoint. Vision also helps define and drive the mission and values of an organization. The mission is the organization's purpose—its function and focus. This present-centered mission statement creates a sense of purpose for employees and customers that will take them into the future with the company. This mission statement should also be short, such as one to two sentences, and should differentiate the organization from others that provide similar products and services. The mission and vision statements that form the organization's story are crucial elements of strategic planning. If they already exist in the organization, the strategic planning process begins with these as a foundation and modifies them only as necessary. If these statements do not already exist, the strategic planning process should likely begin with their creation.

TABLE 17-1. Comparison of Business and Strategic Planning

Type	Characteristics	Purpose
Business planning	Possible use for decisions to start, expand, or terminate a business; short term (1–5 years)	Determine program feasibility; guide investment decisions
Strategic planning	Organization-wide scope; external viewpoint—how the organization controls and interacts with its environment; long term (5–20 years)	Determine what business the organization ought to be in, give a framework for more detailed planning and decisions; ensure that the organization is taking the correct steps

TABLE 17-2. SWOT Analysis Considerations

Internal strengths and weaknesses	External opportunities and threats
Quality of pharmacy service	Changes in market and customer type
Profitability	Regulations that may help or hinder business
Competence and ability of pharmacy staff	Availability of reimbursement for services
Customer service	Extent of competition from other pharmacies
Efficiency of pharmacy operations	Political issues affecting health care delivery

There is often a preplanning phase to define the necessary steps to organize the strategic planning effort. Strategic planning is a financial investment in terms of personnel time and consultant costs, and therefore, these costs should be weighed against the value to be gained by the effort. The value of a well-conducted strategic planning process will greatly exceed its costs, but a superficial or hurried exercise will not result in positive value. Preplanning should define the objectives for the planning effort, the individuals to be involved, the location of the process, and the time needed for the endeavor. For most strategic planning of significant affect, outside advisors are brought in to provide external perspectives and ensure that the process is objective and thorough.

In the actual planning phase of strategic planning, the activity starts with the destination, or vision, in mind. Then the starting point must be determined through situation analysis, and ideas must be generated about how to progress from the current state to the intended vision state. Situation analysis includes evaluation of past performance, including financial indicators and customer satisfaction, and helps define the present. Planners identify goals for the organization and preferred strategies to accomplish the goals. Finally, objectives should be determined that will help reach the goals. These are intermediate points that, when met, will help gauge progress toward the goal. These key milestones ensure the journey is indeed on track.

A strategy should lead an organization to gain advantage relative to its competitors. An often-used exercise in strategic planning is an analysis used by leaders to identify the organization's unique **s**trengths, **w**eaknesses, **o**pportunities, and **t**hreats—a SWOT analysis (Table 17-2). This type of analysis requires a clear understanding of competitors because each SWOT element is considered relative to the competition. Knowing any distinct advantages from which a strategy can be derived is helpful. Likewise, knowing any weaknesses that may make the organization vulnerable can help direct which opportunities should and should not be pursued. Comparing the results of the situation analysis with the vision helps clarify the nature of the gap between the two. The goals identified in strategic planning must help bridge that gap by minimizing threats and mitigating weaknesses while capitalizing on the organization's strengths and opportunities.

To operationalize the strategy, one must ensure that the short-term objectives require assignment of administrative responsibility, timeline, and budget. Communicating the plan to all team members and, with its implementation, beginning to monitor its progress are also important. Failure to implement the plan is due most often to lack of time, unavailability of resources, or failure to measure progress. Planning must be a continuous process to ensure that the organization appropriately adjusts its plan and actions in response to environmental changes significantly affecting the plan.

17-6 Marketing of Goods and Services

Community pharmacies have successfully marketed products and customer service to patients. Marketing for clinical services may have success using these same techniques (Table 17-3), such as fliers (i.e., printed materials) placed inside prescription bags, radio and television advertisements, billboards, and promotion

TABLE 17-3. Marketing of Clinical Pharmacy Services

Barriers in the community pharmacy	Methods to overcome barriers
Patients are unwilling to pay out of pocket.	Target specific populations with service need.
Patients doubt their need for clinical services.	Incorporate new, innovative marketing ideas.
Patients are unaware of pharmacists' roles beyond dispensing.	Take part in local and national pharmacy and disease state promotional campaigns.

at local health fairs. Additional methods might include a tailored marketing approach for targeted patient populations and relationship-building efforts with patients and families. Pharmacists can market services by creating and maintaining mutually rewarding relationships with select groups of patients and partners. This approach is known as *relationship marketing,* which uses—and goes beyond—the traditional four "Ps" of marketing (product, price, promotion, and place). To evaluate targeted market segments, a pharmacy should consider patient access, obstacles to market entry, size of the market, potential revenue and profit, and patients' attitudes and behaviors.

In today's electronic age, digital marketing has become a mainstay for promotion. In addition to social media presence, an email subscriber list can be very useful to increase awareness with the relevant market. For a small fee, a company will help gather email addresses for database entry with permission from the customer. Customers can choose to subscribe or unsubscribe at any time. Many patients look online for information rather than using a printed telephone directory as in years past. For example, posting information online and sending an email regarding an upcoming flu shot clinic or a sale on short-dated over-the-counter products may prove beneficial.

A clinical service that pharmacies often promote is medication therapy management (MTM), which encompasses the assessment and evaluation of a patient's complete medication regimen rather than an individual product. The service is independent of, but may occur in conjunction with, the provision of a medication. MTM services may improve the reliability of health care delivery, prevent medication errors, and enable patients to be more active in their care. Patients may self-refer for this service, or they may be identified and referred by a provider or health plan. MTM services are typically offered by appointment for ambulatory patients but may be provided on a walk-in basis. Face-to-face interactions optimize the ability to observe visual cues to patient health problems, but in certain situations (e.g., homebound patients), telephone interaction may be necessary. Providing this service in accordance with the Health Insurance Portability and Accountability Act, which requires patient confidentiality to be maintained at all times, is important. The MTM service should be provided in a semiprivate or private area by a pharmacist whose time can be devoted to the patient. The number of reviews required to manage a patient's care will vary among patients and will be determined by the complexity of the individual's medication-related problems. Although the patient's payer may limit the extent of health plan benefits with respect to payment for MTM services, the pharmacist may still provide the service on a fee-for-service basis. Therefore, internal and external promotion by the pharmacy is an important consideration to increase revenue to the pharmacy.

17-7 Accounting and Financial Management

Given the relative expense of medications when compared to other health care supplies, having robust accounting, reporting, and analysis capabilities in pharmacy practice management is imperative. Pharmacy leaders must also keep patient safety and quality of care at the forefront of any drug cost-management strategies. They have responsibility for oversight of all pharmaceutical contracting, procurement,

BOX 17-3. Cost-Management Program Elements

- Pharmacy activities: Purchasing and contracting, inventory management and storage, waste reduction
- Charging and reimbursement: Coding, indigent care and 340b programs, payer mix, infusion center
- Interdisciplinary activities: Formulary management, protocol development, physician support

receiving, inventory control, security, and diversion prevention across the organization. This oversight includes alternative distribution channels used during shortages, outsourced sterile products, and reverse distribution, which is the collection of damaged, outdated, or unsold goods and delivery back to the supplier or manufacturer. External benchmarks that account for cost and quality can be useful in aiding leaders to identify and implement cost-reduction strategies. Four main factors drive drug expense: utilization, price, mix, and innovation. Utilization increases are due to increased number of users or days of treatment and so on. Price is simply the unit price of existing drugs. The mix changes when newer medications are used instead of older, less-expensive medications. The blend of mix and utilization increases medication expense when innovative therapies become available for indications previously untreatable by medications.

Financial audits and various analyses are required to ensure appropriate, accurate, and timely documentation of revenue and expenses. Using these data, pharmacy leaders may explore opportunities to implement medication-related services that could improve the financial health of the organization, such as ambulatory infusion areas or retail pharmacies.

An important aspect of managing pharmacy financials is ensuring the best possible pricing through optimal contracting. The three primary mechanisms to purchase pharmaceuticals at discounted prices are facility contracts, group purchasing organization contracts, and wholesaler own-use contracts. Of course, appropriate optimization of generic product utilization is a key factor in managing drug costs. The cost-management strategies that are purely within the pharmacy's control, such as inventory decisions and purchasing contracts, are typically the easiest to implement (Box 17-3).

The growth in spending on inpatient drugs exceeds the growth in spending on retail drugs. Because of delays in updating the pharmaceutical cost index, Medicare reimbursement to pharmacies is not keeping pace with rapidly increasing drug prices. Most hospitals receive a single, diagnosis-related group payment for all nonphysician services, including drugs, provided during an inpatient admission. Hospitals must absorb the loss whenever reimbursement rates cannot match inpatient costs.

17-8 Budgeting

A budget is a detailed plan noting how resources will be acquired and used during a specific period of time. It provides a benchmark to which actual results can be compared. As an example, a retail pharmacy can compare its actual prescription sales in a period to its budgeted prescription sales as a measure of effectiveness. As with any plan, sometimes a situation changes and managers must adjust when faced with a crisis, such as an unanticipated increase in expenses. Managers must gather data in these situations and analyze relevant information to create an action plan. After a crisis passes, managers need to support the staff in returning to normal operations and improving morale. Attention should also be given to assessing any blind spots that may signal future crises before they occur.

Given that market demand for goods or services drives production, managers often begin forecasting by considering the sales or revenue budget projections (Table 17-4). Retail pharmacies base estimates on past dispensing data for sales and volume of prescriptions, with consideration for any trends that might influence future prescription volumes filled in their pharmacies. Hospital pharmacies review patient acuity levels and census information when considering future production needs. Merchandising and manufac-

TABLE 17-4. Key Factors for Consideration in Forecasting Sales (Revenue)

Factor	Considerations
Economic trends in industry	Changing demographics of pharmacy customers
	Changing environment among competing pharmacies
	Changing goods and services offered by pharmacies
Past sales and trends	Recent history of specific organization
	Recent history of entire industry
General economic trends	Assessment of whether a recession or slowdown is expected
	Assessment of whether the economy is growing and how fast
Legal and political events	Switches of prescriptions to over-the-counter items
	New laws affecting sales of goods or services
Other factors	Changing prevalence of a particular illness
	Expectations of a particularly cold winter

turing pharmacies project sales of their goods. Online and mail-order pharmacies predict the number of patients visiting their Web sites and project a certain capture rate that will make a purchase.

An important element of projecting revenue to a retail pharmacy is a consideration of how much the various pharmacy benefits managers (PBMs) will pay the pharmacy for services. A PBM is a third-party administrator contracted by employers, health care plans, unions, and government entities to manage prescription drug programs on behalf of health care plan beneficiaries. PBMs originated several decades ago as processors of prescription drug claims for health care plans, but their role has recently increased because of coverage expansions and increased prescription drug spending. This situation caused commercial health care plans and self-insured employers to outsource the management of their prescription drug spending to PBMs. The PBMs determine the pharmacies to be included in prescription drug plan networks and the amount the pharmacies will be paid. The plan sponsors may agree to require plan beneficiaries to use a mail-order pharmacy for certain medications (often a pharmacy owned and operated by the PBM). The PBM determines which medications will be covered by the plan formulary and may receive rebates from drug manufacturers for inclusion in the plan.

Another consideration is the reimbursement from government programs such as Medicaid, which uses the lowest average manufacturer price (AMP) as the basis for generic drug reimbursement. However, the AMP-based reimbursement is often below a pharmacy's cost to acquire drugs. This inadequate reimbursement results in a net loss to the pharmacy for those prescriptions, which can be devastating if the pharmacy serves a high number of Medicaid patients.

Based on the projected revenue and forecasted volumes, an expense budget detailing how the pharmacy will carry out its operations to meet the demand for its goods and services is required. These budgets contain detailed plans for the use of material, labor, and overhead required to produce a product and provide a service.

Budgeting in pharmacy requires an assessment of current trends in both drug pricing and utilization as well as the ability to project significant changes in these factors in the future (Box 17-4). Numerous methodologies are used for general budgeting. With regard to pharmaceuticals, price and utilization patterns tend to change in varying degrees on the basis of the respective health care sector, such as retail, hospital, or physician practice settings. Industry experts evaluate expected changes in drug patents, new drug or indication approvals, and use in practice to forecast future drug expenditures. The majority of a drug budget is typically based on the cost of 50 to 60 drugs. Pharmaceutical prices very likely will continue to rise and represent a majority of health system pharmacy budgets.

Another type of budget is a capital budget, which plans for the acquisition of capital assets such as equipment and buildings. For both operational and capital budgets, preparing and communicating the

BOX 17-4. Components of Budgeting for Annual Drug Expense

- Collect data from past drug purchases and usage as well as workload and productivity data for analysis.
- Identify high-priority medications accounting for top 50–60 drugs in annual spending and project increases.
- Build new agents into the budget projection.
- Account for nonformulary and lower-priority medications.
- Establish cost-containment plan accounting for patent changes, new protocols, or interchanges.
- Cast budget and maintain drug monitoring vigilance throughout the year.

budget helps set expectations and achieve the desired outcome. Performance targets for the financial operations of an organization must be shared with all levels of the organization, perhaps to varying degrees, so that all team members' activities are focused on the same goals. Assessing the actual results compared to a budget can help managers evaluate the performance of not only the organization as a whole but also individuals and departments. Sometimes, budgets are used as an incentive for individuals to perform well and be paid for that performance.

17-9 Risk Management

In health care and pharmacy practice, patients may have unintended outcomes. All drugs have inherent risks that may result in nonpreventable adverse effects. These are reactions that include intolerances; side effects; and allergic reactions, including anaphylaxis. In addition, preventable adverse drug effects sometimes occur when a medication is prescribed, transcribed, dispensed, administered, or monitored in error. These preventable adverse drug effects are often intercepted before reaching the patient, but unfortunately, some errors reach the patient and may or may not significantly affect the patient's well-being. High-risk medications are those that carry a greater risk for fatality in the event of an error, and some are used in high-risk situations (Table 17-5). Sentinel events are those that cause significant harm to patients and, in some cases, may require reporting to state or other regulatory officials. The Joint Commission defines a sentinel event as any unanticipated event in a health care setting resulting in death or serious physical or psychological injury to a patient or patients, not related to the natural course of the patient's illness.

Transparency with the patient and the family in these cases is of mutual benefit in terms of patient understanding and legal retribution. Large organizations likely have one or more persons in a risk management

TABLE 17-5. Examples of High-Risk Medications and Processes

High-risk medications	High-risk processes
Concentrated electrolytes	Sterile compounding
Chemotherapy	Management of chemotherapy
Insulins	Insulin pump programming
Anticoagulants	Management of anticoagulation therapy
Neuromuscular blockers	Chemotherapy compounding
Opioids	Preparation of pediatric medication doses
Medications with a low therapeutic index	Prescribing of complex medication therapies

department to address patient effects and concerns in conjunction with the health care team. In smaller health care settings such as free-standing pharmacies, the pharmacist is the individual who talks with the patient and the family and helps them navigate next steps when a medication misadventure has transpired.

Patients may be particularly vulnerable to medication-related problems when their health care setting changes, when their payer status changes, or when they change physicians. Because of the complexity and risk in the provision of health care, coordinating care across the continuum to facilitate the appropriate delivery of services is imperative. Transitions of care refer to patient movement between health care providers, locations, or different levels of care within a location as the patient's condition changes. This transition represents a subpart of the broader concept of care coordination. Transitions of care provide a set of actions designed to provide continuity for the patient and family, such as education and logistical arrangements, as well as coordination of the various health care professionals. Pharmacists can identify and prevent problems during transitions of care, reducing medication errors and thereby reducing readmission rates and lengths of hospital stays.

Errors involving medication reconciliation can occur throughout the continuum of care. Medication reconciliation is the process of creating the most accurate list possible of all medications a patient is taking and comparing that list against the physician's orders, with the goal of providing the correct medications to patients at all health care transition points. Reports of these and other errors can be crucial in the identification and correction of process problems to improve the safe care of patients. Data and metrics are used in this area to guide internal quality improvement initiatives and payer incentives. In addition, this type of quality data is often publicly reported to better inform consumer decisions.

Another aspect of risk management is ensuring that proper safety standards are in steady compliance. Pharmacy leaders must ensure continued compliance with all national, state, and local regulations surrounding medications. The more common agencies include state boards of pharmacy, The Joint Commission (TJC) (https://www.jointcommission.org), Drug Enforcement Administration (DEA) (https://www.dea.gov), Centers for Medicare and Medicaid Services (CMS) (https://www.cms.gov), American Society of Health-System Pharmacists (ASHP) (https://www.ashp.org) for technician training programs and health system residencies, and American Pharmacists Association (APhA) (https://www.pharmacist.com/residency-accreditation) for community pharmacy residencies.

The hallmark of health care is to do no harm. Pharmacists largely function as gatekeepers to avoid medication harm as a result of prescribing errors, although dispensing errors can also occur. In recent years, a growing number of health care systems have created dedicated pharmacist positions to serve in medication safety roles. These pharmacists are experts in concepts of human factors engineering and system-based process improvement. Under the direction of the pharmacy leader, they develop a strategic plan for medication safety, which includes special attention to high-risk medications and processes. Technology plays a large role in preventing, and sometimes causing, medication errors. Compelling the use of functions that prevent errant data entry is preferred, particularly in high-risk situations.

A crucial component of any medication safety program is the development and maintenance of a positive culture of safety. Staff members who observe peers being reprimanded or even fired for mistakes leading to significant errors will not likely report errors of which they become aware. Leaders must assure their teams that the focus is on improving the system to prevent errors rather than punishing individuals for an honest mistake. Certainly, if dangerous patterns emerge with an individual after counseling and coaching, additional measures may need to be sought.

In conclusion, pharmacists provide unique expertise in various health care organizations because of their experience with both clinical and business issues. A key function of any leader is building his or her support team and providing goals and directives along with motivation and guidance. To ensure that a leader is moving the team in the right direction, the leader should always make the organization's vision and mission statement a priority. Although short-term goals are helpful, long-term goals as defined by a formal strategic plan are crucial to an organization's longevity. Pharmacy leaders must regularly assess health care trends and identify any organizational gaps that would prevent continued success in light of a changing external environment. Organizations rely on pharmacy leaders to serve as stewards of not only a major portion of health care finances, but also of safe medication use in various patient populations.

17-10 Questions

1. What are the four "Ps" of marketing?
   - A. Product, placement, promotion, plug
   - B. Product, price, position, push
   - C. Product, promotion, persuasion, placement
   - D. Product, price, promotion, place

2. Which of the following statements about the application of relationship marketing is true?
   - A. Relationship marketing encourages focus on selected groups of customers.
   - B. Relationship marketing does not encompass the four Ps of marketing.
   - C. Pharmacists are the only pharmacy team members who need to ensure that service quality is maintained.
   - D. Market niches are often too broad for a pharmacy to serve effectively.

3. In which of the following ways do pharmacy leaders typically influence health system operations? (Mark all that apply.)
   - A. Physicians' prescribing habits
   - B. Supply chain expense
   - C. Admission denials
   - D. Information technology

4. Screening prospective candidates for a pharmacy position should begin by
   - A. comparing the candidates to recent retirees.
   - B. comparing the candidates' experience to the job description.
   - C. comparing the candidates' current salary to the hiring manager's salary.
   - D. comparing the candidates' national origins.

5. Which of the following is usually the best type of question to ask a candidate during a job interview?
   - A. True or false
   - B. Open-ended
   - C. Multiple choice
   - D. Yes or no

6. Which of the following statements is true?
   - A. Business planning is the overarching guide for an entire organization.
   - B. Strategic planning is focused on a specific program's feasibility.
   - C. Strategic planning is the overarching guide for an entire organization.
   - D. Business planning is about broad, long-term organizational success.

7. Which of the following is an analytical technique often used in strategic planning?
   - A. SWAT
   - B. SWAP
   - C. SWOT
   - D. SWOP

8. A company's mission statement should
   - A. briefly note the company's purpose and focus.
   - B. provide a lengthy explanation of a company's services.
   - C. explain the company's approach to charitable giving.
   - D. briefly note recent national recognitions the company received.

9. Drug expense is mainly driven by which of the following? (Mark all that apply.)
   - A. Price
   - B. Utilization
   - C. Risk
   - D. Innovation

10. Which of the following factors should be considered when projecting a pharmacy budget? (Mark all that apply.)
    - A. Capital equipment
    - B. Sales/revenue
    - C. Supply expenses
    - D. Nursing expenses

11. Which of the following is considered a preventable adverse drug effect?
    - A. Side effect
    - B. Hives
    - C. Nausea and vomiting
    - D. Sentinel event

12. Pharmacy leaders have primary responsibility for compliance with which of the following agencies? (Mark all that apply.)

A. DEA (Drug Enforcement Administration)
B. CIA (Central Intelligence Agency)
C. ATF (Bureau of Alcohol, Tobacco, Firearms, and Explosives)
D. FDA (Food and Drug Administration)

13. A formulary is an important tool in a health system because of its role to

A. provide the U.S. Food and Drug Administration with Phase IV post-marketing feedback.
B. control drug costs.
C. test investigational drugs.
D. allow pharmaceutical representative access.

14. The mix of pharmacists and technicians is an important consideration because

A. too many pharmacists is not an efficient use of resources.
B. pharmacists are a less-expensive resource.
C. technicians can provide broader clinical service.
D. pharmacists should spend less time doing drug therapy management.

15. When are pharmaceutical expenses typically reduced?

A. Generics are converted to brands.
B. Shortages of raw materials occur.
C. Group purchasing arrangements are used.
D. The U.S. Food and Drug Administration approves new indications.

16. Pharmacy budget information should typically be

A. kept completely confidential.
B. posted to a public Web site.
C. shared with staff who can affect budget targets.
D. developed with little data or input.

17. Staff retention efforts are beneficial because

A. turnover increases productivity.
B. turnover decreases productivity.
C. turnover keeps trainers productive.
D. turnover gives hiring managers new tasks.

18. Which of the following items should typically be included in a job description? (Mark all that apply.)

A. Duties
B. Skills required
C. Racial preferences
D. Qualifications

19. An organization should develop which of the following documents first?

A. Vision and mission statement
B. Strategic and business plan
C. Budget projection
D. Situation analysis

20. Trends for inpatient drug spending are mainly

A. lower than retail drug spending.
B. outpacing levels of reimbursement.
C. stable and not changing.
D. decreasing to lower levels.

17-11 Answers

1. D. Only this item lists all four of the Ps as discussed in the text.

2. A. Relationship marketing involves specifically targeted types of patients and uses the four Ps of marketing for a narrow niche area. All pharmacy team members must work to maintain service quality.

3. A, B, D. Pharmacy leaders work with prescribers to effectively manage drug supply expenses and use information technology systems. They do not have direct involvement with denying patient admissions.

4. B. Noting whether the applicant has performed jobs in the past similar to the current job is important. Recent retirees and the candidate's national origins are not relevant to the hiring process. Although salary parity to similar-level positions within the organization is important, the hiring manager's salary is not relevant to the screening process.

5. B. Open-ended questions are ideal because they allow the interviewer to hear more from the candidate. The other types of questions typically produce short responses where little is learned about the candidate.

6. **C.** Strategic planning is the primary direction for an organization's long-term success, whereas business planning is a component of the strategic plan and usually assesses a specific program's feasibility.

7. **C.** A SWOT analysis identifies strengths, weaknesses, opportunities, and threats.

8. **A.** The mission statement should be brief and note the company's purpose and focus. Although national recognitions are impressive, they do not state the mission. The approach to charitable giving is an important, but unrelated, discussion.

9. **A, B, D.** The expense of drugs can be affected by pricing; the extent the drug is used for known purposes; or innovative, new purposes. Risk does not significantly affect drug expense.

10. **A, B, C.** Pharmacy budgets must take into account equipment needs (capital), revenue projections, and drug expenses. Nursing expenses are not relevant.

11. **D.** Preventable adverse drug effects are errors that can be serious, such as sentinel events. Side effects, hives, and nausea and vomiting are examples of nonpreventable adverse drug effects.

12. **A, D.** The Drug Enforcement Administration provides oversight of controlled substances; therefore, pharmacy leaders must ensure that their pharmacy is in compliance with DEA regulations. The Food and Drug Administration issues drug labeling and other requirements that must be followed to assure safe use of medications. The other agencies do not directly relate to pharmacy practice.

13. **B.** A formulary is a list of medications that the organization has agreed to use after review of effectiveness, safety, and cost. The other responses do not directly relate to the formulary.

14. **A.** Staff should be mixed to ensure that skills are available in the proper proportion to perform the necessary duties at a reasonable cost. Although technicians cannot provide broad clinical services, they are a less expensive resource that can perform many tasks; therefore, hiring the proper proportion of technicians allows pharmacists to spend more time performing drug therapy management.

15. **C.** Group purchasing generally brings a lower price to all members of the group. However, expenses generally rise when a new indication is approved or drugs are in shortage. Expenses are reduced when brands are converted to generics.

16. **C.** After careful review of data and input from stakeholders, an organization should share its budget internally with the staff, who can take actions to keep drug expenses in line with the budget projection.

17. **B.** High turnover results in time lost to training new individuals and can decrease productivity. In general, trainers and hiring managers are sufficiently busy and prefer to develop existing staff members rather than constantly hire and train new staff members.

18. **A, B, D.** Job descriptions should explain the duties of the position as well as the skills and qualifications needed. Racial preferences can be discriminatory and should not be included in a job description.

19. **A.** The vision and mission statement serve as the initial framework from which the strategic and future business plans are derived. Budget projections and other analyses are performed once an organization's vision and mission are well established.

20. **B.** Drug spending is increasing at a rate faster than the rate of reimbursement, which is, in many cases, decreasing.

17-12 Additional Resources

American Society of Health-System Pharmacists. ASHP guidelines on medication cost management strategies for hospitals and health systems. *Am J Health-Syst Pharm.* 2008;65:1368–1384.

American Society of Health-System Pharmacists. ASHP guidelines: minimum standard for pharmacies in hospitals. *Am J Health-Syst Pharm.* 2013;70:1619–1630. Available at: http://www.ajhp.org/content/70/18/1619.

American Society of Health-System Pharmacists. ASHP guidelines on the recruitment, selection, and retention of pharmacy personnel. *Am J Health-Syst Pharm.* 2003;60:587–593.

American Society of Health-System Pharmacists. ASHP statement on the roles and responsibilities of the pharmacy executive. *Am J Health-Syst Pharm*. 2016;73:329–332. Available at: http://www.ajhp.org/content/73/5/329?sso-checked=true.

Amin R, Badgett C. Importance of pharmacists in transitions of care. Academy of Managed Care Pharmacy. Available at: http://amcp.org/Newsletter.aspx?id=16223. Accessed January 11, 2018.

Gettman DA. Budgeting. In: Zgarrick DP, Alston GL, Moczygemba LR, et al., eds. *Pharmacy Management Essential for All Practice Settings*. 4th ed. McGraw-Hill; 2016:359–374.

Mansur JM. Medication safety systems and the important role of pharmacists. *Drugs Aging*. 2016;33:213–221.

Medication reconciliation to prevent adverse drug events. Institute for Healthcare Improvement Web site. http://www.ihi.org/Topics/ADEsMedicationReconciliation/Pages/default.aspx. Accessed January 11, 2018.

Medication Therapy Management in Pharmacy Practice; Core Elements of an MTM Service Model, Version 2.0. March 2008. American Pharmacists Association and National Association of Chain Drug Stores Foundation. Available at: https://www.pharmacist.com/sites/default/files/files/core_elements_of_an_mtm_practice.pdf. Accessed January 9, 2018.

NORC, University of Chicago. Trends in hospital inpatient drug costs: issues and challenges. Final report to American Hospital Association and Federation of American Hospitals. Washington, DC; 2016. Available at: https://docs.fah.org/website/documents/Trends_in_Hospital_Inpatient_Drug_Costs_Issues_and_Challenges_%281%29.pdf.

PBMs: what is a PBM? National Community Pharmacists Association Web site. http://www.ncpanet.org/advocacy/pbm-resources/what-is-a-pbm-. Accessed January 11, 2018.

PIC pharmacist in charge. HealthCare Consultants Web site. https://pharmacy-staffing.com/pic-pharmacist-in-charge/. Accessed January 11, 2018.

Schumock GT, Donnelly AJ. Strategic Planning in Pharmacy. In: Zgarrick DP, Alston GL, Moczygemba LR, et al., eds. *Pharmacy Management Essentials for All Practice Settings*. 4th ed. New York, NY: McGraw-Hill; 2016: Chapter 4.

State and federal issues affecting community pharmacy. Pharmacy Times Web site. http://www.pharmacytimes.com/publications/career/2008/careers_2008-08/careers_2008-08_8010. Accessed January 11, 2018.

Transitions of care measures. Paper by the National Transitions of Care Coalition Measures Work Group, 2008. Available at: http://www.ntocc.org/Portals/0/PDF/Resources/TransitionsOfCare_Measures.pdf. Accessed January 9, 2018.

White SJ. Recruiting, interviewing, and hiring pharmacy personnel. *Am J Health-Syst Pharm*. 1984;41:928–934.

Wood KD, Offenberger M, Mehta BH, et al. Community pharmacy marketing: strategies for success. *Inov Pharm*. 2011;2(3): Article 48.

Pharmacy Law and Regulatory Affairs

18

LUCY J. ADKINS AND MICAH J. COST

18-1 KEY POINTS

- Two federal laws significantly affect pharmacy practice: the Food, Drug, and Cosmetic Act (FDCA) and the Controlled Substances Act (CSA).
- State pharmacy law regulates the practice of pharmacy in a state and sets out the requirements for becoming licensed in that state. Along with individual state versions of the FDCA and the CSA, each state has a state pharmacy practice act and state board of pharmacy rules and regulations.
- The current legal system comprises six different types of law—statutory, case, civil, criminal, substantive, and procedural—and each type has characteristic enactment, jurisdiction, and procedures.
- The following are the five principal types of statutory law of general interest to pharmacy practice, in descending order of authority: Constitution, treaty or international agreement, statute, regulation, and ordinance.

18-2 STUDY GUIDE CHECKLIST

The following topics may guide your study of this subject area:

- ☐ Overview of the governing framework for pharmacy practice at the state and federal levels
- ☐ Key concepts related to American law
- ☐ An overview of the American legal system
- ☐ Description of the origin, definition, and differentiation of different types of law
- ☐ Functions of the executive, legislative, and judicial branches of government
- ☐ Process of creating a law
- ☐ Examples of legal actions taken against practicing pharmacy professionals in civil, criminal, professional liability, and administrative law.

18-3 Glossary

The legal system and profession have their own "language" just as the health care system and professions use medical terminology. Some words used in legal matters, several of which have a distinctly different and very specific meaning other than how they are used in everyday conversation, are defined in Box 18-1.

BOX 18-1. Glossary of Selected Legal Terms

admissible. A term used to describe evidence that may be heard by a jury and considered by a judge or a jury in civil and criminal cases.

appeal. A request, usually made after a trial, asking another court to decide whether the trial court proceeding was conducted properly.

bail. The release of a person charged with an offense prior to trial date under specified financial or nonfinancial conditions designed to ensure the person's appearance in court when required.

bill. A draft version of a potential law presented to a legislature for consideration of amendments and enactment.

bond. A written agreement by which a person agrees to perform a certain act (e.g., appear in court, fulfill the obligations of a contract) or abstain from performing an act (e.g., committing a crime) that typically requires a sum of money to be held with the condition that failure to fulfill the obligation will result in the forfeiture of the money; the amount of money put up to guarantee the bond.

code. A collection or compendium of laws adopted by a state or nation; also referred to as code of law or legal code. For example, the U.S. Code (USC) consolidates and codifies the general and permanent laws of the United States by categories of subject matter.

commonwealth. A term used by the states of Kentucky, Massachusetts, Pennsylvania, and Virginia as part of their official name (e.g., The Commonwealth of Kentucky).

counsel. A lawyer or a team of lawyers, also known as *legal counsel*. The term is often used during a trial to refer to lawyers in a case. See "lawyer."

damages. Money that a defendant pays to a plaintiff in a civil case that the plaintiff has won; money to compensate the plaintiff for loss or injury.

enact. To establish by legal and authoritative act; to make a bill into law.

expert witness. A person with specialized training and experience about a particular subject who testifies in a case to offer an opinion on an issue in the case based on their specialized knowledge.

felony. A crime that carries a penalty of more than 1 year in prison.

indictment. An official written statement charging a person with a crime, primarily for a felony.

interrogatories. A form of discovery where written questions are to be answered in writing and under oath. Interrogatories are submitted to a party in the case by the party seeking discovery.

jurisdiction. The legal authority of a court to hear and decide a certain type of case; the geographic area over which the court has authority to decide cases.

lawyer. A person licensed to practice law and who advises clients on their legal rights and obligations and represents clients in legal proceedings. An attorney is usually, but not always, a lawyer who acts for another in business or legal matters. Some lawyers refer to themselves as *Attorney at Law*. In everyday language, "lawyer" and "attorney" are often used interchangeably.

misdemeanor. A criminal offense less severe than a felony, generally punishable by a fine only or by imprisonment of less than 1 year.

parties. The plaintiff(s) and defendant(s) in a lawsuit.

probation. A criminal sentence in which the offender is placed under court supervision for a specified period of time but is allowed to remain in the community; a situation or period of time in which a criminal is allowed to stay out of prison if he or she does not commit another crime or breach other court-imposed conditions.

promulgate. To put (e.g., a regulation) into effect; to make known or public.

recede. To withdraw a legal action or plea; to move back or away.

redress. A means of obtaining a remedy; compensation (as damages) for a wrong or loss.

relief. Money damages or any other remedy the plaintiff seeks in a complaint.

sentence. A judgment of the court imposing punishment upon a defendant for criminal conduct.

serve. To deliver or publish a notice or process as required by law; to make legal service upon the person named in a process; to inform or notify by a legal service.

statute. A law passed by a legislature.

stay. The postponement or halting of a judicial proceeding or judgment.

BOX 18-1. Glossary of Selected Legal Terms *(Continued)*

tort. A wrongful act causing injury to the person, property, or reputation (other than a breach of contract) for which relief may be obtained in the form of damages. A tort is also a violation of a duty (e.g., malpractice, not exercising due care) imposed by law, but it is not a crime and is tried in a civil court.

trier of fact. The judge in a bench trial (i.e., no jury involved) or jury in a jury trial that carries the responsibility of determining the issues of fact (weighing the strength of evidence and credibility of witnesses of a debatable issue) in a case; also called *factfinder, finder of fact,* and *trier.*

verdict. A jury's decision on the factual issues in a civil or criminal case.

18-4 Federal and State Laws Governing Pharmacy Practice

Federal Law

Health care in the United States is subject to extensive governmental regulation. The pharmacy profession, compared to many other health care professions, is subject to even greater regulation because of the profession's role in managing the nation's legal drug supply.

Regulation of the practice of pharmacy and the sale of health care products (e.g., drugs, medical devices) comes from the federal (U.S.) and individual state governments. The federal government significantly regulates pharmacy and health care products through two federal laws: the Food, Drug, and Cosmetic Act (FDCA) and the Controlled Substances Act (CSA). The FDCA is administered and enforced by the U.S. Food and Drug Administration (FDA), and the CSA is administered and enforced by the U.S. Drug Enforcement Administration (DEA). The FDCA and CSA are critical federal laws with which a pharmacist must be familiar.

The principal purpose of the FDCA is to regulate the many aspects of the sale of foods, drugs, cosmetics, and medical devices. It addresses issues associated with these products, including the process for FDA approval of drugs and medical devices before their sale in the United States.

The CSA has as its principal purpose the control of the sale of drugs that have a potential for abuse and addiction (i.e., controlled substances). The act addresses a number of issues involving controlled substances, such as registration of distributors and prescribers, schedules (the federal government defines five categories of abuse and addiction potential), limitations on sales, and recordkeeping requirements.

Other important federal laws are the Health Insurance Portability and Accountability Act of 1996 (HIPAA) that is published in *Public Law* at P.L. No. 104-191, which regulates the privacy and security of an individual's health information, and the Poison Prevention Packaging Act of 1970 (PPPA) that is published in the *Code of Laws of the United States* at 15 USC 1471–74, which sets requirements for the packaging of certain household substances, including oral prescription drugs, in child-resistant containers.

State Law

State laws occasionally overlap with federal laws, but each jurisdiction has its unique powers to create laws (Table 18-1) wherein individual states have enacted laws related to the federal FDCA and CSA. Although there are similarities between the federal FDCA and CSA and the related state laws, differences may exist depending on the state. In some cases, the federal FDCA and CSA specifically require or permit states to enact related laws. Under the federal FDCA, states are required to enact laws that license and regulate drug wholesalers, and many states have achieved this federal mandate by including the requirements in the state board of pharmacy's rules and regulations. Under the federal CSA, a limited number of controlled substances, such as a codeine-containing cough suppressant, may be sold by a pharmacy without a prescription. However, the CSA allows individual states to determine whether the sale of such products without a prescription is permitted in a state. Some issues are not addressed in federal law but are exclusively addressed in state law. One such issue is the substitution of generic drug products for

TABLE 18-1. Powers of Federal and State Governments

Federal government	Shared power	State government
Amend the Constitution	Establish courts of law	Ratify amendments to the Constitution
Govern U.S. territories; admit new states	Maintain law and order	Establish local governments
Regulate interstate commerce	Collect taxes	Regulate in-state commerce
Regulate international trade	Borrow money; issue bonds	Establish and regulate corporations
Establish postal system	Charter and regulate banks	Establish and maintain schools
Set standards for weights and measurements	Define crimes and punishments	Issue licenses for marriage, driving, and professions
Maintain armed forces	Make and enforce laws	Take measures for public health and safety
Declare war	Punish criminals	Regulate alcoholic beverages
Establish international treaties and foreign policy	Build roads and transportation systems	Create traffic laws
Protect copyrights and patents	Claim private property for public use	Conduct elections
Print money	Provide for the general welfare	Assume powers not delegated to the federal government or prohibited to the states

brand-name drug products. Each state has enacted laws governing when and how generic substitution may be performed by a pharmacist.

Federal laws do not regulate professions; such regulation is based in state law. Thus, issues such as educational preparation and other requirements for being licensed as a pharmacist are contained in state law and not federal law. Similarly, the requirements for operating a pharmacy, including use of pharmacy technicians, dispensing of prescriptions, and recordkeeping, are contained in state law. Note, however, that the CSA and DEA regulations do impose many requirements on the dispensing of prescriptions for controlled substances and the records that must be maintained by the pharmacy for controlled substances.

Each state creates its own pharmacy practice act and board of pharmacy rules and regulations. The pharmacy practice act is a statute enacted by a state's legislature and generally addresses the following matters:

- Creates the profession of pharmacy in the state and declares pharmacy to be a profession
- Defines the scope of practice for pharmacists, pharmacy technicians, and student pharmacists
- Defines terms associated with the profession and practice of pharmacy
- Creates the state board of pharmacy and establishes the responsibilities of the board
- Sets penalties for violations of the pharmacy practice act and other laws
- Establishes requirements for licensing of pharmacists, pharmacies, pharmacy technicians, manufacturers, and wholesalers
- Addresses miscellaneous matters, such as peer review by pharmacists, if applicable in the state

Typically, the pharmacy practice act is relatively brief compared to the depth and scope of state board of pharmacy rules and regulations. The details of many matters mentioned in the pharmacy practice act are provided in the rules and regulations, which generally address the following aspects:

- Define terms that are not included in the pharmacy practice act
- Establish the procedures, requirements, and fees for licenses
- Set standards for operation of a pharmacy
- Establish professional standards for pharmacists, pharmacy technicians, and pharmacy interns
- Establish requirements for the many aspects of providing pharmaceutical care, dispensing prescriptions, and maintaining records, which may be divided into different sets of standards for different practice settings, such as community pharmacy, institutional (hospital) pharmacy, and nuclear pharmacy

- Set requirements for continuing education
- Establish standards for sterile product preparation and pharmacy compounding
- Address miscellaneous matters, such as operation of a state's controlled substances monitoring database (also known as a prescription drug monitoring program) in some states

18-5 Basics of American Law

Origin of American Law

The origin of American law is *common law*. Common law represents the set of principles based on common usage and custom in England at the time the American colonies were founded in 1776. Rather than developing a new legal system and body of law, the colonists adopted the English common law. The Constitution of the United States is an exception to this general adoption of English common law, reflecting the desire of the colonists to have both independence from England and their own form of government. Much of the common law as the colonists knew it has now been *codified* (the process of incorporating judicial decisions and legislation into an official code) into federal and state statutes.

The common law involves more than the original English principles; it also includes that body of law created by the courts through judicial opinions. The judicial system creates law through court decisions on cases brought before the courts. This judicially created law, and the precedents that come from this law, become part of the common law. The common law continues to evolve even today as cases are decided, but for some legal matters the original common law is still used.

Law Defined

The following definition of law as found in Black's Law Dictionary, Tenth Edition, reads:

> "1. The regime that orders human activities and relations through systematic application of the force of politically organized society, or through social pressure, backed by force, in such a society; the legal system. 2. The aggregate of legislation, judicial precedents, and accepted legal principles; the body of authoritative grounds of judicial and administrative action. . . ."

To paraphrase this definition, law may be described as the whole system or set of rules made by a government that govern conduct; a specific rule made by a government that can be enforced in courts by sanctions and consequences; or a rule of conduct or action that a nation's citizens agree to follow for legal, judicial, and administrative matters.

Types of Laws

Different types of law exist within the legal system. A brief summary of six types—statutory, case, civil, criminal, substantive, and procedural—will aid understanding of the content and application of laws.

Statutory and case law

Statutory law is established by enactments (e.g., statutes, regulations, ordinances) of lawmaking bodies (e.g., legislature, administrative agency, city council, county commission). Five principal types of statutory law are shown in descending order of authority:

- Constitution
- Treaty or international agreement
- Statute
- Regulation
- Ordinance

A constitution is a very broad statement of the powers of the government and its branches. Constitutions exist at the federal and the state levels of government. Constitutions are the highest level of law and are sometimes referred to as the *law of the land*. All other laws, regardless of type, must not conflict with a constitution. If a law does conflict with a constitution, it is said to be *unconstitutional* and consequently unenforceable.

The next level of law below a constitution is a treaty or other form of international agreement. Treaties are agreements between or among different nations and between or among the individual states. Treaties supersede all other types of law except for a constitution.

Statutes are those laws passed by the federal Congress or by a state legislature. Statutes must be consistent with both constitutions and treaties, but they supersede regulations. A statute does not become effective (become a law) upon being passed by the legislature. It must be approved by the President of the United States for a federal statute or by the state governor for a state statute. If the President or governor does not agree with what the legislature has passed, the President or governor may exercise the power of veto (rejection). If a veto occurs, the legislature may vote to override the veto.

Regulations, sometimes referred to as rules, are laws promulgated (enacted) by federal and state administrative agencies and regulatory boards. Pharmacists, pharmacy technicians, and student pharmacists are affected directly by the regulations of a state board of pharmacy and state department of health. The federal government oversees regulations for the Centers for Medicare and Medicaid Services (CMS), the FDA, and the DEA.

Ordinances are laws enacted by local lawmaking bodies such as a city council or county commission. Ordinances address a wide range of matters necessary to govern the affairs of a city or county such as building codes, construction permits, and fines. For example, before the enactment of state and federal statutes limiting the sale of ephedrine and pseudoephedrine products, several cities, in an effort to control the proliferation of clandestine methamphetamine laboratories, had enacted ordinances that placed limitations on the sale of these products that were involved in illicit methamphetamine manufacturing.

Case law is created by judicial decisions or rulings that provide ongoing contributions to the common law. A significant principle of case law is the doctrine known as *stare decisis* (to abide by decided cases). This doctrine holds that decisions made in previous cases are to be followed in subsequent similar cases. Departure from precedents may occur in certain situations. Previous decisions may from time to time be overturned or reversed by higher courts for a variety of reasons. The facts of a current case may differ from the facts presented in the case through which the precedent was established. Finally, note that decisions of federal and state administrative agencies may also establish law (see Section 18-8).

Civil and criminal law

Civil law governs conduct between individuals and, in some cases, between individuals and federal or state government. The concept of civil law is that an individual commits a *wrong* against another individual. Within the civil law is the law of contracts, property, and torts.

Criminal law regulates the conduct of individuals within the context of society as a whole. The concept of criminal law is that when an individual commits a crime, the individual commits a wrong against society, and not just one individual within the society.

Substantive and procedural law

Substantive law is that body of law defining and providing for the rights of individuals. For example, a patient may sue a pharmacist for negligent conduct (an error or omission by the pharmacist) that caused injury to the patient.

Procedural law establishes the process for enforcing one's rights or for obtaining redress (i.e., means of seeking a remedy) when the rights of the individual are violated. An example of procedural law is a statute of limitation. A statute of limitation sets the time limit within which a lawsuit must be filed. The length of time can vary by state. For example, in the state of Tennessee, a personal injury lawsuit, such as one caused by a pharmacist dispensing the wrong medication, must be filed within 1 year from the date when the individual discovers, or in the exercise of reasonable care should have discovered, the injury.

18-6 Overview of the Legal System

The authors of the U.S. Constitution decided to use *federalism* as a constitutional principle to give local communities the right to make their own laws while ensuring that the laws created are still constitutional. This sharing of power is intended to ensure that the central government is powerful enough to be effective, yet not so powerful as to threaten states or citizens (Table 18-1). The legal system was also fashioned with the principle of shared power through three distinct branches at the federal and state levels of government: legislative, executive, and judicial (Figure 18-1). This *branch system* was established as a *system of checks and balances* (Table 18-2), wherein each branch is given power that tends to balance (and serves as a check on) the power given to the other branches.

Legislative Branch

The legislative branch creates laws. By creating laws, the legislative branch initiates the operation of the legal system. At the federal level of government, the legislative branch is the U.S. Congress, which is divided into the House of Representatives and the Senate. Each state has its own legislature, which also consists of a House of Representatives and a Senate.

In addition to creation of laws, the legislative branch establishes administrative agencies because it does not have sufficient expertise and time to address all areas of interest. The administrative agency may

FIGURE 18-1. Government Branches, Jurisdictions, and Functions

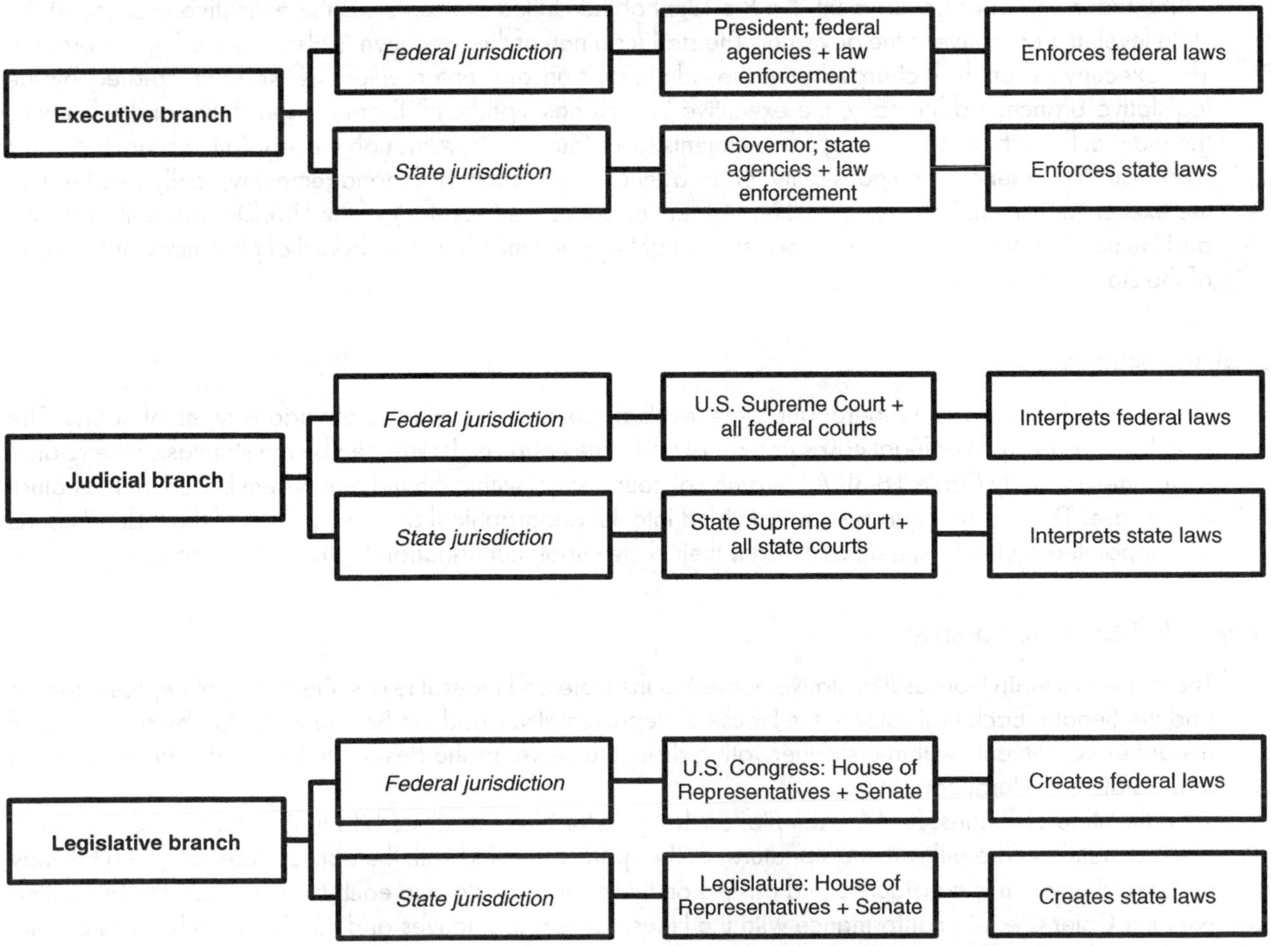

TABLE 18-2. Checks and Balances by the Branches of Government

Government branch	Duty or authority	Check and balance	Branch checking and balancing
Legislative	Create statutes	President can exercise veto.	Executive
Executive	Enforce statutes	Congress can override a presidential veto by 2/3 majority.	Legislative
Judicial	Interpret statutes and Constitution	President nominates federal judges and justices.	Executive
Executive	Enforce statutes	Senate confirms or rejects presidential nominations of federal judges and justices.	Legislative
Executive	Enforce statutes	Congress can impeach the president.	Legislative
Legislative	Create statutes	Courts can invalidate unconstitutional statutes.	Judicial
Judicial	Interpret statutes and Constitution	Statutes can supersede case law.	Legislative

Criminal Law, University of Minnesota Libraries Publishing, 2015.

promulgate regulations only in the specific areas in which it has expertise, and it cannot exceed its limits of authority granted by the legislature.

Executive Branch

At the federal level of government, the President of the United States heads the executive branch. At the state level, the executive is the governor. The staff (cabinet) of the executive is also included in this branch. The executive branch is charged with the administration and enforcement of the laws created by the legislative branch. Additionally, the executive branch has significant fiscal responsibility and influences the judicial branch by nominating appointments to various courts. Although the legislative branch creates administrative agencies, responsibility for an agency's operation and management typically resides with the executive branch. For example, the President appoints the Secretary of the U.S. Department of Health and Human Services. The governor of a state might appoint members to a board of pharmacy or the head of the state department of health.

Judicial Branch

The judicial branch at the federal and state levels of government consists of various types of courts. The jurisdiction and types of legal cases of federal and state courts is determined by the statutes of the related governmental body (Table 18-3). A hierarchy of courts exists within the judicial system based on the nature of the case. The federal court system is divided into 12 geographical districts. Judges of the federal courts are appointed by the President and begin their duties upon confirmation by the U.S. Senate.

How a Bill Becomes a Law

There are two main Houses (legislative bodies) at the state and federal levels: the House of Representatives and the Senate. Each legislator in the House of Representatives and the Senate is elected by a majority of his or her constituents within his or her voting district to serve for the designated term of service as stated in the state or federal constitution.

In the state of Tennessee, for example, each legislator may introduce bills in the House in which he or she is a member. The bill with the signatures of the sponsors is filed with the appropriate clerk. No bill may be passed unless it is considered and passed on three separate days in each House. Once the bill is filed with the Chief Clerk in conformance with the House of Representatives and the Senate rules, it is considered as passed on first consideration. On the following day, the bill is passed on second consideration

TABLE 18-3. Selected Differences of Federal and State Court Jurisdictions

Federal courts	State courts
Federal crime or offense	Crime or offense of a state statute
Constitutionality of a law	Personal and worker injury lawsuits
Patent and copyright violations	Motor vehicle traffic violations
Foreign government or treaty disputes	Family law (divorce, adoption, child custody)
Bankruptcy proceedings	Contract disputes (goods, services, real estate)
Disputes between state governments	Civil court cases
Immigration issues	Probate cases (wills, estates)
Mail or federal tax fraud	Murder; physical or sexual assault
Kidnapping or auto theft across state lines	Drunk or drugged driving
Robbery of a federally insured bank	Malpractice lawsuits
Possession of prescription drugs without a prescription	Illicit drug use or possession (shared with federal)

and referred by the Speaker of the House of Representatives or Speaker of the Senate to the appropriate standing committee.

Once the bill is referred to committee, several actions are necessary to bring it out of committee:

1. The sponsor presents the bill and receives a motion to have the bill recommended for passage by receiving a majority vote of the committee members.
2. After 7 days in a committee without action being taken, the bill may be recalled from committee by a majority of the members of the Senate or House of Representatives.
3. If the bill is not considered controversial in nature, it is placed on the committee consent calendar and then reported as "recommended for passage" if an objection is not raised.
4. In the House of Representatives committees, if the sponsor fails to appear before the committee at the scheduled hearing on two occasions and the sponsor fails to request that the bill be rescheduled, the bill is returned to the Chief Clerk's desk where it is held.
5. In the Senate committees, if the sponsor fails to appear before the committee at the scheduled hearing on any occasion and has failed to request that the bill be rescheduled, the bill is returned to the Chief Clerk's desk for the purpose of being withdrawn from the Senate.

The committee chairs report the bills being recommended for passage to the scheduling committee, which is the House of Representatives Committee on Calendar and Rules or the Senate Calendar Committee. The bill is then referred by these committees to the respective calendars according to the rules of the House of Representatives and the Senate. The bill is then open to debate and amendment by the entire House of Representatives or Senate body considering it. This is the third consideration of the bill, and it may be passed with or without amendment by a majority of the members to which the body is entitled. If the bill is passed by a majority of members, the bill automatically goes to the Chief Engrossing Clerk, where it is retyped and transmitted to the other body for consideration. Identical, or companion bills, must be passed by both Houses. If a bill is passed by one House and is amended in the other, the bill goes back to the House where it was originally passed for action on the amendment. The first House may vote to concur or not to concur. If the first House concurs in the amendment(s), the bill follows through for the governor's approval. However, if the first House refuses to concur, the bill goes back to the House where the amendment originated, and it considers whether to recede (withdraw) or refuse to recede from its position in adopting the amendment(s). If there is a refusal to recede, that House must appoint conference committees, consisting usually of at least three members of each House, to meet and attempt to reconcile the differences between the two Houses on the bill or to recommend a course of action agreeable to both Houses.

After being passed by both Houses, the bill is submitted to the Chief Engrossing Clerk who prepares (i.e., enrolls) the bill in the exact form passed by both Houses and in a format suitable for approval by the two speakers and the governor. The speakers then sign the enrolled copy, and it is automatically transmitted to the governor for action.

The governor may sign the bill, veto it, or allow it to become law with his or her signature. The governor is allowed 10 days (except Sundays) after a bill is presented to him or her to approve or veto the bill. If no action is taken within that period, the bill becomes law without his or her signature. The governor also has constitutional authority to reduce or disapprove any sum of money appropriated in any bill while approving other portions of such bill. If the governor has vetoed a bill or reduced or disapproved an appropriation within a bill, the veto can be overridden (or reduced or disapproved sums of money can be restored) by a majority vote of the membership to which each body is entitled under the state's constitution.

Finally, the Secretary of State's office assigns a public chapter number to each bill passed into law after which it is published and incorporated into the state's legal code. In broad generalities, a similar process is followed at the federal level.

Anatomy of a Civil Lawsuit and Trial

A civil lawsuit is brought by a citizen seeking redress (a remedy) for injury caused by another citizen or by a government entity. A lawsuit is initiated by the plaintiff (the person injured) by filing a *complaint* against the defendant (the person alleged by the plaintiff to have caused the injury). The plaintiff's lawyer files the complaint in the proper court. The complaint is then served (delivered) to the defendant, an action referred to as *service of process*. After receiving the service of process, the defendant must file an *answer* to the complaint within an established period of time.

A court date is assigned by the court. The defendant may delay the trial date by filing a motion for a continuance. This action allows the defense lawyer more time to prepare for the trial. During this time, both parties enter into a process known as *discovery*. Discovery involves such activities as the taking of depositions and the parties' submission of *written interrogatories* to each other. Written interrogatories are questions submitted for written answers given under oath. Discovery is conducted to learn as much as possible about the case before going to trial. Eventually, if pursued by the plaintiff, or if an out-of-court settlement is not reached between the parties, the lawsuit will go to trial.

The trial begins, if it is a jury trial, with the selection of the jury through a process known as *voir dire*. Voir dire is a preliminary examination of a prospective juror by a judge or lawyer for both sides to determine whether the prospective juror is qualified and suitable to serve on the jury. For a nonjury trial, where the judge serves in the role of the jury, voir dire is not necessary and the trial begins immediately.

Lawyers for the plaintiff begin with *opening statements* stating what the evidence will present, and statements by the lawyer for the defendant follow. Opening statements are used to relate to the trier of fact, whether that be a judge or jury. After opening statements are completed, the plaintiff presents evidence by calling witnesses to provide testimonial evidence and introduction of documentary evidence. Documentary evidence in a lawsuit involving a pharmacy may include medical records, prescriptions that have been filed in the pharmacy, package inserts to prescription drugs, and other documents. The plaintiff will also use *expert witnesses* to establish that the error or omission of the defendant breached the applicable standard of care and caused the plaintiff's injury.

Direct examination occurs when a witness is called to the stand and provides evidence in the form of testimony. Each party has the opportunity to *cross-examine* all of the witnesses called by the other party. Following cross-examination, the party that originally called the witness is allowed to conduct *redirect examination* to rebut or clarify evidence brought forth by the cross-examination. Then the other party will have the opportunity to *recross-examine* the witness. This process will continue for as long as the lawyers desire to question the witness.

Not all evidence sought to be introduced at a trial will be allowed. Very specific rules for the introduction of evidence exist to determine whether evidence is admissible. For example, the rules generally will not allow the introduction of *hearsay* testimony. Hearsay testimony is a statement made by a person who, for whatever reason, is not present in court, and the testimony is now being offered in court by a person who heard the statement by the person not present.

After the plaintiff has completed the presentation of evidence, the defendant presents evidence in the same manner. The process of direct, cross-, redirect, and recross-examination will occur again.

Following the presentation of all evidence by both parties, each lawyer will deliver a *closing statement*, which summarizes the evidence presented. The content of opening and closing statements is not considered as evidence. In a jury trial, the judge *charges* the jury at the conclusion of closing statements. Through the charge, the judge will instruct the jury on, among other things, the law applicable to the case and the way the jury must go about reaching its conclusion. After closing statements and charging of the jury, the trier of fact (the jury in this case) retires to deliberate and to reach a decision. Once a decision is reached, either party has the right to appeal the decision.

For the plaintiff to be successful in a lawsuit, the alleged facts must be proved by a *preponderance of the evidence*. This burden of proof will be met if the plaintiff is able to provide sufficient evidence to "tip the scales in favor" of the plaintiff. This burden of proof is substantially less than that required of prosecutors in criminal matters.

Anatomy of a Criminal Lawsuit and Trial

A criminal lawsuit and trial is initiated against a person being charged with (accused of) committing a crime. A person may be charged by an indictment, which is a decision of a grand jury that the person should be criminally prosecuted. A prosecutor presents to the grand jury evidence of a crime and the person believed to have committed the crime.

If the grand jury finds probable cause that a crime was committed by the person, then the grand jury will return an indictment against the person. The indictment will be accompanied by an order that the person to be prosecuted appear before a court of law or, in the alternative, an arrest warrant may be issued. A person also may be charged directly by the government in certain situations, such as when a police officer arrests a person while that person is in the process of committing a crime.

Criminal charges may be for a misdemeanor or a felony offense. Felonies are those crimes punishable by a term of imprisonment of 1 or more years, whereas misdemeanors lead to imprisonment for less than 1 year. Misdemeanors and felonies are handled virtually in the same manner for a trial.

For a charge initiated by an indictment or by the government directly, a determination must be made as to whether the person (the defendant) will be held in custody until the trial. Depending on the nature of the crime alleged and the defendant's circumstances (e.g., the defendant might attempt to flee the country, the defendant has prior convictions), the defendant may be held in custody until the trial. Alternatively, the defendant may be released until the trial if the court determines that such action is appropriate. The court may release the defendant on his or her own recognizance, or it may place a number of conditions upon the release. Conditions may include posting bond for an amount set by the court, being placed under house arrest, being required to wear an electronic tracking device, or surrendering a passport.

If a person is charged directly by the government, rather than through an indictment, a preliminary hearing is the first step in the process. If the defendant is not represented by a lawyer at the time of the preliminary hearing, the defendant will be advised of the right to have a lawyer, and a plea will not be requested. If represented by a lawyer, the defendant may enter a plea at the preliminary hearing.

If a person is charged through an indictment, arraignment is the first step in the process. The preliminary hearing to determine probable cause is not necessary because a grand jury has already made a determination that probable cause exists. Arraignment is the court appearance at which the defendant will enter a plea. The U.S. Constitution guarantees that all defendants facing time in jail have the right to a lawyer. If they cannot afford one, a public defender will be appointed.

Three pleas—guilty, not guilty, or nolo contendere (no contest)—are available to the defendant. Nolo contendere has the same effect as a plea of guilty except that the defendant is not admitting to the facts charged. If the plea is guilty or nolo contendere, a trial is not necessary and the penalty is established by the court or by the prosecutor with subsequent approval by the court.

Guilty pleas are most often the result of *plea bargaining*. The plea bargain is a process where the prosecutor and the defense lawyer negotiate an outcome on the basis of the strengths and weaknesses of each side's case. If a bargain is struck, the defendant will have the opportunity to accept or reject it.

The essential component from the defendant's standpoint is the agreed-upon penalty. The prosecutor will have to make the plea of guilty attractive to the defendant possibly by lessening the potential penalty for the crime charged. The risky aspect of the plea bargain is that the court may reject the bargain. Some judges will tell the defendant before he or she enters the plea that the bargain has been rejected. Others will allow the defendant to withdraw the plea if the bargain has been rejected. Still others will simply allow the defendant to take a chance that the court will accept the plea and agreed-upon punishment.

If the defendant pleads not guilty, then a trial date will be set. The defendant's defense will rest on one or more common theories. Basic theories are (1) that the defendant did not commit the acts charged; (2) that the acts committed do not constitute a crime; and (3) that the defendant committed the acts, but for a variety of reasons, such as self-defense, he or she is not liable for them.

Before the trial begins, the prosecutor and defense lawyer will enter into extensive discovery. Basically, each party has the right to know what evidence, particularly as to witnesses, the other party will use at trial. This process avoids either party being surprised at trial. Following discovery, the trial will begin and generally follow the same process as described for a civil trial. Likewise, the defendant may appeal a conviction to an appellate court.

In the criminal trial, the prosecution must convince the jury beyond a reasonable doubt that a crime was committed and that the defendant committed the crime. If the jury has a reasonable doubt that the defendant committed the crime alleged, then it must find the defendant not guilty, resulting in an acquittal. The defense lawyer's goal is to cast reasonable doubt on the prosecution's case.

If the jury does not have reasonable doubt, then the verdict will be guilty of committing the crime charged, referred to as a *conviction* of the crime charged. Upon conviction, the court will set a sentencing date, at which time the penalty for the crime will be imposed.

Sentencing is typically based on a number of factors such as the previous crime record of the defendant and factors that tend to cast either a positive or a negative light on the defendant. At the sentencing hearing, the court will allow the defendant to make a statement in an effort to lessen the penalty. If the defendant believes the penalty is too harsh, a request may be filed with the court to reconsider. As with a conviction, the defendant can appeal the sentence to the appellate court.

Another possible outcome of a criminal lawsuit and trial is judicial diversion. Judicial diversion (sometimes referred to as pre-trial diversion) may occur after a defendant is charged with committing a crime. The court may place a defendant on *probation* for a defined period of time. If the defendant behaves properly during probation, the criminal charges will be dismissed and the record of the charges expunged (erased) from the court's records. Although the defendant's lawyer will request judicial diversion, the prosecutor may or may not be agreeable. Whether it will be granted to the defendant will depend on the nature of the crime and if the defendant has any prior criminal convictions. This method of disposing of criminal charges is highly attractive to a defendant because the records are expunged and a record of a conviction is never entered.

Although judicial diversion does not result in conviction under the criminal law, it is still considered a conviction under a variety of health care licensing and related laws. For example, state boards of pharmacy, the DEA, and the U.S. Department of Health and Human Services all consider judicial diversion to be a conviction for purposes of their respective laws and regulations. Although the criminal record of the crime may have been expunged, judicial diversion may have to be disclosed and reported to various health care regulatory agencies.

18-7 Professional Liability

Professional liability is another word for *malpractice*. Errors or omissions by a pharmacist, pharmacy technician, or student pharmacist could result in professional liability. Some examples include dispensing the wrong drug or the wrong strength of the proper drug, placing incorrect directions on the prescription label, failing to warn the patient about side effects or contraindications of a drug, providing too many refills of a drug, and failing to detect an allergy or drug interaction through a review of a patient's history.

The most common theory of liability used to establish professional liability is negligence. A negligence-based lawsuit requires the plaintiff to prove four elements:

1. The pharmacist owed a duty to the patient.
2. The act (error), or failure to act (omission), on the part of the pharmacist breached the duty owed.
3. The act (error), or failure to act (omission), by the pharmacist was the proximate cause of the injury.
4. The patient suffered actual injury or harm.

If the plaintiff is unable to prove any one of these four elements, then the plaintiff will not be successful.

The first element, duty owed, asks whether the pharmacist was obligated to do, or refrain from doing, some act for the patient. For example, the pharmacist has a legal duty—is legally obligated—to dispense the correct medication. Sometimes, whether a duty exists is not clear and may vary from state to state.

Once a duty is established, the next step is to inquire if the pharmacist breached the duty—the second element. For example, if the pharmacist dispenses a medication other than the medication prescribed, then the pharmacist has breached the duty to correctly dispense medications.

The third element—proximate cause—is often the most difficult element for the plaintiff. Two separate questions are asked with proximate cause. First, was the error or omission by the pharmacist the *cause-in-fact* of the patient's injury? Second, was the injury suffered by the patient foreseeable to the pharmacist? If the patient can prove that the error or omission was the cause-in-fact and that the injury was foreseeable to the pharmacist, then the element of proximate cause will be present. For the proximate cause to be considered valid, the patient must prove both cause-in-fact and foreseeability.

The fourth element is simply that the patient was injured. This element may be proven in a number of ways, primarily through physician reports of the treatment of the patient for the injury suffered. The quantity and severity of the injury is extremely important because it will be used to establish the amount of compensation to be paid to the patient. Compensable injury is not limited to physical harm, but it may also include mental harm.

Whether a duty is owed and, if owed, whether it was breached are determined by identifying the *recognized standard of care* for the profession in the community, or similar community, in which the defendant practices. The question asked is "What would the reasonably prudent pharmacist have done under the same or similar circumstances?" The plaintiff will use pharmacists as expert witnesses who will testify that the error or omission of the defendant pharmacist did not meet the standard of care. In turn, the defendant pharmacist will use other pharmacists as experts who will testify that the standard of care was met. Ultimately, the trier of fact (jury or judge) will determine the standard of care applicable and whether the standard of care was breached.

In addition to arguing that the standard of care was not breached, the defendant pharmacist may use one or more of a number of defenses to a charge of negligence. These defenses include contributory negligence, comparative negligence, and assumption of the risk.

Contributory or comparative negligence is used to claim that the patient's own negligence caused, or at least contributed to, the injury. Contributory negligence, if established, completely invalidates the plaintiff's legal claim and ends the trial. Comparative negligence, in contrast, requires the jury to apportion the relative degrees of fault between the patient and the pharmacist. This distribution of fault determines the amount of the recovery, that is, compensation for the injury. For example, if a jury finds the appropriate amount of damages for an injured patient to be $100,000 and finds that the patient was 25% responsible for the injury because of the patient's own negligence, then the award would be reduced to $75,000. The doctrine of comparative negligence must be adopted individually by states.

Assumption of the risk is used when the patient was fully informed of the possibility for injury and is now arguing that the pharmacist was negligent, most often in relation to sharing with the patient the risks and benefits of a particular therapy. The use of informed consent is one mechanism for establishing that the patient was informed of the risk and assumed the risk.

Of special importance in relation to pharmacy practice is the liability theory of *negligence per se* which is used when the pharmacist has breached the standard of care by violating a statute or regulation. For example, pharmacists may dispense prescription drugs only pursuant to a valid prescription order. If the pharmacist sells a patient a prescription drug without a prescription and the drug injures the patient, then the charge would be negligence per se because the pharmacist violated a statute or regulation by dispensing the drug without a prescription.

Legally, the difference arises when the plaintiff attempts to prove the four elements of a negligence charge. To prove that the pharmacist had a duty and breached the duty, the plaintiff proves that the pharmacist violated a statute or regulation. Because some statutes and regulations establish duties, a violation of these statutes or regulations may be considered as a breach of a duty and a breach of the standard of care. In practical terms, proving the violation of such a statute or regulation also proves the first two elements of the general negligence theory. However, the plaintiff must then prove that actual injury occurred and that the violation of the statute or regulation was the proximate cause of the injury.

18-8 Administrative Law

In simple terms, *administrative law* is the body of law governing the operation of administrative agencies. The law governing administrative agencies is important to pharmacists because federal and state agencies have significant influence on the daily practice of pharmacy. First, pharmacists and pharmacies are licensed by state boards of pharmacy. Pharmacies dispensing controlled substances are required to obtain a Certificate of Registration from the DEA. Second, the state boards of pharmacy, the DEA, and other federal and state agencies have rules that specify how certain aspects of practice must be conducted. For example, the DEA has regulations establishing requirements for dispensing a prescription for a controlled substance.

Agencies also govern a particular area by *disciplinary* actions against licensees for violation of laws applicable to the profession, trade, or business. A disciplinary action by a state board of pharmacy begins with the delivery of a *notice of hearing and charges* to the pharmacist involved. Disciplinary actions brought by the DEA begin with an *order to show cause*. A notice or order can initiate the formal disciplinary process.

In administrative law, the agency bringing the charges is referred to as the *petitioner* rather than the plaintiff, and the licensee against whom the charges are brought is referred to as the *respondent* rather than the defendant. The following is an example of administrative hearings based on one state's administrative law, but federal and other state administrative laws are similar.

Upon receipt of a notice of hearing and charges, the licensee (pharmacist) may respond to the charges by filing a written answer with the agency. In addition to stating the charges being brought, the notice will set a date, time, and location for the hearing. The notice will also inform the respondent of the right to be represented by a lawyer and to present evidence and cross-examine witnesses. The respondent may appear before the agency and present a defense without the presence of a lawyer, but such action may not be advisable because the state's case against the pharmacist will be presented by a lawyer.

Although a hearing date will be set in the original notice, the hearing date may be continued if good cause can be shown. While awaiting the hearing date, the respondent will be preparing for the hearing through discovery. The respondent may also be negotiating with the lawyer for the government to settle the charges to avoid the time and expense of a hearing—the administrative equivalent of the plea bargain.

If such a settlement is reached, the terms of the settlement will be set forth in writing in a *consent order* or an *agreed order*. The consent order will state the factual background involved (findings of fact), the law or laws violated (conclusions of law), the policy reasons, and the disciplinary action to be imposed. All agency disciplinary orders must contain these elements.

Upon final drafting of the consent order and signing by the respondent, the consent order is presented to the agency for approval. In considering whether to approve the consent order, the agency must base the decision solely on the written consent order. No testimony or other evidence may be presented to the agency to aid in its decision. If the agency rejects the consent order, the respondent may attempt to amend the order, but most likely a hearing will be necessary.

In the administrative law context, such a hearing is a *contested case hearing*. These hearings are conducted in similar fashion to civil trials but with a few differences. If the agency has members, such as members of a state board of pharmacy, then the members serve as the trier of fact at the hearing. In such a hearing, an administrative law judge will be assigned to conduct and oversee the hearing. Although the administrative law judge will not decide whether the charges are proved and what disciplinary measure to impose, the judge will rule on motions, questions of law, and objections raised during the hearing. A very important difference from a civil jury trial is that, unlike civil jurors, the agency members may ask questions of the witnesses following the conclusion of questioning by the lawyers.

At the end of the hearing, the judge charges the agency members like a judge charges a civil jury. The agency members deliberate and decide whether the charges have been proved and, if proved, the disciplinary measure to be imposed. Because contested case hearings are civil in nature, the burden of proof on the lawyer for the government is that of a preponderance of the evidence (evidence that tips the scales in favor of the state) and not that of beyond a reasonable doubt.

Also, unlike in a civil jury trial, the agency members do not retire to a jury room to deliberate, but rather must do so in the presence of the respondent. If the decision of the agency members is adverse to the respondent, then a motion for reconsideration or stay can be filed with the agency. If the agency does not grant these motions, then the respondent can appeal the decision through the judicial system.

If the agency does not have members or if the agency is not authorized to conduct hearings, then an administrative law judge sitting alone will hear the evidence and issue an *initial order* within 90 days of the hearing. Similar to a hearing before agency members, the judge may ask questions of witnesses, but the judge does not have to deliberate and reach a decision in the respondent's presence. The initial order will become a final order if it is not appealed to the agency within a specified time. If the respondent is not satisfied with the resulting final order, an appeal can be taken in the same fashion as an appeal of a final order by agency members.

18-9 Conclusion

Recognizing that pharmacy laws are the result of various governmental functions, knowledge of the operation of state and federal governments can be beneficial to interacting with governmental officials and participating in the legislative process through advocacy. Participating in the legislative process has become an important professional responsibility as governmental influence on the delivery of health care services, including pharmacy services, continues to expand.

Law is constantly changing by the actions of several sources—the U.S. Congress, the state legislative branch, federal and state courts, and administrative agencies. Foremost among the state agencies for pharmacists is the board of pharmacy, which directly addresses pharmacy practice through its regulations and disciplinary proceedings. Pharmacists, pharmacy technicians, and student pharmacists must routinely devote time to review existing, changed, and new laws that affect the daily practice of pharmacy and the patients served by the pharmacy profession.

18-10 Questions

1. Which of these laws regulates many aspects of the sale of foods, drugs, cosmetics, and medical devices?

A. Poison Prevention Packaging Act
B. Food, Drug, and Cosmetic Act (FDCA)
C. Controlled Substances Act (CSA)
D. Health Insurance Portability and Accountability Act (HIPAA)

2. Which federal agency administers and enforces the Food, Drug, and Cosmetic Act (FDCA)?

A. Drug Enforcement Administration (DEA)
B. Food and Drug Administration (FDA)
C. Centers for Medicare and Medicaid Services (CMS)
D. Federal Trade Commission (FTC)

3. Which federal agency administers and enforces the Controlled Substances Act (CSA)?

A. Drug Enforcement Administration (DEA)
B. Food and Drug Administration (FDA)
C. Centers for Medicare and Medicaid Services (CMS)
D. Federal Trade Commission (FTC)

4. What is the purpose of the Controlled Substances Act (CSA)?

A. Protect the privacy and security of individual health information
B. Protect the packaging of household substances
C. Package prescription-controlled substances in child-resistant containers
D. Control the sale of those drugs that have been found to have a potential for abuse and addiction

5. What is the purpose of the Health Insurance Portability and Accountability Act (HIPAA)?

A. Protect the privacy and security of individual health information
B. Protect the packaging of household substances
C. Package prescription-dispensed controlled substances in child-resistant containers
D. Control the sale of those drugs that have been found to have a potential for abuse and addiction

6. What is the purpose of the Poison Prevention Packaging Act of 1970?

A. Protect the privacy and security of individual health information
B. Require that certain household products, including oral prescription drugs, be packaged in child-resistant containers
C. Control the sale of those drugs that have been found to have a potential for abuse and addiction
D. Serve as a checks and balances system for the U.S. government

7. Which of the following is *not* true regarding state pharmacy practice acts?

A. Create the profession of pharmacy in the state and declare pharmacy to be a profession
B. Define the scope of practice for pharmacists, pharmacy technicians, and student pharmacists
C. Establish licensing requirements for pharmacists, pharmacies, pharmacy technicians, manufacturers, and wholesalers
D. Establish the procedures, requirements, and fees for licenses

8. What is the origin of law in America?

A. Substantive law
B. Common law
C. Criminal law
D. Civil law

9. Which of the following is *not* a required responsibility of a state board of pharmacy?

A. Set standards for operation of a pharmacy
B. Establish requirements for dispensing prescriptions and maintaining records
C. Negotiate pharmacy reimbursement rates for prescription drugs
D. Establish standards for sterile product preparation and pharmacy compounding

10. Which of the following is *not* a type of law that exists within the American legal system?

A. Statutory law
B. Anecdotal law
C. Procedural law
D. Criminal law

11. With respect to statutory law, which of the following is ordered correctly from most powerful to least powerful (e.g., descending order of authority)?

A. Statute, ordinance, regulation, constitution, treaty or international agreement
B. Ordinance, regulation, statute, treaty or international agreement, constitution
C. Constitution, treaty or international agreement, statute, regulation, ordinance
D. Regulation, constitution, treaty or international agreement, ordinance, statute

12. Which of the following is considered the highest level of law and is often referred to as the *law of the land*?

A. Constitution
B. Statute
C. Regulation
D. International agreement

13. *Stare decisis* means to abide by decided cases; therefore, decisions made in previous cases are to be followed in subsequent cases. The term *stare decisis* falls under what type of law?

A. Civil law
B. Case law
C. Criminal law
D. Procedural law

14. What is the primary purpose for the three separate branches of government (legislative, executive, and judicial) at the state and federal levels?

A. To give the various agencies power and authority
B. To establish a checks and balances system
C. To enforce the established laws
D. To have responsibility for operation and administration

15. Which branch of government establishes various administrative agencies and gives the agencies power and authority to govern a specific area?

A. Judicial
B. Executive
C. Administrative
D. Legislative

16. Which branch of government is charged with the administration and enforcement of laws created by the legislative branch?

A. Judicial
B. Executive
C. Administrative
D. Legislative

17. Which of the following is *not* one of the elements a plaintiff must prove in a negligence-based lawsuit against a pharmacist, pharmacy technician, or student pharmacist?

A. Duty owed
B. Injury to the patient
C. Proximate cause to the injury by error or omission
D. Findings of fact

18. What is the primary measure of whether or not a duty is owed or a duty is breached?

A. Anecdotal evidence
B. Recognized standard of care
C. Individual testimony
D. Patient harm

19. Which of the statements correctly identifies administrative law?

A. Brought by a private citizen seeking redress for injury caused by another private citizen
B. Body of law created by the courts through judicial opinions
C. Body of law governing the operation of administrative agencies
D. Initiated by a person being charged with (accused of) committing a crime

20. In what instance would a consent order be used by an administrative agency?

A. To negotiate with the lawyer for the government to settle the charges and to avoid the time and expense of a hearing
B. To settle a civil trial brought by a private citizen seeking redress for injury caused by another private citizen
C. To prove errors or omissions by a pharmacist, pharmacy technician, or student pharmacist in the case of professional liability
D. To present evidence of a crime and the particular person or persons believed to have committed the crime to the grand jury

18-11 Answers

1. **B.** The principal purpose of the Food, Drug, and Cosmetic Act (FDCA) is to regulate the many aspects of the sale of foods, drugs, cosmetics, and medical devices.
2. **B.** The Food and Drug Administration (FDA) administers and enforces the FDCA.
3. **A.** The Drug Enforcement Administration (DEA) administers and enforces the CSA.
4. **D.** The purpose of the Controlled Substances Act (CSA) is to control the sale of those drugs that have been found to have a potential for abuse and addiction.
5. **A.** The purpose of the Health Insurance Portability and Accountability Act (HIPAA) is to protect the privacy and security of a person's health information.
6. **B.** The Poison Prevention Packaging Act of 1970 requires certain household products, including oral prescription drugs, to be packaged in child-resistant containers.
7. **D.** State pharmacy practice acts do not establish the procedures, requirements, and fees for licenses. The state board of pharmacy is responsible, in most cases, to establish the procedures, requirements, and fees for licensure.
8. **B.** The origin of American law is common law.
9. **C.** A state board of pharmacy is not required to negotiate pharmacy reimbursement rates for prescription drugs. Pharmacy reimbursement is typically left up to state agencies of insurance and commerce.
10. **B.** The six types of law in the American legal system include statutory, case, civil, criminal, substantive, and procedural law. Anecdotal law is not a type of law.
11. **C.** The five principal types of statutory law of general interest to pharmacy practice, in descending order of authority, are Constitution, treaty or international agreement, statute, regulation, and ordinance.
12. **A.** The Constitution is considered the highest level of law in the United States and is often referred to as the *law of the land.*
13. **B.** The term *stare decisis* falls under case law and relates to decisions made in previous cases that should be followed by subsequent similar cases.
14. **B.** The branch governmental system was established as a system of checks and balances, wherein each branch is given power that tends to balance (and serves as a check on) the power given to the other branches.
15. **D.** The legislative branch creates laws, which initiates the operation of the legal system. This authority allows the legislative branch to establish various administrative agencies and gives the agencies power and authority to govern a specific area.
16. **B.** The executive branch is charged with the administration and enforcement of the laws created by the legislative branch. Although the legislative branch creates administrative agencies, responsibility for an agency's operation and administration typically resides with the executive branch.
17. **D.** A negligence-based lawsuit requires the plaintiff to prove the following four elements: a duty was owed to the patient, an error caused the duty to be breached, the act was the proximate cause of the injury, and the patient suffered actual injury or harm.
18. **B.** Whether or not a duty is owed or whether it was breached is determined by identifying the recognized standard of care for the profession in the community, or similar community, in which the defendant practices.
19. **C.** Administrative law is the body of law governing the operation of administrative agencies, such as federal and state agencies that have significant influence on the daily practice of pharmacy.
20. **A.** An administrative agency would use a consent order to negotiate with the lawyer for the government to settle the charges and to avoid the time and expense of a hearing.

18-12 Additional Resources

Anonymous. The branches of government. In: *Criminal Law*. Minneapolis, MN: University of Minnesota Libraries Publishing; 2015. Available at: http://open.lib.umn.edu/criminallaw/chapter/2-2-the-branches-of-government. Accessed April 4, 2018.

Difference between civil and criminal cases. FindLaw-Thomson Reuters Web site. http://litigation.findlaw.com/legal-system/state-court-cases.html. Accessed April 4, 2018.

Federal vs. state courts—key differences. FindLaw-Thomson Reuters Web site. http://litigation.findlaw.com/legal-system/federal-vs-state-courts-key-differences.html. Accessed April 4, 2018.

Garner BA, ed. *Black's Law Dictionary*. 10th ed. St. Paul, MN: Thomson Reuters; 2014.

Prabhat S. Difference between civil and criminal cases. June 22, 2017. DifferenceBetween.net Web site. http://www.differencebetween.net/miscellaneous/difference-between-civil-and-criminal-cases/. Accessed April 4, 2018.

Roehrich R. Difference between federal and state government. November 21, 2016. DifferenceBetween.net Web site. http://www.differencebetween.net/miscellaneous/politics/difference-between-federal-and-state-government/. Accessed April 4, 2018.

Biostatistics

19

JUNLING WANG

19-1 KEY POINTS

- In statistics, a *population* includes all entities that one is interested in at a given time.
- A *sample* is a collection of entities that are part of a population.
- A frequency distribution typically includes four statistical measures: frequency, cumulative frequency, relative frequency, and cumulative relative frequency.
- The mean, the median, and the mode are the three most commonly used measures of central tendency.
- A test result can be evaluated using four measures of probability estimates: sensitivity, specificity, predictive value positive, and predictive value negative.
- For each parameter of interest, the investigator can compute two estimates: a point estimate and an interval estimate.
- The *null hypothesis* is the hypothesis to be tested. The null hypothesis is a statement presumed to be true in the study population. The *alternative hypothesis* complements the null hypothesis. It is a statement of what may be true if the process of hypothesis testing rejects the null hypothesis.
- The *p* value for hypothesis testing is the probability of seeing a test statistic that is as extreme as or more extreme than the value of the test statistic observed.
- Regression analysis focuses on the assessment of the nature of the relationships with an ultimate objective of predicting or estimating the value of one variable given the value of another variable. Correlation analysis is related to the strength of the relationships between two variables.
- One way to evaluate the regression equation is to calculate the coefficient of determination, which describes the relative magnitude of the scatter of data points about the regression line. The coefficient of determination ranges from 0 to 1.
- The sample estimate of the correlation coefficient is designated as *r*, and the population parameter for the correlation coefficient is designated as ρ. The value of the correlation coefficient ranges from −1 to 1.
- The chi-square test is the most frequently used test when an investigator is working with frequency or count data and when the variables are categorical.
- Nonparametric tests apply when the data are merely rankings or classifications.

19-2 STUDY GUIDE CHECKLIST

The following topics may guide your study of this subject area:

- ☐ Basic concepts: variable, types of variables, population, sample, and simple random sample
- ☐ Descriptive statistics: grouped data, measures of central tendency, and measures of dispersion
- ☐ Evaluation of screening tests: sensitivity, specificity, predictive value positive, and predictive value negative
- ☐ Concepts related to confidence interval: point estimate, interval estimate, reliability coefficient, precision, and margin of error
- ☐ Basic concepts related to hypothesis testing: research hypothesis, statistical hypothesis, null hypothesis, alternative hypothesis, test statistic, rejection region and nonrejection region, significance level, type I and type II errors, *p* value, and one-sided and two-sided tests
- ☐ Regression and correlation: independent and dependent variables, method of least squares, evaluation of the regression equation, correlation model
- ☐ Chi-square tests: observed and expected frequencies
- ☐ Nonparametric tests: advantages, disadvantages, and sign test
- ☐ Limitations of statistical analysis

Editor's Note: Much of the material in the chapter is a summary of work done by Wayne W. Daniel (Daniel WW. *A Foundation for Analysis in the Health Sciences.* 8th ed. Hoboken, NJ: Wiley; 2005).

19-3 Some Basic Concepts

One important part of research is to draw conclusions on the basis of limited amounts of data. Statistical analysis can facilitate the achievement of this goal. The following basic concepts are important to understanding statistics:

- ***Data:*** The raw material that researchers use for statistical analysis is data. In statistics, data can be defined as numbers. These numbers can be the result of measuring (e.g., height, weight, blood pressure) or counting (e.g., the number of patients discharged from a hospital on a given day). Each of these numbers is a *datum,* and all numbers taken together are *data.*
- ***Biostatistics:*** *Statistics* can be defined as a field of study that focuses on (1) the collection and analysis of data and (2) the drawing of inferences about a collection of data when only a part of the data is available for analysis. Statistical analysis can help researchers distinguish random variation from real differences when drawing conclusions. In the case of medical and biological data, statistics are most commonly referred to as *biostatistics.*
- ***Sources of data:*** Data for statistical analysis may be obtained from one or more of the following sources:
  - ***Routinely kept records:*** Organizations typically keep records of day-to-day activities. For example, hospital discharge data provide a wealth of data on the organization's patient care activities.
  - ***Surveys:*** If the data required to answer a research question are not available from routinely kept records, one may need to carry out a survey. For example, one may conduct a survey on patients' transportation costs.
  - ***Experiments:*** Often, the data required to answer a research question are available only as a result of conducting an experiment. For instance, a pharmacist may wish to determine whether pharmacy-based medication therapy management services can improve patient compliance with diabetes medications.
  - ***External sources:*** The data required to answer a research question may exist as published reports, research literature, data banks that are commercially available, or databases that are in the public domain.
- ***Variable:*** A *variable* is a characteristic that takes on different values for different possessors. Some examples of variables include ages of patients vaccinated in a community pharmacy and the heights of patients in a clinic. Different types of variables exist:
  - ***Quantitative variable:*** A *quantitative variable* is a variable whose amount can be measured (e.g., height, blood pressure, age).
  - ***Qualitative variable:*** A *qualitative variable* is a variable whose attributes can be measured. An example of a qualitative variable is sex, which can be female or male. A pharmacist may be interested in counting the number of female and male patrons who visit the pharmacy. These counts are also called *frequencies.*
  - ***Random variable:*** Whenever one measures the height, weight, or blood pressure of an individual, the result is typically called the *value of a variable.* When the values are determined by random factors and cannot be exactly predicted in advance, the variable is called a *random variable.* One example of a random variable is adult height, which cannot be exactly predicted at birth.
  - ***Discrete random variable:*** A *discrete random variable* is characterized by interruptions or gaps in its values. In other words, values are absent between particular values. One example of a discrete random variable is the number of admissions to a hospital in a given time period. The value of this variable cannot be, for example, 3.5 or 1.07 but rather must be a whole number such as 4 or 1.
  - ***Continuous random variable:*** A *continuous random variable* does not have interruptions or gaps in its values, or it can assume any value within an interval between any two of its values. Two individuals' weights may be very close together, but theoretically one can always find another person with a weight falling somewhere in between. In some situations, continuous variables may be recorded as discrete because of the limitations of available measuring instruments. Height, for instance, although a continuous variable, can be measured to the whole inch.

- ***Population:*** In statistics, a *population* includes every member of all entities that one is interested in at a particular time. A population of values includes every member of all the possible values of a random variable that one is interested in at a particular time. A population may be infinite or finite. If a population of values has an endless number of values, the population is infinite. In contrast, if a population of values has a fixed number of values, the population is finite.
- ***Sample:*** A *sample* is a collection of entities that are part of a population. Suppose one's population consists of all patients who filled prescriptions through a chain pharmacy in a given month. If one measures the weights of only a portion of those patients, that portion of patients becomes the sample.
- ***Simple random sample:*** A *simple random sample* is a sample selected from a population such that every possible sample of the same size has the same chance of being drawn. The process of drawing a simple random sample is called *simple random sampling.*

19-4 Descriptive Statistics

In terms of steps for data analysis, a deliberate approach is recommended, which involves first descriptive and then analytic analyses. The main descriptive statistical analysis techniques are described as follows.

Grouped Data

One can group values or observations into class intervals—a set of contiguous, nonoverlapping intervals—so that each observation in the data set belongs to one and only one interval. A commonly used rule of thumb is that one should have between 6 and 15 class intervals.

When grouping data, an investigator counts the number of observations falling into a certain class interval. The investigator can then produce a frequency distribution that typically includes four statistical measures: frequency, cumulative frequency, relative frequency, and cumulative relative frequency. *Frequency* is the number of observations falling in a particular class interval. *Cumulative frequency* is the sum of all observations within a certain interval and within all preceding intervals. *Relative frequency* is the proportion of observations within a certain class interval. *Cumulative relative frequency* is the sum of the proportion of observations within a certain class interval and within all preceding intervals. Table 19-1 shows an example of a frequency distribution.

Measures of Central Tendency

The mean, the median, and the mode are the three most commonly used measures of central tendency. The *mean* is calculated by summing all values for a variable and dividing the total by the number of values for

TABLE 19-1. A Frequency Distribution of the Ages of 100 Individuals

Class intervals (years)	Frequency	Cumulative frequency	Relative frequency	Cumulative relative frequency
10–19	10	10	0.1429	0.1429
20–29	15	25	0.2143	0.3571
30–39	15	40	0.2143	0.5714
40–49	10	50	0.1429	0.7143
50–59	15	65	0.2143	0.9286
60–69	5	70	0.0714	1.0000
Total	70		1.0000	

the variable. The *median* is the value in a data set for which the number of values less than or equal to the median is equal to the number of values greater than or equal to the median. When an odd number of values exists, the median is the middle value when all data are ordered. When an even number of values exists, the median is the average of the two middle values in the ordered array. The *mode* is the most frequent observation in a set of observations. If all observations are different within the data set, there is no mode. A set of values can have more than one mode.

Measures of Dispersion

Measures of dispersion reflect variability in a set of values.

The range

One way to measure dispersion is to use the *range,* which is the difference between the largest value and the smallest value in the data.

Variance

The *variance* measures the scatter of the observations about their mean. When computing the variance of a sample, one subtracts the mean from each observation in the set, squares the differences obtained, sums all squared differences, and divides the total by the number of values in the set minus 1.

Standard deviation

The unit for variance is squared. If the investigator wishes to use the same concept as the variance but express it in the original unit, a measure called *standard deviation* can be used. Standard deviation equals the square root of the variance.

The coefficient of variation

The standard deviation is useful as a measure of dispersion, but its use in some situations may be misleading. For example, one may be interested in comparing the dispersion of two variables measured in different units, such as serum cholesterol level and body weight. The former may be measured in milligrams per 100 milliliters, and the latter may be measured in pounds. Comparing them directly may produce erroneous findings.

The coefficient of variation can be expressed as the standard deviation as a percentage of the mean, which is given by

$$\text{coefficient of variation} = \frac{s}{\bar{x}}(100)$$

where s is the standard deviation and $\bar{x}$ is the mean of the variable. Because the mean and standard deviation have the same units of measurement, the units cancel out when computing the coefficient of variation. Thus, the coefficient of variation is independent of the unit of measurement.

19-5 Evaluation of Screening Tests

In the health sciences, investigators often need to evaluate diagnostic criteria and screening tests. Clinicians frequently need to predict the absence or presence of a disease depending on whether test results are positive or negative or whether certain symptoms are present or absent. A conclusion based on the test results and symptoms is not always correct. There can be false positives and false negatives. When an

TABLE 19-2. Elaboration of Individuals Cross-Classified on the Basis of Disease Status and Test Results

	Test results	
Disease status	**Positive**	**Negative**
Disease	a	b
No disease	c	d

Adapted from Daniel, 2005.

individual's true status is negative, but the test result shows positive, the test result is false positive. When an individual's true status is positive, but the test result shows negative, the test result is false negative. A test result can be evaluated using four measures of probability estimates: sensitivity, specificity, predictive value positive, and predictive value negative:

- ***Sensitivity:*** The sensitivity of a test is the probability of the test result being positive when an individual has the disease. Using notations in Table 19-2, one can show that this probability equals $\frac{a}{a+b}$.
- ***Specificity:*** The specificity of a test is the probability of the test result being negative when an individual does not have the disease. Using the notations in Table 19-2, one can show that this probability equals $\frac{d}{c+d}$.
- ***Predictive value positive:*** The predictive value positive of a test is the probability of an individual having the disease when the test result is positive. Using the notations in Table 19-2, one can show that this probability equals $\frac{a}{a+c}$.
- ***Predictive value negative:*** The predictive value negative of a test is the probability of an individual not having the disease when the test result is negative. Using the notations in Table 19-2, one can show that this probability equals $\frac{d}{b+d}$.

19-6 Estimation

In the field of health sciences, although many populations are finite, including every observation from the population, the sample is still prohibitive. Therefore, an investigator needs to estimate population parameters, such as the population mean and the population proportion, on the basis of data in the sample. For each parameter of interest, the investigator can compute two estimates: a point estimate and an interval estimate. A *point estimate* is a single value estimated to represent the corresponding population parameter. For example, the sample mean is a point estimate of the population mean. An *interval estimate* is a range of values defined by two numerical values. With a certain degree of confidence, the investigator thinks that the range of values includes the parameter of interest. The composition of a confidence interval can be described as

$$\text{estimator} \pm (\text{reliability coefficient}) \times (\text{standard error})$$

The center of the confidence interval is the point estimate of the parameter of interest. The reliability coefficient is a value typically obtained from the standard normal distribution or t distribution. If the investigator needs to estimate a 95% confidence interval, for instance, the reliability coefficient indicates within how many standard errors lie 95% of the possible values of the population parameter. The value obtained by multiplying the reliability coefficient and the standard error is referred to as the *precision* of the estimate. It is also called the *margin of error*.

Confidence intervals can be calculated for the population mean, population proportion, difference in population means, difference in population proportions, and other measures. The first two are discussed here.

Confidence Interval for Population Mean

When estimating the confidence interval for a population mean, after calculating the sample mean, the investigator needs to determine the reliability coefficient. When the sample size is large (a rule of thumb is greater than 30), reliability coefficients can be obtained from the standard normal distribution. When an investigator needs to estimate 90%, 95%, and 99% confidence intervals, the corresponding reliability coefficients are 1.645, 1.96, and 2.58, respectively.

For example, in a study of patients' punctuality for their appointments, a sample of 35 patients was found to be on average 17.2 minutes late for appointments with a standard deviation of 8 minutes. The 90% confidence interval for the population mean is calculated as [15, 19.4]. This confidence interval can be interpreted using the following practical interpretation: the investigators are 90% confident that the interval [15, 19.4] contains the population mean.

Confidence Interval for Population Proportion

To estimate the population proportion, an investigator first needs to draw a sample of size n from the population and compute the sample proportion, $\hat{p}$. Then the confidence interval for the population proportion can be estimated using the same composition as given for a confidence interval. When both np and $n(1 - p)$ are greater than 5 (p is population proportion), the reliability coefficients can be estimated from the standard normal distribution.

19-7 Hypothesis Testing

Both hypothesis testing and estimation examine a sample from a population with the purpose of aiding the researchers or decision makers in drawing conclusions about the population.

Basic Concepts

Null hypothesis and alternative hypothesis

When conducting research, an investigator typically has two types of hypotheses: a research hypothesis and a statistical hypothesis. A *research hypothesis* is the investigator's theories or suspicions that need to be subjected to the rigors of scientific testing. A *statistical hypothesis* is a hypothesis stated in a way that can be tested using statistical techniques. In the process of hypothesis testing, two statistical hypotheses are used: the null hypothesis and the alternative hypothesis. The *null hypothesis* is the hypothesis to be tested and is typically designated as H_0. The null hypothesis is a statement presumed to be true in the study population. As the result of hypothesis testing, the null hypothesis is either not rejected or rejected. Typically, an indication of equality (=, ≥, or ≤) is included in the null hypothesis. The *alternative hypothesis* complements the null hypothesis. It is a statement of what may be true if the process of hypothesis testing rejects the null hypothesis. The alternative hypothesis is typically designated as H_A. Usually, the alternative hypothesis is the same as the research hypothesis.

A word of caution regarding the null hypothesis is warranted here. When hypothesis testing does not reject the null hypothesis, it does not mean proof of the null hypothesis. Hypothesis testing indicates only whether the available data support or do not support the null hypothesis.

Test statistic

The *test statistic* is a numerical value calculated from the data in the sample. The test statistic can assume many different values, and the particular sample determines the specific value that the test statistic assumes. The test statistic can be considered as the decision rule. The value of the test statistic determines whether to reject the null hypothesis.

Values that the test statistic can assume are divided into two groups that fall into two regions for hypothesis testing: the rejection region and the nonrejection region. The values in the nonrejection region are more likely to occur than the values in the rejection region if the null hypothesis is true. Therefore, the decision rule of hypothesis testing is that if the value of the test statistic is within the rejection region, then the investigator should reject the null hypothesis and vice versa.

Significance level

The critical values that separate the rejection region from the nonrejection region are determined by the level of significance, which is typically designated by α. Thus, hypothesis testing is frequently called *significance testing*. If the test statistic falls into the rejection region, then the test is said to be significant.

Type I and type II errors

Because significance level determines the critical values for separating the rejection and nonrejection regions of a test, an investigator obviously has a probability of committing errors when conducting hypothesis testing. There are two types of errors for hypothesis testing (Table 19-3). When the null hypothesis is true, but the statistical decision is to reject the null hypothesis, the investigator has committed a type I error. If the null hypothesis is not true, and the statistical decision is not to reject the null hypothesis, then the investigator has committed a type II error. The probability of a type I error is the level of the significance for the test, which is α. The probability of a type II error is typically designated as β. Another concept often used in statistics is *power*, which is the probability of rejecting a false null hypothesis.

In hypothesis testing, the level of significance, or α, is typically made small so that there is a small probability of rejecting a true null hypothesis. Typical levels of significance for statistical tests are 0.01, 0.05, and 0.1. However, the investigator exercises less control over the probability of a type II error. Keep in mind that the investigator never knows the true status of the null hypothesis. Therefore, to have a lower probability of committing any errors, investigators take more comfort when a null hypothesis is rejected.

TABLE 19-3. Type I and Type II Errors

	Statistical decision	
Status of null hypothesis	**Not to reject H_0**	**Reject H_0**
True	Correct decision	Type I error
False	Type II error	Correct decision

Adapted from Daniel, 2005.

The *p* value

The *p* value for hypothesis testing is the probability of seeing a test statistic that is as extreme as or more extreme than the value of the test statistic observed. Reporting the *p* value as part of the results is more informative than reporting only the statistical decision of rejecting or not rejecting the null hypothesis.

One-sided and two-sided tests

When the rejection region includes two tails of the distribution of the test statistic in testing a hypothesis, it is a two-sided test. If the rejection region includes only one tail of the distribution, then it is a one-sided test. In other words, if both sufficiently large and sufficiently small values of a test statistic lead to rejection of the null hypothesis, then the investigator needs a two-sided test. If only sufficiently large or small values of a test statistic can lead to rejection of the null hypothesis, then the investigator needs a one-sided test.

Hypothesis Testing for a Population Mean

When testing a hypothesis for a population mean, an investigator uses a *Z* statistic or a *t* statistic, depending on whether the sample size is large (this may remind readers of the determination of the reliability coefficient for the confidence interval). When the sample size is small, the investigator should use the *t* statistic.

Hypothesis Testing for a Population Proportion

When one tests a hypothesis for a population proportion and when the sample size is large, the investigator should use a Z statistic.

19-8 Simple Linear Regression and Correlation Analyses

Regression and correlation analyses are used when analyzing the relationship between two numerical variables. Regression and correlation are closely related, but they serve different purposes. Regression analysis focuses on the assessment of the nature of the relationships with an ultimate objective of predicting or estimating the value of one variable given the value of another variable. Correlation analysis is related to the strength of the relationships between two variables.

The Regression Model

Independent variable and dependent variable

In a simple linear regression, two variables are of interest: the independent variable *X* and the dependent variable *Y*. Variable *X* is usually controlled by the investigator, and its values may be preselected by the investigator. Corresponding to each value of *X* are one or more values of *Y*. When the investigator conducts simple linear regression analysis, the objective is to estimate the linear relationship between the independent and dependent variables. The investigator needs to first draw a sample from the population and then plot a scatter diagram of the relationship between the two variables by assigning the values of the independent variable to the horizontal axis and the values of the dependent variable to the vertical axis. An example of such a diagram is the relationship between age and the forced expiratory volume (liters) among a group of children between 10 and 16 years of age (Figure 19-1). It is clear from this diagram that the older the children are, the greater the forced expiratory volume. In other words, a linear relationship may exist between the two variables.

FIGURE 19-1. A Scatter Diagram for the Relationship between Age and the Forced Expiratory Volume

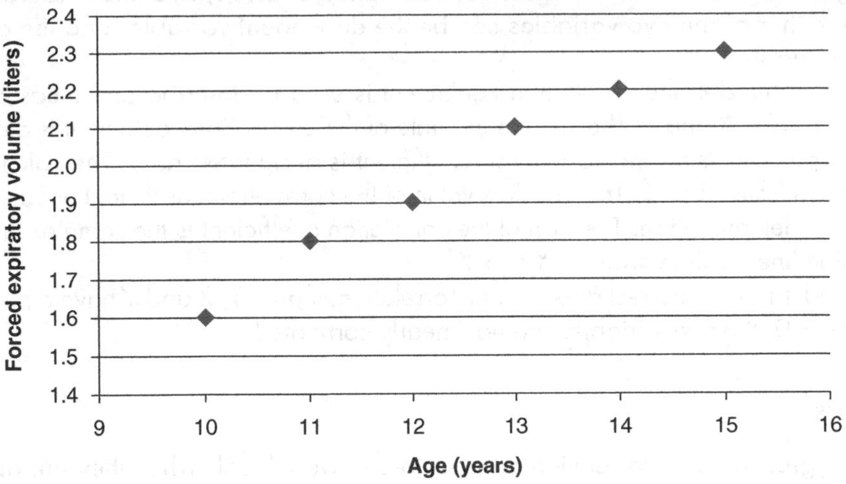

Estimation of the linear line

The method usually followed to obtain the linear line is known as the *method of least squares,* and the line obtained is the *least squares line.*

The general format of the least squares line is $\hat{y} = a + bx$, where a is the sample estimate of the intercept of the line, and b is the sample estimate of the slope of the line. The population parameters for the intercept and the slope of the line are designated α and β, respectively. The estimated least squares line for the linear relationship depicted in Figure 19-1 is given by

$$\hat{y} = 0.23 + 0.14x$$

where a, the intercept of the line, has a positive sign, suggesting that the line crosses the vertical axis above the origin, and b, the slope of the line, has a value of 0.14, suggesting that when x increases by 1 unit, y increases by 0.14 unit.

Evaluation of the regression equation

After the regression equation is estimated, the investigator must evaluate whether the estimate of the slope of the line adequately describes the relationship between the independent and dependent variables. One way to evaluate the regression equation is to calculate the coefficient of determination, which describes the relative magnitude of the scatter of data points about the regression line. The coefficient of determination ranges from 0 to 1. The closer the coefficient of determination is to 1, the closer the observations lie to the regression line. The coefficient of determination for the preceding example is 0.98.

Use of the regression equation

With an estimated linear line, the investigator can then predict the value of the dependent variable when given a value for the independent variable. For example, if $X = 11$,

$$\hat{y} = 0.23 + 0.14(11) = 1.77$$

The Correlation Model

Different from the regression model, which often preselects the values of the independent variable, the correlation model selects a sample of the observation units and then measures the values of the two variables X and Y for each unit of observation. In other words, the two variables X and Y have equal footing. Therefore, in the framework of correlation analysis, two linear regression models may be estimated: either of the two variables can be the dependent variable, and the other becomes the independent variable.

In a correlation model, the correlation coefficient is used to describe and measure the relationship between the variables X and Y. The sample estimate of the correlation coefficient is designated as r, and the population parameter for the correlation coefficient is designated as ρ. The value of the correlation coefficient ranges from -1 to 1. The absolute value of the correlation coefficient equals the square root of the coefficient of determination. The sign of the correlation coefficient is the same as the sign of the slope of the regression line for the variables X and Y.

If $\rho = 1$, X and Y have a perfect direct linear correlation. If $\rho = -1$, X and Y have a perfect inverse linear correlation. If $\rho = 0$, the two variables are not linearly correlated.

Some Precautions

Simple linear regression and correlation analyses are powerful tools when they are appropriately used. However, the investigator may get useless and meaningless information when these analyses are not used properly. The following few precautions should be kept in mind. First, in simple linear regression and correlation analyses, the variables X and Y are measured on the same unit of association. Therefore, discussing the association between the weights of some individuals and the heights of some other individuals would be meaningless.

Second, even when the analysis identifies a strong linear relationship between the two variables, that relationship should not be mistaken as evidence of cause and effect. In that situation, the relationship may be causal, but a third factor may also possibly directly or indirectly affect both the independent and the dependent variables.

Third, an investigator should guard against extrapolation. In other words, the regression equation may not be used to predict the values of the dependent variable outside the range of the values of the independent variable. The reason for this precaution is that the relationship between the variables may not be the same (e.g., nonlinear) outside the range of the values of the independent variable.

19-9 Chi-Square Tests

The chi-square test is the most commonly used test when an investigator is working with frequency or count data and when the variables are categorical. A pharmacy investigator may have a number of pharmacy patrons using different types of insurance at the pharmacy: private insurance, Medicaid, Medicare, and others. These are count data. The investigator may be interested in comparing the insurance status between his or her pharmacy and another pharmacy. Another researcher might be concerned with the rates of compliance with diabetes medications between females and males. The chi-square test is suitable for these scenarios because the variables are categorical.

Two sets of frequencies matter for a chi-square test: observed frequencies and expected frequencies. The *observed frequencies* are the number of observed individuals or other entities that fall into the various categories of the variable of interest (e.g., health insurance status). For example, among 100 pharmacy patrons, 30 might be privately insured, 40 might have Medicare, 20 might have Medicaid, and 10 might not have any insurance. The *expected frequencies* are the number of individuals who fall into the various categories of the variable of interest if the null hypothesis is true. For this example, if the null hypothesis is that individuals are equally likely to be in any one of the four insurance categories, 25 individuals are expected to have each of the four types of insurance.

The quantity of X^2 measures the degrees of agreement between the observed frequencies and the expected frequencies: the poorer the agreement, the greater the quantity of X^2. Therefore, a large enough X^2 value would lead to rejection of the null hypothesis. When the null hypothesis is true, X^2 follows a chi-square distribution, which determines the critical values that separate the rejection region from the nonrejection region.

A word of caution about the chi-square test is needed. When the expected frequencies are too small, a chi-square test would not be appropriate. For example, some writers have suggested that all expected values should be greater than 5 or 10. Otherwise, an alternative test, such as Fisher's exact test, should be used.

19-10 Nonparametric Tests

Most of the statistical tests that have been described so far are parametric statistics, with the exception of the chi-square test. For parametric tests, the investigators are interested in estimating or testing hypotheses about population parameters, such as the population mean or the population proportion. Additionally, not emphasized earlier, the investigator must know the form of the population distribution from which the sample is drawn.

Nonparametric tests have at least the following two advantages compared to parametric tests. First, nonparametric tests apply when the data are merely rankings or classifications. Rankings and classifications may not represent a measurement level strong enough for parametric tests. Second, nonparametric tests tend to be more easily and quickly applied than are parametric tests.

Nonparametric tests also have disadvantages. When the data can be analyzed with parametric tests, using nonparametric tests is a waste of data. Additionally, when the sample size is large, conducting a nonparametric test can be too time consuming.

One type of nonparametric test is the sign test, which focuses on the median of the distribution. The only requirement for using the sign test is that the variable be continuous. The raw data used in the calculation of the test statistic for the sign test are plus and minus signs.

For example, the appearance scores among a group of girls with mental retardation are 4, 5, 8, 8, 9, 6, 10, 7, 6, and 6. Researchers are interested in determining whether the median appearance score among them is 5.

Using a sign test, researchers count the number of values greater than 5 as the number of pluses and the number of values less than 5 as the number of minuses. Values equal to 5 are dropped from further analysis as is typically done for the sign test. Therefore, this example has eight pluses and one minus. If the median for the distribution is indeed 5, one would expect to see an equal number of plus and minus signs. The probability of seeing as many pluses and minuses as in this example can be calculated on the basis of a binomial distribution. The probability turns out to be 0.039 for this test. At the level of significance of 0.05, the statistical decision is to reject the null hypothesis that the median of the distribution is 5.

19-11 Limitations of Statistical Analysis

Statistical analysis can be crucial to helping decision makers and researchers in decision-making processes. However, statistical significance should not be considered definitive, and statistical conclusions should be taken as only one piece of information needed for decision making. Other relevant information, such as safety, cost, and accessibility of a program, should also be considered. Additionally, keeping in mind the difference between statistical significance and clinical significance is important. Although statistical significance is tested objectively using hypothesis testing, clinical significance is assessed subjectively by a patient, a caregiver, or a medical professional. As an example, certain points of blood pressure reduction resulting from an intervention program might be statistically significant according to hypothesis testing. However, if patients, doctors, and caregivers do not perceive patients as having benefited, concluding that the amount of blood pressure reduction is clinically significant would be difficult.

19-12 Questions

1. Which of the following statements about statistics is true?

A. Data used in statistical analysis have to include all entities in a population.
B. If an investigator has a research question, she or he has to collect original data.
C. Statistical analysis draws conclusions on the basis of data from the whole population.
D. Statistics can help distinguish random variation from real differences when drawing conclusions.

2. Which of the following statements is *not* true for variables?

A. A continuous random variable has interruptions or gaps in its values.
B. Height is a quantitative variable.
C. Blood pressure can be a random variable.
D. Weight is a continuous variable.

3. Which of the following is *not* true about frequency distribution?

A. An observation in a data set can belong to more than one interval.
B. Frequency as a statistical measure can be included in a frequency distribution.
C. Relative frequency as a statistical measure can be included in a frequency distribution.
D. Cumulative relative frequency as a statistical measure can be included in a frequency distribution.

4. Which of the following is *not* true about central tendency?

A. A set of values may not have mode.
B. When there is an odd number of values, the median is equal to the middle value when all data are ordered.
C. Mean and median are equal.
D. A set of values may have more than one mode.

5. Which of the following is *not* a measure of central tendency?

A. Median
B. Mean
C. Range
D. Mode

6. Which of the following measures of dispersion is independent of the measurement unit?

A. Range
B. Variance
C. Standard deviation
D. Coefficient of variation

Use the data from this table for Questions 7–10.

The following table shows 100 individuals cross-classified according to disease status and test results.

	Disease		
Test results	**Present**	**Absent**	**Total**
Positive	30	40	70
Negative	20	10	30
Total	50	50	100

7. What is the sensitivity for the test?

A. 30/50
B. 10/50
C. 30/70
D. 10/30

8. What is the specificity for the test?

A. 30/50
B. 10/50
C. 30/70
D. 10/30

9. What is the predictive value positive for the test?

A. 30/50
B. 10/50
C. 30/70
D. 10/30

10. What is the predictive value negative for the test?

A. 10/30
B. 10/50
C. 30/50
D. 30/70

11. Which of the following statements is true?

A. For a population parameter, an investigator cannot produce both a point estimate and an interval estimate.
B. The lower limit of a confidence interval is also called the precision of the test.
C. The reliability coefficient is always determined from a *t* distribution.
D. The reliability coefficient for the confidence interval can be determined on the basis of the standard normal distribution only when certain conditions are met.

12. Which of the following statements is *not* true about statistical hypotheses?

A. The null hypothesis is a statement presumed to be true in the study population.
B. The alternative hypothesis is typically the same as the research hypothesis.
C. A statistical test can prove or reject a null hypothesis.
D. A statistical test has to have a null hypothesis.

13. Which of the following statements is true?

A. If the test statistic falls into the nonrejection region, the test is said to be significant.
B. The rejection region can be on only one tail of the distribution.
C. Researchers typically prefer higher levels of significance.
D. A test statistic can assume different values when different samples are drawn from the population.

14. Which of the following statements is *not* true for type I and type II errors?

A. A statistical test always has either a type I or a type II error.
B. A type I error cannot occur at the same time as a type II error.
C. An investigator exercises less control over the probability of a type II error than a type I error.
D. A type I error occurs when a false null hypothesis is not rejected.

15. Which of the following statements is *not* true?

A. It is *not* appropriate to estimate a linear regression equation for any two variables.
B. A negative slope of a linear regression means the higher the independent variable, the lower the dependent variable.
C. A positive intercept suggests that the regression line crosses the vertical axis above the origin.
D. The investigator typically has control over the values of the dependent variable.

16. Which of the following statements is *not* true?

A. The coefficient of determination ranges from 0 to 1.
B. The correlation coefficient ranges from 0 to 1.
C. The sign of the correlation coefficient is the same as the sign of the slope of the regression equation.
D. The absolute value of the correlation coefficient equals the square root of the coefficient of determination.

17. Which of the following statements is true?

A. Regression analysis can determine whether two variables have a causal relationship.
B. Correlation analysis can determine whether two variables have a causal relationship.
C. If there is a linear relationship between two variables, the relationship outside the range of the values of the independent variable is not necessarily linear.
D. A linear regression model can be used to predict the value of the dependent variable for any values of the independent variable.

18. Which of the following statements is true?

- **A.** When two variables are correlated, only one regression model can be estimated from them.
- **B.** Investigators can preselect values for both variables for a simple linear correlation analysis.
- **C.** Investigators can preselect values of the dependent variable for a simple linear regression analysis.
- **D.** Investigators have some control over the independent variable for a simple linear regression analysis.

19. Which of the following statements is *not* true about the chi-square test?

- **A.** The chi-square test is a nonparametric test.
- **B.** The test statistic of a chi-square test follows a chi-square distribution when the null hypothesis is true.
- **C.** The chi-square test always applies when the data are counts or frequencies.
- **D.** The rejection and nonrejection regions of the chi-square test are determined on the basis of the chi-square distribution.

20. Which of the following statements is true?

- **A.** Parametric tests are always preferred over nonparametric tests.
- **B.** When a sample size is large, a nonparametric test has the advantage of being more easily and quickly applied than a parametric test.
- **C.** The investigator needs to know the form of the population distribution to use a nonparametric test.
- **D.** The sign test takes into consideration only the positive and negative signs of the data.

19-13 Answers

1. D. Statistical analysis can help researchers distinguish random variation from real differences when drawing conclusions.

2. A. A continuous random variable does not have interruptions or gaps in its values, or it can assume any value within an interval between any two of its values.

3. A. In a frequency distribution, each value belongs to one and only one interval. A frequency distribution typically includes four statistical measures: frequency, cumulative frequency, relative frequency, and cumulative relative frequency.

4. C. Mean and median are two different measures of central tendency, and they are not always equal.

5. C. Range is a measure of dispersion.

6. D. The coefficient of variation can be expressed as a percentage of the mean. Because the mean and standard deviation have the same units of measurement, the units cancel out when the coefficient of variation is computed.

7. A. The sensitivity of a test is the probability of the test result being positive when an individual has the disease.

8. B. The specificity of a test is the probability of the test result being negative when an individual does not have the disease.

9. C. The predictive value positive of a test is the probability of an individual having the disease when the test result is positive.

10. A. The predictive value negative of a test is the probability of an individual not having the disease when the test result is negative.

11. D. When the sample size is large (a rule of thumb is greater than 30), reliability coefficients can be obtained from the standard normal distribution.

12. C. When hypothesis testing does not reject the null hypothesis, it does not mean proof of the null hypothesis. Hypothesis testing indicates only whether the available data support or do not support the null hypothesis.

13. D. The test statistic is a numerical value calculated from the data in the sample. The test statistic can assume many different values, and the particular sample determines the specific value that the test statistic assumes.

14. D. When the null hypothesis is true, but the statistical decision is to reject the null hypothesis, the investigator has committed a type I error.

15. D. The independent variable is usually controlled by the investigator, and the investigator may preselect its values.

16. **B.** The value of the correlation coefficient ranges from −1 to 1.

17. **C.** The relationship between the variables may not be the same (e.g., nonlinear) outside the range of the values of the independent variable.

18. **D.** The independent variable is usually controlled by the investigator, and the investigator may preselect its values.

19. **C.** When the expected frequencies are too small, a chi-square test would not be appropriate.

20. **D.** The sign test takes into consideration only the positive and negative signs of the data. The raw data used in the calculation of the test statistic for the sign test are plus and minus signs.

19-14 Additional Resource

Daniel WW. *A Foundation for Analysis in the Health Sciences.* 8th ed. Hoboken, NJ: Wiley; 2005.

Clinical Trial Design

20

BRADLEY A. BOUCHER

20-1 KEY POINTS

- Observational research may be prospective or retrospective.
- Experimental research is usually prospective.
- Experimental designs should seek to minimize bias, confounding variables, and random error.
- Cohort studies may be prospective, cross-sectional, or retrospective.
- Retrospective studies are ideally able to identify an association between variables.
- Well-designed randomized controlled trials (RCTs) can establish a cause-and-effect relationship between variables.
- Evidence-based medicine requires the critical appraisal of medical literature and the adoption of scientifically rigorous, relevant information into clinical practice.

20-2 STUDY GUIDE CHECKLIST

The following topics may guide your study of this subject area:

- ☐ Differences between observational and experimental studies
- ☐ Similarities and differences between major experimental trial design types
- ☐ Differences between parallel and crossover randomized controlled trials
- ☐ Key aspects of RCTs to consider in reviewing published studies
- ☐ Three major blinding categories used in randomized controlled trials
- ☐ Difference between *per protocol* and *intention-to-treat* data analysis techniques
- ☐ Four major steps for critically appraising medical literature
- ☐ Practical methods to assist practitioners in staying current with medical literature
- ☐ Definition of evidence-based medicine
- ☐ Major steps in practicing evidence-based pharmacy

20-3 Introduction

Clinical research refers to studies conducted in humans seeking to answer a question regarding health care. It includes studies evaluating medical disease prevention, diagnosis, and treatment. Data derived from well-planned and well-executed clinical research studies are extremely important in advancing patient care. Although the basic principles of clinical research design techniques and processes are not particularly difficult to comprehend, actually conducting studies is a complex enough process that entire textbooks are devoted to trial design as well as to data processing and interpretation. Many health care practitioners lack the time and expertise to design and execute studies themselves without additional training, and practitioners may even be inadequately prepared to interpret published clinical data. Regardless, understanding the basics of clinical research design is essential for all practitioners to practice evidence-based medicine. Critical appraisal of medical literature and judicious use of new knowledge will aid clinicians in providing the best possible care to the patients they serve.

This chapter introduces the reader to the basic concepts of clinical research; clinical trial design, including the major types of clinical trials; and many of the key aspects of randomized controlled trials. The chapter also addresses the basic principles for evaluating the primary literature and the techniques for reviewing such data and implementing useful findings in clinical practice.

20-4 Fundamentals of Research Design and Methodology

There are two basic types of clinical research: observational research and experimental research. A brief description of each type follows:

- ***Observational research:*** In this type of research, the investigator observes what is occurring without intervening. Typically, descriptive statistics are used to summarize the study results. This method includes measures of central tendency (e.g., arithmetic mean, median, mode) and measures of variability (e.g., range, standard deviation, variance). Observational research may be retrospective or prospective. Retrospective studies involve looking back from the present, whereas prospective studies begin at the present time and observe study variables of interest from the present forward. One specific type of observational research that is very important within medicine is the case report. A case report retrospectively describes a specific clinical case or a limited number of cases. Case reports cannot establish a causal relationship but may often be the first evidence of a previously unknown or unrecognized relationship. Other observational clinical study designs are as follows:
  - ***Case series:*** This type of study is similar to a case report although it reports on a group of patients with similar clinical presentations or exposure to a particular treatment or condition compared with a single case or limited number of cases. A case series may be either retrospective or prospective. The lack of a control group and randomization limits the determination of a causal relationship and rigorous statistical analysis, respectively.
  - ***Cohort study:*** A cohort study selects participants on the basis of one or more specific characteristics and compares them over time to either a different set of patients or the rest of the general population that serves as the control group. In either case, the study group of interest is exposed to the test treatment or condition at the beginning of the evaluation period, whereas the other group is not exposed. Cohort studies are essentially the same as randomized controlled trials (discussed below) except for the absence of randomization. A cohort study can be conducted prospectively, in which case participants are selected on the basis of the study characteristics of interest and then observed following exposure until the conclusion of the study. Cohort studies can also identify

participants retrospectively, in which case participant records are used to identify and prospectively evaluate individuals with the selected characteristics thereafter. Yet another design is to study prospectively one group of patients possessing the study characteristics and having been exposed to the test treatment and to compare that group to a historical participant group evaluated retrospectively. A well-designed cohort study can provide convincing evidence of an association between study variables. However, the inability to randomize patients to one group or another is a major source of bias inherent in conducting cohort studies because the participant groups may not be comparable. *Bias* denotes systematic error within clinical investigations. Bias is distinct from *confounding variables*. The latter term is used to describe variables that are not systematically introduced into the study but that may affect the outcome of interest in clinical studies. Generally speaking, confounding variables cannot be controlled in clinical studies completely (e.g., use of concurrent medications during the course of a study).

- ***Case-control study:*** Case-control studies are similar to cohort studies in that one group of participants has a disease and is compared to a control group that does not have the disease. However, a best attempt is made to find patients within the control group who match the participants with the disease or condition on the basis of a predefined set of characteristics such as age or sex. Another difference is that case-control studies are always retrospective.

- ***Experimental research:*** In this type of research, a specific intervention or exposure to a condition is evaluated in a study group and typically compared with a control group. Experimental research is usually prospective in nature but it may use historical controls or controls from medical literature for the comparator group. Familiarity with the terminology of experimental clinical study designs is useful from several vantage points. One aspect is the ability to efficiently plan and conduct clinical research on the basis of accepted methodologies by motivated investigators. Perhaps more important for most clinicians is the ability to interpret medical literature as previously noted. Upon identification of the methodology used within a published study, the clinician should be able to readily conceptualize how a study was conducted.
  - ***Randomized controlled trial (RCT):*** In this type of trial, study participants are prospectively assigned randomly to one or more treatment or control groups upon meeting the inclusion criteria for the study. A well-designed and well-executed RCT provides evidence of a causal relationship between the intervention being investigated and the primary study outcome. The two most common design subtypes of RCTs are known as parallel and crossover.
    - ***Parallel RCT:*** In this study design, participants are randomized to one of the treatment or control arms of the study. Control groups may receive standard treatments, no treatment, usual care, or placebos. *Placebos* are inactive substances that are often used in clinical drug studies. Typically, study participants receive the assigned treatment or control for the entire trial in a parallel RCT (see Figure 20-1). Outcome responses for each treatment or control group are then compared at the conclusion of the study *between* patients assigned to each study group. Conditions being evaluated can be acute or chronic, which is one of the reasons that parallel RCTs are the most common prospective RCT design.
    - ***Crossover RCT:*** In this design, the study participants receive one or more of the treatments or controls for a predefined period during the course of the study. Participants are then switched or "crossed over" to one or more of the other treatment or control arms (see Figure 20-2). In this instance, outcome responses are compared *within* the same participants, resulting typically in less variability. Although crossover RCTs are efficient for evaluating causal effects of one treatment over another treatment within the same participant, a major limitation is that only stable, chronic, or episodic conditions can be studied. Examples of such conditions include glaucoma, epilepsy, and migraines. Even with chronic or episodic conditions, however, a return to the same baseline state is needed to use a crossover design. This return frequently requires a period of no treatment or usual treatment between study periods to avoid a carryover or residual effect as one treatment ends and the next one begins. This time period is referred to as a "washout" period.

FIGURE 20-1. Example of Parallel Design

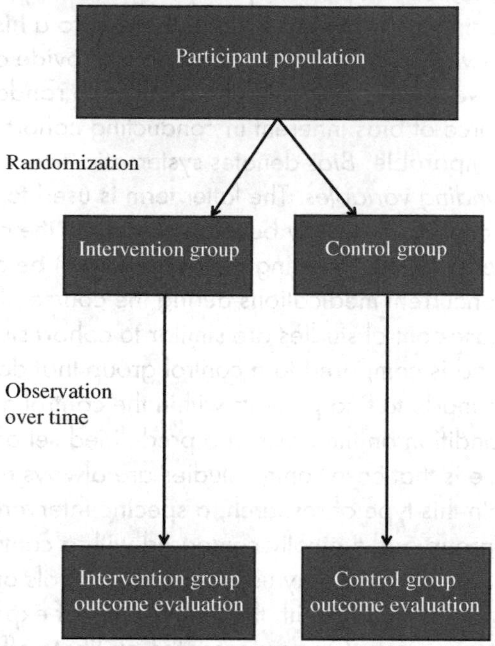

FIGURE 20-2. Example of Crossover Design

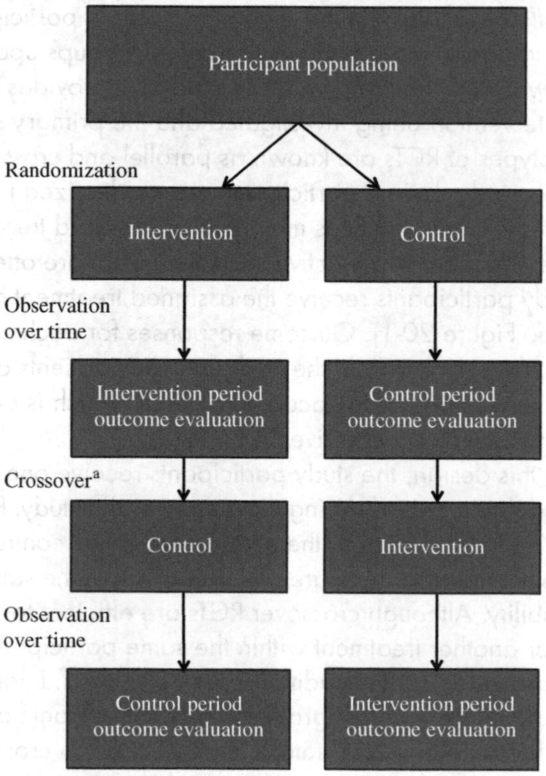

a. May include washout period.

Key Aspects of Randomized Controlled Trials

RCTs have a high weighting in the ranks of medical literature. See Figure 20-3 for a diagram illustrating general considerations regarding scientific rigor of particular study designs. Understanding the basics of RCT design will aid in interpreting the results and applying new literature to study practice. This section reviews key considerations of RCT design. Many of the principles covered here may also be applied to other types of trials.

Sampling and randomization

Sampling of a population is necessary in RCTs because enrolling every patient within a population with a particular disease state or condition in the study is not feasible. Key aspects of sampling are as follows:

- Study participants must be representative of the population to which the results of the study are to be applied.
- Patients enrolled in the study must meet all of the predetermined study inclusion criteria, and conversely, they must not have any of the characteristics listed as exclusion criteria.

Clinicians should consider the aforementioned inclusion and exclusion criteria when applying the study results to avoid extrapolating those results to patients who may not be representative of the population being evaluated. Alternatively, one can infer that similar findings will be observed in other patients who meet such criteria within the probabilities emanating from inferential statistics used to analyze the study data. One of the basic principles of inferential statistics is that patients sampled from a particular population of interest have an equal chance of being randomized or assigned to one of the study groups or another. As such, systematic error can occur when study participants are not properly randomized into the study groups, which can lead to potentially misleading and incorrectly interpreted study results because of bias in patients being assigned to one group or another. Randomization does not ensure that study participant characteristics (e.g., sex, weight, race) are equally divided between study groups. A process known as *stratification* can be used to accomplish the latter. Stratification is a grouping that occurs before randomization, although grouping of patient characteristics can be performed retrospectively. In this latter instance, the process is often referred to as *subgroup analysis*.

Blinding

In clinical trials, *blinding* refers to the process whereby some or all of the participants are unaware of the treatment being received by the study participants. Blinding is an important strategy for decreasing bias

FIGURE 20-3. Hierarchy of Literature Evidence

Trial design	Scientific validity
Systematic reviews and meta-analyses	
Randomized controlled trial	
Cohort study	
Case-control study	
Case series	
Case report	

within any clinical trial. The underlying purpose of blinding is that study volunteers or patients may knowingly or unknowingly alter the study outcome data if they know which treatment or treatments they are receiving. Similarly, study investigators may bias data collection on the basis of the perceived benefits of the treatment or the lack of benefits they are observing if they are aware of the treatment the volunteers or patients are receiving or not receiving, respectively. Nevertheless, certain clinical studies may not be suitable for blinding because of safety or ethical concerns (e.g., administration of investigational treatments through compassionate-use protocols, severely ill patients). Regardless of blinding type, the processes must be in place to break the blind if needed for safety reasons. When no blinding is used, studies are referred to as *open-label* trials. Generally accepted blinding definitions are as follows:

- ***Single blind:*** Patients are unaware of which treatment they are receiving.
- ***Double blind:*** Neither the study patients nor the investigators are aware of the treatments. This method is the traditional gold standard within clinical research focused on treatment efficacy because this design has the greatest potential for minimizing bias from the study participants and investigators.

Maintaining study blinding can be challenging or virtually impossible irrespective of careful study planning and design. Such challenges can be overcome to some extent by using a group of blinded investigators—who are independent of the unblinded investigators or personnel directly interacting with the study participants—to gather the safety and efficacy data. Regardless of the blinding strategies used, investigators should provide details, to the greatest extent possible, on their maintenance of blinding for any trials published in medical literature.

Sample size

Selection of sample size is an extremely important issue in designing randomized controlled trials. Inadequate numbers of study participants will decrease the statistical power of any clinical trial. In this instance, patient numbers may be insufficient to report a statistically significant difference between the study treatments although in actuality a difference does exist. Thus, *statistical power* is the probability of avoiding a false-negative study result. Conversely, the recruitment of an excessive number of study participants may be very inefficient despite being more than adequately powered statistically. Specifically, recruiting an excessive number of patients may take much longer than is necessary, and it may substantially increase the study budget, thereby making the study unfeasible to conduct. Generally, the greater the expected difference between the study treatments, the fewer the number of study participants who will be needed to demonstrate a statistically significant difference between the groups. Furthermore, fewer study participants will be needed when less variability exists in the study outcomes being measured from one participant to another. Statistical power can be calculated by investigators and biostatisticians on the basis of estimates of the expected differences and variability between the study groups and should be included in any published report of the study results.

Controls

In the context of RCTs, controls are the comparator to the treatment of interest. In a crossover study design, patients serve as their own control. As previously noted, control groups may receive standard treatments, no treatment, usual care, or placebos in both RCT crossover and parallel designs. Ideally, the placebo should have dosage form properties (e.g., color, shape, taste) that are identical to the active treatment dosage forms to avoid compromising study blinding. The potential for a "placebo effect" should always be considered. This occurs when the placebo has an effect on the study outcome despite receipt of an inactive substance. Use of placebos may not be suitable for all RCTs because of ethical considerations. In those instances, an active or usual treatment would be used as the control.

Follow-up

Any RCT must follow the study participants over a sufficient period of time to demonstrate adequate safety or efficacy data or both. The length of follow-up is determined by the following:

- The period of time intended for patients to receive the study intervention
- Long-term safety concerns
- The study objectives and outcome measures (e.g., pain scale, overall survival)

During the treatment and follow-up study periods, not all participants may remain in the study. More specifically, participants may drop out of the trial, for a number of reasons, and investigators must plan how to handle the partial data in addition to the study sample size determination as previously noted. The two major analysis approaches are as follows:

- ***Intention to treat:*** This method includes all patients as a member of their respective study group, regardless of completion of the protocol since they began the study and were randomized. Data up to the point of withdrawal are used in the analysis.
- ***Per protocol:*** This method excludes data from participants with significant deviations from the protocol.

Importantly, the two analytical techniques are not mutually exclusive. Often investigators will report results from both techniques that allow the reader of the report to compare potential differences directly.

20-5 Principles of Evaluation for Medical Literature

Critical appraisal is an objective, systematic review of medical literature. The critical appraisal of original research articles can be time consuming; however, the skills required are not difficult to develop and are highly important to pharmacy practitioners. Critical appraisal of the literature can be broken down into four steps:

- Search the literature for relevant evidence.
- Determine the applicability of the study.
- Evaluate basic study design.
- Critically evaluate the validity of the study results.

The following series of questions will aid in evaluating the design of a clinical trial and the validity of the results.

- Did the trial address a focused research question in terms of the following?
  - Population studied
  - Intervention given
  - Outcomes considered
- Did the authors use the correct type of study design?
- Was the assignment of participants randomized?
- Were all of the participants who entered the trial appropriately accounted for as well as those not enrolled in the study?
- Were participants and study personnel blinded? If not, were appropriate efforts made to blind the study treatments, or was there appropriate justification for not blinding?
- Did the groups have similar baseline characteristics at the start of the study?
- Aside from the experimental interventions, were the groups treated equally?
- How large was the treatment effect?

- How precise was the estimate of the treatment effect?
- Can the study results be applied to the local population?
- Were all clinically important outcomes considered?
- Are the benefits worth the harm and costs?

20-6 Principles of Research Design and Analysis in Practicing Evidence-Based Pharmacy

Evidence-based medicine is the process of finding, appraising, and using contemporaneous research findings systematically. This process then serves as the basis for clinical decisions. The following steps can be applied broadly to the interdisciplinary practice of medicine, including the practice of pharmacy:

- Formulate a clear clinical question from a patient's problem.
- Search the literature for relevant clinical articles.
- Evaluate and critically appraise the evidence for validity usefulness.
- Implement useful findings in clinical practice.

Applying current evidence to clinical practice necessitates critical appraisal of the literature. Incorporating the following into routine practice will aid the reader of medical literature in reaching sound clinical decisions:

- Regularly review and keep up to date with relevant medical literature.
- Familiarize yourself with clinical practice guidelines that apply to your area of practice.
- Critically appraise literature to determine validity of study results and applicability to practice.

20-7 Questions

1. Which of the following are descriptive statistics commonly used in characterizing data from observational studies? (Mark all that apply.)

A. Arithmetic mean
B. Normality
C. Mode
D. Range

2. Which of the following clinical study design characteristics is consistent with a case report?

A. Observational
B. Prospective
C. Randomized
D. Controlled

3. Clinical research generally seeks to answer questions for which of the following health care areas? (Mark all that apply.)

A. Disease prevention
B. Diagnosis
C. Treatment
D. Reimbursement

4. Which of the following statements is *true* regarding observational research design characteristics?

A. Participants are blinded.
B. They can be retrospective or prospective.
C. Randomization of participants is preferred.
D. They establish a causal relationship between variables of interest.

5. Which of the following research design types are considered experimental research? (Mark all that apply.)

A. Cohort study
B. Randomized controlled trial
C. Case-control study
D. Retrospective epidemiologic study

6. Cohort studies are the same as controlled trials except for which of the following study design characteristics?

A. Evaluation of causal relationship between study variables
B. Randomization of study participants
C. Exposure to a test treatment or condition
D. Option for use of historical control groups

7. Which of the following clinical trial designs evaluates intrasubject effects between two or more study treatments?

A. Crossover
B. Parallel
C. Case series
D. Cohort

8. Which of the following disease states are suitable for a crossover study design? (Mark all that apply.)

A. Glaucoma
B. Migraine headaches
C. Epilepsy
D. Hypertension

9. Blinding of subjects is an important process within controlled trials to minimize which of the following?

A. Confounding variables
B. Systematic error
C. Bias
D. Variability

10. Randomization is a key process within controlled trials to ensure which of the following?

A. Validity of inferential statistics
B. Avoidance of placebo effect
C. Avoidance of carryover effect
D. Normal distribution of study outcome

11. Which group of individuals is unaware of the subject treatment in a double-blind study?

A. Subjects only
B. Subjects and investigators
C. Investigators and data analysis personnel
D. Data analysis personnel and subjects

12. Which of the following are characteristics of stratification? (Mark all that apply.)

A. Is conducted before randomization
B. Ensures equal distribution of subject characteristics between groups
C. Requires larger number of subjects
D. Can be used in parallel or crossover studies

13. Which of the following is *true* regarding sample size in randomized controlled trials?

A. Increased sample size reduces statistical power.
B. Increased sample size is needed for a crossover design versus a parallel design.
C. Decreased sample size is needed when the expected difference in outcome between groups is large.
D. Decreased sample size is needed where large variability exists in the study outcome being measured.

14. Which of the following groups can serve as a control in a randomized clinical trial? (Mark all that apply.)

A. Standard treatment
B. Placebo
C. Historical
D. Usual care

15. Which of the following are acceptable techniques for managing data from those patients who withdraw from a study before completing the study protocol? (Mark all that apply.)

A. Analyzing the data using an intention-to-treat method
B. Analyzing the data using a per-protocol method with categorization of withdrawal subject characteristics including reason for withdrawal
C. Analyzing the data using both intention-to-treat and per-protocol methods
D. Analyzing the data from those subjects completing the protocol following purging of withdrawal subject information from the study database

16. Which of the following are steps in the critical appraisal of the literature relative to a published study? (Mark all that apply.)

A. Evaluating the validity of the study results
B. Searching for other studies published by the authors
C. Determining applicability of the study
D. Evaluating the basic study design

17. Which of the following questions aid in evaluating a clinical trial? (Mark all that apply.)

A. Were all confounding variables avoided in the study?
B. Did the study groups have similar baseline characteristics?
C. How large was the treatment effect?
D. Are the benefits worth the harm and costs?

18. Which of the following are essential vehicles for practitioners in keeping up to date with new literature? (Mark all that apply.)

A. Review articles
B. Clinical practice guidelines
C. Attendance at continuing education courses
D. Case reports

19. Which of the following are critical steps in practicing evidenced-based medicine? (Mark all that apply.)

A. Search the literature for relevant clinical articles.
B. Regularly converse with colleagues on their approach to a clinical problem.
C. Evaluate and critically appraise the clinical studies for validity and usefulness.
D. Formulate a clear clinical question relative to a particular patient problem.

20. Which of the following are potential confounding variables? (Mark all that apply.)

A. A subject's concurrent medications
B. Medical complications that occur during study period
C. Study dropouts
D. Exclusion of patients with severe forms of the disease being studied

21. Which of the following are used to calculate a sample size? (Mark all that apply.)

A. Desired statistical power
B. Estimated effect size
C. Probability of the results affecting clinical practice
D. Variability and experimental error

22. In a randomized controlled trial that follows a parallel design, which of the following is *true*?

A. Patients serve as their own control.
B. All patients end up receiving all of the interventions in random different orders, depending on group assignment.
C. Only patients who complete the entire protocol are included in the final analysis.
D. Patients are assigned to groups that receive a particular treatment over time; the only planned difference in the groups is the intervention.

23. The intention-to-treat analysis includes data from which patients?

A. All patients regardless of whether they completed the protocol
B. Only patients who complete a specified protocol
C. Only patients who complete the protocol with favorable outcomes
D. None of the patients who did not complete the entire trial

24. The duration of follow-up for a randomized clinical trial is determined for which of the following? (Mark all that apply.)

A. Outcome to be measured
B. Long-term safety concerns
C. Duration of time required to see an effect
D. Study budget

25. The four steps to the practice of evidence-based medicine include which of the following? (Mark all that apply.)

A. Formulate a clear clinical question from a patient's problem.
B. Search the literature for relevant clinical articles.
C. Evaluate and critically appraise the evidence for validity usefulness.
D. Implement useful findings in clinical practice.

20-8 Answers

1. **A, C, D.** Arithmetic mean, mode, and range are descriptive statistics. Normality is used in inferential statistics and is the exception.

2. **A.** Case reports are always observational. Prospective designs, randomization, and controls are all study design characteristics commonly used with randomized controlled trials and are not associated with case reports.

3. **A, B, C.** Clinical research generally seeks to answer questions related to disease prevention, diagnosis, and treatment. Reimbursement is a payment issue not normally addressed in clinical trials.

4. **B.** Observational studies can be retrospective or prospective. Observational studies lack randomization, are unblinded, and are unable to establish a causal relationship between variables of interest.

5. **B.** Experimental research designs include randomized controlled trials. Observational studies include cohort and case-control studies as well as retrospective epidemiologic studies.

6. **B.** Cohort studies do not randomize study participants. Cohort studies do share commonality with controlled trials in that they evaluate causal relationships between study variables, involve exposure to a test treatment or condition, and may occasionally use historical control groups.

7. **A.** Intrasubject effects are analyzed in crossover study designs. Parallel, case series, and cohort designs analyze intersubject effects.

8. **A, B, C, D.** Crossover study designs can be used only for stable, chronic, or episodic conditions. Glaucoma, migraine headaches, epilepsy, and hypertension meet this criterion.

9. **C.** Blinding of subjects is an important process within clinical trials to minimize bias. It does not minimize confounding variables, systematic error, or variability.

10. **A.** Randomization is a key process within clinical trials to ensure the validity of inferential statistics used in analyzing the study results. It does not avoid the placebo effect or the carryover effect or ensure a normal distribution of the study outcome.

11. **B.** Subjects and investigators are unaware of the subject treatment in a double-blind study. In a single-blind study, only the subjects are unaware of the subject treatment. A triple-blind study refers to the blinding of all persons who come in contact with the study procedures or data.

12. **A, B, C, D.** Stratification ensures equal distribution of selected subject characteristics between groups. It requires a larger number of patients and can be used in both parallel and crossover study designs. Stratification is performed before randomization.

13. **C.** Decreased sample size is needed when the expected difference in outcome between groups is large. Increased sample size increases statistical power and is needed when there is large variability in the study outcome being measured. Decreased sample size is needed for a crossover study design because patients are serving as their own controls.

14. **A, B, D.** Randomized controlled trials can use standard treatment, usual care, and placebo as controls. Historical controls cannot be used in a randomized clinical trial.

15. **A, B, C.** Patients who withdraw from a study before completing the study protocol can be managed by analyzing data using an intention-to-treat method or both an intention-to-treat method and a per-protocol method or by categorizing patients according to reason for withdrawal using a per-protocol method. Purging data from the study database upon withdrawal from the study and including only subjects completing the protocol is inappropriate.

16. **A, C, D.** General steps in the critical appraisal of the literature relative to a published study include evaluating the validity of the study results, determining applicability of the study, and evaluating the basic study design. Searching for other studies published by the authors is not generally a step in appraising the literature.

17. **B, C, D.** Asking if the groups have similar baseline characteristics, determining the extent of the treatment effect, and asking if the benefits of the treatment are worth the harm and costs are all aids in evaluating a clinical trial. Determining if all confounding variables were avoided in a study is not an aid in evaluating a clinical trial.

18. **A, B, C.** Important vehicles for practitioners relative to keeping up to date with new literature include review articles, clinical practice guidelines, and attendance at continuing education events. Case reports are generally not an important method for keeping up to date with new literature.

19. **A, C, D.** Critical steps in practicing evidence-based medicine include searching the literature for relevant clinical articles, evaluating and critically appraising the clinical studies for validity and usefulness, and formulating a clear clinical question relative to a particular patient problem. Regularly conversing with colleagues on their approach to a clinical problem is not a part of practicing evidence-based medicine.

20. **A, B, C.** Potential confounding variables include a subject's concurrent medications, medical complications that occur during the study period, and study dropouts. Exclusion of patients with severe forms of the disease being studied is not a confounding variable because it can be controlled.

21. **A, B, D.** The desired statistical power, estimated effect size, and variability and experimental error are all used to calculate a sample size. The probability of the results affecting clinical practice is not generally used in calculating sample size.

22. **D.** In a randomized controlled trial that follows a parallel design, patients are assigned to groups that receive a particular treatment over time; the only planned difference in the groups is the intervention. Patients do not serve as their own control. In general, patients receive only one study treatment depending on group assignment. And all patients are accounted for in the final analysis, including patients who do not complete the study protocol.

23. **A.** The intention-to-treat analysis includes data from all patients regardless of whether they completed the protocol.

24. **A, B, C.** The duration of follow-up for a randomized clinical trial is determined by the outcome to be measured, the long-term safety concerns, and the duration of time required to observe an effect. The study budget is not a scientific factor in determining the duration of follow-up.

25. **A, B, C, D.** Formulating a clear clinical question from a patient's problem, searching the literature for relevant clinical articles, evaluating and critically appraising the evidence for validity usefulness, and implementing useful findings in clinical practice are all steps in the practice of evidence-based medicine.

20-9 Additional Resources

Aparasu, RR, Bentley JP. *Principles of Research Design and Drug Literature Evaluation*. Burlington, MA: Jones and Bartlett Learning; 2015.

Dawson B, Trapp RG. *Basic and Clinical Biostatistics*. 4th ed. New York, NY: Lange Medical Books/McGraw-Hill; 2004.

Friedman LM, Furberg CD, DeMets DL. *Fundamentals of Clinical Trials*. 3rd ed. New York, NY: Springer; 1998.

Greenhalgh T. *How to Read a Paper: The Basics of Evidence-Based Medicine*. London: BMJ Books; 2001.

Guyatt GH, Sackett DL, Cook DJ. Users' guides to the medical literature. II. How to use an article about therapy or prevention. *JAMA*. 1994;271(1):59–63.

Rosenberg W, Donald A. Evidence-based medicine: an approach to clinical problem solving. *BMJ*. 1995;310(6987): 1122–1126.

Spilker B. *Guide to Clinical Trials*. New York, NY: Lippincott Williams and Wilkins; 1991.

Ethics in Health Care Practice 21

ANNETTE M. MENDOLA

21-1 KEY POINTS

- Health care decisions in the United States are guided by the principles and virtues of bioethics.
- The principles of bioethics are autonomy, beneficence, nonmaleficence, and justice. The virtues of bioethics are compassion, discernment, trustworthiness, integrity, and conscientiousness.
- Pharmacists in the United States are guided by the Code of Ethics for Pharmacists. They are expected to do the following:
  - Promote the good of every patient.
  - Exhibit respect for patients' values, beliefs, and culture.
  - Deal with their patients with honesty.
  - Maintain their professional competence.
  - Demonstrate respect for other health care professionals.
  - Place patients' needs ahead of personal gain.
- Ethical dilemmas are situations in which every known course of action conflicts with a person's sense of moral obligation. Resources for addressing moral dilemmas and uncertainty include codes of ethics, medical ethics committees, and trusted colleagues.
- Pharmacists have a duty to avoid conflicts of interest. Conflicts of interest occur when people or organizations have multiple interests and are in a position to make decisions that give them an unfair advantage.
- When providing a product or service would violate a pharmacist's values, a plan that respects everyone involved must be found—for example, a plan that transfers the duties to another pharmacist who is willing to provide the service.
- Ethical practices in patient care include the following:
  - Ensuring that patients are fully informed about their prescribed medications
  - Counseling patients on the safe and appropriate use of their medication
  - Keeping patient information confidential
  - Maintaining awareness of the warning signs of prescription drug abuse
- Ethical practices in business include the following:
  - Promoting drugs on the basis of patients' needs rather than a desire to profit from the sale of the product
  - Dispensing prescription drugs to only those patients who are authorized to possess such medications
  - Hiring and promoting employees with fairness and transparency and supervising and evaluating junior colleagues carefully
- Ethical practices in research include the following:
  - Recruiting, screening, and accepting patients for participation in a clinical study with honesty and integrity
  - Informing the patient about the purpose of the study, the risks associated with it, and the right to discontinue participation
  - Respecting the intellectual property of others, conducting research and quality control procedures with integrity, and reporting and interpreting the data honestly

21-2 STUDY GUIDE CHECKLIST

The following topics may help guide your study of this subject area:

- [ ] The principles of bioethics and the way to use them to guide ethical decision making in health care
- [ ] The virtues of bioethics and the way to use them to build moral character
- [ ] The Code of Ethics for Pharmacists and the way to use it (along with input from ethics committees and trusted colleagues) to address ethical dilemmas and uncertainty
- [ ] Ethical problems posed by conflicts of interest
- [ ] Guidelines for resolving conflicts between patients' right to receive pharmacy services and pharmacists' moral convictions
- [ ] Principles of ethical patient care, particularly those concerning end of life, antibiotic stewardship, and addictive medications
- [ ] Principles of ethical business practice, especially regarding the promotion, sale, and distribution of drugs and equipment and the treatment of junior colleagues
- [ ] Principles of ethical research, including those concerning research design, reporting of results, role of Institutional Review Boards, and treatment of research subjects

21-3 Introduction

As members of the health care team and system (see Chapter 13), the primary set of principles that guide ethical practice of pharmacy are the principles of medical ethics. Some professional duties are not obligations of all individual pharmacists, but are responsibilities of the profession as a whole. This chapter concentrates on the ethical framework for pharmacy practice in the United States. Pharmacists who were educated and have practiced in other countries will likely find that expectations for ethical practice described here are similar to those in other countries. Although fundamental ethical principles are widely accepted, there may be differences in how those principles are interpreted, as well as differences in how dilemmas that result from conflicting ethical principles are resolved.

21-4 Principles of Biomedical Ethics

Health care decisions in the United States are guided by the principles and virtues of bioethics, which are grounded in the fundamental theories of Western ethics. The principles and virtues of bioethics provide the basis for the codes of ethics and professional oaths for the various health care professions, including pharmacy, nursing, medicine, and social work.

Principles

The four principles of bioethics are autonomy, beneficence, nonmaleficence, and justice. Ethically sound decisions reflect consideration of each of these principles.

Autonomy is grounded in the fundamental duty of respect for persons. The foundation for the principle of autonomy is the ability of each person to make choices for herself or himself. (The word comes from the Greek for "self-governing.") Respect for autonomy is shown by respecting a patient's privacy and confidentiality, by obtaining informed consent (or informed refusal) for medical care and participation in research, and by telling the truth.

The profound value placed on individual freedom in the United States is reflected in the emphasis of autonomy in health care here. Although respect for individual persons is valued all over the world, pharmacists trained in other countries may find the degree to which individual choice is emphasized in American health care somewhat surprising.

Beneficence is the obligation to promote the well-being of others—particularly those who have been entrusted into your care. It requires knowledge of one's area of expertise, the patient and his or her situation, and the social context in which the provider and patient encounter each other. It also requires good interpersonal and communication skills. Providers can have duties of beneficence to patients, their families, and other members of the health care team.

Nonmaleficence, often expressed as "do no harm," refers not only to deliberate, malicious harm but also to harm that results from inefficiency, poorly designed systems, carelessness, and performance of tasks beyond one's level of expertise. Duties of nonmaleficence can include supervising assistants and students, minimizing foreseeable harms from poor processes, and maintaining one's knowledge and skills.

Justice maintains that benefits, burdens, and resources should be distributed fairly and equitably. Although this duty may be most evident regarding goods such as medications, it extends to the manner in which professionals allocate their time and attention, to the manner in which subjects are selected for clinical trials, and to procedures for settling disputes. The principle of justice requires providers to be aware of the health and health care disparities in the situations in which they practice and to act responsively to this knowledge.

Virtues

Ethically sound decisions in health care reflect a balance of the four principles of bioethics. Another tool for cultivating ethically sound behavior is the use of the virtues of biomedical ethics. Virtues are the character traits, or moral habits, that are grounded in moral principles. Some suggest that "doing the right thing" comes more naturally when one cultivates good moral habits in addition to thinking about moral principles and considering their application to a situation. We develop good character by striving to cultivate these traits in our everyday life and by thinking about what people with good moral character (such as trusted mentors) would do in a situation.

The five virtues of biomedical ethics are compassion, discernment, trustworthiness, integrity, and conscientiousness.

Compassion

Compassionate people are able to recognize the suffering of others and respond empathetically. They actively watch for unspoken needs and unexpressed concerns. They are kind. Compassion should be extended to patients, colleagues, and oneself.

Ask: Do I understand this patient's concerns? Am I making him or her feel safe and understood?

Discernment

Discernment is the ability to reach appropriate decisions without being unduly influenced or distracted by peripheral considerations, fears, personal preferences, or outside pressure.

Ask: Am I responding to the patient's feelings, needs, and fears, or to my own?

Trustworthiness

Trustworthiness requires being honest with others and acting transparently and with good motives. To be a trustworthy person is to merit the confidence of others.

Ask: Am I being open, or am I tempted to conceal something I know or have done?

Integrity

Integrity involves the willingness to act consistently on one's moral commitments, even when uncomfortable or in the presence of personal risk.

Ask: Am I living up to my own standards for myself?

Conscientiousness

To be conscientious is to place the appropriate weight on the competing duties in a situation. Conscientious people have a sense of when to compromise and when to insist on a course of action. They try to do the right thing for the right reasons and to use the right amount of effort for the situation at hand.

Ask: Am I looking for solutions that respect everyone's interests? Am I giving in when I should be standing up, or being rigid when I should be flexible?

21-5 Code of Pharmacy Ethics and Oaths

Codes of ethics and professional oaths translate the principles and virtues of a profession into guidelines for ethical behavior for its members. The specific behaviors expected of pharmacists in the United States are embodied in the Code of Ethics for Pharmacists, which was developed by the American Pharmacists Association (APhA) in 1994 and is endorsed by all the other major American pharmacy associations.

The eight ethical principles of the code, with a brief comment on the professional behaviors associated with each, are as follows:

1. ***A pharmacist respects the covenantal relationship between the patient and pharmacist.*** Society trusts that pharmacists will conduct themselves as professionals—that they will use their particular set of knowledge and skills to promote the welfare of patients. Pharmacists honor that trust by promising to work together with other members of the health care team to help patients achieve optimum benefit from their medications. This covenant, expressed in the Oath of a Pharmacist (see Box 21-1) is the basis of the pharmacist–patient relationship.
2. ***A pharmacist promotes the good of every patient in a caring, compassionate, and confidential manner.*** Pharmacists serve patients with respect and compassion by responding to their medication needs promptly and courteously, by protecting their health and welfare needs, and by keeping their health information private.
3. ***A pharmacist respects the autonomy and dignity of each patient.*** Pharmacists approach each patient on the patient's own terms—that is, with respect for the patient's values, belief system, and culture—and with appropriate consideration for the patient's level of health literacy and any language barriers or disabilities of the patient. They avoid prejudging a patient on the basis of stereotypes or unfounded generalizations. Pharmacists promote self-determination by encouraging patients to ask questions and to participate in decisions about their health.
4. ***A pharmacist acts with honesty and integrity in professional relationships.*** To act with integrity means to be consistently guided by one's moral and ethical convictions. Practicing with integrity requires openness and transparency in one's actions. Thus, pharmacists have a duty to serve their patients with honesty and with full exercise of their moral and ethical compass.
5. ***A pharmacist maintains professional competence.*** Professional competence entails not only the initial qualifications to become licensed as a pharmacist but also the maintenance of those qualifications through systematic renewal of knowledge and skills. To be competent, pharmacists must also be free of any type of impairment that would affect their judgment and put the public at risk. Thus, competence includes maintaining one's own physical and mental health and seeking appropriate care when needed. Similarly, pharmacists have an ethical duty to avoid the use of alcohol, drugs, or any other substance that would impair their competence to practice their profession. They also have an ethical duty to ensure that any impaired colleague is prevented from engaging in practice until the impairment has been appropriately addressed (see Chapter 13, Section 13-10).
6. ***A pharmacist respects the values and abilities of colleagues and other health professionals.*** Two specific professional behaviors are embodied in this principle. First, pharmacists are expected to

BOX 21-1. Oath of a Pharmacist

"I promise to devote myself to a lifetime of service to others through the profession of pharmacy. In fulfilling this vow:

- I will consider the welfare of humanity and relief of suffering my primary concerns.
- I will apply my knowledge, experience, and skills to the best of my ability to assure optimal outcomes for my patients.
- I will respect and protect all personal and health information entrusted to me.
- I will accept the lifelong obligation to improve my professional knowledge and competence.
- I will hold myself and my colleagues to the highest principles of our profession's moral, ethical, and legal conduct.
- I will embrace and advocate changes that improve patient care.
- I will utilize my knowledge, skills, experiences, and values to prepare the next generation of pharmacists.

I take these vows voluntarily with the full realization of the responsibility with which I am entrusted by the public."

American Pharmacists Association, 2007.

recognize when their knowledge and abilities are inadequate to meet a particular patient's needs and either seek consultation from colleagues (other pharmacists or members of other health care professions) or refer the patient to the care of another, more qualified practitioner. Second, pharmacists are expected to recognize and respect the fact that other health care professionals may differ in their approach to patient care, depending on their individual beliefs and values. Pharmacists should avoid any behavior that raises questions in the patient's mind about the competence of other health care professionals because of such differences.

7. ***A pharmacist serves individual, community, and societal needs.*** Although the primary obligation of a pharmacist is to individual patients, the specific knowledge and skills that pharmacists possess may produce obligations to address particular needs of the community by participating in advocacy, research, and public education. This principle encourages pharmacists to volunteer their services when opportunities arise. It also includes the need to train and mentor future pharmacists and junior colleagues.
8. ***A pharmacist seeks justice in the distribution of health resources.*** Pharmacists are occasionally faced with the need to make decisions regarding the allocation of limited supplies of drugs and devices. Such instances may give rise to ethical dilemmas for the pharmacist. In making such allocations, pharmacists should balance the needs of patients and those of society.

Oaths are pledges that professionals make when they are inducted into their profession. Much like vows of marriage, these oaths are promises one makes when entering into a new role—to serve in that role faithfully.

The Oath of a Pharmacist, which was approved by APhA in 2007, expresses the values spelled out in the Code of Ethics for Pharmacists.

21-6 Ethical Dilemmas

Ethical dilemmas are situations in which every known course of action conflicts with a person's sense of moral obligation. In such situations, there is no single, agreed-upon right course of action, though there are many wrong courses of action. Although true ethical dilemmas are rare, being prepared for how to resolve them is wise.

Ethical dilemmas faced by pharmacists usually fall into the following categories:

- Conflicts between the needs of individual patients and those of society
- Conflicts that arise when drugs (or procedures) prescribed for patients violate a pharmacist's religious or cultural views
- Conflicts that arise when a patient's religious or cultural views (or those of a patient's parents or caregivers) result in the rejection of needed treatment
- Conflicts in rationing scarce resources
- Conflicts that require balancing the need to maintain patient confidentiality with the need to protect other individuals
- Conflicts that arise in the course of conducting clinical research (balancing patient needs against those of a research protocol)

Several resources should be helpful in addressing ethical dilemmas and uncertainty:

- ***Codes of ethics:*** Professional codes of ethics—such as the Code of Ethics for Pharmacists—are tools for reasoning out ethical dilemmas. They are not intended to be catalogs of moral information that professionals can simply consult for answers, because ethically difficult situations inevitably require moral judgment. Rather, they help professionals resolve dilemmas by guiding their reasoning with the fundamental ethical commitments of the profession.

- ***Ethics committees:*** In 1992, the Joint Commission on Accreditation of Healthcare Organizations (a nongovernmental accrediting organization) issued a mandate that hospitals in the United States establish a "mechanism" to provide ethics education and ethical guidance for its constituents. Most hospitals responded by developing ethics committees, usually composed of diverse members of the health care team (including pharmacists) and sometimes including community members. Hospital ethics committees may be consulted to help resolve ethically difficult situations.
- ***Trusted colleagues:*** Pharmacists at any stage of practice should remember the value of talking with trusted mentors and peers. Honest discussions about situations that cause moral uncertainty and moral distress help clarify moral uncertainty, ease moral distress, and build moral community.

21-7 Conflicts of Interest

Conflicts of interest (COI) can arise is a variety of settings (Box 21-2). These COI occur when people or organizations have multiple interests and are in a position to make decisions that give them an unfair advantage. Many such conflicts involve dual relationships, as when a family member is also a business associate. Dual relationships and other COI have great potential to interfere with professional judgment and integrity. Note that a COI exists even if no one actually takes unfair advantage of the situation. Such conflicts should be avoided when possible and managed with integrity and transparency when unavoidable.

Strictly speaking, COI do not pose ethical dilemmas because they do not produce situations in which the right thing to do is morally unclear or every option violates the individual's moral code. Rather, the right course of action is usually clear and in line with the individual's moral code but out of line with her or his personal or financial interests. However, COI do produce morally dangerous situations because human beings have a natural tendency to put their own interests first. For this reason, pharmacists and other professionals have duties to avoid COI whenever possible, including situations in which such conflicts are likely to develop. Moreover, they should avoid even the appearance of COI because the mere appearance of a conflict can cause distrust.

Employers' requirement of a COI disclosure statement from employees is a common practice today. Such a statement discloses any financial or personal interests or entanglements of the employee that might

BOX 21-2. Examples of Conflicts of Interest

- Pharmacists who own their own pharmacy, or who are rewarded on the basis of the profitability of a pharmacy that they manage, are often faced with choices between what is in their best interest financially and what is in the best interest of the patient, either financially or therapeutically.
- Pharmacists who own shares in a pharmaceutical company may be biased in their evaluation of the quality and therapeutic merit of that company's products as opposed to the same or similar products from other vendors. This situation would represent a potential conflict of interest in cases where such pharmacists serve on the pharmacy and therapeutics committee of hospitals or other health care organizations.
- Pharmacists who are paid by pharmaceutical companies to give drug-related presentations are faced with a similar ethical problem. They may tend to speak more favorably about a particular medication, or minimize the risks associated with it, for fear of not receiving future opportunities to present and get paid for it. Similarly, pharmacists who conduct medication-related research that is paid for by a pharmaceutical company also have possible conflicts of interest.
- Pharmacists who are in a position to make hiring decisions, or to recommend individuals for consideration for employment, may have a personal interest in recommending a family member or close friend or associate for employment, irrespective of her or his qualifications. Furthermore, pharmacists who find themselves in a position of supervising employees who are relatives or close associates may lack the objectivity to be effective managers.

compromise his or her objectivity. When requested to complete such statements, pharmacists must be completely honest and forthright. Any problems that the employer or potential employer may have with conflicts thus identified can then be addressed and resolved.

When COI are unavoidable, pharmacists and other professionals have a duty to recognize the conflict and take steps to manage it. This can include cooperating with boards and committees that are designed to help manage COI, such as the institutional review boards that review research involving human subjects. For this reason, a duty of the profession (but not of all individual pharmacists) is to assist peers in managing unavoidable COI by serving on such committees.

21-8 Conscientious Objection

The principle of autonomy, or respect for people, extends to all people in any role: patients, health care professionals, family members, and members of the community. In diverse societies, the duty to respect the moral commitments of all members can result in ethical conflict. When this occurs in the realm of pharmacy, it often involves either reproduction or end of life. Examples of services that may result in ethical conflict include the following:

- Dispensing prescriptions for contraceptives or for medications that may have abortifacient effects
- Dispensing medications to assist terminally ill patients who meet certain criteria to end their lives (physician-aid-in-dying, physician-assisted suicide, or death with dignity; legal in California; Colorado; Montana; Oregon; Washington; Washington, DC; and Vermont, as of 2017)
- Preparing or dispensing drugs for execution of convicted criminals by lethal injection

Conscientious objection is the refusal to perform a service or provide a product on the grounds that doing so would violate one's moral integrity. When providing a product or service would violate a pharmacist's moral or religious belief, a course of action that respects the rights, dignity, and moral commitments of all involved must be found. A common solution to this conflict involves the transfer of duties to another pharmacist who is willing to provide that service.

Merely disagreeing with a practice or finding it morally problematic is not sufficient grounds to appeal to conscientious objection. Refusing to provide the services of one's profession for reasons of conscience is a serious action, and one that is not to be taken lightly. Pharmacists may not invoke conscientious objection to use their position to compel others to comply with their beliefs or to discriminate against patients. Pharmacists who feel morally obligated to refuse to perform a task that would normally be part of their work should take steps to ensure that their refusal does not jeopardize any patient's right to receive products and services in a timely manner and according to his or her own informed choices. This process includes informing their supervisors of their need for accommodation before accepting employment (or as soon as reasonably possible after the belief develops), cooperating with plans to ensure that patient care is not disrupted, and refraining from discussing the conflicting beliefs with patients. Supervising pharmacists have the obligation to develop and implement systems and practices that support respect for people by accommodating both the pharmacist whose conscience forbids particular practices and the patient who believes he or she should receive pharmaceutical services without unreasonable barriers.

21-9 Duties and Dilemmas in Practice

Ethical issues and dilemmas in pharmacy practice can arise in spheres of patient care, business practice, supervision and education of students and trainees, environmental concerns, and research and development.

Patient Care

Patient care is at the center of a pharmacist's practice. Providing patient-centered care means providing pharmacy services in a way that respects the patient and promotes her or his well-being. This type of care includes the following:

- Ensure that patients are fully informed about their prescribed medications, including the positive effects they should expect to receive, the way to take medications correctly and safely, and the side effects and symptoms that signal the need to seek medical attention.
- Encourage questions and provide information in a manner that is readily understandable to the patient, so that he or she can make informed health care choices. This communication can include soliciting information from the patient about any difficulties he or she has with dosing, scheduling, or delivery methods of the prescribed medications.
- Keep patient information confidential.

Some specific domains in patient care are detailed below.

End-of-life care

Care of patients who are known to be at the end of life has been changing in the United States. Patients are now encouraged to consider what is most important to them at end of life and to select treatment goals and modalities accordingly, rather than accepting (or pursuing) treatment without regard for its outcome. Documents (advance directives, advance care plans, living wills) that outline the treatment one would be willing to undergo, and the quality of life one would be willing to accept, are common. Because incapacity resulting from accidents or illness can happen unexpectedly and at any age, people are encouraged to think about who would make medical decisions for them if they become unable to do so for themselves (surrogate decision makers, health care agents, durable powers of attorney for health care).

It follows from the principle of autonomy that fully informed patients who are in possession of decision-making capacity have the right to decline treatment—even life-sustaining treatment. It follows from the principle of beneficence that patients who are suffering should be cared for with sensitivity. Palliative care, which focuses on relief of distressing symptoms at any stage of illness, has become widely used in the United States in recent years, as has hospice, which focuses on the comfort of terminally ill patients who are no longer pursuing curative treatment. Additionally, as of 2017, physician-assisted suicide for terminally ill patients is legal in six states and the District of Columbia, and other states are likely to consider approving this measure in the future.

Because palliative care, hospice, and physician-assisted suicide all make use of prescription medications, pharmacists are wise to consider their own beliefs, values, and emotional needs regarding participating in end-of-life care. Such reflection can help guide decisions about where one chooses to practice and what pharmaceutical services one is ethically comfortable providing for patients at end of life. This is one area in which some pharmacists' personal values may conflict with patient care, and conscientious objection may be considered.

Medications with addictive potential

At present, the United States is experiencing crisis levels of deaths from, and addiction to, opioids and other drugs. The risk that a patient may be trying to acquire opioids for illegitimate purposes must be balanced against the needs of patients who suffer from genuine physical pain. This entrenched and multifaceted problem produces responsibilities for many parties, including pharmacists. Pharmacists can advise prescribing providers about how they can manage their patients' pain without increasing their patients' risk of developing or exacerbating addiction. To provide this service, pharmacists must keep current about effective prescribing practices in pain management, such as national and statewide guidelines for the treatment of chronic pain. Pharmacists, without falling prey to prejudicial cultural stereotyping, should develop an awareness of warning signs that a patient may be trying to acquire drugs illicitly. Systems to detect drug abuse and diversion, such as computerized statewide or regional networks for prescription drug monitoring programs (controlled substances databases) should be used routinely. Requirements and procedures for prescription drug monitoring programs vary by state.

Interprofessional practice

As a member of an interprofessional team, a pharmacist has a duty to respect the knowledge and skills—and the roles—of other members of the team. The pharmacist has a corresponding duty to contribute fully to the deliberations and decisions of the team. In this context, any disagreements about treatment should be discussed respectfully among team members in an effort to achieve the best outcome for the patient. Care should be taken not to undermine patients' confidence in other team members. Likewise, any concerns about another professional's competence (including concerns about impairment) should be handled promptly through appropriate channels. Every member of the team should be guided by the patient's best interest.

Antibiotic stewardship

Overuse and overprescription of broad-spectrum antimicrobials can profoundly damage the human microbiome and has likely contributed to the proliferation of multidrug-resistant organisms. Increasingly, hospitals are adopting programs and practices to promote antibiotic stewardship to address this problem. The objectives of these programs are to optimize patient outcomes, prevent damage to patients' microbiome, and reduce health care costs. Pharmacists play a key role in promoting wise use of antimicrobial medications, whether or not they practice in an institution that has a formal antibiotic stewardship program.

Business Ethics and Pharmacy

Pharmacists whose jobs involve the business of pharmacy have corresponding responsibilities in the realm of business ethics. Ethical business practice in pharmacy is grounded in placing the needs of patients ahead of personal gain. Principles concerning conflicts of interest, discussed above, are particularly germane in this arena. Some specific areas are discussed in the following subsections.

Drug promotion

Pharmacists are ethically bound to promote a drug product only for the indications for which it has been approved by the U.S. Food and Drug Administration or for which there is ample evidence in the professional and scientific literature (off-label use or off-label indications). Any attempt to misrepresent the therapeutic merits of a drug product is unethical. Pharmacists are further obligated to inform patients about any clinically significant adverse effects (including side effects and drug interactions) that are known to occur with a drug, so that patients can adequately evaluate the risks associated with that drug. Drugs should be promoted on the basis of patients' needs rather than a desire to profit from the sale of the product. The same duty applies to the promotion and sales of nonprescription medications, dietary supplements, and durable medical equipment. Communication used in promoting a product should be at a level that is understandable and appropriate for the individual patient.

Drug sales

As a matter of ethics as well as law, a pharmacist may dispense prescription drugs only to a patient who has a valid prescription for that drug or to another individual or entity who is authorized to possess prescription medications. The ethical duty is to avoid doing harm to the public (or to individuals) by making dangerous drugs available to them without prescriber authority and supervision. Pricing practices related to the sale of drugs and equipment should be guided by a sense of fairness. Taking advantage of a drug scarcity to make an excessive profit would be a violation of this ethical principle.

Employment practices

Pharmacists who are responsible for hiring, evaluating, and promoting employees must do so with fairness and transparency. Ethical employment practices include careful supervision to protect the public from error and to encourage professional development of employees. It may also include providing for employee safety in practice settings that have the potential for danger.

Education, Training, and Supervision

Mentoring junior colleagues—new hires, new graduates, pharmacy technicians, and pharmacy students—is both a duty and a privilege. Perhaps the most important way pharmacists can mentor colleagues is by serving as good role models with their own practice.

As in other domains of practice, pharmacists should avoid dual relationships with junior colleagues because these relationships produce conflicts of interest and can foster exploitation. Similarly, junior colleagues should be evaluated honestly and fairly, both to foster their own development and to protect those they serve. Careful supervision is a fundamental component of this practice, as is watching out for one's own biases (see Chapter 13, Section 13-11).

Finally, pharmacists should advocate for their junior colleagues. In the workplace and in educational settings, pharmacists should look out for junior colleagues' well-being. As educators, pharmacists should collaborate with other professionals and encourage their students' professional development. Again, modeling professional behavior, including self-care, is the most fundamental component of mentoring.

Environmental Effect

The health of the natural world significantly affects human health. Pharmaceutical practice has a significant effect on the environment; thus, responsible practice must consider the effect of drugs and health-related products on the natural world. Related duties may include providing environmentally safe disposal of drugs and health-related products, supporting environmentally friendly business practices, and raising awareness in students and trainees of the environmental effects of inappropriate dumping of medications in sewage systems and landfills (see Chapter 13, Section 13-8).

Research Ethics

Pharmacists and others who participate in research involving human subjects must balance the needs and interests of research participants against the need to maintain the reliability of a research protocol. The potential for ethical tension between these interests and notable ethical lapses in the treatment of human subjects in the past have given rise to the field of research ethics.

Research participants, as such, are research *subjects*, though they are frequently also patients. The distinction is important because the goal of research is to advance medical knowledge, whereas the goal of treatment is to benefit the individual patient. *Therapeutic misconception* occurs when patients who enroll in clinical trials as subjects hoping that the study drug will benefit them are not fully aware that they may not benefit from the study at all. Careful informed consent can help avoid therapeutic misconception.

Protecting the rights and safety of research subjects involves honesty and integrity in recruiting, screening, and accepting subjects for participation in a clinical study. This process requires particular care for members of vulnerable populations, such as children, the elderly, pregnant women, prisoners, and those with mental illness or cognitive impairment. Subjects (or, if a subject cannot give consent, the subject's surrogate) must be informed about the purpose of the study and its source of funding, the risks associated with it, and the nature of their participation. They should be made aware of their right to discontinue participation without penalty. All identifiable information about individual subjects must be kept confidential and may not be disclosed without their consent. Informed-consent documents should be thorough and written at an appropriate level of health literacy and should be carefully reviewed with subjects (or their surrogates) before they agree to participate.

Research involving human subjects must be approved by an institutional review board (IRB). IRBs protect the welfare of research subjects by reviewing the research design and materials. Although not a duty of every pharmacist, serving on IRBs is a duty of the profession, given the scope of knowledge that pharmacists possess.

Additional ethical responsibilities in research include respecting the intellectual property of others (including both strangers and collaborators), conducting research and quality control procedures with integrity, and reporting and interpreting the results of statistical data with scrupulous honesty. As in other areas of practice, conflicts of interest between one's personal financial goals and the good of the public should be avoided and should be managed with transparency when they are unavoidable.

Certain areas of clinical research may conflict with the moral commitments of some pharmacists (e.g., research involving stem cells, abortifacients, human genomics). Ultimately, the decision to participate in such research is an individual choice.

21-10 Questions

1. Which of the following statements is correct regarding the differences in ethics among different nations or societies?

A. Ethical values in the United States are no different than those in other countries.
B. Ethical values in the United States are very different from those in most other countries.
C. Cultural differences play no role in ethical differences.
D. Ethical values are shaped in part by the local culture.

2. Which of the following is part of the virtue of *trustworthiness?*

A. Responding empathetically to the needs of patients
B. Compromising when appropriate
C. Telling the truth
D. Distributing resources fairly

3. Which of the following statements is correct regarding the Code of Ethics for Pharmacists?

A. It outlines legal duties for pharmacists in the United States.
B. It is a catalog of moral information that pharmacists consult for specific answers to moral dilemmas.
C. It includes the principle of *loyalty* to one's employer.
D. APhA developed it to guide ethical behavior by outlining the fundamental ethical commitments of the profession of pharmacy.

4. Which of the following statements about *conflicts of interest* is correct?

A. Conflicts of interest are inherently unethical.
B. Dual relationships are rarely a source of conflicts of interest if everyone involved is careful.
C. Conflicts of interest arise when persons or organizations have multiple interests and are in a position to make decisions that give them an unfair advantage.
D. Conflicts of interest arise when people or organizations take unfair advantage of their position.

5. Which of the following statements best describes the covenantal relationship between a pharmacist and a patient?

A. It is a written contract, signed by both.
B. It ensures the economic security of the pharmacist.
C. It is based on mutual trust.
D. It requires pharmacists to ignore their moral convictions.

6. Which of the following involve the duties of *beneficence* for pharmacists? (Mark all that apply.)

A. Maintaining professional competence
B. Doing whatever the patient asks
C. Using good personal and communication skills
D. Protecting patients from bad news

7. Which of the following statements is true regarding *professional competence*?

A. It is the same as cultural competence.
B. It includes professional knowledge but not skills or values.
C. It is an ethical obligation of all pharmacists.
D. It is determined by professional licensure.

8. When a pharmacist becomes aware that another pharmacist has an impairment that would affect her or his professional abilities, which of the following is the ethical duty of the first pharmacist in this situation?

A. Report the other pharmacist to the police.
B. Inform the State Board of Pharmacy.
C. Respect the other pharmacist's professional autonomy, and take no action.
D. Take whatever action is necessary to prevent the other pharmacist from harming a patient.

9. When the availability of a drug is scarce, which of the following is the best ethical course of action for a pharmacist?

A. Distribute the drug on a first-come, first-served basis until the supply is exhausted.
B. Keep all the supply for distribution to the pharmacist's own customers or patients.
C. Place the needs of the broader community ahead of the needs of the pharmacist's own patients.
D. Balance the needs of society and individual patients in making decisions regarding allocation of the drug.

10. Which of the following best describes patient counseling by a pharmacist?

A. Both a legal and an ethical duty
B. An ethical duty but not a legal duty
C. A legal duty but not an ethical duty
D. Neither a legal nor an ethical duty

11. When communicating information about the risks of a drug, a pharmacist has an ethical duty to do which of the following?

A. Withhold the information, so as to avoid alarming the patient.
B. Disclose the information to the patient but assure the patient that the risks are minimal.
C. Disclose the information, and discuss the risks and benefits with the patient.
D. Disclose the information, and discuss the risks without reviewing the benefits.

12. Ethical dilemmas are best described by which of the following statements?

A. They typically have a clear-cut solution.
B. They can and should be avoided by pharmacists.
C. They involve choices between two alternatives, both of which conflict with one's sense of moral obligation.
D. They invariably lead to poor outcomes.

13. When a pharmacist's moral or religious convictions are in conflict with the medical needs of a patient, which of the following is the best course of action?

A. The pharmacist has an absolute right to refuse treatment.
B. The pharmacist has an absolute duty to provide the treatment.
C. The pharmacist should delay making a decision regarding treatment for that patient until the issue can be reviewed by an ethics committee.
D. The pharmacist should refer the patient to another pharmacist who is willing to provide the care.

14. What is the purpose of a medical ethics committee?

A. Regulate biomedical research
B. Help health care professionals in dealing with ethical difficulties
C. Prescribe a course of action that is final and binding
D. Provide legal advice

15. Which of the following situations is *least* likely to pose a conflict of interest?

A. A pharmacist recommends his son-in-law for employment.
B. A pharmacist who serves on a hospital's pharmacy and therapeutics committee owns a considerable amount of stock in a pharmaceutical company.
C. A pharmacy store manager whose annual bonus is tied to total sales considers introducing a line of dietary supplements for which there is little documentation of therapeutic value.
D. A pharmacist whose retirement investments are all in mutual funds serves as the pharmacy purchasing officer for a large hospital.

16. Which of the following statements concerning *conscientious objection* is true?

A. Conscientious objection is a violation of a pharmacist's duty to treat patients with respect.
B. Conscientious objection is a mechanism to nudge patients and their families toward making ethically sound choices.
C. Conscientious objection can be invoked at any time and for any reason.
D. Conscientious objection involves the transfer of duties to another pharmacist when performing a service or providing a product would cause profound harm to one's moral core.

17. Which of the following statements concerning clinical research is correct?

A. The purpose of clinical research is the benefit of research subjects.
B. Ethical clinical research emphasizes the reliability of a research protocol more than the rights of study patients.
C. Although ethics are involved in conducting clinical research, ethical issues very rarely arise.
D. Ethical issues commonly arise in conducting clinical research.

18. Which of the following statements is correct about ethical issues regarding end-of-life care?

A. Physician-assisted suicide is a legal right of all U.S. citizens.
B. It follows from the principle of beneficence that end-of-life care must involve aggressive attempts to sustain life.
C. Use of palliative care requires the review of an ethics committee.
D. It follows from the principle of autonomy that fully informed patients who have decision-making capacity have the right to decline life-sustaining treatment.

19. Which of the following statements regarding interprofessional teamwork is true as an ethical action of a pharmacist?

A. Withhold certain patient information from other members of the team.
B. Raise concerns or disagreements with other members of the team.
C. Disregard the views of another member of the team.
D. Inform a patient that he or she questions the competence or judgment of other members of the team.

20. Which of the following expectations are true for foreign-educated pharmacists who practice in the United States?

A. They must surrender their own moral convictions and beliefs.
B. They must embrace the Code of Ethics for Pharmacists developed by the American Pharmacists Association.
C. They must disregard the needs or wishes of individual patients in cases where those needs or wishes conflict with the pharmacist's moral convictions.
D. They must practice higher ethical standards than pharmacists who graduated from U.S. pharmacy schools.

21-11 Answers

1. **D.** Although considerable similarity exists worldwide in pharmacists' ethical values, some differences are based on local culture.
2. **C.** *Trustworthiness* pertains to being truthful and transparent about your actions.
3. **D.** The Code of Ethics for Pharmacists is not a catalog of specific answers to ethical problems, but rather outlines the fundamental ethical commitments of the profession of pharmacy.
4. **C.** When someone has multiple interests in a situation and is in a position to make decisions that gives her or him an unfair advantage, a conflict of interest exists.
5. **C.** The pharmacist's covenantal relationship with patients is based on mutual trust between pharmacists and patients.
6. **A, C.** *Beneficence* involves maintaining professional competence and good personal and communication skills, as well as having an understanding of the social context in which the pharmacist and patient encounter one another.
7. **C.** All pharmacists have an ethical duty to remain competent.
8. **D.** Protecting patients from potential harm is the first duty of a pharmacist who is aware that another pharmacist is functioning while impaired.
9. **D.** From an ethical viewpoint, both the needs of a pharmacist's individual patients *and* the needs of the broader community should be considered.
10. **A.** Patient consultation is required both by the Code of Ethics for Pharmacists and by law.
11. **C.** A pharmacist has an ethical duty to ensure that a patient is appropriately informed about both the risks and the benefits of any drug prescribed for that patient.
12. **C.** Ethical dilemmas are so named because they involve choices between two alternatives, both of which conflict with one's sense of moral obligation.
13. **D.** A particular pharmacist's moral or religious convictions may not be used as a basis for withholding treatment from a patient. In such cases, a pharmacist may fulfill her or his ethical responsibilities by referring the patient to another pharmacist who is willing to provide the care.
14. **B.** A bioethics committee helps clinical researchers and health care professionals think through ethical dilemmas. Such committees do not exist to regulate biomedical research or to provide legal advice.
15. **D.** From among the choices presented, the one that represents the least potential conflict of interest is that of a pharmacy purchasing officer who does not own stocks in the companies whose products are under consideration for purchase.
16. **D.** If performing a service or providing a product (such as filling a valid prescription for physician-assisted suicide for a terminally ill patient) would violate a pharmacist's conscience, she or he may use proper channels to transfer these duties to another pharmacist.
17. **D.** Ethical issues frequently arise in the course of conducting clinical research.
18. **D.** The principle of autonomy stipulates that informed patients who are capable of making decisions have the right to decline any treatment, including life-sustaining treatment.
19. **B.** It is a pharmacist's ethical duty to take steps to avert patient harm. Therefore, the pharmacist must raise disagreements with other health care professionals in situations where their actions appear likely to result in maleficence (patient harm).
20. **B.** All pharmacists practicing in the United States are expected to be familiar with and abide by the Code of Ethics for Pharmacists developed by APhA.

21-12 Additional Resources

American College of Clinical Pharmacy. Ethical issues related to clinical pharmacy research. *Pharmacotherapy.* 1993;13(5): 523–530. Available at: http://onlinelibrary.wiley.com/doi/10.1002/j.1875-9114.1993.tb04322.x/pdf.

American College of Clinical Pharmacy. Pharmacists and industry: guidelines for ethical interactions. *Pharmacotherapy.* 2008;28(3):410–420. Available at: https://www.acpe-accredit.org/pdf/Guidelines_for_Ethical_Interactions.pdf.

American Pharmacists Association. Code of ethics for pharmacists. Adopted by the membership of the American Pharmaceutical Association, Washington, DC, October 27, 1994. Available at: http://www.pharmacist.com/code-ethics.

American Pharmacists Association. Oath of a pharmacist. Approved by the American Pharmacists Association, Washington, DC, 2007. Available at: http://www.pharmacist.com/oath-pharmacist.

Beauchamp TL, Childress JF. *Principles of Biomedical Ethics.* 7th edition. New York, NY: Oxford University Press; 2012.

Cohen, H. The impaired pharmacist. *US Pharmacist.* 2010;35(9):1. Available at: https://www.uspharmacist.com/article/the-impaired-pharmacist.

Evans EW. Conscientious objection: a pharmacist's right or professional negligence? *Am J Health-Syst Pharm.* 2007;64(2):139–141.

National Association of Boards of Pharmacy. Stakeholders' challenges and red flag warning signs related to prescribing and dispensing controlled substances. 2015. Available at: https://nabp.pharmacy/wp-content/uploads/2016/07/Red-Flags-Controlled-Substances-03-2015.pdf.

Veatch RM, Haddad A, Last EJ. *Case Studies in Pharmacy Ethics.* 3rd ed. New York, NY: Oxford University Press; 2017.

Professional Communications 22

JEREMY THOMAS

22-1 KEY POINTS

- Key components of interpersonal communication are the sender, the receiver, and the message.
- Pharmacists should identify barriers to communication and seek to resolve those barriers.
- Pharmacists should identify patients with low health literacy and develop appropriate visual or written materials.
- Open-ended questions will provide the pharmacist with more information than traditional closed-ended questions.
- A medication history includes allergies, current and past medications, adverse reactions, over-the-counter medications, and adherence.
- Using the "Three Prime Questions" for patient counseling allows the pharmacist to focus on medication information that is unknown to the patient.
- Active listening and empathetic responding are the foundations of the pharmacist–patient relationship.
- Employing assertiveness when dealing with a difficult situation will help the pharmacist maintain open lines of communication.
- Pharmacists must be aware of their own culturally determined values and behaviors and those of other cultures.
- Documenting pharmacist activities is a critical step in providing patient care, both for dealing with potential litigation concerns and for reinforcing roles for pharmacist-provided patient care.
- By assessing a patient's progression through the stages of behavior modification, the pharmacist can assist in improving medication adherence.
- Preparing to communicate with other health care providers will support a more efficient and effective interaction.

22-2 STUDY GUIDE CHECKLIST

The following topics may guide your study of this subject area:

- ☐ Be aware of the barriers to communication and the way a pharmacist's verbal and nonverbal language affect the conversation.
- ☐ Be familiar with the "Single Health Literacy Screening Question," and know how to use it.
- ☐ Be able to use the "Three Prime Questions" for patient counseling.
- ☐ Be familiar with the components of a medication history.
- ☐ Recognize how the principles of behavior change relate to medication adherence.
- ☐ Be familiar with one's own cultural biases, and recognize how they might influence interactions with patients.

22-3 Introduction

Because the role of the pharmacist has transitioned from a task-centered practice to a patient-centered practice, effective communication skills are essential for providing patient care. The pharmacist must develop a trusting relationship with the patient that is based on open communication, cooperation, and mutual decision making, which will lead to a partnership with a common goal of improving health outcomes.

Communication between health care providers and patients serves two functions:

- It establishes an ongoing relationship between the health care provider and the patient.
- It provides an exchange of information that will allow the health care provider to assess a patient's health condition, manage treatment, and evaluate effects on quality of life.

An effective relationship allows the pharmacist to help the patient meet the mutually agreed-on health outcomes that improve the patient's quality of life. The goal is not to induce the patient to do as he or she is told but to help the patient reach the intended outcomes. Communication is a means of reaching an outcome, rather than the end itself.

22-4 Components of Interpersonal Communication

Interpersonal communication involves the following components:

- Generation of a message by an individual
- Transmission of the message from one individual to another
- Reception of the message
- Interpretation of the message

The message can be information, ideas, thoughts, emotions, and so on. The sender can transmit the message through oral (talking); nonverbal (using body posture, hand movements, facial expressions, etc.); and written forms. The receiver interprets the message and assigns a meaning to it.

Numerous communication barriers exist in the pharmacy patient-care setting and can affect interpersonal communication. They include but are not limited to the following:

- Environmental barriers (pharmacy counter, noise, crowds, lack of privacy)
- Personal (low self-confidence, shyness, internal monologue, lack of objectivity, cultural differences)
- Patient barriers (inaccurate perception of the pharmacist's role, the health care system, or the patient's medical condition)
- Administrative and financial barriers (high prescription volume, few support staff members, staff members not paid to talk)
- Lack of time

Feedback is a process by which the receiver can communicate his or her understanding of the message back to the sender. The original sender now becomes the receiver of the feedback or message. Feedback can mean giving a simple nonverbal gesture or asking the patient to repeat a complex set of instructions. Pharmacists can use feedback to ensure that the correct meaning of the message was interpreted.

22-5 Health Literacy

According to Healthy People 2010 (https://www.healthy people.gov/), health literacy is "the degree to which individuals have the capacity to obtain, process, and understand basic health information and services needed to make appropriate health decisions." Health literacy is framed in the context of health care, while general literacy is defined as the basic skills to read, write, and compute without regard to context. One study of health literacy found that 42% of patients could not read and comprehend directions for administering a medication on an empty stomach. Low health literacy can affect people from all ages, races, incomes, and education levels. Many patients who have low literacy levels (approximately half of Medicare and Medicaid recipients read below the fifth-grade level) may try to hide the problem from their health care provider because they are too ashamed or intimidated to ask for help.

Vulnerable populations include the following:

- Elderly people (age 65 or older)
- Minority populations
- Immigrant populations
- Low-income individuals
- People with chronic mental or physical health conditions

Pharmacists should seek to identify patients with low health literacy and develop appropriate visual or written materials.

A simple method for identifying patients with low health literacy is the Single Health Literacy Screening Question:

"How confident are you filling out medical forms by yourself?"

1-Extremely 2-Quite a bit 3-Somewhat 4-A little 5-Not at all

Scores of 3 or greater indicate inadequate health literacy.

Pharmacists should develop appropriate visual or written materials for patients with low health literacy. Health literacy best practices include limiting written information given to patients, using plain (or lay) language in written and verbal communication, and using the teach-back method to confirm patient understanding of shared information. The teach-back method involves asking the patient to repeat the instruction the pharmacist has just provided to the patient. Pharmacists should use patient tools and education developed for those with low health literacy (sixth-grade or below reading level).

The United States Pharmacopeia (USP) has created the USP Pictogram Library, which includes 81 pictograms that can be used to illustrate medication instructions and precautions.

22-6 Patient Interviewing and Counseling

Interviewing and counseling are two common communication skills the pharmacist must possess. The patient interview allows the pharmacist to obtain patient-specific information, which will help the pharmacist formulate a therapeutic plan, enhance patient satisfaction, and provide better patient care. Effective interviewing is a learned skill. The following are key points to consider when interviewing a patient:

- When opening the interview, always introduce yourself and state the purpose of the interview.
- Ask permission of the patient to speak about his or her health care in front of others (family members, friends, etc.).

- Appear professional, interested, confident, and relaxed to put the patient at ease during the interview.
- Establish and maintain a rapport with the patient by being personal.
- If necessary, take notes, but do not lose focus on the patient.
- Control the flow of information by asking only one question at a time.
- Politely redirect the patient to the line of questioning if he or she veers off topic.
- Give the patient ample time to recall information. Gently prod, but do not waste time if the patient cannot remember.

The use of open-ended questions is very helpful when gathering patient information. Open-ended questions are phrased in a manner that cannot be answered by a "yes" or a "no." An example of an open-ended question is, "How did the doctor tell you to take this medication?" This type of question requires the patient to provide much more information than just a "yes" or a "no." In contrast, the closed-ended question, "Did the doctor tell you how to take this medication?" can be answered with a "yes" or a "no."

When closing the interview, summarize to the patient the information you have gathered and explain the plan. Ask the patient if he or she has any questions.

The medication history is an interview with which the pharmacist should be familiar.

Medication History

Obtaining an accurate medication history is a vital skill that the pharmacist must employ. A medication history is much more than a list of medications the patient is taking. It includes allergies, past medications, adverse effects, and over-the-counter (OTC) medications. A comprehensive medication history should be conducted as follows:

- ***Allergies:*** What, when, where, outcomes
- ***Current prescription medications:*** Drug name, purpose, dose and frequency, duration, assessment of effects
- ***Past medication usage:*** Drug name, purpose, time period of use, reason for discontinuation
- ***Adverse drug effects:*** Medication, type of effect
- ***Use of OTC drugs, dietary supplements, and vitamins:*** Drug name, purpose, dose and frequency, duration, assessment of effects
- ***Other substances (tobacco, alcohol, illicit drugs):*** Amount, frequency, duration
- ***Adherence:*** Missed doses, reasons for nonadherence

Patient Counseling

Pharmacists are expected to counsel patients on the use of prescription medications. The Indian Health Service has developed a series of open-ended questions that elicits information the patient already has about his or her medications so the pharmacist can focus his or her efforts on providing information the patient lacks or correcting any misconceptions the patient may have about his or her medications. These questions, called the "Three Prime Questions," are listed below along with the information each question is designed to cover:

- ***"What did the doctor tell you the medicine is for?"*** Name of medication, purpose of medication
- ***"How did the doctor tell you to take the medication?"*** Dosing schedule, additional instructions, length of therapy, storage
- ***"What did the doctor tell you to expect?"*** Expected outcomes, precautions, possible side effects

22-7 Active Listening and Empathy

Active listening is a crucial component in professional communication. Whether one is gathering information from a patient regarding an adverse drug effect or taking a drug information request from another health care provider, listening is vital to the communication process.

Listening is an active process. It first involves the act of will. An individual must be willing to listen. Next, listening requires complete and undivided attention. In addition, the effective listener does not judge or evaluate the communication, problem, or feelings of the other person. This is not to say the pharmacist does not evaluate a clinical issue pertaining to the patient. However, if practicing active listening and empathy, the pharmacist will not evaluate the character of a person on the basis of the merits of the clinical issue.

Following are tips for effective listening:

- Stop talking.
- Eliminate distractions.
- Establish appropriate eye contact.
- Read nonverbal cues.
- Listen to *how* something is said.
- Provide feedback.

Empathetic responding is a by-product of active listening. Empathy means that one actually shares the experience of another. To be empathetic, one must identify with the affective experience of another. By communicating to patients that he or she acknowledges the patient's feelings, which are a result of a particular experience, the pharmacist is able to establish a caring, trusting relationship. Active listening and empathetic responding are the foundations of the pharmacist–patient relationship.

22-8 Assertiveness and Problem-Solving Techniques

Assertiveness is the direct expression of ideas, opinions, and desires. The pharmacist needs to behave assertively in a variety of settings, whether dealing with patients, other health care providers, administrators, or technicians. Assertiveness is not to be confused with aggressiveness. Aggressive behavior seeks to "win" in a conflict. Aggressive behavior does not respect the rights of others and often interrupts or dominates a conversation.

Assertive behavior can be characterized by the following:

- Directly expressing ideas, opinions, and desires
- Showing respect for self and others
- Being willing to openly and honestly communicate feelings, opinions, and needs
- Not violating the rights of others

Several problem-solving techniques have been identified to aid the pharmacist when interacting with individuals in a difficult situation. Each of these techniques is described as follows with an example:

- ***Fogging:*** Acknowledging possible truth from someone while ignoring any implied judgments about oneself:
  Patient: "$90! That's outrageous! You're trying to rip me off."
  Pharmacist: "Yes, this is an expensive medication. If you would like, I can call your doctor and discuss some less expensive alternatives."

- ***Being a broken record:*** Using calm repetition:
  Patient: "The doctor wrote this; you have to fill it!"
  Pharmacist: "I cannot fill this prescription as it is written." (Repeated over and over.)
- ***Using negative inquiry:*** Actively prompting feedback to use the information while prompting the critic to be more assertive and less dependent on manipulative ploys:
  Patient: "That is impossible! I can't give myself an insulin shot."
  Pharmacist: "What is it about giving yourself an insulin shot that bothers you?"
- ***Sorting issues:*** Separating several issues that are sandwiched together:
  Patient: "Why didn't you tell me he had cancer? We all play golf together. I thought we shared everything."
  Pharmacist: "We do share many things as golfing friends, but I am also his pharmacist. And as a pharmacist, I owe him confidentiality."
- ***Disarming anger:*** Offering an honest contract to someone who is exhibiting a lot of anger (writing it down is often helpful):
  Patient: "You gave me the wrong prescription! How could you do this? Do you know what I would have done to you if I would have taken the wrong medicine?"
  Pharmacist: "I didn't realize that an error occurred. Please start from the beginning, and I will write down all of the details."
- ***Selectively ignoring:*** Discriminatory attendance or nonattendance to specific content from another individual:
  Patient: "I'm not sure I can take this medication correctly without some further instructions. Let's have dinner tonight, and we can talk about this some more."
  Pharmacist: "I can explain the instructions to you now. What confuses you?"

22-9 Cultural Influences on Communication of Health Information

Because of the cultural diversity of the United States, pharmacists must be aware of their own culturally determined values and behaviors and be aware of other cultures. *Culture* is defined as a complex pattern of shared meanings, beliefs, and behaviors that are learned and acquired by a group of people during the course of history.

Culture can influence how people view others who are different from themselves. Because of the interactive role the pharmacist has with the patient, the health care team, and the community, pharmacists must strive to avoid certain negative viewpoints of other cultures:

- *Ethnocentrism* is the belief that one's own culture is superior while expressing contempt for another culture.
- *Prejudice* is a preconceived judgment or opinion of another person that is based on direct or indirect experiences.
- *Stereotypes* are fixed perceptions of a particular group or culture that reject the existence of individuality within that group or culture.

These biases can hamper the pharmacist's ability to obtain vital patient information and reach an accurate assessment of the patient.

Pharmacists should also be aware of how different cultures may interpret their communication. Conversation style varies from culture to culture. Some groups may prefer a more direct and to-the-point style, whereas others may prefer a more indirect style with an abundant amount of words. Health beliefs, family relationships, and communication style vary from culture to culture. To promote more effective communication, pharmacists should seek to identify these cultural differences in the patient population they serve and the health care providers with whom they work.

22-10 Group Presentation Skills

Pharmacists are frequently asked to present drug information in a small group setting. These groups may consist of laypersons with a particular disease, such as diabetes; a group of nurses who need to learn how to administer a new medication; a group of physicians requesting prescribing information for a complex medication; or a group of high school students interested in becoming pharmacists.

Before preparing the presentation, the pharmacist should assess the knowledge level of the group and design a presentation that is based on that assessment. For a group of laypeople, the effective presenter would avoid the use of jargon and speak in easy-to-understand lay terms. For a group of physicians, the pharmacist would prepare a presentation with up-to-date scientific evidence attesting to the validity of the information presented.

Time constraints should also be considered. Attempting to provide a large amount of material in a short time frame will only confuse and overwhelm the audience. The use of audiovisual aids can help enhance the overall effectiveness of the presentation but should not be a distraction. If appropriate, the pharmacist should involve the audience by asking questions to the group to encourage participation. Studies have shown that participants in an interactive presentation retain more information than do passive listeners. Allowing time for and encouraging questions from the audience at the end of the presentation is also important.

22-11 Documentation of Pharmacists' Recommendations and Consultations

Pharmacists document patient-care activities for numerous reasons, such as the following:

- To organize thought processes
- To provide continuity of care
- To obtain reimbursement
- To meet accreditation and quality assurance (The Joint Commission on accreditation of health care organizations, state) requirements
- To meet legal requirements (Omnibus Budget Reconciliation Act, state laws)
- To deal with litigation concerns
- To reinforce and create roles for pharmacists

The most common and universally recognized format for documenting patient information is the SOAP (subjective, objective, assessment, and plan) note:

- ***Subjective:*** The subjective portion contains information provided by the patient or the patient's caregivers. It includes complaints or symptoms reported by the patient in his or her own words (chief complaint), a recent history that pertains to those symptoms (history of present illness), the patient's past medical history, the home medication history, allergies, the patient's social and family history, and a review of symptoms.

- ***Objective:*** The objective portion contains data obtained from the patient that can be measured objectively. Such information includes vital signs, physical findings or physical examination results, laboratory test results, serum drug concentrations, diagnostic test results, and a computerized medication profile.
- ***Assessment:*** The assessment portion contains a record of the pharmacist's critical thinking and analysis. It is based on the information available in the subjective and objective portions of the note. If a new problem is identified, adding "newly identified" is common. Likewise, for existing problems, adding "worsened," "stable," or "resolved" is common. Many times, the rationale for the assessment includes published guidelines and recent literature.
- ***Plan:*** The plan portion contains the actions that were or will be taken to resolve the identified problems. The pharmacist should add detailed notes in recommendations involving drug therapy. He or she should provide the medication name, dose, route, frequency, and duration. Included in the plan is the follow-up necessary to ensure the problem is resolved. This follow-up includes monitoring parameters and the interval for the next assessment.

Patient records should always include the date and time of the documentation. The pharmacist should sign his or her name at the end of the SOAP note. Using medical terms is customary when documenting patient care. When writing in the medical record, the pharmacist should be sensitive, accurate, and brief. Do not place blame or state a cause-and-effect relationship. Be aware of litigation, because the patient record is a legal document.

22-12 Principles of Behavior Modification

Adhering to a new medication regimen often requires behavior change. For many patients, starting a new medication regimen can be as difficult as beginning a new exercise program, changing their diet, or ceasing smoking. The more complex the medication regimen, the more difficult may be the change. The goal of the pharmacist is not to force change but to assist patients in moving from being ambivalent to having the will to change. The transtheoretical model of change describes change as a process that occurs over time. The stages of the model are described in the following subsections.

Stage 1: Precontemplation

In this stage, people are not intending to take action in the future, which is usually measured as the next 6 months. People may be in this stage because they are uninformed about the consequences of their behavior. Interventions by the pharmacist at this stage should focus on nonjudgmental advice and information to patients considering change.

Stage 2: Contemplation

In this stage, people are thinking about changing and intending to change in the next 6 months. They are aware of the benefits of changing but also see the challenges or costs associated with the change. Interventions during this stage should aim at encouraging the patient to verbalize the benefits of change and ways to overcome the barriers to change.

Stage 3: Preparation

In this stage, people are intending to take action in the immediate future, which is usually measured as the next month. These individuals have made a conscious decision to take action toward change. Pharmacists can assist patients in this stage by providing specific strategies for success.

Stage 4: Action

In this stage, people have made specific overt modifications in their lifestyles within the past 6 months. Relapse is common at this stage. Continued positive reinforcement is critical to help prevent major relapses.

Stage 5: Maintenance

In the maintenance stage, people are working to prevent relapse, but they do not apply change processes as frequently as do people in action. They are less tempted to relapse and increasingly more confident that they can continue their change.

22-13 Communication with Other Health Care Providers

As a vital member of the health care team, pharmacists frequently interact with other health care providers. Pharmacists most frequently interact with physicians and nurses regarding medication therapy or drug-related problems. When interacting with other health care providers, pharmacists should use professional language instead of lay language as used with patients. Before communicating with other health care providers, the pharmacist should prepare for the interaction. This preparation includes gathering relevant patient information (name, date of birth, current medications, other relevant health information), a complete description of the drug-related problem, specific recommendations to resolve the problem, and possible literature citations and evidence-based guidelines to support recommendations. Usually, the information can be presented in the SOAP note format described in section 22-11. Most health care providers are familiar with the SOAP note format of documentation and communication.

22-14 Questions

1. Which of the following is the best description of feedback?

A. The pharmacist asks a patient, "Do you understand what I'm saying?"
B. The pharmacist tells the patient, "I understand what you are trying to say."
C. The "receiver" repeats back to the "sender" the former's understanding of the message.
D. Feedback is a typical technique that is used in everyday interactions.

2. Acknowledging possible truth from someone while ignoring any implied judgments about you describes which of the following assertive skills?

A. Sorting issues
B. Negative inquiry
C. Disarming anger
D. Fogging

3. What information should be covered through the first prime question during patient counseling?

A. Dosing schedule
B. Storage recommendations
C. Purpose of the medication
D. Possible side effects

4. What information should be covered through the second prime question during patient counseling?

A. Name of the medication
B. Expected outcomes
C. Possible side effects
D. Dosing instructions

5. What information should be covered through the third prime question during patient counseling?

A. Purpose of the medication
B. Storage recommendations
C. Possible side effects
D. Length of therapy

6. Generally, what key word should be used to ask an open-ended question?

A. Can
B. How
C. Will
D. Did

7. In general, what key word would *not* allow you to ask an open-ended question during a patient interview?

A. Do
B. How
C. When
D. What

8. The cultural bias, prejudice, can be defined as which of the following?

A. The belief that one's own culture is superior while expressing contempt for another culture.
B. A preconceived judgment or opinion of another person that is based on direct or indirect experiences.
C. A fixed perception of a particular group or culture that rejects the existence of individuality within that group or culture.
D. A complex pattern of shared meanings, beliefs, and behaviors that are learned and acquired by a group of people during the course of history.

9. Which of the following is a health literacy best practice for providing materials to patients with low health literacy?

A. Developing written materials on a tenth-grade reading level.
B. Using medical terminology when communicating verbally.
C. Using pictures to illustrate medication instructions.
D. Verifying patients understand instructions only if they look confused.

10. Which of the following best describes assertive behavior?

A. Talking over others.
B. Arguing your point to prove you are right regardless of how it affects others.
C. Directly expressing ideas, opinions, and desires.
D. Interrupting when others make illogical points.

11. During a medication history, which of the following is the most appropriate way to inquire about medication allergies?

A. "Do you have any allergies?"
B. "Tell me about any allergies you may have."
C. "What prescription medications are you allergic to?"
D. "Have you ever had an allergic reaction to any medications?"

12. Which of the following best describes the type of information that you should obtain when inquiring about a past medication?

A. Drug name, time frame for taking the drug, and cost of the medication
B. Drug dose, type of allergic reaction, and physician who prescribed drug
C. Drug name, purpose, time period of use, and reason for discontinuation
D. Reason for discontinuation, dispensing pharmacy, and side effects

13. Which of the following best describes the most complete medication history?

A. Allergies, current OTC products, current dietary supplements, and past medications
B. Past medications, current medications, adverse effects, and allergies
C. Illicit drug use, current medications, past medications, and allergies
D. Allergies; current prescription medications; past medications; adverse effects; current OTC medications, dietary supplements, and vitamins; and any alcohol, tobacco, or illicit drug use

14. Which of the following best describes the type of information that you should obtain when inquiring about a current medication?

A. Drug name, purpose, time period of use, and reason for discontinuation
B. Drug name, purpose, dose and frequency, duration, and assessment of effects
C. Drug name, date started, dose, outcomes, and cost
D. What, when, where, and outcomes

15. Which of the following best describes the type of information that you should obtain when inquiring about alcohol, tobacco, or illicit drug use?

A. Amount, frequency, and duration
B. Type, cost, and amount
C. Amount, duration, and name
D. Duration and age

16. Which of the following should the subjective portion of the SOAP note contain?

A. Recommendations, new medications, follow-up, and patient education
B. An evaluation of the findings based on gathered information
C. The way the patient feels, reported information from the patient, and observations that the patient makes about himself or herself
D. The health care team's observations, physical findings, and lab results

17. Which portion of the SOAP note does the following statement best fit?

"Recommend acetaminophen 500 mg every 6 hours as needed for headache. Do not exceed 4,000 mg per day. Return to the pharmacy in 1 week to reassess headache. If headache continues, will refer patient to physician."

A. Subjective
B. Objective
C. Assessment
D. Plan

18. Which portion of the SOAP note do the following vital signs (taken by a nurse) and lab results best fit?

BP: 164/98 mmHg; Pulse: 86; Temp: 98.7°F; Resp: 18; Wt: 163 lb

Labs—K: 4.5; Na: 135; Cr: 1.2; BUN: 17

A. Subjective
B. Objective
C. Assessment
D. Plan

19. Which of the following can be a barrier to active listening and appropriate communication in a community pharmacy setting?

A. Reading of nonverbal cues
B. Lack of privacy
C. Appropriate eye contact
D. Provision of feedback

20. Which of the following statements is true of health literacy?

A. Health literacy is defined as the basic skills required to read and write.
B. Most Medicare and Medicaid recipients read above a ninth-grade level.
C. Low health literacy can affect people from all ages, races, incomes, and education levels.
D. Most patients will report they have low health literacy.

21. ____________ is the belief that one's own culture is superior while expressing contempt for another culture.

A. Stereotype
B. Ethnocentrism
C. Cultural awareness
D. Prejudice

22. At which stage, in the transtheoretical model of change, is an individual thinking about changing and intending to change in the next 6 months?

A. Precontemplation
B. Contemplation
C. Action
D. Preparation

22-15 Answers

1. C. Feedback is a process by which the receiver can communicate his or her understanding of the message back to the sender. Although not used in everyday interaction, this technique can prevent many miscommunications.

2. **D.** Fogging allows the individual to address issues of importance without delving into any implied judgments made because of the stress of the situation.

3. **C.** The first prime question is "What did the doctor tell you this medication is for?"

4. **D.** The second prime question is "How did the doctor tell you to take this medication?"

5. **C.** The third prime question is "What did the doctor tell you to expect from this medication?"

6. **B.** A question beginning with "how" cannot be answered with a "yes" or a "no."

7. **A.** A question beginning with "do" can be answered with a "yes" or a "no."

8. **B.** Choice A is ethnocentrism, choice C is stereotype, and choice D is culture.

9. **C.** The use of pictures can help patients understand medications if they have difficulty comprehending written instructions.

10. **C.** Assertive behavior is not aggressive or disrespectful of others.

11. **B.** Choices A and D are closed-ended questions. C is not the best choice because patients may also be allergic to OTC medications, foods, or dietary supplements.

12. **C.** Choice C provides the most complete and useful information regarding a past medication.

13. **D.** Choice D provides the most complete and useful information regarding the patient's current and past medication use.

14. **B.** Choice B provides the most complete and useful information regarding a current medication.

15. **A.** Choice A provides the most complete and useful information regarding alcohol, tobacco, or illicit drug use.

16. **C.** The subjective portion contains information provided by the patient or the patient's caregivers.

17. **D.** The plan portion contains the actions that were or will be taken to resolve the identified problems.

18. **B.** The objective portion contains data obtained from the patient that can be measured objectively.

19. **B.** A lack of privacy can distract from communication. All other answers can enhance communication.

20. **C.** Low health literacy can affect people from all ages, races, incomes, and education levels.

21. **B.** Ethnocentrism is the belief that one's own culture is superior while expressing contempt for another culture.

22. **C.** At the contemplation stage, an individual is thinking about changing and intending to change in the next 6 months.

22-16 Additional Resources

Beardsley RS, Kimberlin CL, Tindall WN. *Communication Skills in Pharmacy Practice.* 6th ed. Baltimore, MD: Lippincott, Williams & Wilkins; 2012.

Berger BA. *Communication Skills for Pharmacists.* 3rd ed. Washington, DC: American Pharmacists Association; 2009.

Chew LD, Griffin JM, Partin MR, et al. Validation of screening questions for limited health literacy in a large VA outpatient population. *J Gen Intern Med.* 2008;23(5):561–566.

Haig KM, Sutton S, Whittington J. SBAR: a shared mental model for improving communication between clinicians. *Jt Comm J Qual Patient Saf.* 2006;32:165–175.

Health Literacy. Centers for Disease Control and Prevention. Available at: https://www.cdc.gov/healthliteracy/learn/index.html. Accessed November 30, 2017.

Jones RM. *Patient Assessment in Pharmacy Practice.* 3rd ed. Baltimore, MD: Lippincott, Williams & Wilkins; 2015.

Rantucci MJ. *Pharmacists Talking with Patients: A Guide to Patient Counseling.* 2nd ed. Baltimore, MD: Lippincott, Williams & Wilkins; 2007.

USP Pictogram Library. United States Pharmacopeia. Available at: http://www.usp.org/health-quality-safety/usp-pictograms. Accessed November 30, 2017.

Social and Behavioral Aspects of Pharmacy Practice

23

LA'MARCUS T. WINGATE

23-1 KEY POINTS

- Individual behaviors affect health outcomes more than any other single factor and are pivotal in maintaining well-being when patients are healthy as well as ill.
- Medication adherence can be measured using both direct and indirect methods. Direct methods are more accurate, but indirect methods are used more often in practice.
- Adherence is affected by several factors including those related to the patient, the health system, type of therapy, medical conditions, and socioeconomic factors.
- Strategies used to facilitate openness with patients are to listen, acknowledge, wonder, recognize, question, and reflect.
- Patients place extremely high value on the perceived degree of personal attention received from the pharmacist.
- Pharmacists are crucial providers during end-of-life care.
- Pharmacists meet patients' expectations in general; however, room for improvement exists in extending care to patients who are not physically in the pharmacy.
- Pharmaceutical care refers to the pharmacist's obligation to meet all of the patient's drug-related needs, to be held accountable for fulfilling those needs, and to help the patient accomplish his or her medical goals by partnering with other health care professionals.
- Core elements of a medication therapy management program are a medication therapy review, a personal medication record, a medication action plan, intervention and referral, and documentation and follow-up.
- The collaborative working relationships model has been used to evaluate the degree of collaboration between physicians and pharmacists. It consists of five stages: professional awareness, professional recognition, exploration and trial, professional relationship expansion, and commitment to collaborative working relationships.
- Three types of characteristics in the collaborative working relationships model that influence collaboration are participant, context, and exchange characteristics.
- The predominant leadership theories are the trait, behavioral, and situational theories, with situational theory being the most accepted.
- The most effective leadership styles demonstrated within situational theory are the transformational, affiliative, democratic, and coaching styles.
- Professional networks can be beneficial in many ways and are pivotal for young practitioners to establish.
- Every pharmacist having at least some degree of involvement in political action to facilitate advancement of the profession is vital.

23-2 STUDY GUIDE CHECKLIST

The following topics may guide your study of this subject area:

- [ ] Demonstrate an understanding of the roles that patients must play in maintaining their health when they are healthy as well as ill.
- [ ] Describe factors that may influence a patient's adherence to medications and what strategies pharmacists may use to enhance adherence.
- [ ] Apply principles of patient-centered pharmaceutical care to facilitate productive communication and maximize satisfaction.
- [ ] Describe the types of roles pharmacists may fulfill in end-of-life situations.
- [ ] Apply principles of the collaborative working relationships model to foster healthy relationships with other health professionals.
- [ ] Compare and contrast the many different types of leadership styles that are available for pharmacists.
- [ ] Describe the benefits of being involved in professional networks, especially with regard to new pharmacists.
- [ ] Understand the importance of being involved in some type of advocacy that helps to advance the profession.

23-3 Overview

The social and behavioral aspects of pharmacy may be underappreciated in many educational curriculums, but these facets of practice are actually quite important with regard to health outcomes and patients' satisfaction. Patients' perception of the amount of personal attention the pharmacist gives them is often a greater factor in determining their satisfaction than is the amount of pharmaceutical care they receive. This chapter provides an overview of several principles including the behavioral decisions of patients, adherence, and end-of-life situations. Additionally, this chapter covers pharmacy as a patient-centered profession, the perceptions of patients and health care professionals regarding pharmacists' capabilities, the role of the pharmacist in patient care, the role of the pharmacist in interactions with other health care professionals, the development of leadership skills, and the importance of involvement in pharmacy organizations.

23-4 The Role of a Patient's Behaviors in Health

There are several types of decisions patients make on a regular basis that can affect their health. These decisions are reflected in patients' behaviors regarding several areas such as tobacco consumption, excessive alcohol intake, poor dietary habits, lack of physical activity, illicit drug use, and unsafe sexual practices. Collectively, these types of modifiable individual risk factors are known as *behavioral determinants* of health. These risk factors are fairly common among individuals in the United States. For example, approximately 25% of adults consume tobacco products and more than one third of adults are obese. The corresponding effect of behavioral determinants on health in substantial. Consumption of tobacco alone is associated with more than 450,000 preventable deaths annually, and being either overweight or obese is directly related to more than 200,000 preventable deaths each year. Likewise, adoption of specific dietary habits such as excessive salt intake, inadequate consumption of omega-3 fatty acids, and excess consumption of dietary trans fats contribute independently to at least 50,000 otherwise preventable deaths annually.

When considered collectively, behavioral decisions at the individual level are the single most important factor affecting population health, even more so than health care. Whereas components of health care such as adequate access to well-trained health care providers, up-to-date medical facilities, and properly managed medications are integral for patients with disease, individual behavioral decisions affect everyone, including those who are relatively healthy at the present moment as well as those who are ill. Notably, personal behaviors can assist in prevention of illness and disease at three levels: primary prevention, secondary prevention, and tertiary prevention.

Primary prevention involves any type of action that is designed to prevent disease even before it occurs, with an emphasis on reducing the number of risk factors an individual has that may predispose him or her to contracting disease. Examples of primary prevention may include obtaining vaccinations and abstaining from smoking. Patients may engage in primary prevention even when they are not acutely ill or have no chronic disease.

Secondary prevention efforts are designed to minimize complications of an illness or disease by initiating treatment during the early stage of disease, oftentimes when a patient is still asymptomatic. An example of secondary prevention could be undergoing screening for blood glucose or blood pressure levels to identify illness at an early stage.

Tertiary prevention efforts focus on minimizing complications after an individual has been diagnosed with disease and trying to maximize quality of life. Examples of activities that could be a part of tertiary prevention for patients with longstanding diabetes include optimizing pharmacotherapy to control HbA1c and prevent microvascular complications and having patients monitor their blood glucose levels and feet on a regular basis. In this example, one can see that once a patient has an established disease, health care providers can recommend appropriate evidence-based medical interventions. However, the patient continues to play a role in maintaining his or her health. The patient must continue to attend medical appointments as appropriate, make wise decisions concerning his or her daily health-related behaviors, and follow any other advice given by health care providers.

23-5 Adherence Principles

Measurement of Adherence and Terminology

Adherence is the term used to indicate the degree to which a patient follows advice and instructions given by a health care professional to help improve or maintain the patient's health. *Persistence* is a related term that indicates the duration of time that a patient takes a medication. In the broadest sense, adherence can refer to several types of behaviors, such as complying with recommendations for diet and exercise and keeping appointments with health care professionals. However, the bulk of what is known about adherence is related to how well patients take medications in relation to instructions received from health care providers.

Several modalities are available for measuring medication adherence, which generally fall into one of two categories: direct methods or indirect methods. *Direct methods* of ascertaining adherence are generally more accurate and include directly observing a patient take a medication, taking a measure of the drug or metabolite in the blood, and measuring a biological marker that is produced by the drug. *Indirect methods* of evaluating adherence include patient surveys, counting the number of pills in a patient's possession, and assessing the number of doses a patient has had using pharmacy claims databases. The direct methods of ascertaining medication adherence are most accurate. Indirect methods of assessment may be less accurate because a patient may not take a medication even if it is in his or her possession. Nevertheless, direct methods are used less often in practice because they are very labor intensive and can be expensive.

The single most common metric used to measure medication adherence is the *medication possession ratio* (MPR). The MPR is derived by determining the number of days for which a patient has medication and dividing this number by the total number of days the patient is being observed. This value can range from 0 to 100%. For example, if a period of 180 days is being evaluated, and it is determined that a patient has enough medication to take prescribed doses on 130 of those days, the MPR is 72.2%. An MPR of least 80% is generally considered to be good and desirable for sufficient therapeutic effects when taking medications.

Factors Affecting Adherence

The *multidimensional adherence model* is one model that can be used in explaining factors that may affect a patient's adherence to medication. Several categories of factors are proposed to play a role in a patient's adherence to medication:

- *Patient-related* factors can include patients' ability to remember to take medications, beliefs regarding the efficacy of medications, or limited knowledge regarding the disease state.
- *Health system* factors that can affect adherence include lack of adequate communication from health care providers, poor relationships between the health care provider and the patient, insurance systems that make access to medication difficult, and high medication costs.
- *Therapy-related* factors include side effects caused by the drug, complex regimens requiring medications to be taken multiple times during the day, frequent changes in the medications prescribed, and previous situations where a patient recalls taking a medication and it may have been ineffective.

- *Socioeconomic* factors affecting adherence include limited health literacy, language barriers, and limited access to pharmacies or other health care providers because of a relative lack of these types of health care providers in close geographic proximity.
- *Condition-related* factors refer to some type of impairment that may impede a patient's ability to take medication properly (e.g., impaired vision, which may impede a patient's ability to read the instructions on a bottle).

Modifying Behavior and Enhancing Adherence

Pharmacists may employ a multitude of strategies when trying to improve a patient's adherence to medications. In general, they should utilize strategies that help address any types of barriers identified that may prevent the patient from taking the medication properly. For example, when a patient has limited knowledge regarding the efficacy of a medication, the pharmacist must educate the patient concerning the benefits of the medication. However, pharmacists can routinely implement certain practices that may help enhance adherence as characterized by the mnemonic SIMPLE:

- *Simplifying regimen characteristics:* Try to reduce the number of pills a patient may take by using an extended-release medication or a pill with more than one drug if possible. In addition, consider the use of pill organizers.
- *Imparting appropriate knowledge:* Pharmacists should make a practice of consistently educating patients regarding the purpose of the drug in language they can understand. Here the emphasis is on the pharmacist talking to the patient.
- *Modifying beliefs and human behavior:* Pharmacists can go beyond informing a patient about his or her disease and medications by evaluating the patient's belief about the disease and medications. Here the emphasis is on the patient being allowed to convey what he or she believes about his or her medications and disease.
- *Patient communication:* Pharmacists should put an emphasis on communicating with a patient even when he or she is not physically in the pharmacy by sending reminders or calling the patient. In some cases, establishing a line of communication with the patient's family may be worthwhile.
- *Leave the bias:* All health care providers, including pharmacists, must resist the fallacy of believing that some patients are relegated to poor adherence on the basis of their race, income, or social history. Instead, providers should believe that all patients are capable of adhering to therapy properly if given the appropriate care.
- *Evaluate adherence:* Pharmacists can help optimize adherence by periodically evaluating how well patients are meeting adherence goals.

23-6 Pharmacy as a Patient-Centered Profession

Dimensions of Patient-Centeredness

The term *patient-centeredness* has been used to characterize the relationship between physicians and patients. Patient-centeredness involves five dimensions, which describe various aspects of the doctor–patient relationship:

- The *biopsychosocial perspective* dimension involves the combination of biological, psychological, and social factors critical not only to the successful treatment of a patient but also to the etiology of the patient's illness.
- The *patient-as-person* dimension of patient-centeredness involves recognizing that a disease affects each person in a different manner; therefore, patient-centered medicine aims to take into account

the individual's experience with an illness and use it to construct a treatment plan that is best for that particular patient.

- The *sharing of power and responsibility* between patients and physicians is also a crucial aspect of the patient-centered approach to medicine.
- The *therapeutic alliance* dimension specifies that a treatment decision takes into account not only the health care provider's wishes but also the desires and perceived barriers of the patient.
- The *doctor-as-person* dimension recognizes that the health care provider is not simply an objective purveyor of information but instead has some type of emotional attachment with respect to his or her patients. The doctor-as-person dimension of patient-centered medicine takes into account the influence that the health care provider has on the patient as well as the influence the patient has on the health care provider.

Recently, though, patient-centeredness has been expanded in the literature to include the relationship between patients and their pharmacists. By definition, pharmacists are expected to be the drug experts; however, their expertise in pharmacology and pharmacotherapy can alienate the patient if patient-centeredness is not successfully incorporated also. Pharmacists' natural inclination is to rely on their in-depth knowledge of pharmacology and medications to counsel patients, yet those in the profession of pharmacy must embrace the idea of openness to achieve patient-centeredness.

Strategies to Facilitate Openness

Openness is an idea that emphasizes the need to treat each patient as an individual. Openness recognizes that social, cultural, and socioeconomic factors differ among patients, and these factors contribute to an individual patient's health care–related behavior. Pharmacists can use six strategies to enhance the openness in their relationships and encounters with patients. The following three strategies can be used in everyday encounters with patients at the pharmacy:

- ***Listen:*** Listening involves being attentive and realizing and understanding that each patient has his or her own story and experience with a particular disease.
- ***Acknowledge:*** Acknowledging each patient as his or her own individual lets the patient know that the pharmacist understands his or her unique needs.
- ***Wonder:*** The strategy of wondering encourages the pharmacist to be inquisitive and to question whether what is happening to the patient is possible.

Recognize, question, and reflect are also important strategies that pharmacists can use to strengthen their relationship with patients:

- ***Recognize:*** Pharmacists should recognize that they may have preconceived notions and values that may influence their interactions with patients.
- ***Question:*** Pharmacists should make a habit of questioning themselves to identify whether they may be allowing preconceived notions to influence the way they interact with patients.
- ***Reflect:*** Pharmacists should reflect on their daily encounters with patients and use these reflections to improve future patient encounters.

23-7 End-of-Life Issues

One time that is especially important for pharmacists to exercise patient-centeredness is during palliative care situations. By definition, *palliative care* uses a holistic patient-and-family-centered approach to relieve the pain and suffering associated with severe illness to achieve the best possible quality of life and comfort under these circumstances. Whereas *hospice care* also focuses on maintaining comfort and improving quality of life, it is differentiated by its use in situations where the patient has a terminal illness and death is thought to be imminent so that curative care is no longer needed. Both hospice and palliative care are given in end-of-life situations and may be rendered in an inpatient setting, a nursing home, long-term care facility, or the patient's residence. During end-of-life situations, pharmacists can expect to be part of a multidisciplinary team that attends to a patient's physical, emotional, spiritual, and psychosocial needs.

Pharmacists can play several important roles on the interdisciplinary teams managing patients' end-of-life situations because of the unique aspects during this phase of care. During this time, many medications may have to be administered via alternative routes of administration. Pharmacists are able to leverage their expertise in compounding to produce parenteral preparations, solutions, patches, and ointments to facilitate administration of medications when oral routes are not available. Additionally, pharmacists may use their compounding skills in formulating oral preparations that require higher dosages than commercially available. Moreover, a patient's normal kinetics and volume of distribution may change during this time, so that a pharmacist's expertise is essential in identifying the appropriate doses of medication. This skill is especially important in regard to pain medications, where pharmacists may be called upon to make frequent dosage conversions for opioid-containing products.

An important decision that should be made in consultation with the patient and his or her family is whether or not to discontinue certain medications that offer no immediate benefit. Discontinuing certain classes of medications such as statins and antihypertensives can decrease the likelihood of patients experiencing an adverse effect without sacrificing comfort or quality of life in this patient population. Recognizing that patients in end-of-life situations may be candidates to receive therapy to manage conditions that arise as a result of ongoing and persistent pain is also prudent. Such conditions include depression, insomnia, and anxiety.

23-8 Perceptions of Patients and Other Health Care Providers Regarding Pharmacists' Capabilities

Patients' Tangible and Intangible Perceptions of Pharmacists' Capabilities

The bulk of the literature dealing with patients' expectations of pharmacists' duties is related to the traditional dispensing process in the community and ambulatory care settings. Tangible aspects of what patients expect from the dispensing process include the amount of time they have to wait for the prescription or the quality of the patient handouts that accompany the medication. Patients base their expectation of the quality of these tangible properties on their prior experiences with pharmacies. Patients also expect intangible aspects such as friendly customer service. Patients form an opinion of the quality of these factors based on what would take place in an ideal setting. Although intangible aspects may be hard to measure, they are very important to patients. Some data suggest that patients place the most value on the "personal attention" they receive from pharmacists. Personal attention includes the following attributes:

- Patients' perceptions of the pharmacists' friendliness
- Prompt attention
- Willingness of the pharmacist to spend time with the patient

In fact, the personal attention of the pharmacist is a greater factor in determining patient satisfaction than the amount of pharmaceutical care patients believe they receive or their perception of the pharmacist's ability to help them manage their disease.

Success of Pharmacists in Meeting Patients' Expectations

In general, pharmacists do well in meeting the expectations of patients related to the dispensing process. Nationally, pharmacists meet the expectations of more than 75% of patients in matters such as telling patients the purpose of the medication, dosing frequency, possible side effects, and drug–drug and drug–food interactions. Aspects related to personal attention that both pharmacists and patients value highly include communicating a desire to help patients, listening closely to patrons, and being easily approachable. However, pharmacists have opportunities to improve some aspects related to personal attention. Many of these aspects involve instances where the patient is no longer physically present in the pharmacy. For example, pharmacists can remind patients to refill their prescription or call to find out how the medication is working.

The general sentiment is that the general public and other health care professionals do not fully appreciate pharmacists' abilities. For example, even though patients trust pharmacists to perform functions related to the traditional dispensing process, many patients consider physicians to be the primary source of information regarding their medications and pharmacists to be a secondary source of information. Moreover, patients tend to believe that physicians rather than pharmacists are the best sources for instructing them on how to take their medications properly, and physicians are the health care professional patients prefer to call if they have questions. Patients tend to believe that physicians are qualified to perform all the tasks they expect pharmacists to be able to perform, in addition to other tasks that they may perceive pharmacists as unqualified to perform, such as telling them when the medication should begin to show pharmacologic effects and what to do if they miss a dose.

Patients' Acceptance of Nontraditional Pharmacy Roles

Pharmacists have worked hard to garner more involvement in patient care. They have progressively ventured beyond providing only traditional dispensing functions and proved that they can provide other cognitive services that are not directly connected with dispensing medications. Several studies have indicated that many patients in the general population would be willing to pay modest amounts out of pocket for a pharmacist to deliver cognitive services such as blood glucose monitoring, private counseling, cholesterol screening, immunizations, education sessions on disease management, or help in selecting over-the-counter medications. However, the proportion of elderly patients willing to pay for these types of services may be lower. One can reasonably assume that if patients are willing to pay for cognitive services, they must believe pharmacists are capable of providing these services. Yet other patients may be unwilling to pay for cognitive services but still believe that pharmacists are capable of providing these services. Therefore, in the current environment, the majority of patients believe that pharmacists are at least somewhat capable of doing more than traditional pharmacy dispensing functions.

Physicians' Perceptions of Pharmacists' Capabilities

Physicians have also progressively accepted an expanded role for the pharmacist. Yet literature indicates that some physicians assume that they should have primary responsibility for many factors related to drug therapy, such as counseling patients about the dose of the drug, the onset of the medication's effect, the length of time the patient should take the medication, and the measures that should be taken if problems arise. Regardless of the setting, physicians expect pharmacists to be knowledgeable about drugs, to educate the patient on his or her medications, and to maintain good medication profiles on patients. In the hospital setting, physicians want pharmacists to be able to educate patients about their medications, monitor the response to drug therapy, and know the indication for a drug. Physicians' greatest expectations of pharmacists in the community setting are for them to be able to help patients obtain refills in a timely fashion and select appropriate over-the-counter medications. However, some studies indicate that a large proportion of physicians express apprehension about pharmacists in the community setting monitoring the outcomes of drug therapy or treating minor ailments. Nevertheless, physicians' acceptance of the expanded role of pharmacists in patient care is becoming more and more common.

23-9 The Role of the Pharmacist in Patient Care

The phrase *pharmaceutical care* explicitly illustrates the role of pharmacists in patient care. Pharmaceutical care can be thought of as a philosophy that "focuses on the responsibility of the pharmacist to meet all of the patient's drug-related needs, be held accountable for meeting those needs, and assist the patient in achieving his or her medical goals through collaboration with other health professionals" (McGivney et al. 2007). *Medication therapy management* (MTM) is a practical method to incorporate pharmaceutical care into the traditional practice of pharmacy. MTM is a set of services that are specific to a particular patient's drug therapy and medical needs. MTM services include, but are not limited to, the following:

- Performing a comprehensive medication review
- Identifying and resolving drug therapy problems
- Addressing issues of compliance
- Functioning as a disease management coach
- Helping select the appropriate medications with the aid of pharmacogenomic profiles

The American Pharmacists Association and the National Association of Chain Drug Stores have identified and updated the core elements that every MTM program should include. These core elements are as follows:

- A medication therapy review
- A personal medication record that lists not only the medications being taken but also their directions for use, their indications, and the prescriber
- A medication action plan
- Intervention and referral
- Documentation and follow-up

Since MTM's recognition in the Medicare Prescription Drug, Improvement, and Modernization Act of 2003, many efforts have been made to quantify not only the type of drug therapy problems encountered and benefits to the patient but also MTM's benefit to the health care system as a whole. The Asheville Project, a community-based MTM program for hypertension and dyslipidemia, demonstrated that the following indicators of cardiovascular and cerebrovascular health were improved over a 6-year period: mean systolic blood pressure, mean diastolic blood pressure, percentage of patients at blood pressure goal, mean low-density lipoprotein cholesterol, and mean serum triglycerides. Patients in the Asheville Project experienced a decrease in the risk of cardiovascular events by 53% when compared to historical controls. Interestingly, participation in the Asheville Project also reduced medical costs associated with cardiovascular or cerebrovascular events by 46.5%. The Asheville Project is not the only example that has exhibited both clinical and economic benefits. Similar programs have shown improvements in Healthcare Effectiveness Data and Information Set (HEDIS) measures for hypertension and dyslipidemia while also achieving significant cost savings and cost avoidances. As the profession of pharmacy continues to embrace the idea and practice of pharmaceutical care in the form of MTM and expand its scope of practice, the role of pharmacy and pharmacists in patient care will become more evident and influential.

23-10 The Role of the Pharmacist in Interactions with Other Health Care Professionals

Barriers to Interaction between Pharmacists and Physicians

Most information concerning pharmacists' interactions with other health care professionals concentrates on the relationship with physicians. In general, the degree of communication between pharmacists and physicians is believed to be suboptimal. Several reasons have been cited for this problem, such as a lack of assurance among pharmacists in their ability to approach physicians, the lack of immediate physical proximity in the case of community pharmacists, and physicians' views that pharmacists sometimes call about matters that the physicians perceive as trivial. Most pharmacists (more than 80%) in the community setting report contacting physicians' offices on a daily basis regarding patients' medication issues; however, most of the time, they speak with the nurse.

Collaborative Working Relationships Model

One prevalent model used in assessing the degree of collaboration between pharmacists and physicians is the *collaborative working relationships model*. This model proposes that the relationship between pharmacists and physicians can evolve through greater levels of collaboration:

- In stage 0, *professional awareness,* minimal interaction occurs between pharmacists and their physician counterparts.
- In stage 1, *professional recognition,* pharmacists begin to initiate contact with physicians in hopes of establishing positive rapport.
- In stage 2, *exploration and trial,* pharmacists continue to initiate contact while physicians give greater consideration to the risks and benefits involved with this communication.
- In stage 3, *professional relationship expansion,* physicians begin to initiate communication with pharmacists.
- In stage 4, *commitment to collaborative working relationships,* both pharmacists and physicians are determined to maintain and strengthen the relationship, and physicians are convinced that pharmacists offer more benefit than risk.

Although much time and effort may be required to develop collaborative working relationships, they are well worth the effort. These types of relationships have led physicians to entrust pharmacists with a great amount of responsibility, including managing patients with chronic disease states such as diabetes, hypertension, or hyperlipidemia.

The collaborative working relationships model proposes three groups of characteristics—participant, context, and exchange—that can contribute to successful collaborative working relationships:

- *Participant characteristics* reflect personal traits, such as the physician's age, experience, years of residency training, and type of practice.
- *Context characteristics* include properties such as the physician's physical proximity to the pharmacist, any academic affiliations, the practice setting, and the volume of patients seen.
- *Exchange characteristics* refer to how proactive the physician believes the pharmacist is in initiating contact, the amount of trust the physician has in the pharmacist, and the degree to which the roles are specified in the relationship between the physician and pharmacist. The exchange characteristics are the most important in helping establish a collaborative relationship between physicians and pharmacists.

Scarce literature is available regarding the relationship of pharmacists with other health care professionals such as nurses. However, the available studies show that these relationships can have positive outcomes in areas such as medication reconciliation. Regardless of the number of studies that have been conducted in this area, pharmacists need to be proactive in contributing their skills to the health care team. This action will not only help the pharmacy profession grow but also will help enhance patient care. When pharmacists see an unfilled opportunity that they have the ability to meet, they should be willing to take a leadership role in accomplishing the task.

23-11 The Development of Leadership Skills

Definition of Leadership

Pharmacists must be leaders on many levels. Believing that those with prestigious positions in pharmacy organizations are leaders is natural. However, every pharmacist, even the staff pharmacist, is a leader at some level because pharmacists are expected to provide leadership for others working with them, such as pharmacy technicians and other staff members. As mentioned previously, pharmacists also have the capability to be leaders in the health care field when they recognize unmet needs in the health care system and are willing to take the lead role in filling those voids. *Leadership* can be defined as the process through which an individual attempts to intentionally influence another individual or group to accomplish a goal.

Definition of Power and Types of Power

Power can be defined as the ability to exert influence on others, and it is derived through various means. *Formal power* is derived as a result of the position one holds within a particular organization. *Reward power* is held as a consequence of being able to reward subordinates. *Punishment power* is derived from being able to discipline others for undesired behavior. *Expert power* is wielded by a person as a consequence of being extremely proficient in the skills, knowledge, and abilities required to perform well in his or her field. A person holds *charismatic power* whenever he or she exhibits certain charismatic traits that cause others to want to follow that person and his or her vision.

Leadership Theories

Some theories that have been developed to help recognize what makes effective leaders are as follows:

- ***Trait theory:*** This theory proposes that people are born with certain traits that predispose them to being a good leader. The traits most consistently evident in determining good leaders are drive, motivation, integrity, self-confidence, intelligence, and knowledge. Nevertheless, relying exclusively on traits to identify potential leaders is discouraged.
- ***Behavioral theory:*** This theory asserts that people are not born as leaders but rather develop leadership capabilities over time. The behavioral theory proposes that two types of leaders exist: task-oriented leaders, who place more emphasis on the task to be accomplished, and follower-oriented leaders, who place greater importance on the well-being of the workers.
- ***Situational theory:*** The most highly regarded leadership theory, situational theory asserts that successful leadership depends on an individual being able to adapt to the surrounding circumstances and to use the appropriate leadership skills for the specific situation. Many types of leadership styles can be used in different situations:
  - The *coercive leadership style* relies heavily on reward and punishment power; it is heavily task oriented.
  - Leaders who rely primarily on charismatic power are said to use the *transformational style,* a style that has proved effective in more situations than any other leadership style.
  - When leaders are heavily follower oriented and use reward power more than punishment power, they are said to be using an *affiliative style* of leadership.

- The *democratic style* of leadership is characterized by leaders wl have a role in the decision-making process.
- In the *pacesetting style,* leaders expect extremely high standards
- In the *coaching style* of leadership, leaders place high value on c they, too, will be able to take on leadership roles in the future.

Overall, the most effective leadership styles are the transformational, affili approaches.

Stages of Leadership

A widely accepted view holds that leadership is developed over time. P leadership role may be in the first phase of leadership, where they are tive as leaders—they are not even aware that they need to work on deve time, individuals may progress to phase two. In this phase, they are cc because they understand that their leadership skills need development b some capacities. Over time, individuals may arrive at phase three, whe At this point, they have learned to be effective leaders but are still co leadership capabilities. Eventually, leaders may reach phase four, wher leadership is second nature to them.

23-12 The Importance of Involvement in Pharr and Regulatory, State, and Federal Issu

Playing a Role in Moving Pharmacy Forward

After graduating from pharmacy school, many new practitioners cease the state, and national pharmacy organizations. Whether the inactivity of r are completely overwhelmed with their new roles as professionals and th this change or because they feel they will not have as central a role as organizations as they did as members in their student chapters is uncle the demographic makeup of professional organizations, the majority c new practitioners (defined as having worked as a licensed pharmacist fc pharmacy professional organizations provides not only an opportunity t to continue the lifelong learning process and, perhaps most important, development.

Establishing Professional Networks

The most obvious benefit of participating in a professional organizatic professional network. White (2007) describes this network as a group one of the following functions:

- Assist in having a professionally challenging and satisfying caree
- Provide insight about how the pharmacy world functions.
- Provide ideas about how to resolve therapeutic or service challen vices organize and process their work, or how new regulations a
- Provide advice about difficult work situations.
- Assist with exploring career options and finding another pharma
- Assist with writing and publishing scholarly literature.

o allow their subordinates to

of their followers.

eveloping followers so that

tive, democratic, and coaching

eople who have just begun in a
aid to be unaware and ineffec-
loping their leadership skills. In
nsidered aware and ineffective
t are still relatively ineffective in
e they are aware and effective.
stantly striving to improve their
e they are effective leaders and

acy Organizations
es

r extensive participation in local,
ew practitioners is because they
e responsibilities that accompany
new practitioners in professional
ar. However, when one looks at
active members are clearly not
5 years or less). Participation in
network but also an opportunity
participate in professional policy

n is the opportunity to develop a
of people who can serve in any

.

ges, how other pharmacy ser-
e being met.

y position.

first be established. Building
ngs and exchanging business
ining contact with the people
meetings or by collaborating
cement of the profession. The
at is important is pharmacists'

s in some ways more difficult
ment. As with any profession,
during the first years of phar-
, continuing education is an
of licensing boards but also
rovide continuing education
ations embedded to in-depth
aspects of pharmacy-oriented
pharmacist a convenient yet

f professional involvement is
as it is often called, allows
ns that govern the practice
ssed into law are not health
policy development process
the profession of pharmacy.
or oppose legislation. Phar-
want to participate in some
f which they are a member.
aspects of pharmacy are
ative practice agreements
mmunizers are examples of
t the state level. However,
t-provided MTM services).
oment process, grassroots

ssession ratio if the
g evaluated and it is
as enough medication to
30 of those days?

ed

3. Providers are encouraged to use the SIMPLE mnemonic as a strategy to identify ways in which adherence can be advanced. Which of the following is most closely aligned with following the "P" component of this strategy?

A. Pharmacists should work to minimize the number of pills patients have to take.
B. Pharmacists should recognize that patients with low income will probably not be able to adhere to medications.
C. Pharmacists can provide patients with pill organizers.
D. Pharmacists should consistently call patients to remind them of refills.

4. Pharmacists may generally use their compounding skills for which of the following during end-of-life situations? (Mark all that apply.)

A. Formulation of ointments, creams, and patches when oral dosage forms are not available
B. No compounding of medications in end-of-life care because of the similarity of these drugs to those used in other situations
C. Formulation of oral medications that may have higher doses than those that are commercially available
D. Preparation of more effective forms of curative treatments such as statins and antihypertensives

5. Patients derive their expectations of tangible factors in the dispensing process, such as expected wait time, from which of the following factors?

A. Consumer report magazines
B. Their beliefs of what the dispensing process should be in an ideal setting
C. Their previous experience with pharmacies
D. Conversations with their friends and family

6. How important is the amount of personal attention that patients perceive they receive in determining their personal satisfaction with pharmaceutical services?

A. Patients do not consider the personal attention that pharmacists give them in determining their personal satisfaction.
B. Patients consider the personal attention that pharmacists give them, but other factors, such as the amount of pharmaceutical care received, are more important in determining their personal satisfaction.
C. Patients consider the personal attention that pharmacists give them, and it plays an equally important part when compared with other factors, such as the amount of pharmaceutical care, in determining their personal satisfaction.
D. Patients consider the personal attention that pharmacists give them, and it plays a greater part than other factors, such as the amount of pharmaceutical care, in determining their personal satisfaction.

7. Which of the following responsibilities do physicians expect of pharmacists in both community and hospital settings?

A. Demonstrate drug knowledge, educate patients on the medications, and maintain updated medication profiles on patients
B. Demonstrate drug knowledge, educate patients on the medications, maintain updated medication profiles on patients, and monitor drug outcomes
C. Demonstrate drug knowledge, educate patients on the medications, and monitor drug outcomes
D. Demonstrate drug knowledge, maintain updated medication profiles on patients, and monitor drug outcomes

8. Which of the following is *not* a reason that has been cited as a hindrance to the development of collaboration between pharmacists and physicians?

A. Pharmacists' lack of assurance in their ability to approach physicians
B. The physical distance between community pharmacists and physicians
C. Physicians' opinion that sometimes pharmacists may call about trivial matters
D. Physicians' opinion that they already know enough about the drug therapy that they have implemented and do not need any help

9. Which of the following correctly shows the stages of the collaborative working relationships model?

A. Professional awareness, professional recognition, exploration, relationship validation, and commitment to collaborative working relationships
B. Professional awareness, professional recognition, exploration and trial, professional relationship expansion, and commitment to collaborative working relationships
C. Professional awareness, professional recognition, exploration and trial, professional advancement, and commitment to collaborative working relationships
D. Professional awareness, professional exchange, exploration and trial, professional relationship expansion, and commitment to collaborative working relationships

10. Which of the following is *not* considered a context characteristic within the collaborative working relationships model?

A. The size of the city or town where the physician and pharmacist practice
B. The physical proximity of the pharmacist and the physician to each other
C. Any academic appointments for the physician
D. The volume of patients seen by the physician

11. Which set of characteristics within the collaborative working relationships model is the most important in facilitating strong collaborative working relationships between pharmacists and physicians?

A. Participant
B. Context
C. Exchange
D. Communication

12. Which of the following is *not* one of the most important characteristics that the trait theory has identified for leaders to possess?

A. Intelligence
B. Motivation
C. Integrity
D. Charisma

13. Which leadership style uses reward power heavily and emphasizes catering to followers?

A. Affiliative
B. Coaching
C. Democratic
D. Coercive

14. Which of the following has *not* been identified as one of the most effective leadership styles?

A. Transformational
B. Coaching
C. Coercive
D. Democratic

15. A *new practitioner* is defined as a pharmacist who has been practicing as a licensed pharmacist for

A. 3 years or less.
B. 7 years or less.
C. 5 years or less.
D. 4 years or less.

16. What patient-centeredness dimension involves the combination of biological, psychological, and social factors in determining not only the successful treatment but also the etiology of a patient's illness?

A. Biopsychosocial perspective
B. Patient as person
C. Sharing of power and responsibility
D. Doctor as person

17. What patient-centeredness dimension refers to coming to a treatment decision that takes into account not only the health care provider's wishes but also the wishes and barriers of the patient?

A. Doctor-as-person
B. Therapeutic alliance
C. Patient-as-person
D. Sharing of power and responsibility

18. What patient-centeredness dimension takes into account the influence of the physician on the patient and the influence of the patient on the physician?

A. Biopsychosocial perspective
B. Patient as person
C. Sharing of power and responsibility
D. Doctor as person

19. Which of the following strategies can be used with patients at the pharmacy to increase openness between the pharmacist and the patient?

A. Listen, acknowledge, wonder
B. Recognize, question, reflect
C. Listen, acknowledge, reflect
D. Listen, question, reflect

20. Which of the following strategies can be used by pharmacists for self-improvement with respect to patient-centered care?

A. Listen, acknowledge, wonder
B. Recognize, question, reflect
C. Listen, acknowledge, reflect
D. Listen, question, reflect

21. What year was medication therapy management first recognized in the Medicare Prescription Drug, Improvement, and Modernization Act?

A. 2005
B. 2007
C. 2004
D. 2003

22. What openness strategy involves being attentive and realizing and understanding that each patient has his or her own story and experience with a particular disease?

A. Acknowledge
B. Recognize
C. Listen
D. Reflect

23. Which core element of medication therapy management is fulfilled by providing each patient with a complete list of the medications he or she is taking, including directions for use, indications, and prescriber?

A. Medication action plan
B. Medication therapy review
C. Documentation and follow-up
D. Personal medication record

23-14 Answers

1. B. Although all of these other factors may influence health outcomes, the behaviors of individuals are the single biggest determinant of morbidity and mortality within a population.

2. A. The MPR is derived by determining the days' supply for which a patient has medication (130) and dividing this by the total number of days being observed (200).

3. D. The "P" in SIMPLE represents patient communication and refers to maintaining consistent communication with patients, even when they are not in the pharmacy.

4. A, C. During end-of-life care, oral administration may not feasible such as when a patient has excessive nausea and vomiting. If oral administration is feasible, pharmacists may be called upon to compound pain medications where doses are higher than those that are commercially available.

5. C. Patients base their expectations of tangible factors involved in the dispensing process on what they have previously experienced in pharmacies.

6. D. Patients place great value on the personal attention they receive from pharmacists, which is influenced by factors such as the perceived friendliness of the pharmacist.

7. A. These are responsibilities that physicians expect pharmacists to fulfill in the community and hospital settings.

8. D. Physicians acknowledge that pharmacists' drug therapy knowledge can help them make medication choices for their patients.

9. B. This is the only choice that shows the stages of the collaborative working relationships model in the correct order.

10. A. Unlike the other choices presented, the size of the city or town where the pharmacist and physician practice has not been found to be significantly related to the degree of physician–pharmacist collaboration.

11. C. The exchange characteristics have been identified as the most important in helping establish strong collaborative relationships between physicians and pharmacists.

12. **D.** According to trait theory, drive, motivation, integrity, self-confidence, intelligence, and knowledge are the most important characteristics for leaders to possess.

13. **A.** Leaders who use the affiliative leadership style rely heavily on reward power and cater to those under them.

14. **C.** The most effective leadership styles are the transformational, democratic, affiliative, and coaching styles.

15. **C.** Many professional organizations, including the American Pharmacists Association, define a new practitioner as someone who has been licensed and practicing pharmacy for 5 years or less.

16. **A.** Patient as person, sharing of power and responsibility, and doctor as person are patient-centered dimensions that involve the interaction between the patient and the health care provider.

17. **B.** Therapeutic alliance involves making a treatment decision that includes the wishes and barriers of the patient.

18. **D.** Doctor as person is the patient-centered dimension that deals with how the patient and physician influence each other.

19. **A.** This is the correct combination of strategies that are used at the pharmacy to increase openness between the pharmacist and the patient.

20. **B.** This is the correct combination of strategies that can be used by pharmacists for self-improvement.

21. **D.** Medication therapy management was first recognized in the Medicare Prescription Drug, Improvement, and Modernization Act in 2003.

22. **C.** Listening is the only openness strategy that includes all of these aspects.

23. **D.** The personal medication record is the core element of medication therapy management that is satisfied by providing the patient with a complete list of his or her medications.

23-15 Additional Resources

American Pharmacists Association and the National Association of Chain Drug Stores Foundation. Medication therapy management in pharmacy practice: core elements of an MTM service model (version 2.0). *J Am Pharm Assoc.* 2008; 48(3):341–353.

Atreja A, Bellam N, Levy SR. Strategies to enhance patient adherence: making it simple. *MedGenMed.* 2005;7(1):4.

Brock KA, Doucette WR. Collaborative working relationships between pharmacists and physicians: an exploratory study. *J Am Pharm Assoc.* 2004;44(3):358–365.

de Oliveira DR, Shoemaker SJ. Achieving patient centeredness in pharmacy practice: openness and the pharmacist's natural attitude. *J Am Pharm Assoc.* 2006;46(1):56–66.

Herndon CM, Nee D, Atayee RS, et al. ASHP guidelines on the pharmacist's role in palliative and hospice care. *Am J Health-Syst Pharm.* 2016;73(17):1351–1367.

Higgins ST. Editorial: 3rd Special Issue on behavior change, health, and health disparities. *Prev Med.* 2016;(92):1–5.

Holdford DA. Leadership theories and their lessons for pharmacists. *Am J Health-Syst Pharm.* 2003;60(17):1780–1786.

Martin A. Fostering career development through involvement in professional organizations. *Am J Health-Syst Pharm.* 2007;64(14):1472–1473.

McGivney MS, Meyer SM, Duncan-Hewitt W, et al. Medication therapy management: its relationship to patient counseling, disease management, and pharmaceutical care. *J Am Pharm Assoc.* 2007:47(5);620–628.

Tarn DM, Paterniti DA, Williams BR, et al. Which providers should communicate which critical information about a new medication? Patient, pharmacist, and physician perspectives. *J Am Geriatr Soc.* 2009;57(3):462–469.

White SJ. Building and maintaining a professional network. *Am J Health-Syst Pharm.* 2007;64(7):700–703.

Medication Dispensing and Distribution Systems

24

BRANDON M. EDGERSON

24-1 KEY POINTS

- Fraudulent prescriptions can be problematic. Appropriately identifying the correct mechanisms for receiving prescriptions is critical.
- A pharmacist must be able to identify several key elements that are required to be present on a medication prescription and to evaluate them.
- A pharmacist must be able to recognize the required elements of a prescription label.
- *Medication reconciliation* is a process for improving communication throughout a patient's continuum of care. Recognizing the key points at which medication reconciliation should occur is important.
- The medication use process has five key phases in which an error can be identified.
- When one is developing a program for medication error prevention, gaining buy-in from those involved in the medication use process is essential. To gain buy-in, one must ensure that those involved do not view the program as punitive.
- Several key strategies can be used to prevent or reduce the likelihood of medication errors. A pharmacist should be able to explain how to use these strategies within an organization.
- Technological advances have been made in the medication use process. Each element of technology can affect different phases of the medication distribution process.
- Several abbreviations have been identified as error prone and should not be used in the medication use process. The pharmacist should be aware of those abbreviations and the way to address them if identified.
- Several medication distribution models can be used. The pharmacist should be able to identify the advantages and disadvantages of each.
- Several technologies have been used to improve medication distribution safety. Each piece of equipment has specific areas within the medication distribution process in which its safety features provide the greatest benefit.
- To determine that the medication distribution process is functioning appropriately or improving, the pharmacist can use several continuous quality improvement techniques to monitor the functionality of the system.

24-2 STUDY GUIDE CHECKLIST

The following topics may guide your study of this subject area:

- ☐ A pharmacist must be familiar with the three requirements for a hard-copy prescription.
- ☐ There are several key elements that a pharmacist must verify when properly preparing a prescription.
- ☐ A patient medication profile is essential to improving communication between health care providers. Know what is included in a patient profile.
- ☐ Being aware of error detection and prevention tools is important.
- ☐ A pharmacist must know the differences between human error, at-risk behavior, and reckless behavior.
- ☐ An effective medication distribution system is used to ensure that medications are efficiently and safely administered to patients in the most readily administered form.
- ☐ A pharmacist must be able to describe the variety of technologies that can be used to improve patient safety.
- ☐ A pharmacist must be able to identify the phases when medication reconciliation should occur.
- ☐ A pharmacist should be aware of the types of error correction plans that have long-term sustainability.
- ☐ An effective medication distribution system will use a proactive quality improvement plan. A pharmacist must be able to describe the steps of a plan-do-study-act (PDSA) model.
- ☐ A pharmacist must be able to describe and identify medications that can be used in an effective medication trigger tool audit.
- ☐ A pharmacist must be able to understand the importance of a risk priority number and be able to calculate it.

24-3 Overview

This chapter provides fundamental information pertaining to the essential elements of properly preparing and dispensing a prescription medication. It details key elements required for a prescription for regulatory and patient safety reasons. After defining the components of a prescription, the chapter moves to topics related to medication toxicity detection, medication error reduction programs, and application of technology to improve patient safety. Within the chapter is key information related to methods of detecting whether a patient has received a toxic dose of a medication and the steps that can be taken to reduce the chances of a medication error. The chapter concludes with methods to ensure continuous quality improvement in the environment of an ever-changing medication distribution system.

24-4 Preparation and Dispensing of Prescriptions

A *prescription* can be defined as an order for a medication written by an authorized prescriber as defined by state law. The authorized prescriber or licensed practitioner uses a prescription to communicate with a pharmacist. A prescription can be received by various mechanisms. The pharmacist can receive the prescription as a hard copy, verbal order, or electronic transmission. After receiving a prescription, the pharmacist must take several steps to ensure the integrity of the prescription:

- ***Hard copy:*** The prescription must meet the Medicaid tamper-resistant prescription requirements. As of October 1, 2008, all Medicaid prescriptions that are handwritten or printed using e-prescribing must contain at least one feature from each of the following three categories of tamper resistance:
  - ***Category 1: Copy resistant.*** The following indicate copy resistance:
    - Void/Illegal/Copy background pantograph with or without Reverse Rx should appear when the prescription is photocopied.
    - Microprint signature line for prescriptions is generated by an electronic medical record; the signature is viewable at 5× magnification or greater.
  - ***Category 2: Erasure or modification resistant.*** Written prescriptions should have an erasure-revealing background; laser-printed prescriptions should be printed on toner-lock paper.
  - ***Category 3: Counterfeit resistant.*** The prescription should have special counterfeit-resistant features:
    - Quantity check-off boxes and refill indicator
    - Security features and descriptions listed on the prescription
- ***Verbal order:*** A verbal or telephone order can be an official medication order or a lab test order. Verbal or telephone orders should be used only in urgent situations when the prescriber is not able to provide the order in another form. When taking a verbal or telephone order, the receiver of the order should immediately write down the order. After writing the order, the receiver should read back the order to the prescriber to ensure accuracy. To reduce the risk associated with verbal orders, many organizations have adopted a policy to allow such orders only in emergency situations. Such policies can include measures such as the following to reduce risk in the verbal order process:
  - Chemotherapy verbal orders are not permitted.
  - Look-alike, sound-alike drugs must have an indication stated.
  - Complex drug names should be spelled by the prescriber to the receiver.
- ***Fax:*** Medication orders can also be received via facsimile. When receiving an order by fax, the receiver must ensure the following key steps are followed:
  - The fax must be of high quality to ensure the legibility of the orders.
  - The pharmacist processing the order should have the ability to verify that the prescriber has prescribing privileges within the institution.

Elements of the Prescription

Several key elements must be evaluated when preparing a prescription. Table 24-1 describes these elements.

Interpretation of the Order

Determining if the order is appropriate

The pharmacist must properly evaluate a prescription for appropriateness. The pharmacist is responsible for ensuring that all necessary information is legible and available. The pharmacist must use clinical knowledge to interpret the intent of the prescriber.

Handling an inappropriate order

The pharmacist is responsible for communicating with the prescriber if a problem with a prescription is identified. After receiving clarification from the prescriber, the pharmacist needs to document the clarification and process the prescription.

Proper Steps in Preparing a Prescription

As a pharmacist begins to prepare a prescription, he or she must take the following safety precautions:

- The prescription should be logged into the pharmacy system with a unique identification number that should be documented on the prescription.
- The date and quantity dispensed should be entered in the system and recorded on the prescription.
- The pharmacist dispensing the prescription should record his or her name or initials on the prescription.

TABLE 24-1. Key Elements of a Prescription

Key element	Characteristics
Patient information	Patient's name
	Patient's date of birth
	Patient's height
	Patient's weight
	Patient's sex
	Patient's allergy information
Date	Date prescription was written
Time	Time the order was written (inpatient medication orders)
Prescriber	Outpatient prescriptions: prescriber's name, address, phone number, Drug Enforcement Administration (DEA) number, and signature
	Inpatient prescriptions: ability to validate the prescriber by a unique identification number
Product information	Unique identification number in multiple dosage forms
	Brand versus generic
Quantity	Quantity or, alternatively, frequency and duration
Outpatient information	Refill information (not specified means no refills)
	Directions for use (should be clear and direct)
Inpatient information	Directions for the pharmacist for labeling and compounding, if needed

Adapted from Tennessee pharmacy laws.

A pharmacy technician is permitted to assist with prescription preparation. The technician selects the correct product on the basis of the label description.

Before dispensing the prescription, the pharmacist must see that a medication label is prepared. Following are the required elements that must be included on the label:

- Name and address of the pharmacy
- Patient's name
- Prescription date
- Prescription's unique identification number
- Product's name
- Product strength
- Quantity dispensed
- Directions for use
- Prescriber's name
- Expiration date
- Pharmacist's initials

24-5 Development and Maintenance of Patient Medication Profiles

A patient's medication profile provides a historical account of a patient's diagnosis, disease states, allergies, and current and past medication records. An accurate patient profile can provide multiple patient safety benefits. In recent years, many advances have been made in electronic systems to assist with maintaining patient profiles. To improve communication among health care providers, The Joint Commission created a National Patient Safety Goal to incorporate medication reconciliation. Medication reconciliation is required to occur when patients are admitted, when they are transferred from one level of care to another, and when they are discharged.

Maintaining a patient's medication profile has several benefits, including the following:

- Improved patient charting
- Safer ability to validate refill information
- Improved communication among health care providers
- Improved documentation of allergy information

Medication Reconciliation

Medication reconciliation is a systematic approach to improving communication of pertinent medication information as a patient transitions through different levels of care within the health care system. Research has shown that significant medication errors have been associated with poor documentation of medication histories. The most common medication errors encountered when medication reconciliation is not performed appropriately are those associated with omission and duplication. The fundamental belief is that appropriate medication reconciliation can ensure the principles of the "five rights":

- Right patient
- Right medication
- Right route
- Right time
- Right dose

In January 2006, as part of the National Patient Safety Goals, The Joint Commission required implementation of medication reconciliation to improve patient safety. The goal, which is available on The Joint Commission's Web site (https://www.jointcommission.org), reads as follows:

"Goal 8: Accurately and completely reconcile medications across the continuum of care.

"8A: Implement a process for obtaining and documenting a complete list of the patient's current medications upon the patient's admission to the organization and with the involvement of the patient. This process includes a comparison of the medications the organization provides to those on the list.

"8B: A complete list of the patient's medications is communicated to the next provider of service when a patient is referred or transferred to another setting, service, practitioner, or level of care within or outside the organization."

Successfully conducting effective medication reconciliation has several key elements:

- ***Collection and verification of medication history:*** An accurate collection of the medication history should be performed when the patient is admitted. Variations from institution to institution exist on who is responsible for collecting the medication history. Depending on the facility's policy, a nurse, pharmacy technician, or pharmacist may be assigned to collect and verify the home medication list. This process should take place within 24 hours of admission. Use of a standard reconciliation form allows the collector to document the following:
  - Name of drug
  - Frequency
  - Date
  - Data source (pill bottle, referral medical order, patient or family report)
- ***Profile development:*** The physician is responsible for reviewing the home medication list and making an informed decision about the orders to include in the patient's profile. In some institutions, the physician documents his or her decision on the reconciliation form. The physician indicates if he or she would like to continue the medication, discontinue the medication, or modify the treatment.
- ***Transfer reconciliation:*** When a patient transfers from one level of care to another or from one institution to another, a transfer reconciliation must be completed. In a transfer reconciliation, the next health care provider must be given a summary of the patient's current medication profile. The physician must use this list to determine how he or she will develop the patient's new medication profile.
- ***Discharge reconciliation:*** Discharge reconciliation is the process of reviewing the original home medication list and the active routine medications on the profile at time of discharge. The collected lists should be used to prepare the final list of discharge prescriptions.

24-6 Identification and Prevention of Medication Errors

Medication Use Process and Medication Errors

Medication errors have always plagued the medication use system. Medication errors can occur during any of the five steps of the medication use process:

- Ordering and prescribing
- Transcribing and documenting
- Dispensing
- Administering
- Monitoring

Increased Attention to Medication Errors

According to Leape et al. (1991), 38% of all medication errors occur during administration. Of these errors, 98% reach the patient and cause 51% of drug-related patient harm.

Recently, medication errors associated with heparin have drawn major media attention. However, this series of incidents was not the first time that medication errors reached the national stage. Medication errors drew national attention in 1999 with the release of the then Institute of Medicine (now the National Academy of Medicine) report *To Err Is Human* (Kohn, Corrigan, Donaldson 1999), which had the following findings:

- Prescription medication errors result in approximately 7,000 deaths annually.
- The financial cost of drug-related morbidity and mortality is near $77 billion a year. The Institute of Medicine concluded that to create an environment that focuses on preventing medical errors, a safer health system must be built that limits health care providers from making mistakes.

Medication Error Prevention Programs

The goal of a sound program of medication error prevention is not only to identify the issues and solution for one isolated medication error but also to implement a process that will reduce the likelihood that the same or a similar event will occur again.

Common flaws

The tendency is to focus on the human component of the error instead of the problems caused by the highly leveraged system. In this type of environment, the following problems are likely to occur:

- Reporting tends to decrease.
- Health care providers tend to view the system as punitive and see reporting errors as placing their employment at risk.

Encouragement of reporting of medication errors

Health care organizations need to promote an environment in which their employees understand that the intent of reporting errors is to gain knowledge on how to minimize the risk of the same error recurring. Since the report *To Err Is Human* was released, the health care environment has begun another paradigm shift to a concept of a *just culture*.

Just Culture

According to the Institute for Safe Medication Practices, the health care environment has begun to move to the middle. The culture has moved from one of blame to a nonpunitive culture and is now settling on a culture at the midpoint—a just culture. Within a just culture, the system implemented by the health care organization should be fair to the health care provider but also seek ways to minimize safety risk.

Outcome Engenuity (2005) has defined three behaviors that may cause errors:

- ***Human error:*** According to the Institute for Safe Medication Practices (2006), "human error involves unintentional and unpredictable behavior that causes or could have caused an undesirable outcome, either because a planned action is not completed as intended or the wrong plan is used to achieve an aim."
- ***At-risk behavior:*** An error associated with at-risk behavior results when an employee modifies a process to achieve a secondary goal. A common example is when patient volume increases and the health care provider deviates from the normal routine to increase patient throughput. Typically,

when this type of behavior is discovered, the health care provider has some incentive to engage in it. The goal of the health care organization is to identify the incentives for this behavior and build a system that takes into account incentives to direct health care providers to the appropriate safe behaviors.

- ***Reckless behavior:*** Reckless behavior occurs when a health care provider intentionally places a patient at risk. This type of behavior is demonstrated when the health care provider makes a decision that does not place the patient's interest first. The health care provider knows the risk but makes a conscious choice to disregard the risk and potential outcome. When this type of behavior is identified, disciplinary action is justified.

Methods of Preventing Medication Errors

Many strategies have been explored to reduce the risk of occurrence of medication errors. Many organizations have incorporated medication error reduction programs into their day-to-day processes. Following are several steps that organizations may use to focus on reducing medication errors:

- ***Incorporating medication error reduction into the strategic plan:*** To gain momentum in building a safer health care arena, organizations must identify medication safety as a top priority. Health care organizations must realize that no quick solution exists to building safer workflow processes. Therefore, as organizations evaluate their strategic plan, some dedication to patient safety must occur. Within the strategic plan, the organization must define its strengths and the barriers to a safer environment. With the identified barriers, the organization must define their risk, identify potential system-based solutions, define potential cost associated with the solution, and establish the timeline in which to incorporate the solution.
- ***Promoting medication error reporting systems:*** As organizations move toward a system to promote medication safety, creating an environment in which medication safety information is freely shared is imperative. Several commercially available software programs for medication error reporting are available, or an organization may choose to develop its own. The idea behind using medication error reporting systems is to identify where potential problems may occur. The intent of these systems is to collect information pertaining to actual errors and near-miss events. A *near-miss event* can be defined as a potential error that is identified before reaching the patient. The information collected from actual medication errors and near misses can be used to identify trends and establish system-based changes to reduce the potential of the same event recurring.
- ***Establishing medication error teams or committees:*** Medication error teams should be established within health care organizations. The medication use process cannot be improved by simply defining a strategic plan. A medication improvement process must incorporate a variety of health care professionals involved in the medication use process. A medication error team should be composed of medical, pharmacy, nursing, informatics, respiratory, biomedical, radiology, and other health care professionals who may be involved in the medication use process. Having the correct representatives review the medication error data allows health care organizations to gain a better understanding of workflow processes and barriers to delivering proper care. By gaining a variety of perspectives and understanding the workflow, the medication error team can establish sound recommendations that take into account the needs of the patients and the concerns of the work environment.
- ***Communicating through patient- and family-centered care:*** In recent years, the health care arena has begun to become more transparent. A patient- and family-centered care facility is one that encourages participation and information sharing among the patient, family, and health care associates. Within this environment, patients and families are encouraged to ask questions and share opinions. When information is shared in a health care facility, medication errors can sometimes be avoided.

TABLE 24-2. Component of Medication Use Processes Affected by Technology

Technology	Component affected
Computerized prescriber order entry	Ordering and prescribing
Bar coding at point of care	Administration
Medication bar coding	Dispensing
Smart pumps	Administration
Automated dispensing cabinets	Dispensing and administration
Robotics	Dispensing

- ***Using technology:*** A variety of technology options is available that can affect medication safety. In selecting technologies, consideration of the component of the medication use process at which the technology is directed is important. Table 24-2 presents several common technologies and gives the component of the medication use process they may affect.
- ***Using decentralized practice models:*** A variety of pharmacy practice models can be used, depending on the needs, design, and staffing options within an institution. A decentralized practice model offers the advantage of availability of the pharmacist within the medication use process. In a decentralized practice model, a pharmacist can intervene at the point of ordering and prescribing by meeting with the prescriber on rounds. Research has shown that the closer the error gets to the administering phase, the more likely it will reach the patient. Therefore, if the pharmacist intervenes earlier and more often in the medication use process, a greater chance exists of preventing an error from reaching the patient.
- ***Eliminating dangerous abbreviations:*** The use of abbreviations has long been a common practice within the health care industry. Because of illegibility, ambiguity, and misinterpretation of the intent of abbreviations, many errors result from this practice. On the basis of these findings, in 2005, The Joint Commission published a list of "do not use" abbreviations (see Table 24-3). This list is recommended for adoption by health care organizations.
- ***Incorporating redundancy checks:*** Creating redundancy within the health care system is one way to improve the medication safety process. Double-check systems have been used for years to verify that health care providers have identified that they are providing the right medication to the right patient

TABLE 24-3. "Do Not Use" Abbreviations

Unapproved abbreviation	Solution
U	Write out *units.*
IU	Write out *international units.*
qd	Write out *daily.*
qod	Write out *every other day.*
MS/MSO_4	Write out *morphine sulfate.*
Leading and trailing zeros	Eliminate trailing zeros (2 mg instead of 2.0 mg); add leading zeros (0.2 mg instead of .2 mg).
@	Eliminate the @, and write *at.*
μg	Eliminate *μg*, and write *mcg.*
cc	Eliminate *cc*, and write *mL.*

Adapted from The Joint Commission (https://www.jointcommission.org/assets/1/18/dnu_list.pdf).

by the right route at the right time and in the right dose. The Institute for Safe Medication Practices also recommends an independent double check. In an independent double check, two health care providers perform the same task independent of each other and then compare the results to verify accuracy. Using this method should reduce the probability of biasing the verifier's response.

- ***Creating a high-alert drug list:*** An institution can define a high-alert drug on the basis of historical data in the literature that outline the risk associated with the use of the product. In addition, the institution may define a high-alert drug on the basis of institution-specific data that have proved that a risk is associated with use of a particular product. Once the institution has defined its high-alert drug list, specific instructions should be established on how to handle products on the list if ordered. Some examples of precautions that might be taken when handling high-alert drugs are double checks, computerized warnings, special labeling, and special storage requirements.
- ***Addressing illegible handwriting:*** Illegible handwriting has been associated with a variety of serious medication errors. Some institutions have implemented special policies to address the readability of patient orders. Some examples of programs are handwriting courses to educate prescribers on the risk associated with poor handwriting. Some institutions have implemented printing-only policies in an attempt to improve legibility. In addition to printing requirements, some organizations require prescriber stamps with a unique identifier so that a prescriber can be quickly identified if an order needs clarification.

24-7 Identification and Prevention of Drug Toxicity

In the health care system, paying attention to identification of medication toxicity is important. Traditionally, medication toxicity has been identified retrospectively during a patient's clinical assessment. Drug toxicity is usually identified during laboratory testing and clinical presentation. However, in this model of addressing medication toxicity, the patient may already be experiencing an adverse effect from the medication.

For a limited number of medications, therapeutic drug monitoring programs can be used to identify potential toxicity. In such a program, potentially serious toxicity can be detected in patients who are not demonstrating any symptoms. Clinical pharmacists can play a vital role in the success of a therapeutic drug monitoring program.

Medication Trigger Tools

Trigger tools are another method for identifying potential toxicity. A trigger tool is an auditing method of detecting an adverse drug effect by detecting "triggers." Some of the common trigger drugs that might be included on a trigger tool would be diphenhydramine, naloxone, and vitamin K. When these drugs are detected during the audit, the investigator is trying to determine the following:

- *Diphenhydramine:* Signs of hypersensitivity or allergic reactions
- *Naloxone:* Potential oversedation
- *Vitamin K:* Over-anticoagulation associated with warfarin therapy

Clinical Alerts

Clinical alerts are designed to allow the health care provider to simultaneously monitor changes in a patient's clinical condition while maintaining workflow. Clinical alerts can be designed to notify the health care provider of sudden changes in laboratory values, changes in medications, potential drug interactions, and a variety of other real-time notifications as needed by him or her. The alerts can be designed to deliver a notification by report, phone, pager, and personal digital assistant. By receiving this information in a timelier manner, the health care provider can respond to the patient's need and ultimately reduce the likelihood of an adverse outcome.

24-8 Distribution System Issues Associated with All Types of Practice Settings

Medication distribution systems involve the process and method by which the medication is distributed to the patient care area for administration by a nurse. Several key steps can maximize the safety and efficiency of a successful medication distribution model.

In the medication distribution model, the goal from a pharmacy perspective is to provide the ordered medication in the most readily administered form. Table 24-4 describes several distribution models and the advantages and disadvantages they offer.

TABLE 24-4. Advantages and Disadvantages of Medication Distribution Models

Distribution model	Description	Advantages	Disadvantages
Inpatient centralized	Majority of distribution functions are carried out in a central location; medication is then delivered to the patient care areas.	Resources can be used more efficiently.	Delays may occur in the delivery of care.
Floor-stock distribution	In this commonly used model, products are prepared in their most readily administered form and safely secured in the patient care area.	Model improves timeliness of administration.	Medication can be obtained before pharmacist review.
Unit-dose distribution	Single patient-specific dose is prepared in a central location and properly labeled with patient-specific information.	Nursing staff can properly administer the dose without additional manipulation.	Medication administration delays may occur because of location of central pharmacy and nursing units.
Cart-delivery distribution	Typically, a 24-hour supply of a patient's current medication profile is prepared and delivered to the nursing unit at one standard time daily.	Full daily supply of patients' medications is delivered to a standardized location on the nursing unit, providing easy access and medication retrieval.	When medication orders are changed or discontinued, the previous orders are not easily retrieved from the nursing unit.
Inpatient decentralized	Majority of the components of the medication distribution process occurs in the patient care area; typically, the pharmacist processes medication orders or verifies orders from the nursing unit.	Clarifications and order correction can occur in a timelier manner; overall medication delivery turnaround time is improved.	Extensive resources are required; increased inventory and increased waste may occur.
Blended or hybrid	Model combines components of both the centralized and the decentralized models; the decision should be based on the infrastructure and philosophy of the distribution model used by the organization.	Model can be designed to include the top advantages of other models.	Extensive resources are required.

Based on Cardinal Health, 2008.

24-9 Role of Automation and Technology in Workload Efficiency and Patient Safety

One of the major recommendations made by the Institute of Medicine (now the National Academy of Medicine) to address the need for reducing medication errors is to incorporate technology into the medication use process. Various technologies are being employed throughout the medication use process. With the variety of technologies available, several debates have occurred on which technologies organizations should use first. The most common recommendation is to use the technology that has the most significant effect at the point where medication errors most commonly occur. The highest volume of medication errors has been reported to occur during the prescribing phase, followed closely by the administration phase. On the basis of these data, the two technologies recommended are computerized prescriber order entry (CPOE) and bar code administration.

Following are several technologies that may be used to improve the safety and efficiency of the medication distribution process:

- ***CPOE:*** Computerized prescriber order entry is a technology that enables a prescriber to communicate an order electronically to an ancillary department. Research has shown that a significant number of medication errors can be attributed to failures within the transcription process. Successful implementation of CPOE systems can significantly reduce an organization's medication error rates. However, implementation of CPOE systems within organizations has been slow. Many failures of CPOE systems can be attributed to an organization's inability or unwillingness to customize the system, which is essential to gaining buy-in from users. When moving down the path to CPOE, the organization must devote sufficient time to planning and must incorporate physicians throughout the process.
- ***Bar code administration:*** When used successfully, bar code technology can significantly reduce medication error rates. Bar coding can be used at the dispensing phase and the administration phase of the distribution process. During the dispensing phase, a bar code system can be used to stock and store inventory correctly and to verify that the correct product is being dispensed. During the administration phase, patients can be given an identification armband with a bar code so that the nurse can verify that he or she has the correct patient. The product-specific bar code can then be used to verify that the patient has an active order that needs to be given at a specific time. This technology should decrease errors associated with wrong drug administration, wrong time administration, and wrong patient administration.
- ***Electronic medication administration records:*** Electronic records have been designed to reduce the risk of errors at the point of administration. With an electronic medication administration record system, the nurse can document administration activities at the bedside. Documenting at the bedside reduces the probability of multiple doses being administered as a result of poor documentation systems.
- ***Automated dispensing cabinets:*** An automated dispensing cabinet (ADC) is a computerized medication storage unit. An ADC allows medications to be securely stored in the nursing unit, thus providing greater access to needed medications near the point of care. Unlike a traditional floor-stock model, which may allow nurses access to medications without a pharmacist's review, an ADC can be designed to interface with the organization's medication ordering system. By using the interface capability, an ADC can provide additional safety checks and reduce risk in the medication administration phase within the distribution process. Some organizations may choose to combine an ADC and bar coding to ensure proper stocking of ADCs as an extra safety feature.
- ***Smart pumps:*** Medication errors associated with intravenous therapy present a high patient safety risk. Typically, these errors are difficult to detect, and usually they reach the patient. With traditional infusion pumps, programming errors are common. Traditional infusion pumps have a 10,000-fold dosing range that increases the likelihood of decimal placement errors, which can be significant.

To avoid medication errors, smart pumps incorporate drug libraries. Libraries include medication standards, which include information about drug concentrations, dosing units, and dose limits. Libraries can be designed to fit the needs of specific patient care areas. A library can be designed for an emergency department, a critical care unit, and a variety of other settings. When the libraries are properly used, they provide an alert to the user if any of the safety limits are exceeded.

- ***Robotics:*** Robotics is used to assist pharmacy departments in improving safety and functionality in the dispensing phase of the medication distribution process. Robotics uses bar code technology to assist pharmacy departments in storing medications, dispensing patient-specific bar-coded doses, and streamlining the credit and return process. Robotic devices have been designed to handle unit-dose oral preparations and preparations of intravenous medications.
- ***RFID (radio frequency identification):*** RFID is a technology that uses electronic tags to relay identifying information to an electronic reader. The primary use in the health care pharmacy arena is in inventory control. Some health care systems have implemented RFID tagging for crash carts, anesthesia carts, and operating room medication kits. The primary purpose is to improve patient safety by enhancing stocking efficiencies and accuracy. Although RFID is more expensive to implement than bar coding, it offers the advantage of proximity scanning, which allows the scanning of inventory without touching each individual item.

24-10 Medication Error Reduction Programs

Each organization must devote the necessary attention to creating a culture of safety. To create a culture of safety, a sound medication error reduction program requires a multidisciplinary focus. With a culture of medication safety, each member of the organization understands the value of participation. The key component of such a program is the ability to gather information in a timely manner to develop system-based action plans. Several key steps are required to initiate a successful reduction program, including the following:

- ***Using an effective report-tracking tool:*** Several commercially available reporting programs are available, or an organization may choose to develop its own program.
- ***Developing action plans:*** An effective program for medication error reduction identifies the root cause of an error and decides on the course of action. A wide variety of actions can be selected. Actions can range from self-correction to complete system design changes. When designing system-based changes, organizations must ensure that the changes made are sustainable. The most effective system-based changes are high-leverage changes that force the end user to make the correct decision. An example of a forced function change would be to require a response to a question to verify that a lab value is in the appropriate range before allowing removal of a medication from an automated dispensing cabinet. The least sustainable system-based change that can be implemented is reeducation.
- ***Identifying best practices:*** An effective medication error reduction program has processes in place to identify whether a best practice standard is available to prevent an error identified by the reported data.

24-11 Continuous Quality Improvement Program

A continuous quality improvement (CQI) program is the proactive monitoring of a process to ensure consistency and quality in its outcome. Several tools can be implemented when establishing a CQI program to monitor a medication safety process.

Plan-Do-Study-Act Cycle

The plan-do-study-act (PDSA) model for improvement has been used successfully in the health care arena. When a medication error team decides to use a PDSA process for improvement, the team must follow the cycle for improvement:

- ***Plan:*** Use a team to establish a plan that is based on the evidence found during the investigation.
- ***Do:*** Implement the plan established by the team with a specific timeline.
- ***Study:*** Once the plan has been implemented, study the findings to identify the success of the plan.
- ***Act:*** Using the information identified, have the team make the necessary adjustments to the plan and repeat the cycle.

Failure Mode Effect Analysis

Another CQI program that can be used to evaluate medication safety is failure mode effect analysis (FMEA). The primary objective of an FMEA is to identify potential failures within the system. An effective FMEA has several steps:

- ***Establish severity:*** After identifying the potential failure, assign a severity score between 1 and 10. A score of 1 represents no danger, and a score of 10 represents critical danger.
- ***Establish an occurrence score:*** The occurrence score is the probability of how often the risk might occur. A score of 1 represents low frequency, and a score of 10 represents high frequency.
- ***Establish a detection score:*** The detection score represents the likelihood of detection if the failure should occur. A score of 1 represents high likelihood of detection, and a score of 10 represents high probability that the failure would go undetected.

When all three scores are determined, a risk priority number (RPN) can be established. The RPN can be used to assist the evaluation team in establishing priorities for action plans. As action plans are implemented, the RPN should be recalculated to determine the effect of changes.

Root Cause Analysis

A root cause analysis is a retrospective analysis of an undesirable event with the purpose of developing an action plan to prevent the undesirable event from recurring. Medication error teams can use root cause analysis to identify system-based failures and develop sustainable action plans to prevent the undesirable event from recurring.

24-12 Questions

1. Which of the following is *not* an acceptable form for receiving a prescription?

A. Hard copy
B. Verbal order
C. Electronic transmission
D. Photocopy

2. As of October 1, 2008, prescriptions are required to meet the Medicaid tamper-resistance regulations. Which of the following is an example that meets the requirement?

A. A state official protective seal should appear.
B. Void/Illegal/Copy pantograph with or without Reverse Rx should appear when the prescription is photocopied.
C. A prescriber-specific identification number should be included.
D. None of the above.

3. For receipt of a verbal prescription, which of the following does The Joint Commission require?

A. Chemotherapy orders should be documented on a chemo order form.
B. The receiver of the order should perform a read back.
C. Within 24 hours, the prescriber should document the order.
D. An organization should create a verbal order form.

4. Before a prescription is dispensed, a medication label must be prepared. Which of the following is *not* a required element?

A. Quantity dispensed
B. Directions for use
C. Patient's date of birth
D. Date

5. Maintaining a patient profile has several benefits. Which of the following is *not* a benefit?

A. Evaluation of prescribing patterns
B. Safer ability to validate refill information
C. Improved communication among health care providers
D. Improved documentation of allergy information

6. In 2006, as part of the National Patient Safety Goals, The Joint Commission required implementation of medication reconciliation to improve patient safety. Medication reconciliation should occur when?

A. When a patient is admitted to a hospital
B. After any medication is discontinued
C. After any diagnostic test is performed
D. When an adverse medication effect is detected

7. What are the three stages at which medication reconciliation should occur?

A. At admission, on transfer, and after dialysis
B. At admission, on discharge, and at clinic visits
C. At admission, on transfer, and on discharge
D. None of the above

8. When a patient goes to a hospital, an admission medication reconciliation process should be performed within how much time from the admission?

A. 12 hours
B. 24 hours
C. 36 hours
D. 48 hours

9. Of the five components of the medication use process, which area has been shown to have the highest rate of medication errors associated with it?

A. Prescribing and ordering
B. Administering
C. Dispensing
D. Monitoring

10. Of the five components of the medication use process, which area has been shown to have the highest likelihood that any error made will reach the patient?

A. Prescribing and ordering
B. Administration
C. Dispensing
D. Monitoring

11. To promote a culture of safety, a health care organization should create an environment that

A. is protective of patient information regarding possible medication errors.
B. identifies which individual is responsible for the error.
C. allows the pharmacy department to be solely responsible for addressing medication safety issues.
D. promotes a nonpunitive environment in which safety information is freely shared.

12. Which of the following statements best describes an organization that functions within a just culture?

A. An organization that deals only with errors attributed to system failures
B. An organization that looks to terminate all employees involved in errors resulting in patient harm
C. An organization that functions with the intent that all errors are self-correcting
D. None of the above

13. Within a just culture, three types of behaviors have been defined during evaluation of medication errors. Which of the following is *not* a recognized behavior?

A. Human error
B. Passive behavior
C. At-risk behavior
D. Reckless behavior

14. Within an organization, which of the following reasons does *not* support the need for including medication safety in the organization's strategic plan?

A. To assist the organization in establishing priorities to address patient safety concerns
B. To identify barriers the organization may be facing in enhancing patient safety
C. To measure the relative safety culture of the organization against competitors
D. To define the potential cost of implementing patient safety technology

15. Which of the following would be a reason for collecting near-miss medication error data?

A. To publish the information on the patient care floors
B. To determine if certain trends exist that might identify a significant system issue
C. To establish a high medication error reporting rate
D. To determine which department has the highest reporting rate

16. An organization establishing a medication error committee should include participants from which department?

A. Pharmacy
B. Medical staff
C. Information systems
D. All of the above

17. Which of the following is *not* considered an effective way to bring about medication safety in an organization?

A. Eliminate the use of dangerous abbreviations.
B. Restrict the use of high-risk drugs.
C. Implement medication safety technology.
D. Improve the communication process between all involved in the medication use process, including family members.

18. Various medication safety technologies are available. According to the research, which of the following should have the greatest effect on reducing medication errors?

A. Automated dispensing cabinets
B. Smart pumps
C. Computerized prescriber order entry
D. Bar coding

19. A *medication trigger tool* has been defined as an auditing method for detecting an adverse effect. Which of the following drugs would *not* be included on a trigger tool?

A. Protamine
B. Vitamin K
C. Acetaminophen
D. Naloxone

20. When conducting an FMEA, determining the RPN is important. What does the RPN measure?

A. Severity, occurrence, and detection
B. Location, detection, and severity
C. Severity, detection, and negligence
D. None of the above

21. The most common medication errors encountered when medication reconciliation is not performed appropriately are those associated with omission and duplication. The fundamental belief is that appropriate medication reconciliation can ensure the principles of the "five rights." Which one of the following is *not* one of the five rights?

A. Right patient
B. Right medication
C. Right route
D. Right hour

22. Medication trigger tools are a method for identifying potential toxicity. A trigger tool is an auditing method of detecting an adverse drug effect by detecting triggers. Which of the following is *not* a common trigger drug?

A. Diphenhydramine
B. Naloxone
C. Vitamin K
D. Acetaminophen

23. What is the PDSA cycle?

A. Prioritize, do, study, act
B. Plan, do, study, act
C. Plan, delegate, study, act
D. Plan, do, self-evaluate, act

24. Which of the following is *not* correct as it relates to RFID?

A. RFID technology is less expensive than bar coding.
B. RFID scanning allows time-saving benefits as it relates to medication kits, etc. (proximity scan versus individual scan with bar code).
C. RFID technology may potentially have higher read-failure rates.
D. RFID technology is less intuitive with respect to patient and medication scanning.

25. Clinical alerts are meant to

A. inform the patient of stable laboratory values.
B. inform the patient of drug interactions.
C. inform the health care provider of stable laboratory values.
D. inform the health care provider of drug interactions.

26. Which of these distribution models allows for the drug to be dispensed without pharmacist verification?

A. Inpatient centralized model
B. Floor-stock distribution model
C. Unit-dose distribution model
D. Inpatient decentralized model

24-13 Answers

1. D. Photocopy. A photocopy is not an acceptable form of a prescription because a photocopied prescription has a greater potential for tampering.

2. B. The Centers for Medicare and Medicaid Services require three elements to meet the tamper-resistant requirement. Within category 1, a Void/Illegal/Copy pantograph meets that requirement.

3. B. When a verbal order is received, The Joint Commission requires the receiver to perform a read back. A read back requires the receiver of a verbal order to write down the order and then read back the order to the prescriber. Performing this action should improve the accuracy of the order.

4. C. The date of birth is not required for a prescription. The quantity, directions for use, and date are all required elements of a prescription.

5. A. A medication profile is designed to improve communication among health care providers. A profile is also a place to retrieve pertinent information regarding allergies and refills.

6. A. Medication reconciliation is required at the point of patient admission, on transfer between changes of level of care, and on discharge.

7. C. Medication reconciliation should occur at admission, on transfer, and on discharge. The process of reconciliation is to review the list of medications that the patient is currently receiving before writing new orders.

8. B. An admission medication reconciliation should be performed as soon as possible when a patient is admitted. However, information may not be readily available. Therefore, the standard allows 24 hours from the time of admission.

9. A. Prescribing and ordering has the highest rate of medication errors. This problem can be associated with errors related to transcription and illegible handwriting.

10. B. Errors made at the administration phase have the highest probability of reaching the patient because it is the last phase before the drug is given to the patient.

11. D. To promote a culture of safety, an organization must promote an environment in which safety information is freely communicated and employees are not punished for participating.

12. D. A just culture looks for the root cause of an error. In a just culture, the evaluation process seeks out system failures, but if a human resource issue is identified, appropriate actions are taken.

13. B. A just culture defines the three behaviors involved in errors as human error, at-risk behavior, and reckless behavior.

14. C. The strategic plan for an organization should incorporate a plan for medication safety. The plan should include potential barriers, priorities for safety initiatives, and a financial plan for implementation.

15. B. Near-miss data can provide an organization with valuable information. Near-miss data can be trended to identify the root cause of potential risk points, which can be used to prevent future errors.

16. D. The key to creating a successful medication error committee is to have a multidisciplinary team approach. Involving multiple disciplines in the action planning process allows the organization to gain expertise in the problem area, which can lead to greater buy-in to action plans.

17. B. Restricting the use of high-risk drugs is not an appropriate action to improve medication safety. Creating a high-alert drug list with specific actions to take when medications on the list are used is a more appropriate action.

18. C. Research has shown that the highest rate of medication errors occurs at the prescribing phase of the distribution process. CPOE works at the prescribing phase and will reduce the rate of errors during the ordering process.

19. C. The trigger tool audit looks for medications that may be ordered to correct problems that result from a potential adverse effect. Naloxone, protamine, and vitamin K fit the criteria.

20. A. An RPN is calculated by determining a severity rating, an occurrence rating, and a detection rating.

21. D. The five rights are right patient, right medication, right route, right time, and right dose.

22. D. Acetaminophen is not a common trigger drug. A trigger drug is prescribed to minimize the harm associated with an adverse reaction. Diphenhydramine is used to minimize hypersensitivity or allergic reaction, naloxone is used to reverse potential over-sedation, and vitamin K is used to reverse over-anticoagulation associated with warfarin therapy.

23. B. The PDSA cycle has the following steps: (1) plan—use a team to establish a plan that is based on the evidence found during the investigation; (2) do—implement the plan established by the team with a specific timeline; (3) study—once the plan has been implemented, study the findings to identify the success of the plan; and (4) act—using the information identified, have the team make the necessary adjustments to the plan and repeat the cycle.

24. A. RFID is more expensive than bar coding. However, it offers the advantage of proximity scanning. Proximity scanning is attractive to institutions using carts and kits. The inventory can be scanned without touching each individual item.

25. D. Clinical alerts are designed to provide health care providers with pertinent patient safety information related to medication changes or lab value changes.

26. B. Floor-stock distribution models will consist of items that have a low-risk safety profile. Such models are also effective for providing low-risk sensitive items to a patient care area.

24-14 Additional Resources

Bates DW. Preventing medication errors: a summary. *Am J Health-Syst Pharm.* 2007;64(suppl 9):S3–S9.

Bond CA, Raehl CL, Franke T. Clinical pharmacy services, hospital pharmacy staffing, and medication errors in United States hospitals. *Pharmacotherapy.* 2002;22(2):134–147.

Cardinal Health. Optimizing the medication use process: improving clinical, operational, and financial performance. Proceedings from the April 2008 Interdisciplinary Conference. San Diego, CA: Cardinal Health; 2008.

Kohn LT, Corrigan JM, Donaldson MS, eds. *To Err Is Human: Building a Safer Health System.* Washington, DC: National Academy Press; 1999.

Koppel R, Metlay JP, Cohen A, et al. Role of computerized physician order entry systems in facilitating medication errors. *JAMA.* 2005;293(10):1197–1203.

Leape LL, Brennan TA, Laird N, et al. The nature of adverse events in hospitalized patients: results of the Harvard Medical Practice Study. *N Engl J Med.* 1991;324(6):377–384.

Marx D. Patient safety and the "just culture": a primer for health care executives. Prepared for Columbia University, New York, NY; 2001. Available at: http://www.chpso.org/sites/main/files/file-attachments/marx_primer.pdf.

Nicol N. Case study: an interdisciplinary approach to medication error reduction. *Am J Health-Syst Pharm.* 2007;64(suppl 9): S17–S20.

Oldland AR, Golightly LK, May SK, et al. Electronic inventory systems and bar code technology: impact on pharmacy technical accuracy and error liability. *Hosp Pharm.* 2015;50(1):34–41.

Oren E, Shaffer ER, Guglielmo BJ. Impact of emerging technologies on medication errors and adverse events. *Am J Health-Syst Pharm.* 2003;60(14):1447–1458.

Our long journey towards a safety-minded just culture—part II: where we're going. *ISMP Medication Safety Alert!* Newsletter. September 21, 2006. Institute for Safe Medication Practices Web site. https://www.ismp.org/newsletters/acutecare/articles/20060921.asp.

Outcome Engenuity. An introduction to just culture. 2005. Available at: https://www.outcome-eng.com/david-marx-introduces-just-culture/.

Pedersen CA, Schneider PJ, Scheckelhoff DJ. ASHP national survey of pharmacy practice in hospital settings: dispensing and administration—2014. *AM J Health-Syst Pharm.* 2015;72(13):1119–1137. Update from 2008 article.

Schneider PJ. Opportunities for pharmacy. *Am J Health-Syst Pharm.* 2008;65(suppl 9):S10–S16.

Survey of automated dispensing shows need for practice improvements and safer system design. *ISMP Medication Safety Alert!* Newsletter. June 16, 1999. Institute for Safe Medication Practices Web site. https://www.ismp.org/newsletters/acutecare/articles/19990616.asp.

Uy RCY, Kury FP, Fontelo PA. The state and trends of barcode, RFID, biometric and pharmacy automation technologies in US hospitals. *AMIA Annu Symp Proc.* 2015;2015:1242–1251. Available at: https://www.ncbi.nlm.nih.gov/pmc/articles/PMC4765644/.

CLINICAL SCIENCES

area 4

EDITOR: *BRADLEY A. BOUCHER*

Evidence-Based Practice 25

JOSEPH M. SWANSON

25-1 KEY POINTS

- A staggering volume of medical literature is published yearly.
- Clinical studies fall into two major categories: treatment and observational.
- The most statistically rigorous clinical trial design is the blinded, randomized, controlled trial.
- Evidence-based medicine approaches a clinical dilemma as an answerable clinical question.
- The Cochrane Collaboration was developed to provide regularly updated reviews of clinically important questions.
- Evidence-based guidelines provide the strength of a recommendation based on the quality of the supporting literature.
- A clinical practice guideline generally consists of abbreviated text containing a recommendation for quick reference by the clinician.
- A clinical practice guideline contains text describing the literature that supports the provided recommendations.
- The lack of a standardized grading scale in clinical practice guidelines makes the reader's initial determination of the way recommendations were developed extremely important.
- The AGREE (Appraisal of Guidelines for Research and Evaluation) II Instrument consists of 23 items organized into six different sections and is used to evaluate the quality of clinical practice guidelines.
- Seven steps are taken to apply clinical practice guidelines to patient care: new evidence, dissemination, acceptance, consensus, development, implementation, and assessment.
- Validation studies are essential for confirming original research findings.
- Validation studies have begun to demonstrate the usefulness of applying clinical practice guidelines to patient care.

25-2 STUDY GUIDE CHECKLIST

The following topics may guide your study of this subject area:

- ☐ Understanding of different literature categories
- ☐ Understanding of the rigor of each category of literature
- ☐ Awareness of the concept of evidence-based medicine and practices and the reason this concept is important to patient care
- ☐ Factors to consider when implementing change to clinical practice based on research published in the medical literature
- ☐ How to find clinical practice guidelines
- ☐ Important considerations when determining whether guidelines are evidence based
- ☐ Variables to consider when using clinical practice guidelines
- ☐ Important factors for evaluating clinical practice guidelines
- ☐ Steps required to incorporate clinical practice guidelines into direct patient care
- ☐ Steps required to keep patient care protocols, pathways, and order sets up to date

25-3 Introduction

The volume of medically related research published each year is staggering. Searching a medical citation database will often produce in excess of 750,000 publications in one year's time. Unfortunately, the vast amount of information produced presents a significant dilemma for clinicians trying to stay up to date in their practice. A single clinician's review and processing of all of the available literature pertaining to his or her practice is impractical—and likely impossible. Thus, a mechanism to inform clinicians about important information related to their clinical practice is imperative.

Interestingly, despite the numerous publications produced yearly, a significant number of unanswered questions still exist for important clinical scenarios. This dilemma may be even more difficult for the practicing clinician, because he or she has nowhere to turn to determine the appropriate action in such cases. This situation is referred to as the *art of medicine.* Unfortunately, patients are at risk of receiving less-than-optimal care in these situations. Again, clinicians' capacity to seek guidance for these troubling clinical scenarios is extremely important.

Even when the clinician is knowledgeable about current literature supporting specific care, patients often do not receive optimal care. Translating evidence produced in the medical literature into clinical practice poses many problems, especially when new data are generated that may alter the best approach to a specific clinical condition. Additionally, conflicting results often produce two or more schools of thought as to the best practice despite adequate evidence of any specific action.

Clinical practice guidelines incorporate the vast evidence for a specific topic and present it in a concise, organized, and easily understandable fashion. Because clinical practice guidelines evaluate the available literature and provide clinicians with a system for understanding the strength of this evidence, they are often referred to as *evidence-based guidelines.*

25-4 Principles of Clinical Practice Guidelines for Various Diseases and Their Interpretation in the Clinical Setting

Literature Categories

When posed with a clinical dilemma, the clinician can turn to colleagues for assistance, or he or she can research the question using various types of literature. The literature available to the clinician ranges widely. Any published literature may be incorporated into practice as long as the strengths and limitations of each are understood and addressed. Following are various types of studies published in the medical literature:

- Randomized controlled trials, which are considered the most statistically rigorous
- Nonrandomized trials
- Observational studies
  - Cohort studies
  - Case-control studies
  - Cross-sectional studies

The ability to apply individual studies directly to patient care can be impaired because of study limitations. Therefore, scientists use other methods to investigate the results identified in individual studies:

- Meta-analysis
- Review
- Systematic review
- Clinical practice guidelines

Clinical practice guidelines are generally broader than the preceding types of literature, provide recommendations specifically to guide patient care, and are developed by leading clinicians in the field. A more detailed description is provided later in this chapter.

Definition of Evidence-Based Medicine

To understand clinical practice guidelines, one must discuss the foundation on which they are built. In the 1950s, the first argument for a methodological approach to medical decision making was presented. It was suggested that incorporation of statistics and probabilities could improve medical decision making. The term *decision analysis* was introduced in the 1970s. In the 1980s, evidenced-based medicine (EBM) and medical decision making (MDM) became more prominent in the medical community. Both address the concern for variations in clinical practice resulting in less than optimal care of patients. These variations are unrelated to a patient's severity of illness but are often associated with other factors, such as geography or socioeconomic status.

Although EBM and MDM have common foundations, the medical community has embraced EBM more than MDM. Thus, EBM forms the basis for the current approach to patient care. EBM approaches a clinical dilemma as an answerable clinical question represented by the mnemonic *PICO:*

- The *P* refers to the patient's problem.
- The *I* addresses the clinical intervention.
- The *C* represents a comparison of the intervention with at least one alternative.
- The *O* is for the desired clinical outcome that is used to compare interventions.

The PICO model is best applied to foreground questions, which are specific knowledge questions that affect clinical decisions. Using the mnemonic provides a semiformal structure that can be applied to any clinical problem. When using PICO, EBM highlights the quality of literature used to support the intervention, and it emphasizes different levels of significance based on the research methods employed in the published study. Additionally, it supports a systematic literature review or meta-analysis when conflicting evidence exists. Unfortunately, conducting a systematic literature review is impractical for the individual clinician. Although a review can be done over a period of time, it does not allow for immediate application of information to a specific patient problem. Performing a meta-analysis is extremely time consuming and is likely not feasible for the practicing clinician. Development of the Cochrane Collaboration was an effort to provide regularly updated reviews of clinically important questions. The reviews are intended for a broad readership that does not have time for an individual, careful, and critical review of the literature. More information on the Cochrane Collaboration is available at http://www.cochrane.org.

The meta-analyses available through the Cochrane Collaboration provide important information to clinicians seeking answers to a very specific question. Clinical practice guidelines emulate the goals of the Cochrane Collaboration, but on a broader scale. This is best represented by the fact that many guidelines are now incorporating systematic reviews into the guideline development process. Using these reviews, guidelines seek to provide evidence-based information to the practicing clinician regarding various aspects of a disease state or clinical condition.

Definition of Clinical Practice Guidelines

According to the Institute of Medicine, *clinical practice guidelines* are "systematically developed statements to assist practitioner and patient decisions about appropriate health care for specific clinical circumstances," and their purpose is "to make explicit recommendations with a definite intent to influence what clinicians do" (Field and Lohr 1992). These statements incorporate key factors such as a systematic review of the literature, clinicians, patients, and specific clinical situations. Each is integral when applying evidence from clinical trials to an individual patient with a specific medical condition.

Essentially two types of clinical practice guidelines exist, the *traditional* form and the *evidence-based* form.

Experts in a specific field develop the traditional clinical practice guidelines. The purpose is to provide recommendations for clinicians, generally in the form of decision trees, flowcharts, tables, and best practice guides. Although these guidelines usually incorporate primary literature into the process, they do not always include a comprehensive review and often do not provide ratings for the strength of recommendations. Thus, varying portions of the guidelines are determined by expert opinion or perceived best practices. Traditional clinical practice guidelines require the reader to trust that the expert guideline developers have sufficiently evaluated the available literature. Additionally, the reader must have faith that the guideline development was free of bias, because that is not always evident in the published document.

Evidence-based clinical practice guidelines take a more systematic approach than do traditional guidelines. They are still developed by an expert panel. However, a major difference is a comprehensive, methodological review of the literature including both qualitative and quantitative (meta-analysis) analyses. This review includes all literature on a specific topic, not only randomized clinical trials but also less rigorous study designs such as retrospective reviews, case studies, and prospective nonrandomized studies. The use of less-than-optimal literature leads to the next important aspect of evidence-based guidelines—evaluation of the strength of supporting literature. Evidence-based guidelines identify the literature supporting specific recommendations. They then apply a grade for the recommendation that is based on the strength of available literature. These types of guidelines can include expert opinions, and if so, this inclusion is clear in the recommendation.

Both types of guidelines may provide insight into important aspects of a clinical condition that the currently published literature does not adequately address. That section is generally titled "Future Research" and is used to stimulate researchers to attempt to answer the important questions included there.

Anatomy of a Clinical Practice Guideline

The anatomy of a clinical practice guideline is fairly simple. A guideline generally contains a description of methodology, an introduction to the disease state, definitions of grading, recommendations, and discussion of evidence supporting those recommendations. Additionally, guidelines often provide suggested clinical pathways for diagnosis and treatment of the clinical condition. The general nature of these pathways is intended to provide a starting point for clinicians to incorporate regional or local practice variations into guideline recommendations, creating a customized pathway. Figure 25-1 provides a generic example. Tables are used to highlight important facts that all clinicians should remember. All guidelines provide a references section that allows clinicians to find original studies supporting recommendations in the guidelines. The references also allow clinicians the opportunity to incorporate inclusion and exclusion criteria of specific studies in local practice.

The general outline of a clinical practice guideline should be included at the beginning of the document. Box 25-1 provides a sample outline of a clinical practice guideline. Guidelines begin with a formal explanation of the intent, scope, and methodology used in the development. Those sections provide the transparency considered so important when evaluating the integrity of a guideline. An introduction highlights the condition and the reasons it is important to clinicians.

Following that section is a brief epidemiology of the condition, if this information was not included in the introduction. Most clinicians are relatively aware of this information, but guidelines can provide the most recent information. If pathogenesis is included in a guideline, it should highlight recently identified information. This information should have some relevance to the clinical condition and therapies that address the newly identified pathogenesis.

Some conditions are preventable. A section describing the prevention of the condition may or may not be relevant. In conditions where prevention is feasible, separate guidelines may focus entirely on this aspect of the condition.

Diagnosis and evaluation of the clinical condition is one of the most important areas of a guideline and likely contains the majority of recommendations. Therapy for the condition is the only section that may contain as much information as the diagnosis section. This section is one of the most important for pharmacists, because it usually contains the relevant literature for medications.

FIGURE 25-1. Generic Example of a Clinical Pathway

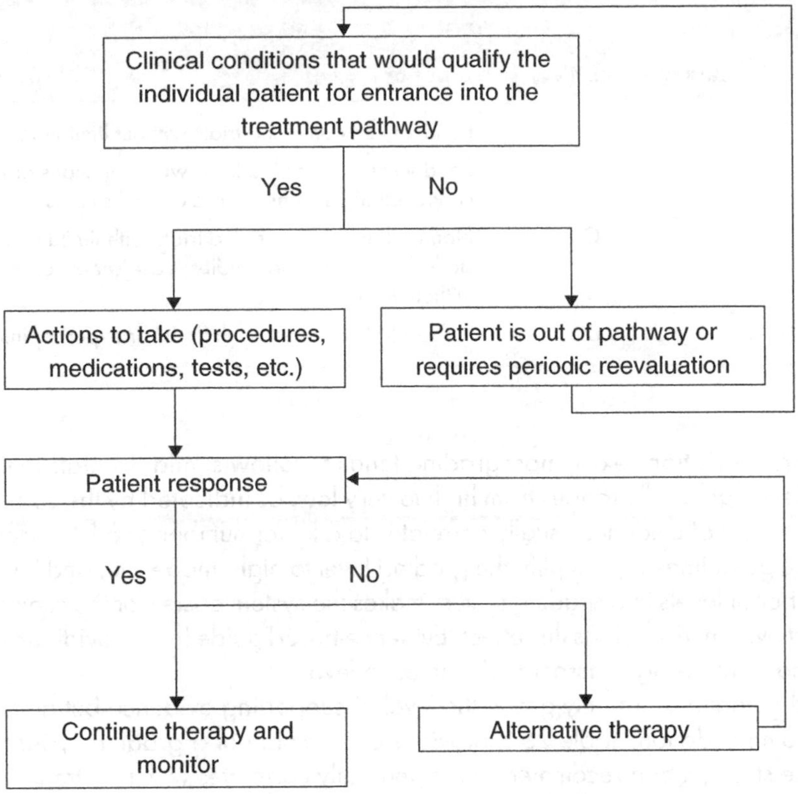

Some guidelines will contain sections that describe how to monitor for response to therapy. These sections can be important to pharmacists because they can contain recommendations for determining medication failure, changing the medication therapy, or identifying medication-related adverse effects.

Some, but not all, guidelines include sections identifying important clinical questions not yet answered and areas for future research. These sections usually guide researchers toward areas of important concern or possible breakthroughs in patient care. Additionally, such sections alert clinicians to future literature that may change practice.

Levels of Evidence

As previously mentioned, clinical practice guidelines provide clinicians guidance for recommendations. The quality of evidence supporting recommendations is described by grading systems. Grading systems are presented in different variations of letters and numbers, depending on the expert panel developing the

BOX 25-1. Outline of a Clinical Practice Guideline

- Summary of the intent and scope of the clinical practice guideline
- Methodology used to develop and prepare the guideline
- Grading system for ranking recommendations in the guideline
- Introduction to the topic
- Epidemiology of the clinical condition
- Pathogenesis of the clinical condition
- Prevention of the clinical condition (if possible)
- Diagnosis and evaluation of the clinical condition
- Therapy for the clinical condition
- Evaluation of response to therapy
- Identification of important clinical questions not addressed in the literature
- Suggestions for future research on the clinical condition

TABLE 25-1. Example of an Evidence Grading System

Quality of supporting evidence	Numbers	Letters	Types of studies
High	1	A	Randomized controlled trials without limitations
Moderate	2	B	Randomized controlled trials with limitations or nonrandomized controlled trials (cohort, case-control studies, etc.) without limitations
Low	3	C	Nonrandomized controlled trials with limitations or noncontrolled studies (observational studies, case series, case reports, etc.) without flaws
Very low	4	D	Noncontrolled studies with flaws or expert opinions

guidelines. Although variations exist, most grading tends to follow similar formats to that in Table 25-1. The quality of evidence generally ranges from high to very low, as indicated by the corresponding letter or number. The higher level of evidence usually correlates to a lower number or a letter appearing sooner in the alphabet. Some guidelines will simplify the grading level to high, moderate, and low. The belief is that restricting the number of levels in a grading system makes the system easier for the clinician to understand. However, no direct evidence supports this effect. Evidence-based guidelines provide an explanation of the grading system and study designs associated with each level.

Evidence-based guidelines not only grade the level of supporting evidence but also usually grade the strength of the recommendation. Table 25-2 provides an example of a grading system for guideline recommendations. The strength of a recommendation generally correlates with the strength of the supporting evidence. However, the strength of the recommendation usually provides a risk-versus-benefit determination. Recommendation strength can range from "recommend implementing the recommendation," usually corresponding to a positive risk-versus-benefit ratio, to "recommend not implementing the recommendation," usually with a negative risk-versus-benefit ratio. These strengths are often represented by letters or numbers, as with the grading of evidence. The symbols used for the recommendation strength are usually different from those used for grading of evidence.

A combination of letters and symbols is often used when providing strength for the recommendation and grading the supporting literature. The use of two different scales provides an easily understandable and concise form of grading. For example, a strong recommendation with strong supporting evidence would likely be graded as a 1A recommendation. Interestingly, no research addresses the most effective method of grading either the recommendation or the supporting evidence.

Although the combination of numbers and letters can effectively communicate the strength of the recommendation, lack of uniformity may cause confusion. Current clinical guidelines have no standardized method of grading the literature and recommendation. Many times, the same number or letter has a different meaning depending on the organization or expert panel. This lack of standardization makes the reader's initial determination of the grading scale used in a specific clinical practice guideline extremely

TABLE 25-2. Example of a Recommendation Grading System

Recommendation strength	Numbers	Letters	Risk vs. benefit
Recommend implementing	1	A	Desirable effects with benefit clearly outweighing risk
Consider implementing	2	B	Desirable effects with benefit appearing to outweigh risk
Consider not implementing	3	C	Possible undesirable effects with risk appearing to outweigh benefit
Recommend not implementing	4	D	Undesirable effects with risk clearly outweighing benefits

important. The GRADE (Grading of Recommendations Assessment, Development, and Evaluation) Working Group was formed with the idea of reaching an agreement on a uniform, logical approach to grading the quality of evidence and the strength of recommendations. If the GRADE approach is universally adopted, all guidelines could provide the same grading regardless of the expert panel developing the guideline. This outcome would allow clinicians to compare and contrast grading of recommendations across the board. It is anticipated that standardized grading could improve compliance by clinicians. Until this occurs, clinicians are expected to review each guideline carefully and determine how the recommendations and supporting evidence are graded. Finally, the clinician needs to sort out the differences in grading levels and supporting evidence produced in different guidelines.

Finding Applicable Guidelines

If a clinician wishes to apply EBM to one of his or her patients, a complete review of the literature is impractical. One of the most efficient methods is to identify a clinical practice guideline that addresses the patient's specific condition. As previously mentioned, a guideline will have recommendations for clinically important conditions. However, where does the clinician go to find the appropriate guidelines? Many would immediately turn to a bibliographic database such as the National Library of Medicine's MEDLINE?/PubMed? at https://www.nlm.nih.gov/bsd/pmresources.html. A search of MEDLINE?/PubMed? may produce the appropriate guideline as long as it is published in an indexed journal. Unfortunately, not all practice guidelines appear in indexed journals. Some are published online, and others may appear in nonindexed journals. A search of this database might miss important, clinically relevant guidelines. Additionally, MEDLINE?/PubMed? does not always provide access to the full text of cited guidelines. Even if the clinician were to find the appropriate guideline, he or she might not be able to access the entire text and thus not be able to evaluate recommendations in the guideline. Fortunately, the clinician has other options. In fact, the Internet offers several choices to access a variety of guidelines. The Web sites listed in Box 25-2 provide access to various guidelines. The National Guideline Clearinghouse is an initiative of the Agency for Healthcare Research and Quality and U.S. Department of Health and Human Services. It is a public resource for evidence-based clinical practice guidelines; it is frequently used to obtain full-text clinical practice guidelines for multiple clinical conditions.

Examples of commonly referenced clinical practice guidelines are included in Table 25-3. As indicated in the table, more than one organization often supports the guideline. Guidelines are generally published in well-respected peer-reviewed journals, and availability ranges from easily accessible online copies to required journal subscription hard copies.

Evaluation of Clinical Practice Guidelines

The evaluation of clinical practice guidelines is important when determining whether to apply recommendations directly to patients, especially when more than one set of guidelines exists for a specific clinical condition. A prime example is the CHEST (American College of Chest Physicians) guidelines for the prevention of venous thromboembolism and the EAST (Eastern Association for the Surgery of Trauma) guidelines for management of venous thromboembolism. Both guidelines address prevention of deep vein thrombosis in traumatically injured patients, but the recommendations of each differ slightly. Therefore,

BOX 25-2. Sources for Obtaining Clinical Practice Guidelines

Agency for Healthcare Research and Quality, National Guideline Clearinghouse, https://www.guideline.gov

Centers for Disease Control and Prevention, https://www.cdc.gov

National Library of Medicine, Health Services/Technology Assessment Text, https://www.ncbi.nlm.nih.gov/books/NBK16710/

Guidelines International Network (requires fee and membership), http://www.g-i-n.net/home

TABLE 25-3. Commonly Used Clinical Practice Guidelines

Guideline	Supporting organization
Antithrombotic Therapy for VTE Disease	American College of Chest Physicians
The Seventh Report of the Joint National Committee on Prevention, Detection, Evaluation, and Treatment of High Blood Pressure	National Heart, Lung, and Blood Institute
Expert Panel Report 3: Guidelines for the Diagnosis and Management of Asthma	U.S. Department of Health and Human Services; National Institutes of Health; and National Heart, Lung, and Blood Institute
ACCF/AHA Guideline for the Management of Heart Failure	American College of Cardiology Foundation and American Heart Association
ADA Clinical Practice Recommendations	American Diabetes Association
Therapeutic Monitoring of Vancomycin in Adult Patients: A Consensus Review of the American Society of Health-System Pharmacists, the Infectious Diseases Society of America, and the Society of Infectious Diseases Pharmacists	American Society of Health-System Pharmacists, Infectious Diseases Society of America, and Society of Infectious Diseases Pharmacists

clinicians caring for trauma patients are responsible for reviewing each set of guidelines and the literature supporting recommendations for each. Then the clinician must determine which recommendations to incorporate in the care of his or her patients.

The Appraisal of Guidelines for Research and Evaluation (AGREE) II Instrument, which is available at https://www.agreetrust.org/wp-content/uploads/2017/12/AGREE-II-Users-Manual-and-23-item-Instrument-2009-Update-2017.pdf, provides a tool for guideline users to assess the methodological quality of clinical practice guidelines. The authors of the AGREE II Instrument state that it is intended for use by the following groups:

- Policy makers—to decide which guidelines can be recommended for use in practice
- Guideline developers—to follow a structured and rigorous development methodology and to use a self-assessment tool to ensure that their guidelines are sound
- Health care providers—to undertake their own assessment before adopting the recommendations
- Educators or teachers—to help enhance critical appraisal skills among health professionals

The AGREE II Instrument consists of 23 items that are organized in six different domains. Each domain addresses a different aspect of a guideline's quality:

- ***Scope and Purpose (3 items):*** This domain deals with the major aspects of the guideline. It focuses on the overall purpose of the guideline, the important clinical questions addressed, and the target patient population.
- ***Stakeholder Involvement (3 items):*** This domain determines the degree to which the guideline represents the views of clinicians using the guideline and the target patient population.
- ***Rigor of Development (8 items):*** This domain investigates the degree to which the development group researched the available evidence. It addresses the processes used to gather, synthesize, and evaluate the available literature. Additionally, it determines the methods used to produce recommendations.
- ***Clarity of Presentation (3 items):*** This domain focuses on the language used in the guideline and the way the authors have formatted the document.
- ***Applicability (4 items):*** This domain addresses the key factors in implementing the guideline, including organizational, behavioral, and cost implications.
- ***Editorial Independence (2 items):*** This domain deals mostly with the developers of the guideline. It evaluates the independence and possible conflicts of interest of the development group.

TABLE 25-4. Example of AGREE II Instrument Scoring for Domain 1

	Item 1	Item 2	Item 3	Total
User 1	2	2	3	7
User 2	3	3	3	9
User 3	3	2	2	7
Total	8	7	8	23
Maximum score	(Strongly agree) × (number of users) × (number of items) Example: 4 × 3 × 3			36
Minimum score	(Strongly disagree) × (number of users) × (number of items) Example: 1 × 3 × 3			9
Standardized score	$\frac{\text{Obtained score} - \text{Minimum score}}{\text{Maximum score} - \text{Minimum score}}$ Example: $\frac{23-9}{36-9}$			51.8%

Based on AGREE II Instrument, 2017.

The 23 items in the six domains are organized so that the user of the instrument can rank his or her evaluation of the guideline. Each item may receive a minimum score of 1 (indicating the user strongly disagrees with the item statement) and a maximum score of 7 (indicating the user strongly agrees with the item statement). All items within a domain are scored, and the total score is tallied for each user review. The total score for each user is added together to determine the obtained score. The maximum score is the number 7 (strongly agree) times the number of items in a domain, times the number of appraisers. The minimum score is calculated in the same way as the maximum, only the number 1 (strongly disagree) is used. The standardized score accounts for all users' input and the maximum and minimum scores possible. Table 25-4 shows a sample score.

25-5 Integration of Scientific and Systems-Based Knowledge into Treatment Protocols and Clinical Practice Guidelines

The two main reasons for directly applying to patients the evidence-based recommendations from clinical practice guidelines are as follows:

- ***Improving patient care:*** In 2000, the Institute of Medicine published a report, *To Err Is Human*, stating that up to 98,000 inpatients die unnecessarily each year. These deaths can be attributed to medical error. This rate is unacceptable and has spurred attempts to improve patient care. Additionally, other reports suggest that Americans do not receive care based on the best available scientific evidence. Incorporating clinical practice guidelines into local practice assists clinicians in identifying the best care. In doing so, patient outcomes are improved. For example, a study demonstrated that applying the community-acquired pneumonia guidelines to patients reduced their length of stay and mortality in the hospital.
- ***Lowering cost:*** Applying clinical practice guidelines to patient care not only improves patient outcomes but also can reduce costs. In the community-acquired pneumonia example, patient charges were reduced. If patients receive better care, they will be more likely to address health concerns

sooner. If clinicians follow guidelines, they will be less likely to miss important clinical issues. Identifying clinical issues sooner permits reduction in medical costs or avoidance of those costs altogether.

Common forms of incorporating clinical practice guidelines into patient care include protocols, pathways, guidelines, and order sets. Although clinicians view each of these methods differently, they can be categorized by how much they restrict clinician decision making:

- ***Protocols:*** A protocol is a plan for a course of medical care of patients. It tends to be the most restrictive form of dictating care. Depending on the protocol, patient care may be completely determined by the protocol. Many clinicians are concerned that protocols remove clinical decision making, thus removing the clinician from the care of patients.
- ***Pathways:*** In contrast, pathways provide a plan for a course of action, which is generally followed, but allows the clinician to make decisions and break from the pathway based on patient-specific factors. They are considered less restrictive than protocols.
- ***Guidelines:*** Although guidelines provide evidence, they leave the decisions completely to the clinician. They provide the most autonomy for clinicians.
- ***Order sets:*** By providing options for clinicians, order sets aim to clue the user into thinking about specific aspects of care. They may be used independently but are often combined with protocols, pathways, or guidelines.

The general process of incorporating newly identified clinical evidence or clinical practice guidelines into direct patient care has several steps, as illustrated in Figure 25-2. Pharmacists should be involved in each step of this process.

The American Society of Health-System Pharmacists developed guidelines addressing the pharmacist's role in this process:

- ***Step 1: New evidence.*** Medical researchers generate new evidence and report the results of specific studies in medical journals. Pharmacists are playing a bigger role in the generation of new evidence now than ever before. However, the role for the pharmacist in integration of new evidence into direct patient care is most prominent in the later steps in the process.
- ***Step 2: Dissemination.*** All health care practitioners are responsible for disseminating newfound knowledge, but pharmacists can be integral in this step. Pharmacists can conduct journal club meetings to highlight important evidence that should be applied directly to patients. Pharmacists

FIGURE 25-2. Process by Which New Research Is Incorporated into Clinical Practice

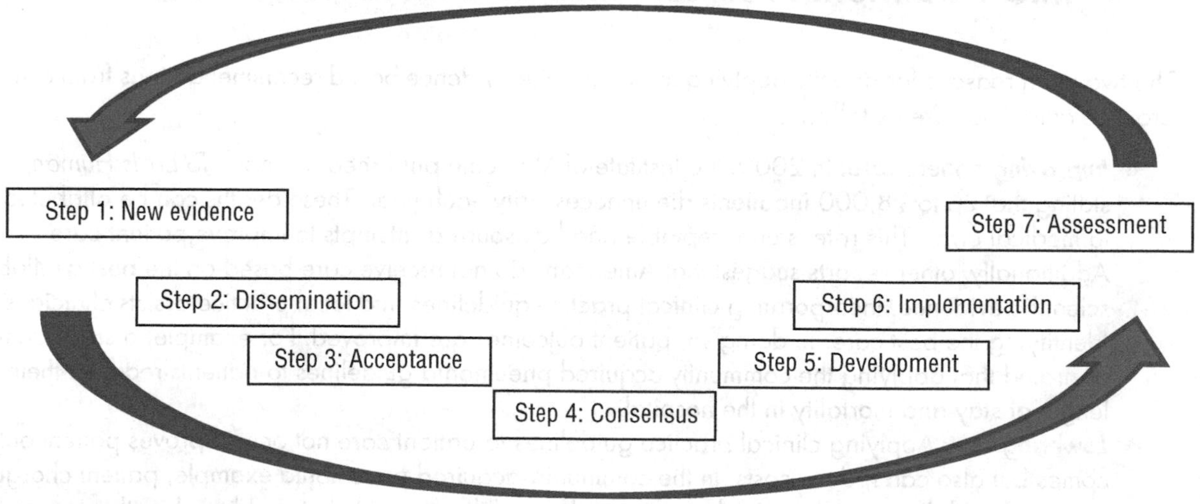

should monitor important guidelines that apply to their practice area. They should help inform other health care practitioners when updates or new guidelines are published.

- ***Step 3: Acceptance.*** Whether new evidence is accepted depends highly on the quality of the evidence. If new evidence clearly provides a great benefit with very little risk, it is usually welcomed by all. More controversy usually arises when the risk-to-benefit ratio is not as clear. The pharmacist's role in acceptance is to highlight the risks and benefits and discuss them with other pertinent health care professionals. Placing the risks and benefits into perspective will facilitate an understanding of new evidence.
- ***Step 4: Consensus.*** To achieve consensus, one must bring local practice leaders together to determine the best method of applying the new evidence to patient care. Pharmacists may be the practice leaders, or they may assist other leaders in this process.
- ***Step 5: Development.*** This step involves the incorporation of the new evidence into a new or currently existing clinical protocol, pathway, or order set. In the hospital setting, development is usually performed by a multidisciplinary team that likely includes a pharmacist.
- ***Step 6: Implementation.*** This step occurs immediately following development. Implementation includes education of all health care practitioners involved in applying the new evidence to the patient. Following the initial education, members of the development team are usually available to help with troubleshooting any problems with the new evidence.
- ***Step 7: Assessment.*** This final step involves measuring the effect of implementing the new evidence by auditing patient outcomes after implementation. An important part of the assessment phase is providing feedback to the development team. Feedback is used to augment or revise the implementation. Additionally, it can identify ways to improve the implementation process, such as providing enhanced education or awareness raising.

The entire process is circular, in that new evidence is constantly generated. Although not all evidence will be incorporated, continual monitoring of newly published evidence is essential to ensure that patients receive the most effective care.

25-6 Evaluation of Clinical Trials that Validate Treatment Usefulness

Research enhancing patient outcomes can greatly improve clinical practice. Although new research is exciting and often quickly adapted to clinical practice, results should be confirmed in independent study to ensure that the initial results were true. Thus, validation of research is extremely important. Validation generally occurs on a single-study basis, meaning that one study shows improved patient outcomes and is validated by a different single study; however, with the increased use of clinical guidelines, studies are being published that validate the entire guideline:

- ***Validation of a single study:*** An example is a study investigating the effects of an aldosterone antagonist on mortality in patients with heart failure. The study documented a 30% reduction in the risk of death compared to placebo. Following this study, a different group of researchers investigated the use of another aldosterone antagonist and were able to achieve a 15% reduction in mortality. This study validated the results from the original research and has formed the basis of aldosterone antagonist use as standard of care in patients with heart failure.
- ***Validation of clinical practice guidelines:*** In 2003, the Canadian clinical practice guidelines for nutrition support in critically ill patients receiving mechanical ventilation were published. These guidelines systematically reviewed the pertinent literature regarding the topic and provided clinicians a set of recommendations. In 2004, a validation of these guidelines was published. Conducting a randomized controlled trial evaluating the numerous recommendations provided in the

practice guidelines is impossible. Therefore, the validation study was a multicentered, prospective observational study of 59 intensive care units (ICUs). The researchers investigated the association between five recommendations in the clinical practice guidelines and adequacy of enteral nutrition. The study concluded that ICUs more consistent with guidelines demonstrated more success with enterally feeding patients.

Unfortunately, two factors often prevent clinicians from confidently implementing promising results:

- ***Lack of validation studies:*** Ensuring that the results found in one study are correct can be difficult. Researchers and clinicians rely on sound study design and statistical evaluation to provide confidence in the results obtained. However, a possibility always exists that the promising results occurred by chance or that some unknown factor contributed to the improved outcomes. If a separate study confirms the initial study's promising results, clinicians have more confidence that the improved outcome is indeed a real effect. Some well-conducted single studies have such a great influence on the medical community that performing a validation study is difficult or impossible. Following are the two main reasons for this difficulty:
  - If one study shows a significant benefit, and the medical community supports the results, a validation study may be considered unethical. Clinicians may believe so strongly in the benefit that a controlled trial may be considered as placing study subjects at unnecessary risk. For this scenario to occur, the original study not only would have to be extremely well conducted, well designed, and controlled, but also would need to have a sufficiently large study population. Alternatively, a multitude of well-conducted but insufficiently powered studies can produce a similar effect.
  - One major barrier to the successful completion of a validation study is physician preference. If a physician believes the original study results are convincing enough, he or she may prefer to withhold patients from enrollment in a validation study, especially if the validation uses a placebo-controlled arm. The physician may want to ensure his or her patients receive the therapy from the original study, hoping that they will receive the benefit originally found.
- ***Conflicting results in validation studies:*** Numerous examples show significant research results being confounded by subsequent studies unable to validate the original results. A prime example is a study investigating the use of low-dose steroids in patients with septic shock. The original study found improved mortality in certain patients receiving low-dose steroids. Unfortunately, a large multicentered study was unable to confirm the mortality benefit identified in the initial study. The results from the second study have produced a dilemma for clinicians wanting to use low-dose steroids in their patients. Whether this treatment will benefit patients is now uncertain.

Despite the difficulties with validating original research, these studies are essential to clinicians who want to ensure their patients receive the best evidence-based care available. When new research has not been validated, the clinician needs to evaluate the risk-to-benefit ratio of the new findings. If the new research is implemented, clinicians have to monitor patients closely for the desired outcome and any potential adverse effects.

25-7 Questions

1. Medically related literature published each year consists of approximately

A. 1,000 publications.
B. 5,000,000 publications.
C. 50,000 publications.
D. 750,000 publications.

2. Which study design is considered the most statistically rigorous?

A. Cohort
B. Case control
C. Randomized
D. Cross-sectional

3. Use of blinding in a clinical trial is expected to

A. decrease bias in the study.
B. increase bias in the study.
C. have no effect on bias.
D. increase and decrease bias in the study.

4. Which of the following best describes a meta-analysis?

A. A qualitative method of combining the results of multiple independent studies and synthesizing the results to arrive at a conclusion about the specific question studied
B. A single-center independent study
C. A quantitative method of combining the results of multiple independent studies and synthesizing the results to arrive at a conclusion about the specific question studied
D. A nonquantitative review of the literature

5. What is the difference between a clinical practice guideline and a review?

A. There is no difference between a review and a clinical practice guideline.
B. Reviews have a broader scope than clinical practice guidelines.
C. Reviews provide recommendations that are specifically designed to guide patient care.
D. Clinical practice guidelines provide recommendations that are specifically designed to guide patient care.

6. Which organization is best known for developing meta-analyses for important clinical conditions?

A. Cochrane Collaboration
B. National Meta-Analyses Group
C. International Society for Meta-Analysis
D. National Library of Medicine

7. Which methodological approach to patient care looks at clinical dilemmas as answerable clinical questions?

A. Medical decision making
B. Decision analysis
C. Evidence-based medicine
D. Standard medical analysis

8. How do evidence-based clinical practice guidelines differ from traditional clinical practice guidelines?

A. A methodological review of the literature is performed for evidence-based guidelines.
B. Traditional clinical practice guidelines provide recommendations that are more specific.
C. Nationally renowned experts develop evidence-based clinical practice guidelines.
D. Traditional clinical practice guidelines are published only online.

9. Which of the following sections of clinical practice guidelines is most important to pharmacists?

A. Introduction
B. Diagnosis
C. Future research
D. Therapy

10. What is the general purpose of sample clinical pathways used in practice guidelines?

A. To dictate exact care provided in the pathway
B. To provide a foundation for customized pathways
C. To reduce thinking by clinicians
D. To change policies of medical insurers

11. If a clinical practice guideline provided a recommendation supported by a well-conducted randomized controlled trial, what number would it likely be graded?

A. 4
B. 5
C. 3
D. 1

12. If a clinical practice guideline provided a D recommendation, what are the experts likely recommending?

A. Recommend not implementing the recommendation.
B. Recommend implementing the recommendation.
C. Consider implementing the recommendation.
D. Consider not implementing the recommendation.

13. Which of the following Web sites contains 1,422 guidelines published from 2011 to 2017 worldwide?

A. http://www.medmatrix.org
B. https://www.cdc.gov
C. http://www.myguidelines.org
D. https://www.guideline.gov

14. Which of the following groups should use the AGREE II Instrument?

A. Patients
B. Hospital policy makers
C. Patients' families
D. No one

15. If three users evaluate a clinical practice guideline using the AGREE II Instrument and are currently looking at Domain 4, Clarity of Presentation (contains three items), what is the maximum possible score?

A. 10
B. 27
C. 63
D. 105

16. If the maximum possible score for an AGREE II Instrument domain is 64, the minimum possible score is 16, and the obtained score is 56, what is the standardized score?

A. 83%
B. 17%
C. 50%
D. 25%

17. Which of the following is a rationale for incorporating clinical practice guidelines into patient care?

A. To reduce physician independence
B. To increase medical errors
C. To increase physician independence
D. To reduce medical errors

18. Which of the following is the final step in incorporating clinical practice guidelines into direct patient care?

A. Acceptance
B. Consensus
C. Assessment
D. Implementation

19. Which of the following best describes a validation study?

A. Original research not previously reported
B. Confirmation of original research by an independent group
C. Laboratory research supporting a clinical trial
D. Recommendation by a clinical expert

20. Which of the following prevents clinicians from implementing new evidence in patient care?

A. Lack of interest
B. Lack of validation studies
C. Confirmatory validation studies
D. Incorporation into clinical practice guidelines

25-8 Answers

1. D. Searching a medical citation database, such as MEDLINE?/PubMed?, by 1-year increments produces approximately 750,000 publications.

2. C. Use of a randomized design decreases the likelihood for other factors to influence the outcome of a clinical trial.

3. A. Blinding reduces bias in the study by preventing those conducting the study to influence the outcomes of the study.

4. C. The definition of a *meta-analysis* is a quantitative method of combining the results of multiple independent studies and synthesizing the results to arrive at a conclusion about the specific question studied.

5. D. A review compiles and synthesizes information about a topic, but a practice guideline provides weighted recommendations that are designed to guide each aspect of care related to that topic.

6. A. The Cochrane Collaboration was established specifically to conduct meta-analyses. The National Library of Medicine is the world's largest medical library and the other organizations are fictitious.

7. C. Evidence-based medicine is based on the "answerable clinical question" and is represented by the mnemonic *PICO* (*P*atient's problem, clinical *I*ntervention, *C*omparison with at least one alternative, and clinical *O*utcome).

8. **A.** Clinical practice guidelines that are not evidence based often represent opinion. Only evidence-based guidelines can ensure that a methodological review of the literature was performed.

9. **D.** Pharmacists are medication experts. Medication therapy is the focus of all pharmacists. Although the sections addressing other issues are very important, they may not pertain to pharmacists as much as the section covering therapy.

10. **B.** Many local pathways will differ from those provided in guidelines. This is acceptable and sometimes preferred. Adapting guideline pathways to local care is very important to address the most effective approach to patient care.

11. **D.** Guidelines generally use a lower number to represent a strong grading.

12. **A.** Similar to grading, recommendations are usually less strong as they move through the alphabet. Thus, a recommendation of choice **A** is usually better than a recommendation of choice **D**.

13. **D.** The Web site of the National Guideline Clearinghouse, https://www.guideline.gov, states that it contains such guidelines.

14. **B.** Neither patients nor their family members would use the AGREE II document to evaluate practice guidelines. However, hospital policy makers should be able to grade the strength of a guideline.

15. **C.** If there are three items, there are 21 possible points per reviewer, because each item has a maximum score of 7. Thus, $3 \times 7 = 21$. If all three reviewers provide the maximum score on each item, there is a total of 63 points. Thus, $3 \times 21 = 63$.

16. **A.** The standardized score = (obtained score − minimum score)/(maximum score − minimum score). If this score is reported as a percentage, it is multiplied by 100. Thus, $(56 - 16)/(64 - 16) = 40/48 = 0.83 \times 100 = 83\%$.

17. **D.** The only beneficial answer is to reduce medical errors. Guidelines do not attempt to reduce or increase physician independence.

18. **C.** The seven steps are new evidence, dissemination, acceptance, consensus, development, implementation, and assessment. Hence, assessment is the final step.

19. **B.** Validation studies duplicate (to some degree) an original study that shows benefit to determine if the benefit can be reproduced, thereby suggesting a true beneficial effect.

20. **B.** Validation studies are important to help determine if the beneficial effect is true or just occurred by chance. Clinicians prefer to wait until a study has been validated before automatically implementing the studied intervention into clinical practice.

25-9 Additional Resources

AGREE Next Steps Consortium. Appraisal of Guidelines for Research & Evaluation II: AGREE II Instrument. London: AGREE Next Steps Consortium; December 2017. Available at: https://www.agreetrust.org.

American Society of Health-System Pharmacists. ASHP guidelines on the pharmacist's role in the development, implementation, and assessment of critical pathways. *Am J Health-Syst Pharm.* 2004;61(9):939–945.

Elstein AS. On the origins and development of evidence-based medicine and medical decision making. *Inflamm Res.* 2004;53(suppl 2):S184–S189.

Field MJ, Lohr KN. A provisional instrument for assessing clinical practice guidelines. In: Field MJ, Lohr KN, eds. *Guidelines for Clinical Practice: From Development to Use.* Washington, DC: National Academies Press; 1992:346–410.

Hargrove P, Griffer M, Lund B. Procedures for using clinical practice guidelines. *Lang Speech Hear Serv Sch.* 2008;39(3):289–302.

Institute of Medicine. Clinical Practice Guidelines We Can Trust. Released March 23, 2011. Available at: http://www.nationalacademies.org/hmd/Reports/2011/Clinical-Practice-Guidelines-We-Can-Trust.aspx.

Institute of Medicine. *To Err Is Human: Building a Safer Health System.* Washington, DC: National Academies Press; 2000.

Schünemann HJ, Best D, Vist G, Oxman AD. Letters, numbers, symbols and words: how to communicate grades of evidence and recommendations. *CMAJ.* 2003;169(7):677–680.

Clinical Pathophysiology

26

THEODORE J. CORY

26-1 KEY POINTS

- *Inflammation* is a reaction of vascularized tissue and is a protective attempt by the body's defense mechanism to remove harmful stimuli and return the tissue to its normal structure or function.
- *Edema* is the abnormal accumulation of fluids in the interstitial spaces of cells or tissues. It is controlled by hydrostatic and osmotic pressure.
- *Hemorrhage* is the loss or escape of blood from the circulatory system, caused by trauma, vascular wall damage resulting from disease, or malfunction of the body's normal mechanism to maintain hemostasis.
- *Thrombosis* is the pathologic process of formation of a blood clot, which is referred to as a *thrombus*.
- *Infarction* is the process of forming an ischemic necrosis in the body tissue or organs. Infarctions most commonly occur in cardiovascular tissue as a result of thrombus formation.
- *Shock* is a serious condition involving decreased perfusion of tissues and organs because of inadequate blood flow.
- *Developmental defects* originate in the embryonic period and are most commonly the result of genetic or chromosomal abnormalities and environmental agents.
- A *neoplasm* is an abnormal mass of tissue attributable to uncontrolled cellular proliferation. Neoplasms can be benign or malignant in nature.
- *Hypertension* is defined as a repeatedly elevated blood pressure exceeding 130 mmHg (systolic) or 80 mmHg (diastolic). Hypertension can be caused by abnormalities of the renin–angiotensin system, dysregulation of the sympathetic nervous system, natriuretic hormone, and endothelial dysfunction.
- *Diabetes mellitus* is an endocrine disease in which the body does not properly produce or use insulin, resulting in hyperglycemia. Chronic hyperglycemia can result in macrovascular complications (i.e., stroke, hypertension, myocardial dysfunction) and microvascular complications.
- *Hyperlipidemia* is an abnormal elevation of fat in the blood, which can lead to coronary artery disease.

26-2 STUDY GUIDE CHECKLIST

The following topics may guide your study of this subject area:

- ☐ Familiarity with the causes and effects of inflammation and repair and the diseases related to these factors
- ☐ Awareness of the different types of hemorrhage, thrombosis, and shock and the risks associated with them
- ☐ Awareness of teratogenicity and the causes of developmental defects
- ☐ Understanding of a neoplasm, the difference between a benign and malignant neoplasm, and the causes of neoplasms
- ☐ Awareness of the fundamental factors that influence not only blood pressure but also cardiac output and systemic vascular resistance and the causes of increases or decreases in these two factors
- ☐ Familiarity with the symptoms, types, and risks associated with diabetes mellitus
- ☐ Awareness of the different types of lipoproteins and the risks of elevated levels

26-3 Basic Principles and Mechanisms of Disease

Inflammation and Repair

Inflammation is the reaction of vascularized tissue in the body to local injury or insult. It is a protective attempt by the body's defense mechanism to remove the harmful stimuli and return the tissue to its normal structure or function. Excessive inflammation can, however, be pathogenic.

Inflammation can be caused by numerous injurious stimuli, including the following:

- Chemical irritants or toxins
- Mechanical or physical trauma
- Altered or damaged cells
- Microorganisms

Clinical signs and symptoms of acute inflammation include the following:

- Redness
- Fever
- Swelling
- Pain

The inflammatory response that is produced by the body involves two distinct components: vascular and cellular.

Vascular component

The vascular component of the inflammatory process begins with the initial injury. Following injury, the body increases blood flow to the site through dilation of the arterioles. Dilation of the arterioles ultimately leads to dilation of the capillaries and venules.

In normal states, the capillaries and venules allow the passage of only small molecules out of the vasculature into the surrounding tissue, retaining macromolecules, such as cells and plasma proteins, inside the vessel.

In acute inflammation, the endothelial lining of the microvasculature is altered, thus allowing increased permeability of macromolecules into the tissue space. With this increased vessel permeability to macromolecules, there is also movement of body fluid, which causes swelling, or *edema,* at the area of injury. In diseases including cancer and lung disease, inflammation can be chronic, resulting in long-term damage to the inflamed site.

Cellular component

Along with vasculature changes that occur during the inflammatory process, numerous cellular changes are also occurring. As fluid is lost into the tissue space, large amounts of red blood cells, white blood cells, and platelets remain behind, causing blood viscosity to increase.

This increase in viscosity causes a phenomenon called *margination.* Margination is a process in which white blood cells, or *leukocytes,* relocate from their normal central location in the bloodstream to the periphery along the endothelium wall.

After margination progresses, leukocytes adhere to endothelial cells, before migrating from the blood to the tissue, where they are responsible for limiting the harmful stimuli and beginning the process of repair.

Mediators of inflammation

Histamine is stored in the granular tissue of mast cells. Once released, histamine produces vasodilation and increased vascular permeability.

Factor XII, also known as Hageman factor, is stored in an inactive form in plasma. Once activated, this plasma protein triggers the activation of four different cascades or systems important to inflammation and repair:

- The *coagulation cascade* leads to thrombin formation, which converts fibrinogen into fibrin, ultimately leading to clot formation.
- The *kinin cascade* leads to the production of bradykinin. Bradykinin is a peptide that causes vascular dilation and increases permeability.
- The *fibrinolytic cascade* involves the conversion of plasminogen into the active protease plasmin. Plasmin has two important functions: degradation of fibrin clots and activation of the complement cascade.
- The *complement cascade* has many important functions. It produces proteins that form the membrane attack complex, which attacks harmful microorganisms. Additional activated proteins in this cascade are mediators of inflammation causing vasodilation, increasing vascular permeability, promoting chemotaxis and phagocytosis, and initiating histamine release.

Arachidonic acid is a fatty acid found in many cell membranes. Two different pathways metabolize arachidonic acid, which results in the production of potent inflammatory mediators.

Prostaglandins and thromboxanes are produced from arachidonic acid through the cyclooxygenase pathway. Prostaglandins induce vasodilation and increase vascular permeability. Thromboxanes facilitate platelet aggregation, which is important to the healing and repair process.

The lipoxygenase pathway results in the production of leukotrienes. Leukotrienes initiate chemotactic activities for white blood cells, cause vasodilation, and increase vascular permeability.

Hemodynamic Disturbances

Hemodynamics is defined as the function of blood flow or circulation and the forces involved. Alterations or disturbances in the normal pattern of blood flow can be harmful to the organs and tissues of the body.

Examples of disturbances in circulation include the following:

- Edema
- Congestion and hyperemia
- Hemorrhage
- Thrombosis
- Embolism
- Infarction
- Shock

Edema

Edema is the abnormal accumulation of fluids in the interstitial spaces of cells or tissues. To understand edema, one must understand the distribution of water between the body's fluid compartments. In the normal adult, approximately 50–60% of lean body weight is composed of water stored in two basic compartments:

- The *intracellular compartment* contains approximately two-thirds of total body water.
- The *extracellular compartment* stores the remaining one-third of total body water.

The extracellular compartment is further divided into the interstitial space and plasma space, which are separated by the capillary wall.

Normal exchange of body water from each compartment is controlled by hydrostatic and osmotic pressure, which are regulated by plasma proteins. Disruption of this normal exchange explains the etiology of edema.

Causes of edema include the following:

- Increased hydrostatic pressure
- Decreased osmotic pressure
- Increased vascular permeability caused by inflammation
- Obstruction of a lymphatic channel
- Sodium retention

Congestion and hyperemia

Congestion and hyperemia are increases in blood volume in a given tissue or vessel.

Congestion is a passive process in which the drainage of blood from a given area is interrupted. An example of congestion can be seen in valvular stenosis. In this disorder, blood volume is increased in the cardiac chamber preceding the valve that is failing to open properly. The process of congestion may become a chronic condition leading to permanent damage of the affected tissue. Varicose veins are also an example of chronic congestion.

Hyperemia is an active process in which blood flow is increased to a given area. An example of this process can be seen in acute inflammation.

Hemorrhage

Hemorrhage is the loss or escape of blood from the circulatory system. Accumulation of this lost blood may be external or enclosed within the tissue space of the body. A *hematoma* is referred to as the accumulation of blood within the tissues and can range in severity from mild (e.g., a bruise) to more severe (e.g., a subdural hematoma).

Petechiae are pinpoint hemorrhages (< 0.3 cm) seen most commonly on dermal or mucosal areas. *Purpuras* are widespread hemorrhages slightly larger (0.3–1 cm) than petechiae and usually are found under the dermal surface. *Ecchymoses* are larger (≥ 1 cm), often blotchy hemorrhages that also are found on mucosal or dermal areas.

Hemorrhages can be caused by trauma; vascular wall damage resulting from disease; or malfunction of the body's normal mechanism to maintain hemostasis, such as clotting. Systemically, the significance of hemorrhages depends on the site, rate, and volume of blood loss.

Thrombosis

Thrombosis is the pathologic process of formation of a blood clot within the circulatory system. The formed clot is referred to as a *thrombus.*

Thrombus formation results from three factors known as Virchow's triad:

- Decreased blood flow
- Injury or abnormality of the endothelial wall of the vessel
- Changes to the normal properties or processes of blood coagulation

Thrombi can form in either the venous or the arterial portion of the circulatory system. Because of high pressures on the arterial side of the system, most thrombi are formed by an abnormality of the vessel wall (e.g., atherosclerosis). However, on the venous side, blood pressure is lower (as compared to arterial blood) and most thrombi are formed because of decreased blood flow.

The effect of thrombus formation can vary depending on the site and extent of occlusion. Thrombi may eventually be broken down by fibrinolysis, causing little harm; they can propagate and cause vessel occlusion, which leads to tissue damage or death; or they can embolize and move elsewhere in the circulatory system.

Embolism

An *embolism* is the lodging of a detached mass, or embolus, from one area of the bloodstream to another. Most emboli are formed from blood clots and are referred to as *thromboemboli.*

Most commonly, thromboemboli are formed within the deep veins of the lower extremities. They eventually become dislodged and flow through the right side of the heart, terminating in the pulmonary arteries and causing severe obstruction. This condition is known as a *pulmonary thromboembolism*.

Emboli can also be found in the arterial system, most commonly originating from the chambers on the left side of the heart. Cardiac abnormalities, such as atrial fibrillation, increase the risk of embolism.

Infarction

Infarction is the process of forming an ischemic necrosis within a tissue or organ. *Ischemia* is a lack of adequate blood supply to an area of tissue. Persistent ischemia can result in necrosis (morphological changes indicative of cell death) in that area.

The etiology of infarction is most commonly associated with thrombus formation in the cardiovascular system, leading to various vascular diseases.

Atherosclerosis is an example of a vascular disease leading to infarction. Atherosclerosis is characterized by thickening of the arterial wall by lipid plaques. Old plaques eventually calcify, narrowing the lumen of the artery, favoring thrombus formation on the plaque surface and obstructing normal blood flow.

Shock

Shock is a serious condition involving decreased perfusion of tissues and organs because of inadequate blood flow. Signs and symptoms of shock can include cold, mottled skin; mental status changes; and oliguria.

The etiology of shock can be divided into four basic groups:

- *Hypovolemic shock* is due to an inadequate volume of circulating blood most commonly caused by hemorrhage or trauma. In hypovolemic shock, cardiac output (CO) is reduced because of decreased venous return and systemic vascular resistance (SVR) is high because of compensatory vasoconstriction.
- *Distributive shock* is also due to an inadequate volume of circulating blood; however, fluid is not actually leaving the body as is seen in hypovolemic shock. Infections (*septic shock*), anaphylaxis (*anaphylactic shock*), and medications (*neurogenic shock*) are common causes of circulatory vasodilation leading to this type of shock. CO usually is normal to elevated and SVR is reduced in distributive shock.
- *Cardiogenic shock* is caused by cardiac malfunction and is most commonly seen in patients suffering myocardial infarction or cardiac arrhythmias. CO is reduced and SVR is increased in cardiogenic shock.
- *Obstructive shock* occurs when normal blood flow is interrupted or obstructed. Pulmonary embolisms and cardiac tamponade are examples of this type of shock. CO is reduced and SVR is increased in obstructive shock.

The goal of therapy in patients with shock is to restore blood flow to organs and tissues until the underlying cause can be corrected.

Shock can potentially progress through three stages:

- ***Nonprogressive stage:*** Reflex neurohumoral mechanisms are activated, and normal circulation is restored.
- ***Progressive stage:*** Tissue and organs remain hypoperfused, thereby increasing damage and decreasing the likelihood of compensation. This condition can be seen in cases with severe blood loss.

- ***Irreversible stage:*** This stage occurs when the body has sustained injuries beyond repair by therapeutic intervention.

Developmental Defects

Developmental defects are those originating in the embryonic period. Most developmental defects are discovered at birth; however, they can affect an individual at any point in the life cycle, from birth to adulthood.

The etiology of developmental defects falls within four general categories:

- The result of genetic or chromosomal abnormalities (intrinsic)
- The result of an environmental agent (extrinsic)
- Multifactorial reasons (intrinsic and extrinsic)
- Unknown or unidentifiable origin (idiopathic)

Developmental defects can be divided into four significant subtypes:

- *Malformations* are defects in normal development as a result of an abnormality of intrinsic cause.
- *Deformations* are defects in the form, shape, or position of a body part resulting from abnormal mechanical forces placed on the fetus during development.
- *Dysplasias* refer to defects attributable to an abnormality in the cellular organization or arrangement.
- *Disruptions* are abnormalities of normal growth and development caused by extrinsic exposures.

Genetic and chromosomal abnormalities

Defects of genetic origin can be classified as numerical or structural.

Numerical abnormalities involve defects caused by missing or extra chromosomes (*aneuploidy*). Aneuploidy has multiple causes; however, it is most commonly caused by nondisjunction (a failure of chromosomes to separate during cell division) during the process of mitosis. Down syndrome (trisomy 21) is the most common numerical abnormality; in Down syndrome, three copies of chromosome 21 are present.

Structural abnormalities involve missing or additional genetic material attributable to deletions, translocations, inversions, and duplications of chromosomal segments. The Philadelphia chromosome seen in some patients with chronic myelogenous leukemia is an example of a structural chromosomal defect. In this defect, translocation of chromosomes 9 and 22 occurs.

Abnormalities caused by environmental factors

Exposure of the developing fetus to environmental agents or substances, often called *teratogens,* may cause developmental defects. In most cases, the exact mechanism by which teratogens cause harm to the developing fetus is complex and depends on the teratogen. Teratogens may include drugs, chemical agents, infectious processes, radiation, and maternal disease states.

Many drugs, including alcohol, and chemical agents are well-known teratogens causing a wide variety of effects. Retinoic acid is an example of a teratogenic drug; it causes craniofacial deformities, cardiovascular anomalies, and neural tube defects.

Microorganisms that are present in the mother are often capable of crossing the placental membrane and subsequently infecting the fetus. Rubella, herpes simplex virus, varicella, and *Toxoplasma gondii* are a few examples of infectious teratogens.

Radiation exposure during pregnancy may cause growth and mental retardation as well as other developmental defects.

Maternal disease processes, such as poorly controlled diabetes mellitus and hypertension, are known to cause deformities such as limb abnormalities and congenital heart defects.

Critical factors affecting teratogenicity include the period of development when exposure occurs, the dosage and duration of exposure to the teratogen, and the genetic makeup of the exposed subject. Exposure of the embryo to a teratogen during the period of tissue and organ formation increases the likelihood of major congenital anomalies.

Both the dosage and the duration of exposure to a given teratogen are important; however, not all teratogens exhibit similar dose–response relationships. A single exposure to a very large dose may be more harmful than multiple exposures to a lower dose of the same teratogen.

Neoplasia

Neoplasia is the overgrowth or abnormal proliferation of cells of a tissue. A *neoplasm,* also known as a tumor, is an abnormal mass of tissue attributable to uncontrolled cellular proliferation.

Related definitions

Many similarities between neoplasms and other disturbances of growth exist, making terminology difficult. The following terms are used in defining growth disturbances:

- *Agenesis* is the failure of organ formation during embryo development.
- *Aplasia* is the failure of organ or tissue development.
- *Hypertrophy* is the enlargement or overgrowth of an organ or tissue because of an increase in cell size.
- *Hyperplasia* is the enlargement in the size of an organ or tissue because of cellular proliferation.
- *Atrophy* is a breakdown or decrease in the size of a given body tissue or organ.
- *Metaplasia* is a change in cell type, usually caused by an adverse stimulus.
- *Dysplasia* is an abnormality in the maturation or differentiation of cells within a tissue.

Characteristics of neoplastic cells

Two types of neoplasms exist—benign and malignant—and they differ in their growth pattern and behaviors.

Benign neoplasms characteristically are slower-growing tumors that tend not to invade surrounding tissue. Benign tumors do not have the ability to spread to other sites of the body.

Malignant neoplasms grow more rapidly than their benign counterparts, often invading surrounding tissue and causing disruption of normal function. Malignant tumors have the ability to metastasize, spreading to another site within the body and forming a secondary tumor.

Metastasis

Some malignant tumors possess the ability to spread to distant sites of the body, usually through invasion of the bloodstream or lymphatic system by the growing tumor. Once entry into the blood or lymph is gained, tumor growth continues, eventually separating into small emboli.

The small emboli are then carried along with the normal flow of blood or lymph until they reach a point where passage cannot occur. When the emboli become lodged, tumor growth resumes until invasion of the surrounding tissue occurs; thus, the tumor gains access to a secondary site.

The lung is one of the more common sites of secondary tumors spread through the bloodstream. This condition is most often seen with malignant tumors at sites of good systemic venous drainage, such as the bladder, prostate, breasts, and colon.

Etiology of neoplasms

Research into the cause of neoplastic growth suggests that alterations, or somatic mutations, in deoxyribonucleic acid (DNA) sequence by carcinogens ultimately result in the disruption of normal cell proliferation and death. *Carcinogens* are physical or chemical agents capable of causing genetic mutations. Examples of known carcinogens are as follows:

- Tobacco and tobacco smoke
- Radiation (e.g., ultraviolet rays from the sun)

- Viruses (e.g., human papillomavirus)
- Asbestos
- Certain pesticides
- Certain heavy metals (e.g., lead)

As previously indicated, the formation of neoplasms involves mutations in the regulatory genes controlling cell growth and elimination, such as proto-oncogenes, tumor suppressor genes, genes that regulate cell death, and DNA repair genes.

Proto-oncogenes

Proto-oncogenes are genes with multiple functions, most importantly coding for proteins that control cell proliferation, differentiation, and elimination. Defective or mutated forms of proto-oncogenes are called *oncogenes*. Oncogenes may result in the uncontrolled production of growth factors, ultimately leading to rapid and unnecessary cell growth.

Several mechanisms exist for the transformation of proto-oncogenes into oncogenes:

- *Point mutation* is a single nucleotide change in the DNA sequence that results in a change in a single amino acid in a protein (see Chapter 3).
- *Gene amplification* is an overexpression of the encoded protein.
- *Chromosomal translocation* is an inappropriate expression of the gene.

Tumor suppressor genes

Tumor suppressor genes are responsible for inhibiting cell growth, division, and death. Mutations of tumor suppressor genes result in a loss of function, thereby causing the cell to ignore normal inhibitory signals.

Tumor suppressor genes are recessive, meaning both normal alleles must mutate before uncontrolled growth can occur.

Apoptosis-regulating genes

Apoptosis is the normal process of programmed cell death resulting in elimination of cells from an organism. Genes regulating apoptosis are responsible for promoting and inhibiting this normal process. Mutation of this gene type may result in the failure of cells to die, thus causing accumulation.

DNA repair genes

DNA repair genes are responsible for correcting errors that may occur during cell duplication.

Effects of neoplasms

Local effects of tumors on their host are often related to the size and location of the tumor and can cause tissue destruction and obstruction. Destruction and obstruction can occur with both benign and malignant tumors.

Systemic effects of tumors may be related to abnormal hormone production, nutritional deficiencies, and infection. Hormonal effects produced by neoplasms in endocrine glands may be life threatening. For example, overproduction of insulin, caused by an adenoma of the pancreas, may result in fatal hypokalemia or hypoglycemia.

Hematological deficiencies, such as anemia, often occur in malignancies. Anemia can occur through many mechanisms. Directly, anemia may be caused by bleeding caused by the invasiveness of the tumor on body tissues and vessels. Metastatic tumor growth can also invade bone marrow, thereby causing a suppression of normal function.

Cachexia is a wasting syndrome resulting in loss of body fat and lean body mass. It often occurs with malignant neoplasms. Cachexia results in a generalized weakness, weight loss, anorexia, and fever for the tumor host.

26-4 Pathophysiology of Disease States Amenable to Pharmacist Intervention

Hypertension

Hypertension, a leading cause of death in the United States, is defined as a repeatedly elevated blood pressure exceeding 130 mmHg (systolic) or 80 mmHg (diastolic). Hypertension is classified as primary (also called *essential*) or as secondary:

- *Primary hypertension* is a much more complex condition in which no specific cause can be identified. Approximately 90–95% of hypertensive cases are considered primary hypertension.
- *Secondary hypertension* is a disorder in which the cause is known. Renal artery stenosis, chronic renal disease, and hyperaldosteronism are a few examples of causes of secondary hypertension.

The maintenance of blood pressure depends on two factors: cardiac output and systemic vascular resistance. Alterations increasing one or both of these factors may lead to hypertension.

Most commonly, hypertension is caused by increases in SVR. Resistance is increased by a reduction in vessel size (vasoconstriction) or increases in blood viscosity or volume. CO is increased by conditions affecting heart rate or stroke volume.

Discussed next are a few factors that may affect CO or SVR, thereby causing hypertension.

Abnormalities of the renin–angiotensin system

Abnormalities of the renin–angiotensin system can result in hypertension. Renin is secreted by the juxtaglomerular cells of the kidney in response to decreases in renal arteriolar pressure or blood flow. Renin is responsible for converting angiotensinogen to angiotensin I.

Angiotensin I is then converted to angiotensin II by an enzyme called *angiotensin-converting enzyme* (ACE). Angiotensin II, a potent direct vasoconstrictor, also stimulates the release of aldosterone (responsible for sodium and water retention). Retention of sodium and water increases blood volume, thereby increasing vascular resistance.

Sympathetic nervous system

The sympathetic nervous system is important in the regulation of normal blood pressure. This process of blood pressure regulation is controlled through stimulation of adrenergic receptors (alpha and beta) by catecholamines. Any disturbance of the sympathetic nervous system may cause hypertension.

Natriuretic hormone

Atrial natriuretic peptide (ANP) is secreted by the atria of the heart in response to increased blood flow. ANP increases urinary excretion of sodium and water, thereby causing a decrease in blood pressure.

In addition to its renal effects, ANP is also thought to affect vascular smooth muscle by inhibiting the sodium-potassium ATPase pump. This inhibition increases the intracellular concentrations of sodium and calcium, thus inducing vasoconstriction.

Endothelial dysfunction

Numerous vasoactive substances are produced in the vascular endothelium. Any dysfunction of the endothelium may lead to alteration of vascular tone, potentially causing hypertension.

Nitric oxide is a potent vasodilator released by the endothelial cells in response to changes in blood pressure. Oxidative stress has been suggested to possibly cause a deficiency in nitric oxide, thus causing hypertension.

Endothelial cells also release a vasoconstricting substance called *endothelin*. Numerous vasoconstricting agents, such as angiotensin II, vasopressin, and norepinephrine, have been suggested to increase the release of endothelin. Overstimulation of the production of endothelin may cause hypertension.

Diabetes Mellitus

Diabetes mellitus is an endocrine disease in which the body does not properly produce or use insulin, resulting in hyperglycemia.

Insulin is necessary for the transport of glucose into cells, where it is stored as glycogen to be used for energy. In normal physiology states, insulin is produced by the beta cells of the islets of Langerhans of the pancreas. Insulin release is adjusted in response to serum glucose levels.

In addition to glucose uptake, insulin stimulates amino acid uptake and, thus, protein synthesis by muscle. It can also stimulate fatty acid storage in adipose tissue.

Diabetes mellitus is classified into two primary types and two secondary types; however, only the primary types will be discussed in detail. The primary types are as follows:

- Type 1 (formerly known as *insulin-dependent diabetes mellitus*)
- Type 2 (formerly known as *insulin-independent diabetes mellitus*)

The secondary types are as follows:

- Gestational diabetes
- Other specific secondary types, including drug-induced types and those related to genetic defects of the beta cell, genetic defects in insulin action, exocrine pancreas disease, endocrinopathies, and infections

Symptoms of diabetes mellitus may include polyuria, polydipsia, polyphagia, fatigue, and weight loss.

Type 1

Patients with type 1 diabetes mellitus have a permanent loss of insulin production. Type 1 accounts for approximately 10% of primary cases of diabetes mellitus.

Most cases of type 1 result from an immune-mediated destruction of beta cells of the pancreas by T-lymphocytes. Hyperglycemia results, caused by an insulin deficiency. The remaining cases are idiopathic in nature, because autoimmunity is not evident in this group.

Current research suggests that both genetic and environmental factors are responsible for triggering autoimmune destruction. Onset of disease occurs most commonly in children and adolescents, although occasionally the disease may not be present until adulthood.

Type 2

Type 2 diabetes mellitus involves a combination of a relative resistance to the action of insulin and a deficiency in its secretion. Type 2 accounts for approximately 90% of primary cases.

Although the specific cause of type 2 diabetes mellitus is not known, research does show that it is not immune mediated. Type 2 is a genetic disease; however, environmental factors are believed to play an important part in its onset and perpetuation.

Complications of diabetes mellitus

Acute

Previously mentioned symptoms of polyuria, polydipsia, and polyphagia are all a result of hyperglycemia and may be seen in patients with type 1 or type 2 diabetes mellitus. Polyuria occurs when the threshold for glucose reabsorption by the kidneys has been exceeded. This condition results in osmotic diuresis, which increases urine output (*polyuria*). As a result of this increase in urine output, dehydration occurs, which stimulates thirst (*polydipsia*). Increased hunger (*polyphagia*) may be a result of significant calorie loss when glucose is lost in the urine.

Diabetic ketoacidosis (DKA) is a potentially life-threatening complication. It occurs more frequently in patients with type 1 disease. DKA occurs when severe beta-cell destruction has occurred without supplementation of exogenous insulin therapy. In the absence of adequate insulin therapy and an increase in counterregulatory hormones, glucose levels begin to increase. Despite this increase, the necessary uptake of glucose cannot occur in muscle tissue, fat, or the liver because of the lack of insulin. As a result of this lack of necessary energy source, a process called *lipolysis* occurs. Lipolysis is the breakdown of lipids, resulting in the production of free fatty acids, which are used for energy, and of ketone bodies. Ketone bodies are produced faster than cells can use them. The accumulation of ketone bodies results in an acidotic state.

Chronic

Macrovascular complications are a significant part of diabetes. Patients with diabetes are at a higher risk of complications, including hypertension, myocardial infarction, stroke, and coagulopathies. The mechanism by which complications affecting the large vessels occur is through atherosclerotic plaque formation. The exact relationship by which diabetes causes atherosclerosis is poorly understood.

Microvascular complications (retinopathy and nephropathy) and neuropathies are often seen in diabetic patients. Diabetes-associated retinopathy is one of the leading causes of blindness in the United States. Diabetic nephropathy is the leading cause of kidney failure in the United States. Renal changes include thickened basement membranes and sclerosis of the glomerular arteries.

Although poorly understood, three mechanisms seen in hyperglycemic states have been proposed as the cause of microvascular complications:

- Formation of advanced glycosylation end products
- Sorbitol formation in cells through the polyol pathway
- Oxidative stress as a result of hyperglycemia

Hyperlipidemia

Hyperlipidemia, by definition, refers to an abnormal elevation of fat in the blood. Cholesterol, triglycerides, phospholipids, and free fatty acids are important lipids found in the plasma of the human body. Because lipids are not water soluble, they are transported in the plasma as lipoproteins. Four major classes of lipoproteins exist:

- *Very-low-density lipoproteins* (VLDLs) are formed and secreted by the liver. They are rich in triglycerides and are eventually converted to low-density lipoproteins.
- *Low-density lipoproteins* (LDLs) are formed by catabolism of VLDLs. LDLs are the major transporters of cholesterol from the liver to tissue.
- *High-density lipoproteins* (HDLs) are often referred to as "good cholesterol." HDLs are secreted by the liver and intestine into the blood, where they take up cholesterol and transport it back to the liver; there it is excreted into bile.
- *Chylomicrons* are formed from exogenous fat sources and solubilized in the intestinal epithelium. They carry lipids to muscle and adipose tissue.

Elevated levels of serum lipids can be related to a number of environmental factors or disease states (e.g., obesity, hypothyroidism, nephritic syndrome). They can also be genetically linked. Hyperlipidemia as a result of a genetic link is referred to as *familial hyperlipidemia.*

Hyperlipidemia is important because it is a modifiable risk factor in the process of atherosclerosis, which commonly causes coronary artery disease. Atherosclerotic plaque formation is thought to occur from the retention of LDLs on the endothelial surface.

Asthma

Asthma is a chronic airway inflammatory disorder characterized by individual acute attacks that are triggered by the environment and by genetic predispositions. It is characterized by obstruction of airflow by bronchospasms, mucus hypersecretion, and inflammation.

Early acute-phase bronchospasm occurs secondary to a hypersensitivity of the bronchioles to an environmental or allergic irritant that initiates an immunoglobulin E immune-mediated response. This acute-phase response is due to the release of histamine and leukotrienes from mast cells, which causes inflammation and airway edema, thereby constricting the airway. Short-acting bronchodilators are usually successful in controlling this acute-phase bronchospasm.

During the acute-phase reaction, cytokines and chemokines are also released. Their release promotes a late-phase inflammatory response. The release of these pro-inflammatory mediators promotes the activation of basophils, eosinophils, neutrophils, and macrophages. Systemic and inhaled corticosteroids are often needed to control this late-phase response.

26-5 Questions

1. Bradykinin, an important mediator of inflammation, is formed following activation of the kinin cascade. What is the principle action of bradykinin?

A. It converts fibrinogen to fibrin, which is important in clotting.
B. It promotes vascular dilation and increases vascular permeability.
C. It degrades fibrin clots and activates complement cascade.
D. Protein production is important in the membrane attack complex.

2. Which of the following mediators of inflammation is stored in the granular tissue of mast cells?

A. Arachidonic acid
B. Leukotrienes
C. Plasmin
D. Histamine

3. Edema is caused by which of the following changes?

A. Decreased osmotic pressure in the plasma
B. Decreased hydrostatic pressure in the capillaries
C. Decreased vascular permeability caused by inflammation
D. Increased excretion of sodium

4. Purpuras are hemorrhages of what size?

A. < 0.3 cm
B. 0.3–1 cm
C. ≥ 1 cm
D. ≤ 0.3 mm

5. Thrombus formation in the venous side of the circulatory system is most commonly attributable to

A. vessel endothelium injury.
B. increased blood flow.
C. decreased blood flow.
D. disseminated intravascular coagulation.

6. Thrombus formation originating in what part of the body often leads to a severe, life-threatening event known as *pulmonary thromboembolism?*

A. Left atrium of the heart
B. Deep veins of the lower extremities
C. Ascending aorta
D. Aortic arch

7. Which of the following occurs in a patient experiencing hypovolemic shock?

A. Cardiac output is decreased, and systemic vascular resistance is increased.
B. Cardiac output is normal, and systemic vascular resistance is decreased.
C. Cardiac output is increased, and systemic vascular resistance is increased.
D. Cardiac output is decreased, and systemic vascular resistance is decreased.

8. What is a developmental defect resulting from an abnormality in the cellular organization or arrangement called?

A. Disruption
B. Malformation
C. Dysplasia
D. Deformation

9. What mechanism is most commonly responsible for causing Down syndrome?

A. Translocation of the Philadelphia chromosome (9 and 22)
B. Deletion of a portion of the short arm of chromosome 5
C. Nondisjunction during meiotic segregation
D. Robertsonian translocation of chromosome 21

10. Of the following findings, which is most likely an indication that a neoplasm is malignant?

A. Invasion into surrounding tissue
B. Necrosis
C. Slow tumor growth
D. Atypia

11. Neoplasms are the result of alterations or mutations in the DNA sequence by carcinogens, which disrupt normal cell regulation. Tumor suppressor genes are an example of a regulatory gene found in the body. Which of the following alterations in the tumor suppressor gene may cause the development of a neoplasm?

A. Mutation of both alleles of the tumor suppressor gene, causing overexpression of the protein product
B. Mutation of one allele of the tumor suppressor gene, causing overexpression of the protein product
C. Mutation of one allele of the tumor suppressor gene, causing inactivation of the protein product
D. Mutation of both alleles of the tumor suppressor gene, causing inactivation of the protein product

12. In addition to directly causing vasoconstriction, angiotensin II stimulates the release of what substance from the adrenal cortex?

A. Dopamine
B. Aldosterone
C. Vasopressin
D. Angiotensin-converting enzyme

13. Which of the following substances released by endothelial cells is a potent vasodilator?

A. Endothelin
B. Vasopressin
C. Dopamine
D. Nitric oxide

14. Which of the following substances released by endothelial cells is a potent vasoconstrictor?

A. Nitric oxide
B. Endothelin
C. Renin
D. Aldosterone

15. Diabetic ketoacidosis occurs most frequently in patients with which type of diabetes?

A. Type 1 diabetes mellitus
B. Type 2 diabetes mellitus
C. Gestational diabetes
D. Drug-induced diabetes

16. Which of the following occurs as a result of an immune-mediated destruction of beta cells?

A. Type 1 diabetes mellitus
B. Type 2 diabetes mellitus
C. Gestational diabetes
D. Drug-induced diabetes

17. The movement of leukocytes from a central location to the periphery of the blood vessel during inflammation is referred to as

A. phagocytosis.
B. margination.
C. sequestration.
D. exudation.

18. Which of the following substances are formed through the cyclooxygenase pathway?

A. Leukotrienes
B. Hageman factor
C. Prostaglandins
D. Histamine

19. What type of shock can be seen in some patients following a pulmonary thromboembolism?

A. Hypovolemic shock
B. Distributive shock
C. Cardiogenic shock
D. Obstructive shock

20. Renin is a substance secreted in response to decreases in renal arteriolar pressure or blood flow. What part of the kidney is responsible for secreting renin?

A. Peritubular capillary endothelial cells
B. Mesangial cells
C. Lacis cells
D. Juxtaglomerular cells

26-6 Answers

1. B. Bradykinin, a product of the kinin system that is derived from high molecular weight kininogen, causes pain, promotes vasodilation, and promotes vascular permeability.

2. D. Histamine, which produces vasodilation and increased vascular permeability once released, is stored in the granular tissue of mast cells.

3. A. Normal exchange of body water from the interstitial space and plasma is controlled by hydrostatic pressure of the capillary blood and osmotic pressure regulated by plasma proteins. If osmotic pressure in the plasma decreases, net fluid movement will be out of the blood into the interstitial space.

4. B. Purpuras are widespread hemorrhages, between 0.3 and 1 cm, found under the dermal surface. They are commonly caused by platelet dysfunctions and vascular injury.

5. C. Thrombus formation is due to three factors known as Virchow's triad: injury or abnormality of the endothelial wall of the vessel, decreased blood flow, and changes in the normal process of coagulation. On the venous side, blood pressure is lower (as compared to arterial blood) and most thrombi are formed because of decreased blood flow.

6. B. The most common source of embolus formation is in the deep veins of the lower extremities. Once the thrombus breaks free, it flows through the right side of the heart, ultimately terminating in the small branches of the pulmonary artery, where it occludes blood flow.

7. A. Hypovolemic shock is due to an inadequate volume of circulating blood, thereby causing a decrease in venous return, which decreases cardiac output. As compensation for the reduced cardiac output, vasoconstriction occurs, thus increasing systemic vascular resistance.

8. C. Dysplasias are defects resulting from an abnormality in the cellular organization or arrangement.

9. C. Most commonly, Down syndrome occurs as an error during cell division. Other causes, although less likely, are mosaicism and Robertsonian translocation of chromosomes 21 and 14.

10. A. Invasion of the tumor into surrounding tissue is a characteristic of malignant neoplasms. Other findings suggestive of malignancy are rapid growth and metastasis of the tumor.

11. D. Tumor suppressor genes are recessive, so both alleles must be mutated for neoplastic growth to occur.

12. B. Aldosterone is responsible for sodium and water retention. Retention of sodium and water increases blood volume, thus increasing vascular resistance.

13. D. Nitric oxide is a potent vasodilator released by the endothelial cells in response to changes in blood pressure.

14. B. Overstimulation of the production of endothelin may cause hypertension.

15. A. Diabetic ketoacidosis is a potentially life-threatening complication most commonly seen in patients with type 1 disease.

16. A. Type 1 diabetes mellitus is a result of an immune-mediated destruction of beta cells by T-lymphocytes, thereby causing insulin deficiency.

17. B. Margination is a process in which white blood cells, or leukocytes, relocate from their normal central location in the bloodstream to the periphery along the endothelium wall.

18. C. Prostaglandins and thromboxanes are produced from arachidonic acid through the cyclooxygenase pathway.

19. D. Obstructive shock occurs when normal blood flow is interrupted or obstructed. In cases of obstructive shock, cardiac output is reduced and systemic vascular resistance is increased.

20. D. Juxtaglomerular cells are responsible for secreting renin. Renin converts angiotensinogen to angiotensin I.

26-7 Additional Resources

Beevers G, Lip GYH, O'Brien E. The pathophysiology of hypertension. *BMJ.* 2001;322(7291):912–916.

Funk JL. Disorders of the endocrine pancreas. In: Hammer GD, McPhee SJ, eds. *Pathophysiology of Disease: An Introduction to Clinical Medicine.* 7th ed. New York, NY: McGraw-Hill; 2013. http://accessmedicine.mhmedical.com/content.aspx?bookid=961&sectionid=53555699.

Kumar V, Abbas AK, Fausto N. Hemodynamic disorders, thromboembolic disease, and shock. In: Kumar V, Abbas AK, Fausto N, eds. *Robbins and Cotran Pathologic Basis of Disease.* 9th ed. Philadelphia, PA: Elsevier Saunders; 2015:113–135.

Nowack JT, Handford AG, eds. *Essentials of Pathophysiology: Concepts and Applications for Health Care Professionals.* 2nd ed. Boston, MA: McGraw-Hill; 1999.

Saseen JJ, MacLaughlin EJ. Hypertension. In: DiPiro JT, Talbert RL, Yee GC, et al., eds. *Pharmacotherapy: A Pathophysiologic Approach.* 10th ed. New York, NY: McGraw-Hill; 2017:45–77.

Triplett CL, Repas T, Alvarez C. Diabetes mellitus. In: DiPiro JT, Talbert RL, Yee GC, et al., eds. *Pharmacotherapy: A Pathophysiologic Approach.* 10th ed. New York, NY: McGraw-Hill: 2017;1139–1182.

Health Promotion, Disease Prevention, and Population Health

27

SHANNON W. FINKS

27-1 KEY POINTS

- Advising patients on health promotion and disease prevention is an integral part of the counseling experience and can greatly affect a patient's physical condition and well-being.
- Pharmacists should ensure that patients are being appropriately screened for high-risk diseases and are up to date with immunizations needed to prevent the spread of disease.
- Pharmacists should encourage patients to engage in healthy lifestyle habits, including consumption of a healthy diet, appropriate type and duration of exercise, and avoidance of tobacco exposure to improve overall health.
- Women of childbearing age should consume appropriate amounts of folic acid to avoid birth defects.
- Risk assessment for atherosclerotic disease should begin at age 20 years and be assessed every 4–6 years in low-risk patients and more often in those at higher risk.
- Risk factors for atherosclerotic cardiovascular disease (ASCVD) should be assessed with intention to modify risks such as hypertension, hyperlipidemia, and blood glucose.
- A 10-year risk calculation of greater than 7.5% is regarded as high enough to benefit from statin therapy and a 10-year risk calculation of greater than 10% may warrant aspirin therapy for primary prevention of atherosclerotic disease.
- Vaccinations are an important preventive health measure that should be addressed for health promotion and disease prevention.
- Pharmacists who are certified to provide vaccinations should be familiar with the current immunization schedule and principles recommended by the Centers for Disease Control and Prevention (CDC).
- Any adverse effect from vaccination must be reported to the Vaccine Adverse Event Reporting System (VAERS, https://vaers.hhs.gov/index).
- Pharmacists should be able to recommend appropriate cancer screenings based on individualized risk for disease.
- Daily aspirin therapy may be considered for colorectal cancer prevention in those with perceived risk for colorectal cancer who are not at risk for bleeding and in those who can commit to taking aspirin long term (i.e., greater than 10 years).
- Prevention of osteoporosis is focused on maximizing peak bone mass and minimizing bone loss over time, including adequate intake of calcium and vitamin D; maintaining an exercise regimen that promotes bone density; and obtaining bone mineral density testing based on age and risk for disease.

27-2 STUDY GUIDE CHECKLIST

The following topics may guide your study of this subject area:

- ☐ Understand dietary components, and be able to communicate with patients regarding daily requirements for healthy adults.
- ☐ Distinguish between overweight and obese adults, and be familiar with dietary and exercise recommendations to achieve healthy weight.
- ☐ Apply appropriate smoking cessation counseling techniques to conversations with patients who smoke or who have smokers in the household.
- ☐ Establish an individual patient's risk for atherosclerotic cardiovascular disease (ASCVD), and appropriately recommend statin and aspirin therapy for primary prevention.
- ☐ Refer to the CDC immunization schedule in recommending appropriate immunizations for both children and adults.
- ☐ Appropriately recommend individual cancer screenings for patients at risk.
- ☐ Recommend appropriate calcium and vitamin D supplementation and exercise techniques for the prevention of osteoporosis in at-risk populations.

27-3 Overview

For a pharmacist, advising patients on health promotion and disease prevention is an integral part of the counseling experience and can greatly affect a patient's physical condition and well-being. In addition, changes in lifestyle can work in conjunction with medications so that the patient obtains the greatest benefit from treatment. Furthermore, effects can also occur at the community and society levels, especially by ensuring that patients are being appropriately screened for high-risk cancer and are up to date with immunizations needed to prevent the spread of disease.

27-4 Promotion of Wellness and Nonpharmacologic Lifestyle Choices

This section stresses the lifestyle modifications needed for healthy living. Such modifications may prevent or delay the onset of diseases such as hypertension, diabetes, hyperlipidemia, and obesity. Typical areas to focus on for counseling are (1) diet, (2) weight management, (3) exercise, and (4) smoking cessation.

Dietary Intake

Patients often feel overwhelmed when adjusting their diet. Many factors can influence the ability of patients not only to understand appropriate nutrition but also to institute such changes at all. Examples of such factors include education level, cost of food, and nutritional habits of other family members. Areas to highlight in dietary counseling include adequate nutritional regimens; fruits and vegetables; whole grains; dairy; appropriate caloric intake; nutritional requirements (carbohydrates, proteins, fats); sodium restriction; potassium; and vitamins and minerals.

Nutritional regimens and benefits of a healthy diet

Although one "best" dietary approach for reducing disease and mortality has not been prioritized, diets such as the Mediterranean diet and the Dietary Approaches to Stop Hypertension (DASH) diet share similar recommendations: the majority of calories should come from fruits, vegetables, whole grains, legumes, and nuts, while intake of red meats and saturated fats should be limited. Both dietary approaches have shown health benefits including reductions in cardiovascular disease morbidity and mortality.

Pharmacists should recommend that nutrients consumed should come primarily from foods—not supplements (Table 27-1). Patients should aim for nutrient-rich foods that provide substantial amounts of vitamins and minerals and few calories. Increased intakes of fruits, vegetables, whole grains, and low-fat dairy should be encouraged.

The U.S. Department of Agriculture Food Guide provides a guide for intake of nutrients based on caloric intake.

Fruits and vegetables

People who eat more fruits and vegetables in their diet have a reduced risk of stroke, diabetes, other cardiovascular disease, and certain types of cancer (oral, pharynx, larynx, lung, esophagus). Increased consumption of fruits and vegetables is associated with lower risk of all-cause mortality such that each serving is estimated to be associated with approximately a 4% lower mortality risk.

Intake should include the five vegetable subgroups: dark green, orange, legumes, starches, and other. Based on a 2,000-calorie diet, the daily requirement is nine servings (4.5 cups).

TABLE 27-1. Recommended Daily Intake of Typical Dietary Nutrient Components

Nutritional components	Recommended intake
Calories	1,800–2,000 kcal/day
Carbohydrate	45–65% of total daily calories
Protein	10–35% of total daily calories
Fat	20–35% of total daily calories
Saturated	< 10% of total daily calories
Trans	Limited
Cholesterol	< 300 mg/day
Fish	8 oz/week
Fiber	14 g/1,000 calories eaten in a day
Sodium	< 2,400 mg/day (< 6 g of NaCl)
Potassium	4,700 mg/day
Whole grains	≥ 3 ounce-equivalents
Fat-free or low-fat dairy	3 cups
Vitamins and minerals	
Vitamin B_{12}	2.4 mcg/day *(especially patients > 50 years of age)*
Folic acid	400–600 mcg/day
Vitamin D	25 mcg/day or 1,000 IU/day
Moderate alcohol consumption	Men ≤ 2 drinks/day Women ≤ 1 drink/day

Whole grains

Whole grains are an important source of fiber. They should be the first ingredient listed in a food, and the words *whole* or *whole grain* should appear before the ingredient's name. By U.S. Food and Drug Administration standards, to be considered whole grain, the product must claim at least 51% whole grain ingredients by weight and be low in fat. Examples of whole grain products include whole wheat, whole oats or oatmeal, whole grain corn, popcorn, brown rice, wild rice, and sorghum. Increased whole grain consumption has been associated with lower total and cardiovascular mortality. Fiber reduces the risk of coronary heart disease and may assist with weight loss and constipation. Fiber-rich foods may lower the risk of diabetes.

Patients should be encouraged to replace refined grains with whole grains such that at least 50% of all grain intake is from whole grain sources. Recommended daily intake is 3-ounce equivalents of whole grain.

Dairy

Dairy includes milk and foods made from milk. Dairy products are a good source of protein as well as calcium, vitamin D, and potassium micronutrients. Dairy products reduce the risk of low bone mass. Recommended daily intake for adults is 3 cups of fat-free or low-fat dairy products. High-fat dairy consumption can lead to weight gain but has not been associated with increases in overall mortality.

Calories

Many Americans consume more calories than needed without meeting recommended daily requirements. Normal caloric intake should be 1,800–2,000 kcal/day. Maintaining caloric balance over time prevents obesity. The healthiest way to reduce caloric intake is to reduce intake of sugar, fats, and alcohol.

Nutritional requirements

Carbohydrates

Recommended intake of carbohydrates is 45–65% of total calories. Fiber is included in this group and consists of nondigestible carbohydrates. Recommended intake is 14 g of fiber per 1,000 calories consumed.

Patients should avoid beverages high in added sugar because individuals who consume these beverages tend to consume more calories. Encourage patients to look at the ingredients list to find out what foods contain added sugars.

Patients should focus on whole fruits (fresh, frozen, canned, dried) and legumes (beans, peas).

Proteins

Recommended intake of protein-rich foods is 10–35% of total calories equaling 5.5 ounces daily. Foods that are rich in proteins include meat, seafood, eggs, legumes, nuts, and seeds. Consumption of processed foods and red meat is associated with increases in death from cardiovascular disease and cancer and should therefore be limited.

Fats

Fats supply energy, and essential fatty acids are needed by the body to serve as a carrier for fat-soluble vitamins (A, D, E, K) and as building blocks of membranes.

Recommended intake is 20–35% of total calories. Less than 10% of total calories should come from saturated fat. Less than 300 mg/day should come from cholesterol. Few Americans consume less than 20% of calories from fat.

Limit trans fat to a minimum. Intake of saturated fat is more excessive than trans fat and cholesterol in the United States. Trans fat is found in processed foods and oils.

Most dietary sources of fat should come from polyunsaturated fatty acids (PUFAs) and monounsaturated fatty acids (MUFAs). PUFAs include omega-6 and omega-3 fatty acids. Omega-6 fats include soybean, corn, and safflower oils. Omega-3 fats include soybean, canola, and flaxseed oils; walnuts; and fish (salmon, trout, herring). Fish consumption may reduce the risk of mortality from coronary heart disease and may reduce the risk of death from cardiovascular disease in people who have already had a cardiac arrest.

Recommend two servings weekly (8 oz/week) of fish. Beware of methylmercury contamination in fish (e.g., swordfish, shark, king mackerel, tilefish), especially during pregnancy.

Sodium restriction

Sodium reduction can lead to lower blood pressure, which can lead to a reduction in stroke, heart disease, heart failure, and kidney damage. Recommend less than 2,400 mg/day of sodium (1 tsp of salt) or less than 6,000 mg of sodium chloride. Further restriction may be warranted in patients who already have hypertension or heart failure. Natural salt content of foods accounts for only about 12% of sodium intake; 77% of sodium consumed is derived from the manufacturing process of foods.

Choose and prepare foods with little salt. After the use of less salt for a time, the taste for salt tends to decrease.

Potassium

Potassium-rich diets can blunt the effects of salt on blood pressure, reduce the risk of developing kidney stones, and possibly decrease bone loss with age. Recommend intake of 4,700 mg/day. Dietary potassium can lower blood pressure and blunt the effects of salt on blood pressure in African Americans and middle-aged and older adults.

Avoid salt substitutes (potassium chloride) in patients with kidney disease.

Vitamins and minerals

People older than 50 years of age should be encouraged to meet the recommended daily allowance for vitamin B_{12} (2.4 mcg/day) because of a reduced ability to absorb naturally occurring vitamin B_{12}. The crystalline form can be absorbed.

Adolescent females and women of childbearing age should eat foods high in iron, such as meat and certain plant foods (e.g., spinach), to avoid possible iron deficiency.

Pregnant women should consume 600 mcg/day of synthetic folic acid in addition to food forms to prevent neural-tube defects, spina bifida, and encephalopathy in a fetus. Women of childbearing age should have a daily intake of 400 mcg/day.

Vitamin D is important for optimal calcium absorption. The acceptable measurement of a patient's vitamin D status is through a 25-hydroxyvitamin D level (normal 35–55 ng/mL). Elderly individuals, dark-skinned individuals, and those with insufficient sunlight exposure need substantially higher vitamin D intake (25 mcg, or 1,000 IU, per day).

Vegetarians should give special attention to their intake of protein, iron, and vitamin B_{12}. If they are not consuming dairy products, calcium and vitamin D intake should be supplemented.

Alcohol and diet

For weight loss, little to no alcohol should be consumed because the calories from alcohol lack essential nutrients.

Alcohol may have beneficial effects when consumed in moderation. Moderate alcohol consumption is defined as less than or equal to 2 drinks/day for males and less than or equal to 1 drink/day for females and lightweight persons. For these purposes, 1 drink = 12 oz of beer, 5 oz of wine, 1.5 oz of 80-proof distilled spirits, or 1 oz of 100-proof distilled spirits.

Excess alcohol can lead to cirrhosis, pancreatitis, and damage to heart and brain. It can increase the risk of motor vehicle accidents, hypertension, stroke, suicide, and some types of cancer. Alcohol should be avoided in pregnancy.

Weight Management

Overweight individuals have higher risk of premature death, diabetes, hypertension, dyslipidemia, cardiovascular disease, stroke, gall bladder disease, respiratory dysfunction, gout, osteoarthritis, and certain cancers.

Monitoring of body fat

Body fat can be monitored using the body mass index (BMI). BMI is calculated as follows:

$$\text{BMI} = \frac{\text{Weight in kg}}{(\text{Height in meters})^2}$$

BMI is a reliable indicator of total body fat, which is related to the risk of disease and death. It is overestimated in patients who are very muscular and underestimated in patients who have lost muscle mass.

The U.S. Department of Health and Human Services uses the following weight status classification:

- Normal BMI = 18.5–24.9 kg/m^2
- Overweight BMI = 25–29.9 kg/m^2
- Obesity I BMI = 30–34.9 kg/m^2
- Obesity II BMI = 35–39.9 kg/m^2
- Obesity III BMI $\geq$ 40 kg/m^2

Waist circumference is a good indicator of abdominal fat, which is a predictor of risk for developing heart disease. Use a tape measure at the level of the patient's navel to measure the waist. For males, a high-risk waist circumference is greater than 40 inches (102 cm), and for females, a high-risk waist circumference is greater than 35 inches (88 cm).

Appropriate weight loss and goals

Modest weight loss (10 lb) is beneficial. Reduction of further weight gain is important:

- 50–100 kcal/day reduction will prevent weight gain.
- 500 kcal/day reduction is a common goal in most weight-loss programs.

The healthiest way to reduce caloric intake is to reduce amounts of sugar, fat, and alcohol. Special attention should be given to portion or serving sizes.

Exercise, as discussed in the next section, is also an important component of weight loss:

- To prevent weight gain, exercise 60 minutes/day with moderate to vigorous intensity.
- To lose weight, exercise 60–90 minutes/day with moderate intensity.

Exercise

Types of activities

There are many ways to exercise, and suitable activities can be found for every patient's lifestyle. See Table 27-2 for some examples.

TABLE 27-2. Examples of Moderate- and Vigorous-Intensity Activities

	Approximate calories/hour for 154 lb person
Moderate physical activity	
Hiking	370
Light gardening or yard work	330
Dancing	330
Golfing (walking and carrying clubs)	330
Bicycling (< 10 mph)	290
Walking (3.5 mph)	280
Weight lifting (light workout)	220
Stretching	180
Vigorous physical activity	
Running (5 mph)	590
Bicycling (> 10 mph)	590
Swimming (slow freestyle laps)	510
Aerobics	480
Walking (4.5 mph)	460
Heavy yard work (chopping wood)	440
Weight lifting (vigorous effort)	440
Basketball	440

U.S. Department of Health and Human Services and U.S. Department of Agriculture, 2005.

Both aerobic exercise and muscle strengthening are beneficial. Aerobic exercises are physical activities that use large muscle groups in a rhythmic manner. Such exercises make a person's heart beat more rapidly, thereby increasing its strength and making it more fit over time.

Resistance exercise (weight training or resistance bands) can reduce osteoporosis as well as increase muscle strength and tone. Resistance training can include 8–10 different exercises with 10–15 repetitions and one to two sets per exercise. Patients should do such exercises at least 2 days of the week. Incorporation of flexibility training is also recommended.

Moderate- to vigorous-intensity exercise is preferred. During moderate-intensity activity, a person should be able to talk but not sing. During vigorous-intensity activity, the person should be unable to say more than a few words without pausing for a breath.

Length of activity

To reduce the risk of chronic disease, individuals should perform moderate-intensity exercise at least 30 minutes/day every day of the week. Benefits in health have been consistently shown if aerobic activity occurs at least 3 days/week.

Muscle-strengthening exercises should be performed to the point at which the individual would have difficulty doing another repetition without help.

For weight training, one set of 8–12 repetitions of each exercise is effective, although two or three sets may be more effective.

Cautions

A health care provider should be consulted in the following situations:

- Men older than 40 years and women older than 50 years before beginning a program of exercise
- Individuals with chronic disease (such as heart disease or diabetes)
- Individuals who have symptoms such as chest pain or pressure, dizziness, or joint pain

Patients with osteoarthritis should do low-impact exercise that has a low risk of joint injury (swimming, walking, and strength training).

Inactive patients becoming active should follow these guidelines:

- Increase the amount of physical activity gradually over a period of weeks to months.
- Remember that adults 65 years of age or older require at least 2–4 weeks to adapt to a new level of activity.
- First increase the number of minutes per session (usually start at 5 minutes), then increase the number of days per week, and then increase the intensity.
- Begin muscle strengthening just 1 day/week at a light or moderate level of intensity. Over time, activity may be increased to 2 days/week.
- Warm up (before exercise) and cool down (after exercise). This time also counts as daily exercise activity.

Benefits of exercise

Exercise reduces abdominal fat and preserves muscle during weight loss. Higher levels of physical fitness result in lower risk of early death, coronary heart disease, stroke, hypertension, hyperlipidemia, diabetes, metabolic syndrome, colon cancer, and breast cancer. Mortality from all causes of death is lower in physically active people.

Physical activity can also assist in managing mild to moderate depression and anxiety. It can help patients lose weight and can prevent weight gain. It can prevent falls and result in better cognitive function. Resistance exercise increases muscular strength, endurance, and muscle mass.

Smoking Cessation

Measuring a patient's exposure to tobacco can be important in clinical care situations. The unit of measure used is the *pack year*. The pack year is calculated by number of packs (20 cigarettes/pack) smoked in a day × years smoked. Hence, a patient who has smoked 2 packs per day for 5 years has a 10 pack-year smoking history. The adverse effects of tobacco are related to the amount of tobacco smoked. People are at risk for adverse effects if they are exposed to secondhand smoke, even if they have never smoked.

Adverse effects of smoking

Smoking adversely affects nearly every organ system. Some health consequences associated with smoking are abdominal aortic aneurysm, coronary heart disease, cerebrovascular disease, peripheral arterial disease, chronic obstructive pulmonary disease, reduced fertility, sudden infant death syndrome, preterm delivery, placental abruption, placenta previa, cataracts, osteoporosis, periodontitis, peptic ulcer disease, and poor wound healing. Avoidance of tobacco and secondhand smoke should be discussed with patients at every opportunity.

Ways to encourage patients to quit

Health care professionals, including pharmacists, can be instrumental in helping patients to quit smoking. Keep in mind the "Five R's":

- ***Relevance:*** Give the patient information that is relevant to his or her situation.
- ***Risks:*** Inform the patient of the risks of smoking.
- ***Rewards:*** Emphasize the rewards of a life without smoking.
- ***Roadblocks:*** Discuss the barriers the patient is experiencing.
- ***Repetition:*** Repeat these interventions whenever the patient is seen.

In counseling patients, pharmacists can also use the "Five A's":

- Ask whether they use tobacco.
- Advise them to quit.
- Assess their readiness.
- Assist them with quitting.
- Arrange for a follow-up.

Nonpharmacologic therapies

Pharmacists are aware of the medications that can be used to assist in smoking cessation, but a number of nonpharmacologic therapies are also available:

- Quitting "cold turkey"
- Tapering the number of cigarettes
- Reading self-help materials
- Entering a formal cessation program
- Using aversion therapy
- Using acupuncture
- Using hypnosis
- Using massage

Withdrawal symptoms

Symptoms peak 48 hours after cessation, gradually dissipate over the next 2–4 weeks, and completely resolve within 1 month. Increased appetite and weight gain may persist for 6 months.

To help a patient avoid postcessation weight gain, do the following:

- Discourage strict dieting while quitting.
- Recommend physical activity.
- Encourage healthy choices.
- Recommend increased water intake.
- Recommend chewing sugarless gum.
- Encourage patients to select nonfood rewards.

Barriers to cessation

Patients will experience barriers in their attempt to cease smoking. Monitor for the following:

- Nicotine withdrawal symptoms
- Fear of failure
- Need for social support
- Depression
- Concern over weight gain
- Sense of deprivation or loss

27-5 Screening and Disease Prevention

Healthy People 2020 (a U.S. Department of Health and Human Services initiative) has four overarching areas in health as goals:

- To attain high-quality, longer years of life, free of preventable disease and premature death
- To eliminate health disparities, achieve health equity, and improve health for all groups
- To protect health throughout all stages of life
- To create social and physical environments that promote health

Pharmacists can have a direct influence in the clinical arena, particularly in preventive services because of their access to the public. These areas include risk assessment for atherosclerotic cardiovascular disease, immunizations, cancer screening, and osteoporosis prevention.

Atherosclerotic Disease Prevention

Atherosclerotic disease is the most common cause of death of Americans and is classified into four main disease subsets:

- Coronary heart disease (CHD) and cardiovascular disease (CVD)
- Cerebrovascular disease
- Peripheral arterial disease
- Aortic atherosclerosis including thoracic or abdominal aortic aneurysm

Prevention offers the public the greatest benefit in reducing the global burden of myocardial infarction, stroke, heart failure, and death caused by the atherosclerotic process.

Screening

Risk assessment for atherosclerotic disease should begin at age 20 years and be assessed every 4–6 years in low-risk patients and more often in those at higher risk (i.e., every 2 years). Risk assessment after age 79 years is not necessary. Risk assessment includes identification and evaluation of traditional risk factors and calculation of a 10-year risk in those who have not developed atherosclerotic cardiovascular disease (ASCVD) to date (i.e., primary prevention).

Identification of traditional risk factors

First, identify major traditional risk factors (both modifiable and nonmodifiable) for atherosclerotic diseases and modify risks where appropriate.

Nonmodifiable risks

- Age (greater than 45 years in men; greater than 55 years in women)
- Gender (males at greater risk until females reach 6th decade of life)
- Ethnicity (African Americans at greatest risk)
- Family history (premature heart disease in a male primary relative less than 55 years of age or female primary relative less than 65 years of age)

Modifiable risks

- Hypertension
- Hyperlipidemia
- Diabetes
- Tobacco smoking

Risk calculators

If patient has two or more traditional risk factors or is greater than 40 years of age, an ASCVD risk score should be calculated to estimate the patient's 10-year risk of suffering an atherosclerotic-related event. For patients with low or very low 10-year risk, or patients who are less than 40 years of age, a lifetime ASCVD risk can be estimated. Each can be estimated by using one of the following risk calculators, which approximate the risk of hard events such as myocardial infarction, stroke, and death:

- ASCVD Pooled Cohort Equation (2013) is preferred by the American College of Cardiology (ACC)/American Heart Association (AHA).
- Framingham (2008 global version) predicts cardiovascular and cerebrovascular events as well as softer endpoints such as heart failure.
- MESA (Multi-Ethnic Study of Atherosclerosis) risk score (2015) includes multiple ethnic backgrounds.
- Reynolds Risk Score (2008) includes hsCRP (high-sensitivity C-reactive protein).

Assessment of systolic blood pressure and cholesterol levels are used by these risk calculators. Therefore, objective measurements such as blood pressure and laboratory results for total cholesterol, high density lipoprotein cholesterol, and low-density lipoprotein cholesterol levels are needed to predict ASCVD risk. Other screening (not included in the above risk calculators) includes assessment of alcohol intake, physical activity, BMI, waist circumference, creatinine clearance, and blood glucose.

Pharmacologic therapy for the primary prevention of ASCVD

A 10-year risk calculation of greater than 7.5% is regarded as high enough risk to benefit from statin therapy, and a 10-year risk calculation of greater than 10% may warrant aspirin therapy for primary prevention of atherosclerotic disease.

Statin therapy

If a patient meets the following criteria, statin therapy is thought to be beneficial for primary prevention (i.e., reducing risk for ASCVD development):

- A patient with LDL-C (low-density lipoprotein cholesterol) greater than190 mg/dL
- A patient age 40–79 years with diabetes and LDL-C greater than 70 mg/dL
- A patient age 40–79 years without diabetes but with an LDL-C greater than 70 mg/dL *and* an ASCVD 10-year risk estimate of greater than 7.5%

In most cases, moderate- to high-intensity statin therapy is warranted, as long as the patient does not have high risk for statin-related adverse drug effects (e.g., age, previous intolerance, drug interactions) or contraindications to drug therapy (i.e., pregnancy). High-intensity statins are those that are expected to reduce LDL-C by more than 50% and include atorvastatin 40–80 mg and rosuvastatin 20–40 mg. Benefit in prevention may be related to effects of the statin other than LDL-C reduction alone.

Aspirin therapy

The U.S. Preventive Services Task Force recommends aspirin at a low dose (i.e., 81 mg/day) for cardiovascular disease prevention for men and women ages 50–70 years who have a 10-year estimated risk for an ASCVD event that is greater than 10%. Aspirin is not currently recommended for patients over 80 years of age because of the lack of evidence of clear benefit in this population.

Do not use aspirin therapy in patients at increased risk of gastrointestinal bleed or hemorrhagic stroke. The U.S. Preventive Services Task Force also recommends not encouraging those who are younger than age 50 years to take a daily aspirin for primary prevention of cardiovascular disease because the risk for ASCVD is not generally high enough to accept the long-term risk for bleeding with aspirin use within this age group.

The effects of aspirin on primary prevention may differ in men and women. Aspirin reduces incidence of myocardial infarction (MI) but not stroke in men and reduces incidence of stroke in women but not MI until the woman is older than age 65 years, at which point it affects stroke and MI equally. Aspirin is beneficial in all patients for secondary prevention, regardless of race.

Modifying Major Risk Factors

Hypertension

Hypertension, or high blood pressure, is a major risk factor for myocardial infarction, stroke, heart failure, and renal failure. Hypertension is known as the silent killer because some patients may not have any symptoms or be aware that they have hypertension. Recently, the diagnostic criteria for hypertension changed and is now defined as a usual blood pressure (BP) of greater than or equal to 130/80 mmHg. These new criteria mean that roughly 45% of all American adults meet the definition for having hypertension.

Screening

- BP should be routinely measured for everyone 18 years of age or older.
- Diagnosis is made on an average of two or more readings on two or more occasions with the following classifications:
  - Normal is less than 120 mmHg systolic and less than 80 mmHg diastolic blood pressures
  - Elevated is 120–129 mmHg systolic and less than 80 mmHg diastolic blood pressures
  - Stage 1 hypertension is 130–139 mmHg systolic or 80–89 mmHg diastolic blood pressures
  - Stage 2 hypertension is greater than or equal to 140 mm Hg systolic or greater than or equal to 90 mmHg diastolic blood pressures
- Goal BP less than 130/80 mmHg is recommended.
- Nonpharmacologic lifestyle modifications (DASH diet, exercise, weight loss, as outlined in Section 27-4) are recommended for everyone for prevention of hypertension and as a part of treatment in adults with elevated and mild hypertension.
- The decision to initiate drug therapy is based on ASCVD risk as well as degree of blood pressure elevation (see Chapter 29).

Blood lipid management

Blood lipid management is an important component of prevention. Healthy lifestyle modification is successful for mild lipid abnormalities. Those patients who benefit most from statin therapy for primary prevention are outlined above. In those who have other lipid abnormalities or in whom statin therapy does not reduce LDL-C as expected, refer to Chapter 29 on hyperlipidemia.

Diabetes management

Patients with diabetes mellitus should be considered at highest risk for an ASCVD event. Their risk should be managed aggressively with lifestyle modifications, statin therapy for prevention, and aspirin therapy if over age 50 years. See Chapter 29 for management of blood glucose.

Immunizations

Immunization offers both individual and public health protection from a multitude of preventable illnesses. Pharmacists play a key role in reminding the public about the benefit of immunizations and in some cases may also be certified to administer immunizations in their work environment. Immunization rates for influenza and pneumococcus remain low despite the fact that approximately 50,000–70,000 adults die annually from these two preventable diseases alone. The Centers for Disease Control (CDC) and its Advisory Committee on Immunization Practices (ACIP) provides recommendations for immunizations for both children and adults. Pharmacists who are certified to provide vaccinations should be familiar with the current immunization schedule and the following principles:

- Current vaccination schedules and recommendations are available online at the National Center for Immunization and Respiratory Diseases (NCIRD) Web site: https://www.cdc.gov/ncird/.
- All patients should be screened for eligibility to receive annual influenza vaccination and pneumococcal vaccination where appropriate.
- Recommended preparation, storage, and route of each vaccination is described in the package labeling and must be followed precisely.
- All providers who administer vaccines must follow directives and maintain records, including type of vaccine and dose; site and route of administration; date of vaccination; date of next vaccination due; the manufacturer and lot number; and name, address, and title of the person administering the vaccination.
- Vaccine information statements from the CDC should be used and given to those receiving vaccinations.
- All providers must report any adverse effects from vaccination to the Vaccine Adverse Event Reporting System (VAERS, https://vaers.hhs.gov/index).

Cancer Screening

Healthy People 2020 and the American Cancer Society focus on screening for breast, cervical, colorectal, and prostate cancers to prevent disease in the area of oncology. A number of nonpharmacological measures to prevent cancer include the following:

- Avoid use of tobacco products (most effective in preventing cancers of the oropharynx, bladder, esophagus, and lung).
- Maintain a physically active lifestyle.
- Maintain a healthy weight.
- Consume a diet rich in fruits and vegetables, whole grains, and low trans and saturated fats.
- Limit alcohol consumption.
- Protect against sexually transmitted illness.
- Avoid excess sun.
- Screen regularly for breast, cervical, and colorectal cancers.

Breast cancer

Screening for breast cancer is likely to be of most value in those who are most likely to develop breast cancer and where early treatment is more effective than later for reducing mortality. Major risk factors include the following:

- History of ovarian, peritoneal (including tubal), or breast cancer
- Family history of above
- Genetic predisposition (if patient's BRCA status is known)
- Previous exposure to radiotherapy to chest between ages 10 and 30 years

Women with the above risks should be referred to a specialist for aggressive risk determination. Women without these risk factors are considered average risk and can be screened according to the American Cancer Society breast cancer screening guidelines as follows:

- Monthly breast self-examination is an option for women starting at age 20 years so that they know how their breasts normally look and feel; women should report any breast changes to a health care provider.
- Mammography should occur at the following intervals:
  - Per individual choice in women ages 40–44 years
  - Annually, starting at age 45 to 54 years
  - Every 2 years after age 55 years
  - Can continue for women older than 70 years as long as they are in good health and life expectancy is greater than 10 years

The U.S. Preventive Services Task Force breast cancer screening guidelines are as follows:

- Statements:
  - Evidence is insufficient to assess benefits and harms of either digital mammography or MRI (magnetic resonance imaging) instead of film mammography as a screening tool.
  - Evidence is insufficient to assess the benefits and harms of clinical breast examination beyond screening mammography in women *over* age 40 years.
- Recommendations:
  - The guidelines recommend against teaching breast self-examination.
  - For women younger than age 50 years, the decision to have mammography scheduled regularly every 2 years should be based on the risk-to-benefit ratio of the individual patient.
  - Mammography is recommended every 2 years, from age 50 to 74 years.
  - Evidence is insufficient to assess the additional benefits and harm of screening women over age 75 years.

Cervical cancer

The following screening guidelines apply:

- Human papillomavirus (HPV) vaccination is beneficial to both males and females by safely protecting against cancers that can result from persistent HPV infection.
- In those who have not been previously vaccinated, HPV vaccination is recommended for females up to age 26 years, for males up to age 21 years, and for males who have sex with males up to age 26 years.
- Cervical cancer screening in females should start at age 21 years, but not before.
- Pap smear cytology testing should occur every 3 years between ages 21–29 years, and additional HPV testing should occur if a Pap test result is abnormal.
- In women ages 30–65 years, either HPV testing is recommended every 5 years or a sole Pap test is recommended every 3 years, based on the patient's individualized choice (U.S. Preventive Services Task Force recommendations).

- Co-testing with cytology and HPV every 5 years or cytology alone every 3 years in women ages 30–65 years is recommended by the American College of Obstetricians and Gynecologists.
- Women age 65 years or older with normal results in the past 10 years can choose to stop cervical cancer screening.
- Women with a history of serious cervical precancer should be tested for 20 years past initial diagnosis, even past age 65 years.
- Women who have had their uterus and cervix removed for reasons not related to cancer should not be tested.
- All women vaccinated against HPV should follow the above screening recommendations.

Colorectal cancer

Men and women age 50 years or older at average risk for developing colorectal cancer should be screened using one of the following tests. If any of these tests are positive, then a colonoscopy should be performed. Those patients who are at an increased or higher risk of colorectal cancer should have screening done before age 50 years and more often. These people include patients with a personal history of colorectal cancer or adenomatous polyps, a history of inflammatory bowel disease, a strong family history of colorectal cancer or polyps, or a known family history of a hereditary colorectal cancer syndrome.

The following tests detect polyps and cancer:

- Flexible sigmoidoscopy every 5 years
- Double-contrast barium enema every 5 years
- Computed tomographic (CT) colonography (virtual colonoscopy) every 5 years
- Colonoscopy every 10 years

The following tests mainly detect cancer:

- Fecal occult blood test (FOBT) every year
- Fecal immunochemical test (FIT) every year
- Stool DNA (deoxyribonucleic acid) test with an uncertain interval

For FOBT and FIT tests, a take-home multiple sample method should be used. FOBT and FIT tests performed during a digital rectal exam in a health care provider's office do not constitute an adequate screening.

Aspirin therapy has been shown to reduce risk for colorectal cancer, but only after long-term use of daily preventive therapy (i.e., greater than 10 years). Daily aspirin therapy (variable dosing is used in clinical trials, however, low-dose aspirin is preferred) may be considered for colorectal cancer prevention in those with perceived risk for colorectal cancer who are not at risk for bleeding and in those who can commit to taking aspirin long term.

Prostate cancer

The American Cancer Society recommends that men have a chance to make an informed decision about whether to be screened for prostate cancer. Men age 50 years and older who are at average risk of prostate cancer and have a life expectancy of at least 10 years should discuss with their physician the benefits and risks of screening. For those at high risk, this discussion should begin at age 45 years. These patients would include African American men or those who have a primary male relative found to have prostate cancer before age 65 years. For those at even higher risk, this discussion should take place at age 40 years. These patients would include men with several family members who had prostate cancer at an early age.

A prostate specific antigen (PSA) test is used for screening purposes. If the PSA is very low (less than 4 ng/mL), the patient may need to be retested only every 2 years; however, men with high PSA levels may need to be tested annually. The U.S. Preventive Services Task Force concludes that the decision to be screened for prostate cancer be individualized in men ages 55–69 years after a discussion with a clinician regarding the benefits and risks of screening. Screening offers only a small potential benefit of reducing the chance of death from prostate cancer.

Osteoporosis

Prevention of osteoporosis is focused on maximizing peak bone mass and minimizing bone loss over time because osteoporotic fracture leads to significant morbidity and increased risk for mortality in Americans. Osteoporosis is defined on the basis of bone mineral density (BMD) measurements at the spine, hip, or forearm by DEXA (dual-energy x-ray absorptiometry):

- Normal
  - T-score of 1 or above
  - BMD within 1 SD (standard deviation) of a "young normal" adult
- Osteopenia
  - T-score between –1 and –2.5
  - BMD within 1 to 2.5 SD of a "young normal" adult
- Osteoporosis
  - T-score –2.5 or below
  - BMD 2.5 SD or more below a "young normal" adult

Screening

Risk factors include advanced age, low dietary calcium and vitamin D intake, smoking, weight less than 127 pounds, menopause, family history of osteoporosis, Caucasian ethnicity, and inadequate physical activity.

The U.S. Preventive Services Task Force recommends screening for the following:

- All women age 65 years or older or age 60 years or older with increased risk of fracture
- All men age 70 years or older

The National Osteoporosis Foundation recommends screening for the following:

- All women over age 65 years and men over age 70 years regardless of risk factors
- Postmenopausal women with risk factors
- Men ages 50–70 years with risk factors
- Women in the menopausal transition if they have a specific risk factor associated with increased fracture risk, such as low body weight, prior low-trauma fracture, or high-risk medication
- Adults who have a fracture after age 50 years
- Adults who have a condition (e.g., rheumatoid arthritis) or are taking a medication (e.g., glucocorticoids in a daily dose greater than 5 mg prednisone or equivalent for 3 months or more) associated with low bone mass or bone loss
- Postmenopausal women stopping estrogen therapy

The North American Menopause Society recommends screening as follows:

- All women over age 65 years regardless of clinical risk factors
- Postmenopausal women with medical causes of bone loss regardless of age
- Postmenopausal women with a fragility fracture
- Postmenopausal women age 50 years or older if they have one or more of the following risk factors:
  - Fracture after menopause (except skull, facial bone, ankle, finger, or toe)
  - Weight less than 127 lb or BMI less than 21 kg/m^2
  - History of hip fracture in parent
  - Current smoker

  - Rheumatoid arthritis
  - Alcohol intake of more than two drinks per day

The American College of Obstetricians and Gynecologists recommends screening as follows:

- Postmenopausal women over age 65 years
- Postmenopausal women under age 65 years with one or more risk factors for osteoporosis
- All postmenopausal women who have had a fracture

The American Association of Clinical Endocrinologists recommends screening as follows:

- All women age 65 years or older
- All adult women with a history of fracture not caused by severe trauma
- Younger postmenopausal women with the following risk factors:
  - Weight less than 127 lb
  - Family history of spine or hip fracture

According to the American Association of Clinical Endocrinologists, screening should occur every 2 years unless a new risk factor presents.

The World Health Organization has helped develop a FRAX (fracture risk assessment tool) score that provides the patient with a 10-year probability of fracture. This score is used in addition to BMD screening. The U.S. National Osteoporosis Foundation recommends offering treatment choices to anyone with a low bone density whose FRAX score for hip fracture is 3% or more or whose risk for other bone fractures is greater than 20%.

Nonpharmacologic therapy to reduce fracture risk

Nonpharmacologic recommendations to reduce fracture risk include the following:

- Ensure adequate intake of calcium and vitamin D:
  - Recommended dietary calcium for women over age 50 years is 1,200–1,500 mg/day. Intakes of calcium greater than 1,200 mg increase risk of kidney stones or cardiovascular disease.
  - Recommended dietary intake of vitamin D is 800–1,000 IU/day, aiming for a 25 (OH) D level of 30 ng/mL or more.
- Decrease or stop alcohol intake:
  - Alcohol intake of three or more drinks per day is detrimental to bone health.
  - Moderate alcohol consumption is associated with a higher BMD and a decrease in hip fracture.
- Perform weight-bearing and muscle-strengthening exercises.
- Stop tobacco use.
- Wear undergarments with hip pad protectors.

27-6 Questions

1. How many grams per 1,000 calories consumed is the recommended intake of fiber?

A. 7 g
B. 14 g
C. 25 g
D. 30 g

2. Which of the following types of fish may be at increased risk of containing methylmercury?

A. Salmon
B. Tuna
C. Trout
D. Swordfish

3. People older than age 50 years should be encouraged to meet the recommended daily allowance for which of the following?

A. Vitamin C
B. Vitamin B_6
C. Vitamin B_{12}
D. Folic acid

4. Which of the following would be an example of one defined alcoholic beverage?

A. 1 glass of wine
B. 1 whisky sour
C. 2 oz of 80-proof whisky
D. 12 oz of beer

5. How long should a person do some sort of moderate-intensity exercise to reduce the risk of chronic disease?

A. 30 minutes/day every day of the week
B. 30 minutes/day 5 days of the week
C. 60 minutes/day every day of the week
D. 60 minutes/day 5 days of the week

6. You have a patient who has smoked 10 cigarettes per day for 14 years. Calculate the patient's pack-year history.

A. 140 pack-years
B. 120 pack-years
C. 7 pack-years
D. 6 pack-years

7. Prevention of cervical cancer is accomplished through which of the following?

A. Pap smear
B. Vaccination
C. Pap smear and vaccination
D. Mammography

8. For which average blood pressure would someone be diagnosed with Stage 1 hypertension?

A. Systolic blood pressure 120–129 mmHg
B. Diastolic blood pressure 85 mmHg
C. Systolic blood pressure greater than 140 mmHg and diastolic blood pressure greater than 90 mmHg
D. Diastolic blood pressure less than 80 mmHg

9. Which of the following represents gender differences in the expected benefit of daily aspirin for primary prevention of ASCVD?

A. It prevents cardiovascular events in men and stroke in women.
B. It prevents stroke in men and cardiovascular events in women.
C. It prevents stroke in both men and women.
D. It prevents cardiovascular and stroke events in both men and women.

10. What is the recommended 25 (OH) D level for a woman older than age 50 years to prevent osteoporosis?

A. Greater than or equal to 10 ng/mL
B. Greater than or equal to 20 ng/mL
C. Greater than or equal to 30 ng/mL
D. Greater than or equal to 40 ng/mL

11. Resistance exercise such as weight training should occur at least how many days of the week?

A. 1 day
B. 2 days
C. 3 days
D. 4 days

12. Pharmacists can refer to which organization for an up-to-date schedule of recommended vaccinations in both children and adults?

A. VAERS
B. American Academy of Pediatrics
C. American Influenza Association
D. Centers for Disease Control and Prevention

13. What is the name of the scoring system used to determine a patient's 10-year risk of developing a fracture?

A. Framingham
B. Fracture risk
C. FRAX
D. Fractile risk

14. Which patient will benefit most from atorvastatin 80 mg daily?

A. An 88-year-old man without diabetes with an ASCVD 10-year risk of 15% and history of myopathies
B. A 55-year-old woman with diabetes and LDL-C 125 mg/dL and a 10-year risk of 9.5%
C. A 65-year-old man without diabetes with a 10-year risk of 7.5% and LDL-C 69 mg/dL
D. A 32-year-old woman with no pertinent medical history and ASCVD score of 6% and LDL-C 90 mg/dL

15. How many servings per week of fish should a person have to reduce the risk of mortality from coronary heart disease?

A. Two servings (4 oz each serving)
B. Two servings (8 oz each serving)
C. Four servings (4 oz each serving)
D. Four servings (8 oz each serving)

16. Most of the sodium consumed (77%) is a result of

A. the addition of salt at the table.
B. the addition of salt during cooking.
C. nature.
D. the manufacturing process of foods.

17. Which of the following dietary minerals can lower blood pressure and blunt the effects of salt on blood pressure in African Americans and middle-age and older adults?

A. Sodium
B. Potassium
C. Magnesium
D. Zinc

18. How often should colorectal cancer screening by colonoscopy occur in men and women older than 50 years if deemed to have an average risk?

A. Every 2 years
B. Every 5 years
C. Every 10 years
D. Every 20 years

19. Screening for prostate cancer in men with average risk of prostate cancer and a high PSA level annually is acceptable as long as they have a life expectancy of how many years?

A. 2
B. 5
C. 10
D. 15

20. The first fasting lipid panel should be obtained at what age and how often if no risk factors are present?

A. 20 years old and every 2 years
B. 20 years old and every 5 years
C. 25 years old and every 2 years
D. 25 years old and every 5 years

27-7 Answers

1. **B.** Recommended intake is 14 g of fiber per 1,000 calories consumed.

2. **D.** In addition to swordfish, methylmercury contamination is common in shark, king mackerel, and tilefish.

3. **C.** People older than age 50 years have a reduced ability to absorb naturally occurring vitamin B_{12} and may require supplementation.

4. **D.** One defined alcoholic beverage is equivalent to 12 oz of beer, 5 oz of wine, or 1.5 oz of 80-proof distilled spirits.

5. **A.** To reduce the risk of chronic disease, one should perform moderate-intensity exercise 30 minutes per day every day of the week.

6. **C.** A pack is 20 cigarettes; therefore, 10 cigarettes equal half a pack, and 0.5×14 years = 7 pack-years.

7. **C.** Prevention of cervical cancer is accomplished through vaccination and screening for disease, not simply with the vaccination alone; patients should receive screening even if they have been previously vaccinated.

8. **B.** Stage 1 hypertension is defined as a systolic blood pressure of 130–139 mmHg or a diastolic blood pressure 80–89 mmHg.

9. **A.** The use of daily aspirin for patients with a 10-year coronary heart disease risk of 10% or more prevents cardiovascular events in men and stroke in women.

10. **C.** The recommended 25 (OH) D level for a woman older than 50 years of age to prevent osteoporosis is 30 ng/mL or more.

11. **B.** Resistance exercise should occur at least 2 days each week.

12. **D.** The Centers for Disease Control and Prevention and its Advisory Committee on Immunization Practices provides recommendations for immunizations for both children and adults.

13. **C.** FRAX is the scoring system used to determine a patient's 10-year risk of developing a fracture.

14. **B.** A 55-year-old woman with diabetes and LDL-C 125 mg/dL and a 10-year risk score of 9.5% meets criteria for benefiting from high-intensity statin therapy.

15. **A.** To reduce the risk of mortality from coronary heart disease, one should consume at least 8 oz of fatty fish per week, which can be divided up into 4 oz servings twice a week.

16. **D.** The manufacturing process is the major contributor in salt consumption.

17. **B.** Dietary potassium can lower blood pressure and blunt the effects of salt on blood pressure in African Americans and middle-age and older adults.

18. **C.** A colonoscopy should occur every 10 years for colorectal cancer screening in patients who have been determined to have an average risk.

19. **C.** Per the U.S. Preventive Services Task Force recommendations for screening for prostate cancer in men with average risk of prostate cancer and a high PSA level, annually is acceptable as long as they have a life expectancy of 10 years.

20. **B.** The first fasting lipid panel, along with other risk assessment, should be obtained at 20 years of age and every 5 years if no risk factors are present.

27-8 Additional Resources

American Cancer Society. American Cancer Society guidelines for the early detection of cancer. Available at: https://www.cancer.org/healthy/find-cancer-early/cancer-screening-guidelines/american-cancer-society-guidelines-for-the-early-detection-of-cancer.html. Last updated July 2017. Accessed November 27, 2017.

Camacho PM, Petek SM, Binkley N, et al. American Association of Clinical Endocrinologists (AACE) and American College of Endocrinology clinical practice guidelines for the diagnosis and treatment of postmenopausal osteoporosis. *Endocr Pract.* 2016;22(Suppl 4):1–42.

Centers for Disease Control and Prevention. Vaccines and immunizations. Available at: https://www.cdc.gov/vaccines/.

Chelmow D. Practice Bulletin No. 168: cervical cancer screening and prevention. *Obstet Gynecol.* 2016;128(4):e111–e130.

Eckel RH, Jakicic JM, Ard JD, et al. 2013 AHA/ACC guideline on lifestyle management to reduce cardiovascular risk: a report of the American College of Cardiology/American Heart Association Task Force on Practice Guidelines. *Circulation.* 2014;129:S76–S99.

Goff DC, Lloyd-Jones DM, Bennett G, et al. 2013 ACC/AHA guideline on the assessment of cardiovascular risk: a report of the American College of Cardiology/American Heart Association Task Force on Practice Guidelines. *Circulation.* 2014;129:S49–S73.

Saslow D, Solomon D, Lawson HW, et al. American Cancer Society, American Society for Colposcopy and Cervical Pathology, and American Society for Clinical Pathology screening guidelines for prevention and early detection of cervical cancer. *CA Cancer J Clin.* 2012;62(3):147–172.

Stone NJ, Robinson JG, Lichtenstein AH, et al. 2013 ACC/AHA guideline on the treatment of blood cholesterol to reduce atherosclerotic cardiovascular risk in adults. *Circulation.* 2014;129:S1–S45.

U.S. Department of Health and Human Services. *2008 Physical Activity Guidelines for Americans: Be Active, Healthy, and Happy!* Washington, DC: U.S. Department of Health and Human Services; 2008. Available at: https://www.health.gov/paguidelines/guidelines/default.aspx#toc.

U.S. Department of Health and Human Services, Office of Disease Prevention and Health Promotion. *Healthy People 2020.* Washington, DC: U.S. Department of Health and Human Services; 2017. Available at: https://www.healthypeople.gov. Accessed November 27, 2017.

U.S. Department of Health and Human Services and U.S. Department of Agriculture. Dietary Guidelines for Americans, 2005. 6th ed. Washington, DC: U.S. Government Printing Office; 2005. Available at: https://health.gov/dietaryguidelines/dga2005/document/pdf/DGA2005.pdf?_ga=2.85038233.1659578818.1515599419-414328588.1515599419.

U.S. Preventive Services Task Force. Prostate cancer screening draft recommendations. Available at: http://www.screeningforprostatecancer.org. Accessed November 27, 2017.

U.S. Preventive Services Task Force. Screening for breast cancer: U.S. Preventive Services Task Force recommendation statement. *Ann Intern Med.* 2016;164:279–296.

Whelton PK, Carey RM, Aronow WS, et al. 2017 ACC/AHA/AAPA/ABC/ACPM/AGS/APhA/ASH/ASPC/NMA/PCNA Guideline for the Prevention, Detection, Evaluation, and Management of High Blood Pressure in Adults. *J Am Coll Cardiol.* 2017. doi:10.1016/j.jacc.2017.11.006.

28

Patient Assessment

NANCY BORJA-HART

28-1 KEY POINTS

- The Pharmacists' Patient Care Process integrates five elements that should be incorporated by pharmacists practicing patient-centered care: collect, assess, plan, implement, and follow-up.
- Comprehensive medical history of a patient includes the patient's chief complaint (CC), history of present illness (HPI), and past medical history (PMH). A problem-focused interview includes addressing a specific problem in relation to location, quality, severity, timing, setting, modifying factors, and associated symptoms. Documentation of the interview is very important to summarize the patient's subjective and objective information as well as the health care provider's assessment of the diagnosis and treatment plan.
- Physical assessment includes *inspection,* which is observing the problem site and related areas; *palpation,* which is touching the area; *percussion,* which involves specific techniques in touching to evaluate tenderness and reflexes; and *auscultation,* which is listening for sounds using a stethoscope.
- Vital signs are the measurement of physiological parameters of the patient to assess weight, respiration, pulse, temperature, and blood pressure. Values different from normal are indications of medical conditions that need to be treated.
- Laboratory values and diagnostic tests are measurements of elements in specimens (i.e., blood, urine, sputum) to evaluate organ conditions. Abnormal values indicate a disease or medical condition that may warrant treatment.
- False-positive and false-negative test results are due to in vivo interference (caused by the pharmacological or the toxicological drug effect) or in vitro interference (caused by the interaction of drugs in specimens).
- Point-of-care home devices are available to screen for prescription and illicit drug use, confirm pregnancy, and assist with self-monitoring patients with diabetes.

28-2 STUDY GUIDE CHECKLIST

The following topics may guide your study of this subject area:

- ☐ Be familiar with the Pharmacists' Patient Care Process developed by the Joint Commission of Pharmacy Practitioners.
- ☐ Identify pertinent information needed for obtaining a comprehensive patient history.
- ☐ Be familiar with the four tenets of physical assessment: inspection, palpation, percussion, and auscultation.
- ☐ Identify normal ranges for common clinical laboratory values and diagnostic tests, and be aware of their clinical use.
- ☐ Be able to calculate body mass index and creatinine clearance.
- ☐ Be aware of over-the-counter point-of-care glucometers, pregnancy tests, hemoglobin A1c (HbA1c) testing, and drug screening.

28-3 Pharmacists' Patient Care Process

In recognizing the need for a consistent process of care in the delivery of patient care services, the Pharmacists' Patient Care Process (PPCP) was developed by the Joint Commission of Pharmacy Practitioners alongside other major pharmacy organizations and key stakeholders. This process requires five elements that should be incorporated by pharmacists practicing patient-centered care: collect, assess, plan, implement, and follow-up (see Figure 28-1).

During the *collect* phase, the pharmacist should gather pertinent subjective and objective information such as medical history, medications (over-the-counter, prescription, dietary supplements), laboratory results, physical assessment findings, vital signs, allergies, social history, socioeconomic factors, preferences and beliefs, and health and functional goals. Many of these topics are covered in this chapter. This information could be gathered from the patient or the patient's medical records. After collecting pertinent information, the pharmacist should *assess* this information to identify issues and optimize pharmacotherapy. Each medication can be reviewed for appropriateness (i.e., Does this patient have gastroesophageal disease warranting omeprazole usage?), effectiveness (i.e., Are the patient's blood sugars controlled?), safety (i.e., Does the patient complain of muscle aches with his or her statin therapy?), and patient adherence (i.e., patient forgets to take his or her blood pressure medicine sometimes). Assessment of the patient's health and functional status, risk factors, health data, cultural factors, health literacy, access to medications, immunization status, and need for other health care services is also important within this domain. The pharmacist should then develop a patient-centered *plan,* working with the patient and/or the caregiver and other health care professionals. The plan should optimize pharmacotherapy by addressing medication-related problems, set goals for clinical measures, engage the patient, and support care continuity. Following plan development, the pharmacist should *implement* the plan in collaboration with other health care professionals, the patient, and/or caregiver. During implementation of the plan, medication therapy can be initiated, modified, discontinued, or administered as authorized; pharmacists can provide education and self-management training, refer patients to other health care professionals as needed, engage in preventive care strategies, and schedule follow-up appointments as needed. Within the *follow-up* process, the pharmacist should *monitor* and *evaluate* the effectiveness of the care plan and

FIGURE 28-1. Pharmacists' Patient Care Process

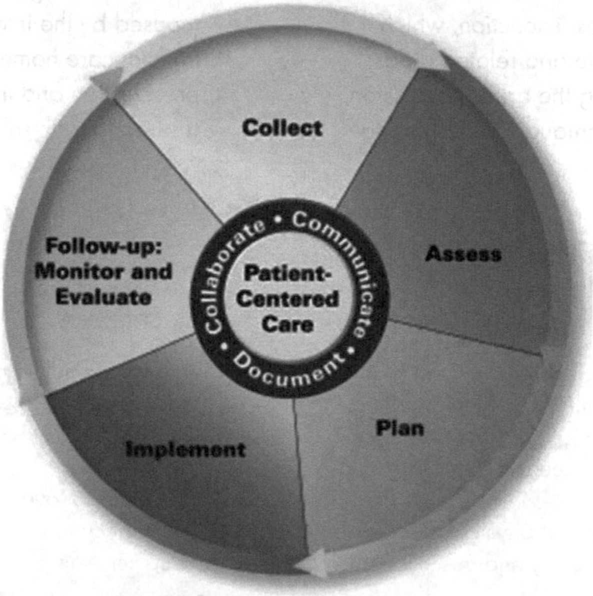

Joint Commission of Pharmacy Practitioners, 2014.

modify accordingly. Laboratory work, vital signs, and patient feedback can be gathered to reevaluate the initial plan.

Overall, the PPCP provides a good framework for pharmacists to provide quality patient care. However, pharmacists must know how to collect pertinent information as it relates to pharmacotherapy. Patient assessment is one of the most important skills that a pharmacist can learn. To provide quality care, pharmacists must be able to communicate appropriately with both the patient and the other health care providers. Collecting pertinent information from the patient is important to obtain the clearest picture possible of his or her health status. Performing physical assessment will help give insight into patients' complaints or unknown issues. Understanding laboratory values and interpreting routine tests allow pharmacists to assess pharmacotherapy issues more effectively. This information can then be documented in specific formats so that other health care providers can use the information to provide the appropriate care.

28-4 Obtaining a Comprehensive Patient History

Obtaining a comprehensive patient history is a vital part of patient care. The medical history may include the following information:

- ***Chief complaint (CC):*** This information establishes the reason for the patient's visit.
- ***History of present illness (HPI):*** This history identifies the onset of the illness and modifying factors.
- ***Past medical history (PMH):*** This information establishes the patient's medical background of disease state and conditions. The history should distinguish between chronic conditions (e.g., diabetes, hypertension) and acute conditions (e.g., recent surgery, injury, or infection). A patient's previous medical record should be included if possible.
- ***Medications, allergies, and immunizations:*** These include all medications taken by any route (e.g., oral, injectable), including prescription drugs, over-the-counter medications, dietary supplements, and treatment remedies. Adverse drug reactions, allergies, and immunization history should also be noted.
- ***Family history:*** This information includes the patient's family medical history, such as diabetes, hypertension, high cholesterol, mental illness, and any genetic disorders as well as causes of death in family members.
- ***Social history:*** This information includes the patient's social activities that may relate to the presented illness (e.g., daily activities, exercise, smoking, alcohol and illegal drug consumption, living conditions). This history also includes people associated with the patient, such as a spouse, children, parents, siblings, and pets.
- ***Review of systems (ROS):*** This information is usually arranged by organ system (i.e. gastrointestinal, respiratory, musculoskeletal) and can include physical assessment tests and findings, vital signs, and observations, such as checks of the site of the chief complaint, organs possibly involved, temperature, blood pressure, and any abnormal mental status.

Problem-Focused Interview

The patient interview should be conducted using mostly open-ended questions and statements. This method allows the patient to elaborate on his or her condition, rather than answering yes or no. Seven basic screening questions may be used in the interview to address the problem:

- ***Location:*** Where is the symptom?
- ***Quality:*** What is it like? Describe it.
- ***Severity:*** How bad is it? How does it interfere with your life?
- ***Timing:*** How long has it been present? When did it start? How often does it occur?

- ***Setting:*** How did it happen? What were you doing when it started?
- ***Modifying factors:*** What makes it better or worse? What did you use to treat it?
- ***Associated symptoms:*** What other things have you noticed?

Closing of the Interview

In closing the interview, the interviewer should do the following:

- Summarize all the gathered information for the patient.
- Discuss the plan and follow-up method.
- Ask for additional questions and concerns.
- Write an organized document.

Documentation

The interview information for each visit should be organized in four identifiable sections to make it easy for providers to follow: **s**ubjective, **o**bjective, **a**ssessment, and **p**lan, also referred to as a SOAP note. SOAP notes can be used for the *plan* process in the PPCP cycle.

- ***Subjective information:*** This section reflects all the information reported by the patient as presented. It includes how the patient feels, his or her observations about the current condition, and current medications (prescription, over-the-counter, dietary supplements) he or she is taking.
- ***Objective information:*** This section includes the health care provider's physical or mental observations, the patient's vital signs, any physical findings, and any laboratory test results. Medications may be listed here if not reported by the patient.
- ***Assessment:*** This section includes the health care provider's evaluation and diagnosis of the case presented. For example, the patient has uncontrolled hypertension (goal less than 130/80 mmHg) and requires additional drug therapy.
- ***Plan:*** This section can include the health care provider's treatment plan and recommendations, the medication prescribed or discontinued, and the patient counseling performed. It should include follow-up visits and monitoring recommendations for the patient.

Interim Interview

Follow-up visits should include an interim interview. The goal of the interim interview is to address four main issues:

- Patient's control over his or her health conditions
- Patient's adherence with his or her medications and treatment plans
- Complications (if any) of the prescribed medication or treatment plans
- Range of symptoms (if any were present initially), if reduced or compounded

28-5 Physical Assessment Techniques, Terminology, and Modifications Caused by Common Disease States and Drug Therapy

Physical assessment of a patient is essential for proper diagnosis. It includes inspection, palpation, percussion, and auscultation.

Inspection

Inspection involves a general observation of the patient, noting abnormal physical appearance or behavior. Observing the body build and nutrition of the patient helps detect obesity as well as cachectic and athletic states in the patient. Any malformations noted during inspection may point to birth defects or the consequence of trauma.

Gait should also be examined in patients, because it could indicate abnormalities such as ataxia, foot drop, and intoxication. Additionally, examination of a patient's gait can be used to monitor carbidopa/levodopa effectiveness in patients with Parkinson's disease.

Palpation

Palpation involves the use of the sense of touch in the evaluation of the patient. It helps the health care provider assess the texture, moisture, temperature, masses, vibrations, and pulsations in the patient's body. Brevity of touch can be used to gather information during the assessment:

- A light touch should be used for skin surfaces.
- Deeper touches should be used to assess organs or masses in the body.

Different areas of the hand are also helpful in palpating the patient:

- Fingertips are best to use for fine, tactile sensation.
- The dorsal surface of the hand can be the most helpful in assessing temperature.
- The palm surface at the metacarpal joints is best to assess vibrations.
- Finger pads are always best for deep palpation, including the palpation of organs.

Two fingers or the whole hand can be used when performing tests that assess strength in a patient.

Although being gentle is important in palpating the patient, pain can signal an important finding. Any areas of the body the patient pinpointed as being tender during the interview should be palpated last.

Percussion

Percussion is used to produce sounds, elicit tenderness, or assess reflexes in a patient. It is also helpful in locating organ borders, identifying organ shape and position, and determining whether an organ is solid or filled with gas.

Percussion may be administered either directly or indirectly:

- During a direct percussion, the finger or hand is used to strike directly against the body.
- Indirect percussion, in contrast, involves tapping a finger against the middle finger of a hand that is held against a specific area of the body.
- Blunt percussion is delivered by striking a fist directly to an area of the body.

Percussion can deliver a variety of sounds that can reveal a lot about the patient's organs:

- A tympanic or drum-like sound may indicate a gastric bubble.
- A hyperresonant or boom-like sound may indicate an emphysematous lung.
- A resonant or hollow sound indicates a healthy lung.
- An example of an area of the body that would deliver a dull or thud-like sound on percussion would be the liver.
- A flat or very dull sound is found in normal muscle tissue on percussion.

Auscultation

Auscultation involves listening for normal and abnormal sounds with a stethoscope. Sounds, including heart, breath, and bowel, can also signify medical conditions, if abnormal.

To perform auscultation, the health care provider must apply the stethoscope to the naked skin. Auscultation is usually carried out last.

28-6 Vital Signs, Laboratory Values, and Diagnostic Tests

Vital Signs

Vital signs are used to measure various physiological functions of the patient. An evaluation of vital signs should be included in every patient case presentation. Vital signs evaluated are patient weight, respiration, pulse, temperature, and blood pressure (Table 28-1).

Following are common laboratory tests using blood specimens that can be extracted from the medication record. See Table 28-2 for further breakdown of normal values and their clinical relevance.

- ***Basic metabolic panel (BMP):*** The BMP provides important information about the current status of the kidneys (blood urea nitrogen [BUN]), electrolytes and acid–base balance (sodium [Na], potassium [K], carbon dioxide [CO_2], chloride [Cl]), blood glucose, calcium levels, and serum creatinine [SCr]). This can be denoted using the shorthand format below:

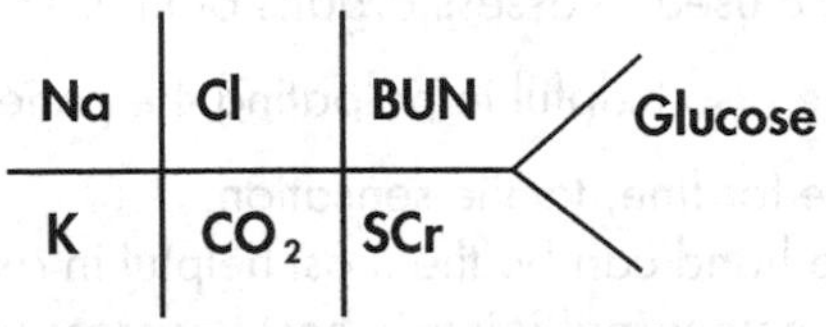

TABLE 28-1. **Vital Signs and their Relevance**

Vital	Measurement (units)	Value	Comments
Weight	Pounds (lb)	n.a.	Normal value is often age dependent.
	Body mass index (BMI; kg/m^2)	Underweight: < 18.5; normal: 18.5–24.9; overweight: 25–29.9; obese: ≥ 30	BMI takes weight (kg) and height (m) into account.
Respiration	Breaths/minute	Adults: 12–20; newborns: 30–60; children: 20–40	Normal value is often age dependent. The respiratory rate increases during periods of stress, metabolic disorders, lung and cardiac disease, and elevated temperature. Some terminology used is as follows: ■ Apnea: absence of breathing ■ Dyspnea: difficult breathing or shortness of breath ■ Orthopnea: difficulty breathing in supine position ■ Tachypnea: rapid breathing ■ Bradypnea: slow breathing ■ Hyperpnea: deep, rapid breathing; hyperventilation ■ Kussmaul breathing: deep, regular breathing with rate slow, normal, or fast ■ Ataxic respiration: unpredictably irregular breathing ■ Cheyne–Stokes respiration: cyclic pattern of apnea and varied breathing

TABLE 28-1. Vital Signs and their Relevance *(Continued)*

Vital	Measurement (units)	Value	Comments
Temperature	Degree Fahrenheit (°F) or degree Celsius (°C)	Normal human: 98.6°F or 37°C; range: 97.6–99.4°F or 36.5–37.5°C	Temperature variation has many causes, including environmental (room temperature) and individual factors (circadian rhythm, exercise, stress, hormones, and age). Temperatures are typically measured either in the ear canal or in the oral cavity. If measured rectally, the temperature will read 1°F higher than if measured orally. If an axillary temperature is taken, it will typically read 1°F lower than a temperature measured orally. When temperature is taken orally, the patient should not chew, smoke, or drink warm or cool liquid around the time the temperature is measured.
Pulse	Beats/minute	Range: between 60 and 100 bpm	Pulse is generally taken at the radial artery. A pulse < 60 beats per minute is indicative of bradycardia. Pulses > 100 beats per minute indicate tachycardia.
Blood pressure (BP)	mmHg	Systolic/diastolic	Normal BP is < 120/80 mmHg. Elevated BP is (systolic) 120–129 and (diastolic) < 80 mmHg. Stage 1 hypertension BP is (systolic) 130–139 or (diastolic) 80–89. Stage 2 hypertension BP is (systolic) > 140 or (diastolic) ≥ 90 mmHg. BP readings may be affected by the patient's medications, white-coat syndrome, emotional state, circadian rhythm, cigarette smoking, caffeine, full bladder, lack of time to adjust to surroundings, and obesity, as well as environmental factors (hot or cold room), equipment, and measuring technique.

n.a., not applicable.

- ***Complete blood count (CBC):*** This test is used to assess for disorders such as infection and anemia. Laboratory values measured include hematocrit (Hct), hemoglobin (Hgb), red blood count (RBC), white blood cell (WBC) count (with or without differential count), and platelet (Plt) count. This can be denoted using the shorthand format below:

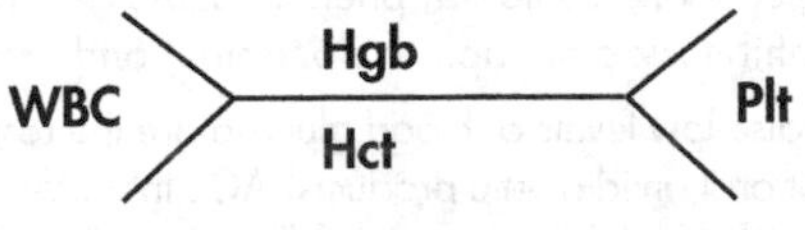

TABLE 28-2. Laboratory Values and Relevance[a]

Test	Normal range	Relevance of level abnormalities
Sodium (Na)	135–145 mEq/L	Low level (hyponatremia) causes hypovolemia. Hypertriglyceridemia and hyperglycemia cause false high Na level. High Na level (hypernatremia) causes hypervolemia.
Potassium (K)	3.5–5 mEq/L	Acidosis, alkalosis, insulin, glucose, and b_2-agonists can change serum K without changing total body level. Low K level can be caused by diuretics and amphotericin B. Hemolysis (hemolytic anemia) can cause a false increase in K. Angiotensin-converting enzyme (ACE) inhibitors, potassium-sparing diuretics, trimethoprim, and heparin can also increase K levels.
Chloride (Cl)	95–105 mEq/L	Increased losses of Cl through the proximal tubule in the kidney results in metabolic alkalosis.
Magnesium (Mg)	1.5–2.2 mEq/L	Vomiting and diarrhea result in decreased Mg levels. Renal insufficiency, hemolytic anemia, and increased intake of antacids result in increased Mg levels.
Calcium (Ca)	8.2–10.8 mg/dL	Alkalosis may increase Ca protein binding, and acidosis may decrease it. These conditions result in low and high free Ca, respectively. Therefore, Ca levels need to be adjusted on the basis of albumin levels.
Phosphate (P)	2.6–4.5 mg/dL	Abnormal levels are associated with malnutrition, diarrhea, and refeeding syndrome.
Blood urea nitrogen (BUN)	8–20 mg/dL	Increased levels are associated with dehydration; protein tolerance (from liver failure); decreased renal perfusion; increased protein breakdown (from gastrointestinal bleeding, injury, burn, fever, or exercise); and medication (corticosteroids or tetracycline). Chloral hydrate can falsely elevate BUN levels. Decreased BUN levels are associated with malnutrition and liver failure. Chloramphenicol and streptomycin can falsely lower BUN levels.
Serum creatinine (SCr)	0.7–1.5 mg/dL	SCr is directly related to muscle mass and muscle metabolism. It measures high in the following: ■ Body builders ■ Protein-rich diet consumers ■ Cases of dehydration ■ Increased temperature ■ Muscular dystrophy ■ Myasthenia gravis ■ Decreased renal secretion or function ■ Liver failure ■ Medication (cimetidine, triamterene, amiloride, spironolactone, trimethoprim, ACE inhibitors, high doses of aminoglycoside antibiotics)
Blood glucose	Fasting: < 100 mg/dL; diagnosis of diabetes if ≥ 126 mg/dL	Blood glucose measurement depends on the fed or fasting state of the patient. Low levels (hypoglycemia) are associated with conditions such as diabetes, pancreatic cancer, and hyperinsulinemia. High levels (hyperglycemia) are associated with conditions such as diabetes, pancreatic cancer, pancreatic injury, and insulin resistance. False high glucose levels are associated with patients taking thiazide; loop diuretics; corticosteroids; diazoxide; sympathomimetic agents (epinephrine, albuterol, terbutaline); glucagon; isoniazid; phenothiazine derivatives; somatropin; thyroid hormones; protease inhibitors; olanzapine; clozapine; and oral contraceptives. False low levels of blood glucose are the result of patients taking high doses or combinations of oral antidiabetic products, ACE inhibitors, disopyramide, fibrates, fluoxetine, monoamine oxidase inhibitors, pentoxifylline, propoxyphene, salicylates, and sulfonamide antibiotics.

TABLE 28-2. Laboratory Values and Relevance[a] *(Continued)*

Test	Normal range	Relevance of level abnormalities
Cholesterol/ lipid profile	Total cholesterol < 200 mg/dL; LDL < 100 mg/dL; HDL ≥ 40 mg/dL (men), ≥ 50 mg/dL (women); triglycerides < 150 mg/dL	Cholesterol measurement depends on the fed and fasting state of the patient. Testing in the fasting state is recommended. The lipid profile is used to calculate the patient's risk for atherosclerotic cardiovascular disease to determine need for dyslipidemia therapy.
Hemoglobin A1c (HbA1c)	< 5.7%	This test measures the percentage of glucose attached to blood hemoglobin in the past 2–3 months. It is used to diagnose diabetes and evaluate diabetes treatment and management.
International normalized ratio (INR)	< 1; desired range for most patients on warfarin 2–3	INR assesses clotting factors made by the liver. It is used in management of coagulation therapy in patients taking medication such as warfarin and other anticoagulation drugs. High levels are associated with medication such as ciprofloxacin, trimethoprim, fluconazole, erythromycin, and omeprazole. Low levels are associated with food rich in vitamin K (leafy greens) and medication (cyclosporine, cholestyramine, barbiturates, and rifampin).
Liver function test		This test assesses the various activities of the liver, synthetic function, and hepatic disease. Assessment of liver function involves the following: ■ INR ■ Cholesterol ■ Aspartate aminotransferase (AST) (8–42 IU/L) ■ Alanine aminotransferase (ALT) (3–30 IU/L) ■ Lactate dehydrogenase (100–225 IU/L) Test levels are affected by the following: ■ Cancer ■ Fatty liver ■ Viruses (human immunodeficiency virus, hepatitis) ■ Chemicals (alcohol) ■ Medications metabolized by the liver (statins, acetaminophen, and others) False elevation of hepatic transaminase is the result of drug toxicity because isoniazid and rifampin produce hepatotoxicity and inflammation.

a. Normal values may vary from lab to lab depending on techniques and reagents used.

- ***Lipid panel:*** This blood test can be used to assess risk for atherosclerotic cardiovascular disease. Laboratory values measured include high-density lipoprotein (HDL), low-density lipoprotein (LDL), very-low-density lipoprotein (VLDL), total cholesterol (TC), and triglycerides (TG).
- ***Liver function:*** This test assesses the various activities of the liver, synthetic function, and hepatic disease. Laboratory values measured include alanine aminotransferase (ALT) and aspartate aminotransferase (AST).

28-7 False-Positive and False-Negative Test Results

Drugs taken by the patient can affect laboratory test results. The mechanism by which drugs affect test results is classified as either in vivo or in vitro interference.

In vivo interference is caused by the pharmacological or the toxicological drug effect (see Table 28-2).

In vitro interference is caused by the interaction of drugs in specimens (urine, blood, tissue) with laboratory testing reagents and may include the following reactions:

- Some β-lactam antibiotics in adequate concentrations may deactivate aminoglycosides if allowed contact time in the test tube, which results in lower levels of measured aminoglycoside.
- Test tubes containing heparin may interfere with measurement of aminoglycoside.
- Test tubes containing fluoride may cause a false increase in BUN level when measured by the Ekatchem assay.
- Glucose and cholesterol levels measured by peroxidase-catalyzed assays are affected by drug-induced hepatotoxicity with bilirubin levels of 10 mg/dL.
- Contact media may change specimen results because of the presence of chemicals or radioactive substances.
- Urine discoloration to orange-red may result if the patient is taking phenazopyridine.
- Urine may change to blue-green or blue if the patient is taking amitriptyline and methylene blue, respectively.
- Proteinuria appears in the urine sample if the patient is taking acetazolamide. This result is a false positive because acetazolamide may cause urine pH to be alkaline and changes the reagent reaction to urine.
- Creatinine measured by the Jaffe assay is affected by cefoxitin to form a chromophore with the reagent.
- Immunoassay antibody reacts with drugs that coexist in the specimen. For example, caffeine cross-reacts with reagents specific for theophylline. Drug metabolites of digitoxin interfere with digoxin assay.
- Laboratory reagents may bind to a drug in the specimen and interfere with the assay of another analyte.
- Wavelength at which an analyte is measured may be affected by the presence of another drug in the specimen.
- Interpretation of data with suspected drug interference should take into account additional factors:
  - Signs and symptoms of case presentation and medical history
  - Comparison of different test results at different times
  - Assessment of the organ in question with a different exam or test

28-8 Common Calculations Related to Patient Assessment

Body Mass Index

Body mass index (BMI) can be used to determine whether a patient would be considered overweight. BMI (kg/m^2) is defined as weight in kilograms divided by height in meters squared (kg/m^2). Patients with a BMI less than 18.5 are considered *underweight.* Normal range is 18.5–24.9. Patients with a BMI between 25 and 29.9 are considered *overweight.* Patients with a BMI of 30 or greater are considered *obese.*

Creatinine Clearance

This calculation provides an estimate of the creatinine clearance (CrCl). It can be used not only to assess kidney function but also to monitor patients on nephrotoxic medications and to assess the need for renal dosing adjustments.

The estimated CrCl using the Cockroft–Gault formula is calculated as follows:

$$\text{Estimated CrCl(mL/minute)} = \frac{[(140 - \text{age}) \times \text{weight in kg}]}{(\text{SCr} \times 72)}$$

The equation must be multiplied by 0.85 if the patient is female. Ideal body weight is used in this equation except if the patient's actual body weight is less than his or her ideal body weight. In that case, the actual body weight should be used. Adjusted body weight should be used for obese patients:

Adjusted body weight (kg) = Ideal body weight + 0.4 (Adjusted body weight – Ideal body weight)

Ideal body weight:

Males: Ideal body weight (kg) = 50 + (2.3 × inches over 5 feet)

Females: Ideal body weight (kg) = 45.5 + (2.3 × inches over 5 feet)

28-9 Over-the-Counter Testing Devices

Blood Glucose Monitors

Blood glucose meters are available for patients with diabetes to use for self-monitoring. These devices measure plasma glucose level.

Many types of monitors are available in the U.S. market, and they vary in size and color, amount of blood sample (microliters), time to show the results (seconds), memory storage capacity, alarms and sounds, strips, accessories (lancet devices, control solutions, recording software), and manufacturer. All monitors are approved for accuracy by the U.S. Food and Drug Administration for home use.

Health care providers should help the patient choose a monitor depending on the patient's dexterity, medication formulary, and budget if paying out of pocket. Patients should receive training on how to use the monitor, how to manage high and low glucose levels, and when to check glucose levels. The American Diabetes Association recommends a fasting blood glucose goal of 80 to 130 mg/dL for patients with diabetes.

Pregnancy Testing Devices

Pregnancy testing devices measure hCG (human chorionic gonadotropin) hormone level in the urine. They are 97% accurate. (Blood tests obtained for laboratory testing are more than 99% accurate.) Results are displayed either as +/– symbols or digital text (pregnant, not pregnant). Most commonly, these tests use a dipstick that is held in the urine stream or dipped into a sample of urine. Ideally, the first urine of the morning should be sampled. Women should test 1 week after a missed period for improved accuracy but can test as early as the first day of a missed period.

Home Testing for HbA1c

Point-of-care testing for hemoglobin A1c (HbA1c) is commonly used in medical offices and in some pharmacies. These tests provide immediate results, usually within 10 minutes. A few kits are available for home testing, specifically Bayer's A1c Now Self Check kit and store brands of this product (CVS, Walmart, and

Walgreens). These meters require minimal blood use, and results are available within 5 minutes. These meters can give patients a snapshot of their blood glucose control within a 3-month time frame. Most patients with diabetes have an HbA1c goal less than 7%.

Drug Screening for Home Use

Home drug screening tests are used to test urine and hair for both prescription and illicit drugs: amphetamine, ecstasy, methamphetamine, barbiturates, benzodiazepine, marijuana, cocaine, opiates, methadone, and steroids.

Results can be obtained immediately (for cocaine and marijuana) or after a few days when samples are sent to the laboratory for analysis. Test results are confidential.

28-10 Questions

1. Goal fasting blood glucose levels for a diabetic patient should be between

A. 80 and 130 mg/dL.
B. 100 and 150 mg/dL.
C. 90 and 200 mg/dL.
D. 60 and 90 mg/dL.

2. The "S" section of SOAP notes should contain which of the following?

A. It contains laboratory results, vital signs, and physical findings found during the patient examination.
B. It includes a summary of the interviewer's plan to treat the patient.
C. It includes prescription and referral.
D. It reflects the information that is given by the patient in his or her own words.

3. Which of the following is *not* an open-ended question?

A. Do you have a neurological disorder?
B. How do you feel?
C. What symptoms do you have?
D. When do you experience pain?

4. A patient's medical history does *not* include which of the following?

A. Chief complaint and history of patient illness
B. Treatment plan
C. Past medical history of patient and family
D. Social history of patient

5. Which of the following is *not* one of the seven basic screening questions used to assess a patient's health problem?

A. Location and quality
B. Severity and timing
C. Current income
D. Setting and associated symptoms

6. Subjective information in the SOAP notes includes

A. laboratory test results.
B. medication taken by the patient.
C. vital signs and physical findings.
D. blood pressure measurement.

7. An interim patient interview does *not* include which of the following parameters?

A. The initial interview with the patient
B. The follow-up interview
C. A check of compliance and complications
D. The outcomes of the treatment plan

8. In the patient's physical assessment, inspection includes

A. observing the patient's general physical and behavior appearance.
B. checking the patient's blood pressure.
C. writing the SOAP notes.
D. obtaining the patient's family history.

9. What should a patient do before a blood pressure check?

A. Rest for at least 5 minutes.
B. Eat a meal.
C. Drink two glasses of water.
D. Refrain from taking medication for 24 hours.

10. A false high sodium level can be caused by which of the following?

A. Hyperglycemia
B. Hyponatremia
C. Hypovolemia
D. Hypervolemia

11. False high potassium is caused by

A. eating diet with leafy vegetables.
B. hemolysis.
C. a high-fat diet.
D. lack of sleep.

12. Which condition below *does not* increase levels of blood urea nitrogen?

A. Dehydration
B. High protein breakdown
C. Burns
D. Malnutrition

13. Which medication class *does not* potentially cause a false high glucose level?

A. Loop diuretics
B. Corticosteroids
C. ACE inhibitors
D. Isoniazid

14. Which medication below is *not* associated with a high INR?

A. Hydrochlorothiazide
B. Fluconazole
C. Omeprazole
D. Ciprofloxacin

15. Which statement is false?

A. Phenazopyridine causes orange-red urine.
B. Tylenol causes white urine.
C. Acetazolamide causes false-positive protein in the urine.
D. Amitriptyline causes blue-green urine.

16. OTC drug screening provides immediate results for

A. barbiturates.
B. benzodiazepine.
C. cocaine and marijuana.
D. steroids.

17. Temperature assessment is best conducted using

A. a light touch with the palm surface.
B. the fingertips.
C. the finger pads.
D. the dorsal surface of the hand.

18. A patient in your pharmacy thinks she may be pregnant and plans to purchase one of the digital testing devices today. Which of the following counseling points is *not* correct?

A. For improved accuracy, test 1 week after a missed period.
B. If you don't believe the test results, a blood test would be more accurate.
C. It is best to use a urine sample taken before bedtime.
D. This test measures hCG levels in the urine.

19. What is a normal blood pressure?

A. Less than 140/90 mmHg
B. Less than 130/80 mmHg
C. Less than 120/70 mmHg
D. Less than 120/80 mmHg

20. Which is a false statement regarding serum creatinine?

A. SCr measures low in body builders and in consumers of a protein-rich diet.
B. Normal SCr level ranges between 0.7 and 1.5 mg/dL.
C. Cimetidine, spironolactone, and ACE inhibitors may cause an increase in SCr.
D. SCr is related to muscle metabolism.

28-11 Answers

1. A. The recommended goal fasting blood glucose levels for a patient with diabetes should be between 80 and 130 mg/dL without symptoms of hypoglycemia.

2. D. The "S" stands for subjective. Hence, the "S" section of SOAP notes should reflect the information that is given by the patient in his or her own words.

3. A. An open-ended question should not allow an answer of yes or no. For example, it should start with how, when, why, and what. Such a question allows the patient to describe more of the symptoms and give a detailed history for proper assessment.

4. **B.** Medical history should include chief complaint, history of patient illness, past medical history of the patient and his or her family, and his or her social history. It will not include the treatment plan; this plan should be in the SOAP notes.

5. **C.** The seven basic screening questions to assess a patient's health problem should include inquiries about the health complaint, such as the physical location of the complaint and quality, severity, timing, setting, and associated symptoms. Current income should not be a screening question to address the physical problem.

6. **B.** Subjective information in the SOAP notes includes the information reported by the patient. Medication taken by the patient will be part of the subjective notes. Laboratory tests, vital signs, and physical or mental observations are part of the objective information.

7. **A.** The interim interview is a follow-up interview of an initial interview. It is conducted to check a patient's compliance, any complications that may have arisen since the initial interview, and the outcomes of the treatment plan.

8. **A.** In the patient's physical assessment, inspection includes observing the patient's general physical and behavior appearance before the next step of examination of vital signs.

9. **A.** In preparing for a blood pressure check, the patient should be in a resting position for 5 minutes. Blood pressure should not be measured immediately after eating a meal or drinking a large amount of liquid. The patient should take his or her medication as prescribed, and the pharmacist should inquire about such medications as part of the patient's clinical assessment.

10. **A.** Hypertriglyceridemia and hyperglycemia cause a false high sodium level.

11. **B.** False high potassium is caused by hemolysis or hemolytic anemia because the cellular content of potassium is higher than extracellular levels. Eating leafy vegetables affects vitamin K, not potassium.

12. **D.** Increased levels of BUN are caused by dehydration, high protein breakdown, and burns—not by malnutrition.

13. **C.** A false high glucose level is associated with loop diuretics, corticosteroids, and isoniazid but not with ACE inhibitors.

14. **A.** A high INR is associated with fluconazole, omeprazole, and ciprofloxacin but not with hydrochlorothiazide.

15. **B.** Tylenol does not cause white urine. Statements A, C, and D are correct.

16. **C.** OTC drug screening provides immediate results for cocaine and marijuana but not for drugs like barbiturates, benzodiazepine, and steroids.

17. **D.** Temperature assessment is best conducted using the dorsal surface of the hand, not the palm, fingertips, or finger pads.

18. **C.** The first urine of the morning should be sampled for improved accuracy because it contains a higher concentration of hCG.

19. **D.** The recommended normal blood pressure should be less than 120/80 mmHg.

20. **A.** The serum creatinine level is high in body builders and in consumers of a protein-rich diet. Answers B, C, and D are correct.

28-12 Additional Resources

Alldredge BK, Corelli RL, Ernst ME, Guglielmo BJ, eds. *Koda-Kimble & Young's Applied Therapeutics: The Clinical Use of Drugs.* 10th ed. Baltimore, MD: Lippincott Williams & Wilkins; 2013.

Barker LR, Burton JR, Zeive PD. *Principles of Ambulatory Medicine.* 7th ed. Baltimore, MD: Williams & Wilkins; 2007.

Bickley LS. *Bates' Guide to Physical Examination and History Taking.* 12th ed. Philadelphia, PA: Lippincott Williams & Wilkins; 2016.

Herrier RN, Apgar DA, Boyce RW, Foster SL, eds. *Patient Assessment in Pharmacy.* New York, NY: McGraw-Hill; 2015.

Joint Commission of Pharmacy Practitioners. Pharmacists' patient care process. 2014. Available at: https://jcpp.net/wp-content/uploads/2016/03/PatientCareProcess-with-supporting-organizations.pdf.

Lee M. *Basic Skills in Interpreting Laboratory Data.* 6th ed. Bethesda, MD: American Society of Health-System Pharmacists; 2017.

Schwartz CR, Garrison MW. Interpretation of clinical laboratory tests. In: Alldredge BK, Corelli RL, Ernst ME, Guglielmo BJ, eds. *Koda-Kimble & Young's Applied Therapeutics: The Clinical Use of Drugs.* 10th ed. Baltimore, MD: Lippincott Williams & Wilkins; 2013:16–41.

Williamson MA, Snyder LM, eds. *Wallach's Interpretation of Diagnostic Tests: Pathways to Arriving at a Clinical Diagnosis.* 10th ed. Philadelphia, PA: Lippincott Williams & Wilkins; 2014.

Clinical Pharmacology and Therapeutic Decision Making 29

G. CHRISTOPHER WOOD

29-1 KEY POINTS

- When making clinical decisions, a pharmacist must consider some key general concepts: the quality of evidence from the medical literature, the assessment of risks and benefits, cost and adherence issues, the way decisions fit within the health care team's plans, and critically, the patient's preferences and health goals.
- Regarding assessment of drug therapy, key aspects include appropriateness and effectiveness of each medication, safety (i.e., adverse effects), potential for interactions, and patient adherence.
- When preparing drug therapy plans, a pharmacist must consider key aspects: optimizing each drug–disease pairing, setting treatment goals, engaging the patient (i.e., getting buy-in), and ensuring appropriate support is in place.
- For follow-up of drug therapy plans, important aspects include coordinating with the patient and the health care team so that patient visits occur in a timely manner; optimizing therapy when appropriate; and documenting and communicating updated plans with the patient and health care team.
- Basic drug therapy management issues are presented for a selection of some of the most common, important disease states in the United States, where drug therapy is a significant part of care. When appropriate, additional information is given on adverse effects and diagnostic tests. Disease state examples include the following:
  - *Neurologic:* Pain, migraine, major depression
  - *Cardiovascular:* Hypertension, congestive heart failure, myocardial infarction, stroke, venous thromboembolism, hyperlipidemia
  - *Respiratory:* Asthma, chronic obstructive pulmonary disease, allergy, cough and cold
  - *Gastrointestinal:* Gastroesophageal reflux disease, peptic ulcer disease, diarrhea, constipation
  - *Endocrine:* Diabetes mellitus, hypothyroidism, glucocorticoid use
  - *Others:* Infectious diseases, renal function, and dietary agents
- Special attention should be paid to narrow therapeutic index drugs that can quickly move between states of being ineffective (i.e., subtherapeutic levels) to effective to toxic (i.e., adverse effects occurring because of supratherapeutic levels).
- Clinicians should be sensitive to working with different cultural groups identified by race or ethnicity, age, sex, sexual orientation, religion, disability, and socioeconomic status. Some areas to consider in providing culturally competent care include health beliefs that may be different from societal norms, language barriers, and differences among groups in drug pharmacokinetics and pharmacodynamics.

29-2 STUDY GUIDE CHECKLIST

The following topics may guide your study of this subject area:

- ☐ Familiarity with the delivery of patient care as described in the Pharmacists' Patient Care Process
- ☐ Effective strategies for educating and communicating with patients and the health care team
- ☐ Ability to research and learn the basics of appropriate drug therapy management for common diseases in the United States using guidelines from major organizations that can be consulted for basic drug therapy decision-making regarding major disease states
- ☐ High level of observation for adverse effects from drugs that may be missed by the patient and other members of the health care team
- ☐ Appropriate documentation of clinical assessments, drug therapy plans, and follow-up depending on the health care setting

29-3 Introduction

As mentioned in Chapter 28, the major U.S. pharmacy organizations, in a collaboration called the Joint Commission of Pharmacy Practitioners, approved the Pharmacists' Patient Care Process (PPCP) in 2014. This process is the profession's latest advancement in providing a model of collaborative (i.e., team-based) patient care that gained major momentum in the 1980s and 1990s, often under the banner of "pharmaceutical care." In this decade, it was recognized that while pharmacists have been performing in more advanced patient-care roles for many years, practice was often highly variable. As such, the PPCP provides a more standardized framework for pharmacists to provide patient care.

The overarching steps in the PPCP are (1) collect information, (2) assess that information, (3) make a drug therapy plan, (4) implement the plan, and (5) follow-up of the effects of the plan. Issues of data collection (i.e., collect information) and communication (i.e., implement the plan) are primarily addressed in other chapters (Chapters 22, 24). Thus, this chapter will focus on some key concepts of assessing clinical information and developing and monitoring drug therapy plans. Examples of common drug therapy issues from selected major disease states seen in the United States will be used to highlight these processes using a head-to-toe format by body system.

29-4 Application of Evidence-Based Decision Making to Patient Care

Drug therapy plans should be developed using evidence-based practice when possible. The medical literature has several categories of evidence from high-quality studies (e.g., large randomized controlled trials) to lower-quality publications (e.g., case reports, observational studies). In addition, various types of reviews (e.g., narrative and systematic reports, meta-analyses) and consensus guidelines are available to help provide guidance on clinical questions (see Chapters 20 and 24 on literature and evidence-based practice, respectively). Regarding any drug therapy decision, clinicians should appropriately weigh the quantity and quality of evidence, the risk–benefit relationship to the patient between improved outcomes and risk of adverse effects, cost and adherence issues that may affect the patient's ability to obtain and continue to use a drug, acceptance by the other members of the health care team, and critically, the patient's health goals.

A common example is the use of aspirin for preventing myocardial infarction (MI), which is clearly a desirable goal but one that is complicated by an increased risk of gastrointestinal (GI) bleeding. There are many factors to consider before starting aspirin for this indication including whether the patient had an MI (i.e., primary versus secondary prevention); the patient's calculated MI risk using the Framingham score; risk factors for bleeding, including a history of GI bleeding; and patient preference. In this case, cost and adherence are less problematic, but these issues can be critical in other situations.

In addition to considering the evidence regarding a drug therapy decision, a number of important aspects of assessment, planning, and follow-up need to be considered. Some critical examples are described in the following subsections.

Assessment

Assess each medication for the following:

- ***Appropriateness:*** Do all drugs have an appropriate condition for which they are being used? Are the optimal drugs being used for each condition? Are any diseases not being treated? Are all doses appropriate for the patient, indication, or organ function status?
- ***Effectiveness:*** Is the patient progressing toward agreed-upon, evidence-based treatment goals (e.g., blood pressure, cholesterol, blood glucose)?

- ***Safety:*** Is the patient having adverse effects? Are drug interactions occurring?
- ***Patient adherence:*** Is the patient actually taking the drug as ordered and if not, why? Cost? Adverse effects? Doesn't understand the need? Administration issues or education? Patient preference?

Planning

Develop plans by doing the following:

- ***Optimize:*** Recommend drug therapy changes based on the assessment of each drug–disease pairing using the criteria above.
- ***Set goals:*** Establish or change goals as needed on the basis of the criteria above.
- ***Engage the patient:*** Provide appropriate education and ensure the patient is on board with the plan.
- ***Support continuity of care:*** Formulate a follow-up plan, and navigate transitions of care if needed.

Follow-up

Provide follow-up by doing the following:

- Work with the patient and other members of the health care team to reassess the patient at appropriate times in the future using the above criteria as appropriate.
- Document progress, and change goals if needed.

29-5 Design of Patient-Centered, Culturally Relevant Treatment Plans

The multicultural population of the United States requires that health care providers be sensitive to working with a broad array of groups. These groups may identify by race or ethnicity, age, sex, sexual orientation, religion, disability, and socioeconomic status. Obviously, establishing a relationship with patients to determine how their cultural identity affects their feelings toward their health care decisions is important. Three areas to consider in delivering culturally competent care are health beliefs, language differences, and racial or other differences that may affect pharmacokinetics and drug response.

Health Beliefs

Clinicians should try to ascertain each patient's beliefs concerning his or her illness and treatment options. Some examples include the cultural stigmas around treating mental illness or HIV (human immunodeficiency virus) infection, refusal of blood transfusions by members of some religions, or reliance on unproven traditional remedies over standard treatments. Clinicians should ask open-ended questions about the patient's health care beliefs in a way that does not introduce personal assumptions or judgment.

Language

In areas of the United States where a language other than English is commonly encountered, clinicians and health care systems should have communication plans for non-English-speaking patients. Having several employees on-site who speak the predominant secondary language would be ideal. Large health care systems often have translation services available. Educational materials also need to be available in appropriate languages. More technological tools are becoming available to aid communication (e.g., Google Translate) and to provide language-appropriate materials.

Differences in Pharmacokinetic and Pharmacodynamic Response

Differences in drug elimination (pharmacokinetics) or response (pharmacodynamics) may be attributable in part to race, sex, and age. For instance, females may have slower renal drug clearance than males. Older patients may have slower renal and hepatic clearance of drugs and may be more susceptible to drug effects and side effects (e.g., opiates, drugs with anticholinergic activity). Alternatively, young patients may have augmented (i.e., faster than normal) renal clearance of drugs. Racial differences in drug response exist in some situations. For hypertension, a primary driver of initial therapy is if a patient is African American or non-African American (see the hypertension subsection in Section 29-6). African American patients also may have different responses to isosorbide dinitrate and hydralazine treatment in congestive heart failure (CHF) and responses to β_2-agonists in asthma. In some cases, a genetic mutation for slow or rapid drug metabolism, or a risk of an adverse effect, is more common in a certain group. For example, some Asian patients are more likely to have a genetic profile that confers susceptibility to severe skin reactions from phenytoin. As precision medicine continues to evolve, additional guidance on these and other issues will emerge.

29-6 Common Drug Therapy Issues from Selected Major Disease States

The following sections will briefly describe some of the most common drug therapy issues from a selection of major disease states encountered in the United States, including the basics of drug selection, efficacy, safety, and other important factors. Specific treatment goals will be included when appropriate. Disease states will be presented by body system in a head-to-toe format with some stand-alone sections as appropriate (e.g., infectious diseases).

Neurologic System

Acute and chronic pain

Treatment goals

Goals are decreased pain and improvement in performing daily activities. Pain scores (e.g., 10-point scale) can provide a method to track pain over time.

Drug selection

Opioids

The mechanism of action (MOA) is an opiate receptor agonist. Many opioids are available, such as morphine, codeine, hydromorphone (Dilaudid), oxycodone (OxyContin), hydrocodone (Vicodin, Lortab), and fentanyl. Dosing equivalency tables between products are widely available. Opioids are used for moderate to severe acute pain and for some forms of chronic pain. However, a major shift is underway in chronic pain management to use fewer opioids when possible because of the opioid addiction crisis. Opioids can be given orally or by intravenous (IV), intramuscular (IM), or topical (patch) route. Doses vary greatly (i.e., potency), but efficacy is similar at equipotent doses. Dosing intervals also vary by drug product. The major differentiating factors in regimens include (1) varying times of onset and duration of action based on the delivery system used (e.g., immediate-release po, extended-release po, IV, patch) and individual drug pharmacokinetics and (2) varying incidence of adverse effects (rash, hypotension) between some agents. Long-acting agents can be used for chronic pain whereas acute pain is typically treated with short-acting agents. Tolerance can develop, necessitating increasing doses. Major adverse effects include sedation, respiratory depression, constipation, rash, hypotension, and addiction. Antihistamines or changing agents can be tried for rash. There are many combination products with acetaminophen.

Therefore, ensure that patients do not exceed the total daily dose of acetaminophen (4,000 mg/day) when using such products. Methadone should be prescribed only by specialists familiar with that agent because of methadone's long and widely varying half-life and its risk of QT-interval prolongation.

Nonsteroidal anti-inflammatory drugs

The MOA of nonsteroidal anti-inflammatory drugs (NSAIDs) is inhibition of prostaglandin production. Many NSAIDs are available over the counter or by prescription. Examples include aspirin, ibuprofen, naproxen, ketorolac, and celecoxib (Celebrex). Acetaminophen is not technically an NSAID, but it is commonly included in this group. NSAIDs are used for mild-to-moderate musculoskeletal and inflammatory pain as well as other types of pain (e.g., headaches, migraines). Some agents (e.g., ibuprofen, acetaminophen) are also used for fever. Aspirin is primarily used for prevention of cardiovascular events. Intravenous formulations of ibuprofen, ketorolac, and acetaminophen are available. Adverse effects include GI bleeding and renal dysfunction with NSAIDs and liver toxicity with acetaminophen at high doses. Ketorolac is limited to 5 days of use. Celecoxib causes less GI bleeding but may increase the risk of MI.

Tramadol

Tramadol has multiple MOAs, including some opiate receptor activity and serotonin and norepinephrine uptake inhibition. It is an oral agent for various types of pain. Adverse effects are similar to those of opioids (less intense) but also include an increased seizure risk.

Adjunctive agents

Adjunctive agents such as pregabalin (Lyrica), gabapentin, some antidepressants, some antiepileptic agents, and transdermal lidocaine can be used for neuropathic pain. The major adverse effects with pregabalin and gabapentin are sedation and other mental status changes that necessitate slowly titrating doses upward as tolerated.

Migraine

Treatment goals

Goals are to relieve pain and the associated symptoms (e.g., nausea).

Drug selection

Initial therapy for mild to moderate migraine includes NSAIDs, acetaminophen, and combination agents with caffeine or butalbital. Opioids can be added. Many serotonin receptor agonists (triptans, e.g., sumatriptan) are available in po, subcutaneous, and intranasal dosage forms and are used for severe cases, mild-to-moderate cases that do not respond to initial treatment, or in patients known to have poor responses to initial treatment. Ergotamine derivatives can be given but may worsen nausea. Migraine prophylaxis in patients with frequent, severe episodes is individualized and may include β-blockers, antiepileptics, and antidepressants.

Major depressive disorder

Treatment goals

Goals are the resolution of depressive symptoms and prevention of suicide attempts.

Drug selection

A large number of antidepressant agents are in the top 200 prescribed drugs in the United States. A very large array of agents is available, including selective serotonin reuptake inhibitors (SSRIs, e.g., fluoxetine), serotonin norepinephrine reuptake inhibitors (e.g., venlafaxine), bupropion, trazodone and nefazodone, tricyclic antidepressants (TCAs), and newer agents such as mirtazapine and vilazodone. No agent or class is clearly superior. Newer classes are generally started first because of fewer adverse effects. Many patients require changes to other agents, addition of second agents for nonresponse, or both. Second-generation antipsychotics (e.g., aripiprazole, quetiapine) may also be added. Drug selection can be affected by adverse effects that vary between drugs and include sedation, GI upset, sexual dysfunction (SSRIs); seizure risk (bupropion); and anticholinergic effects (TCAs).

Other notable adverse effects from neurologic agents

Movement disorders

Dopamine receptor antagonist drugs (e.g., haloperidol and other antipsychotic or phenothiazine agents, metoclopramide) may cause extrapyramidal symptoms (EPS). EPS can be treated with anticholinergic agents, a change to newer generation antipsychotic agents, or both.

Cognitive changes

Sedative-hypnotic drugs (e.g., benzodiazepines, nonbenzodiazepine hypnotics such as zolpidem) can cause sedation and retrograde amnesia. Hypnotic agents have been associated with altered sleep behavior such as sleepwalking. Anticholinergic drugs (e.g., first-generation antihistamines, TCAs, GI antispasmodics, benztropine) can cause confusion, short-term memory impairment, sedation, visual disturbances, and hallucinations. Elderly patients are at greater risk for more of these side effects.

Key points regarding diagnostic tests

- *Computed tomography (CT) scan of the head* is a radiographic test that valuates a number of potential abnormalities, including ischemia (e.g., stroke), bleeding (e.g., traumatic brain injury), or masses (e.g., tumors).
- *Magnetic resonance imaging (MRI) scan of the head* is a nonradiographic test generally similar to a CT scan but preferred in some types of imaging. MRI provides better imaging of soft tissue, whereas CT images bone better. Radiocontrast dye, if used with either test, can be nephrotoxic. Patients with metal implants generally cannot undergo MRI.
- *Lumbar puncture* analyzes the cerebrospinal fluid (CSF) for meningitis.
- *Electroencephalography (EEG)* assesses for seizure activity.

Cardiovascular System

Hypertension

Treatment goals

The blood pressure goal is less than 130/80 mmHg in most adults. Another goal is the prevention of cardiovascular events such as stroke and MI.

Drug selection

Initial drug selection is from four major drug classes (thiazide diuretics, angiotensin-converting enzyme inhibitors [ACEIs] and angiotensin receptor blockers [ARBs], calcium channel blockers [CCBs], β-blockers) and is primarily influenced by other conditions that may be treated with antihypertensive agents, and if the patient is African American. For African American patients, initial therapy should include a thiazide or a CCB. Non–African American patients can be started on a thiazide, CCB, ACEI, or ARB. ACEIs and ARBs may be preferred in younger patients (less than 60 years old), whereas a thiazide or CCB may be preferred in older patients. Many patients require combination therapy with drugs from these primary drug classes. A number of other secondary agents and classes are available, such as α-blockers; clonidine; hydralazine; and the newer agent, aliskiren.

Considerations when treating other conditions

- ***Chronic kidney disease (CKD) or diabetes:*** Treatment should include an ACEI or ARB, which can provide protection against further kidney damage.
- ***Coronary artery disease (including post-MI):*** A β-blocker and an ACEI or ARB are first-line agents (decrease mortality).
- ***Stroke:*** An ACEI or ARB is a first-line agent.
- ***Congestive heart failure (CHF):*** An ACEI or ARB and a β-blocker are first-line agents (decrease mortality). Spironolactone and loop diuretics are also commonly used. Carvedilol (Coreg) is a mixed α- and β-blocker commonly used for CHF.
- ***Atrial fibrillation:*** A β-blocker or non-dihydropyridine CCB (diltiazem or verapamil) is used to provide rate control. Alternatively, amiodarone may be used for rhythm control but is associated with numerous adverse effects including pulmonary fibrosis and thyroid dysfunction. Anticoagulation is also used in most patients to prevent thromboembolic stroke (e.g., warfarin or a newer agent such as apixaban, dabigatran, rivaroxaban).

Notable adverse effects

All agents can cause hypotension, which can lead to dizziness, falls, and syncope. Diuretics can cause excessive urination, hypokalemia, hypomagnesemia, metabolic alkalosis (especially loop diuretics), and hypocalcemia (loop diuretics only). CCBs can cause peripheral edema and constipation. Non-dihydropyridine CCBs can cause bradycardia and heart block and can worsen CHF. ACEIs and ARBs can cause angioedema and hyperkalemia and can worsen renal function (though they are often renally protective). ACEIs can also cause cough. β-blockers can cause fatigue, bradycardia, heart block, and bronchoconstriction in patients with lung disease (avoided with selective agents such as metoprolol). Note: Some drugs can increase blood pressure including NSAIDs, oral decongestants, glucocorticoids, and stimulants used for weight loss or attention deficit hyperactivity disorder.

Congestive heart failure

Treatment goals

Goals are to reduce symptoms (dyspnea, fatigue, peripheral edema), slow disease progression, and prolong survival.

Drug selection

Loop diuretics are used to reduce acute fluid overload. Several agents reduce mortality and are considered first-line agents including ACEIs and ARBs, β-blockers (primarily metoprolol, carvedilol, bisoprolol), and aldosterone antagonists (spironolactone). β-blockers are started at low doses to avoid acute worsening of symptoms. Hydralazine plus isosorbide dinitrate is recommended for African American patients who cannot receive an ACEI or ARB. Eplerenone is an alternative to spironolactone that does cause endocrine adverse effects (e.g., gynecomastia). Digoxin can be added in patients not controlled with first-line agents, but it is associated with higher mortality if drug levels are elevated. Common adverse effects are described in the hypertension subsection earlier in this section. Additional notable issues include the need to slowly titrate β-blockers to avoid worsening CHF symptoms, hyperkalemia with spironolactone, risk of toxicity with digoxin (arrhythmias, central nervous system [CNS] and GI side effects), headache from isosorbide dinitrate, and lupus from hydralazine.

Myocardial infarction

Acute treatment of MI is highly complex and related to a number of factors including time from onset of symptoms, non-ST-segment elevation versus ST-segment elevation, occurrence of a revascularization procedure (percutaneous coronary intervention, coronary artery bypass surgery) versus fibrinolysis, and other risk factors. Various combinations of antiplatelet agents (aspirin, clopidogrel, prasugrel, ticagrelor) are used with acute anticoagulation (e.g., IV heparin, subcutaneous enoxaparin). Long-term therapies that have been shown to decrease mortality after MI include antiplatelet agents (various regimens based on initial management [e.g., stents] and other factors); β-blockers; high-intensity statins; and often an ACEI or ARB, an aldosterone antagonist, or both.

Ischemic stroke

Thrombolysis with alteplase is recommended in selected patients within 4.5 hours of symptom onset. The major adverse effect with alteplase is bleeding. Aspirin should be started within 24–48 hours. Anticoagulation with IV heparin or other agents is generally not recommended. Secondary stroke prevention primarily involves controlling risk factors such as hypertension and diabetes.

Venous thromboembolism (deep venous thrombosis and pulmonary embolism)

Acute treatment is either an IV heparin infusion titrated to a goal partial thromboplastin time (PTT), subcutaneous low-molecular-weight heparin (LMWH), or subcutaneous fondaparinux (Arixtra). Heparin and LMWHs can cause an immune-mediated thrombocytopenia (heparin-induced thrombocytopenia) that can be life threatening. Follow-up venous thromboembolism (VTE) therapy is for at least 3 months with oral anticoagulation. Newer agents may be preferred over warfarin because of less monitoring and, in some cases, less bleeding. However, newer agents are expensive, and warfarin is still widely used. Some female hormone drugs such as oral contraceptives can increase the risk of VTE.

Hyperlipidemia

Treatment goals

Goal levels for low density lipoprotein (LDL) cholesterol and treatment intensity vary by age and risk factors such as preexisting cardiovascular (CV) disease, diabetes, and calculated CV risk. Secondary treatment goals include non-LDL cholesterol and triglycerides in some patients.

Drug selection

HMG-CoA (3-hydroxy-3-methylglutaryl coenzyme A) reductase inhibitors (i.e., statin drugs) are first line. Non-statin drugs such as ezetimibe or bile acid sequestrants may be added in selected situations. Fenofibrate and niacin are falling out of favor. Common significant adverse effects from statin therapy include myopathy and elevation of liver transaminases.

Key points regarding diagnostic tests

- *Electrocardiogram (ECG)* is a tracing of electrical activity of the heart. It is used to diagnose a number of arrhythmias, ischemic events (e.g., MI), or other abnormalities.
- *Echocardiogram* is an ultrasound test of the heart that detects a number of abnormalities, including valvular disease, and the type and severity of heart failure.
- *Stress tests* include various types of tests that evaluate for cardiac ischemia or other abnormalities.
- *Troponin* is a blood test to help determine if a myocardial infarction is occurring.
- *Partial thromboplastin time (PTT)* and *international normalized ratio (INR)* are the most common indicators of anticoagulation. Therapeutic heparin is monitored with PTT, and warfarin is monitored with the INR.

Respiratory System

Asthma

Major asthma guidelines describe a stepwise treatment approach for patients not responding to initial therapy. Some key points in the treatment steps for adults include (1) using a short-acting β_2-agonist (SABA prn); (2) adding a low-dose inhaled corticosteroid (ICS); (3) if more control is needed, increasing the ICS dose, adding a long-acting β_2-agonist (LABA, many available, e.g., salmeterol), or both; and (4) if a high-dose ICS plus LABA is not effective, adding an oral corticosteroid, considering omalizumab for patients with allergies, or both. Educating patients on proper inhaler technique for asthma and chronic obstructive pulmonary disease (COPD) is important to ensure medication efficacy.

Chronic obstructive pulmonary disease

The Global Initiative for Chronic Obstructive Lung Disease (GOLD) guidelines are widely known and grade patients by illness severity. Some key points in the treatment steps include (1) beginning initial therapy with an SABA prn plus a long-acting bronchodilator, which can be either a LABA or a long-acting anticholinergic (e.g., tiotropium); (2) adding a second long-acting bronchodilator from the other drug class not currently used; and (3) considering the addition of theophylline or, if the patient has chronic bronchitis, roflumilast. Nonselective β-blockers can worsen bronchoconstriction in asthma or COPD.

Allergy

Treatment is based on symptoms. For sinus drainage, first-generation antihistamines such as diphenhydramine (Benadryl) cause more sedation and anticholinergic adverse effects and are shorter acting than newer generation agents such as loratadine (Claritin), cetirizine (Zyrtec), and fexofenadine (Allegra). However, first-generation drugs have a faster onset of action. Antihistamine nasal sprays and eye drops have fewer systemic adverse effects. Oral nasal decongestants are available but can cause tachycardia, hypertension, and CNS stimulation. Specifically, pseudoephedrine sales are often subject to special regulation (e.g., storage behind the counter, entry into patient registry for purchase). Nasal decongestant sprays are also available but are recommended for only short-term use (less than 72 hours) to avoid rebound congestion. Dextromethorphan is the only over-the-counter (OTC) cough suppressant. CNS disturbances can occur with high doses. Guaifenesin is a widely used OTC agent to thin pulmonary secretions. OTC nasal corticosteroids are available and are effective for nasal allergies, though with a long onset of action (i.e., days to weeks).

Cough and cold

Treatment for adults is based on symptoms and is similar to allergy (see subsection earlier in this section). Antihistamines and decongestants are not recommended for children younger than 6 years of age.

Key points regarding diagnostic tests

- *Peak expiratory flow rate* is used for monitoring asthma severity. It can be self-administered with a handheld device.
- *Spirometry* is used for monitoring COPD. Several parameters are monitored, including forced expiratory volume in one second (FEV_1).
- *CT scan of the chest* is used for diagnosing pulmonary embolism.

Gastrointestinal System

Gastroesophageal reflux disease

Mild gastroesophageal reflux disease (GERD) can be treated with antacids prn or histamine 2–receptor antagonists (H2RAs). Moderate to severe GERD is treated with proton pump inhibitors (PPIs). Weight loss and avoidance of food triggers are also helpful. Concerns with long-term use of PPIs include the risk of *Clostridium difficile*–associated diarrhea and hypomagnesemia. Some drugs can cause esophagitis, including tetracycline antibiotics and bisphosphonates used for osteoporosis. β-blockers, CCBs, and caffeine can decrease lower esophageal sphincter tone and worsen GERD.

Peptic ulcer disease

Treatment of peptic ulcer disease (PUD) is based on the severity of symptoms (e.g., mild dyspepsia to active bleeding) and etiology. *Helicobacter Pylori*–associated ulcers require combination antibiotic therapy (e.g., clindamycin plus either metronidazole or amoxicillin) plus a PPI for 10–14 days. NSAID-induced ulcers are treated with H2RAs or PPIs, and the NSAID is stopped or changed to celecoxib. PPIs or misoprostol can be used to prevent NSAID-induced ulcers in selected patients.

Diarrhea

Treatment involves elimination of causative factors if possible (e.g., diet) and oral replacement of fluids and electrolytes if needed. Medical evaluation is needed if symptoms are severe (e.g., dehydration, bloody stools) or last more than 48 hours, or if fever is present. Otherwise, OTC loperamide is the simplest therapy for most patients. Drug therapy may also include diphenoxylate and atropine; bismuth subsalicylate (turns stools black, avoid in aspirin allergy); or bulk-forming agents such as psyllium, calcium polycarbophil, and methylcellulose. Probiotics and antibiotics are used only in selected situations. Drugs that can cause diarrhea include antibiotics and magnesium supplements and antacids.

Constipation

Initial treatment includes lifestyle and dietary changes. A number of drug therapy options come from several drug classes including bulk-forming agents (listed previously), emollients and stool softeners (docusate), lubricants (mineral oil), stimulants (bisacodyl, senna), hyperosmotics (e.g., lactulose, sorbitol, MiraLAX), and magnesium or phosphate saline laxatives. Newer agents such as lubiprostone (Amitiza), linaclotide (Linzess), or opioid antagonists such as methylnaltrexone (Relistor) are used for chronic or opioid-induced constipation in selected patients. Drugs that can cause constipation include opiates, calcium supplements and antacids, anticholinergics, muscle relaxants, and CCBs.

Drug-induced hepatic dysfunction

A large number of drugs have the potential to cause hepatic dysfunction. These drugs include acetaminophen (greater than 4,000 mg /day), amiodarone, statins, older anticonvulsants (e.g., phenytoin, carbamazepine, valproic acid), azole antifungals (e.g., fluconazole), and some tuberculosis drugs (notably, isoniazid).

Key points regarding diagnostic tests

- *Hepatic transaminases*—aspartate aminotransferase (AST) and alanine aminotransferase (ALT)—in elevated levels indicate cellular liver damage. AST may be higher than ALT in alcohol-induced liver disease.
- Alkaline phosphatase and bilirubin are present in elevated levels in cholestatic liver disease.

Endocrine System

Diabetes mellitus

Treatment goals

Goals are individualized on the basis of a number of factors; however, a hemoglobin A1c less than 7% is reasonable in many nonpregnant adults. Preventing long-term complications such as CV events, blindness, neuropathy, and renal failure are also treatment goals.

Drug selection

Drug selection is complex depending on a number of patient factors. Guidelines are available from several major medical organizations. Type 1 diabetes is less common and requires insulin therapy. The major adverse effect with insulin is hypoglycemia. Type 2 diabetes is more common, and the first-line agent is metformin. The most common adverse effects with metformin include GI distress and rare but serious lactic acidosis. Often, two to four drug regimens are required and many agents can be added to metformin on the basis of various factors. Some examples of agents that can be added include insulin, sulfonylureas (e.g., glyburide), pioglitazone, dipeptidyl peptidase–4 inhibitors (e.g., sitagliptin), and glucagon-like peptide-1 receptor antagonists (e.g., liraglutide). Notably, pioglitazone can cause fluid retention and cause or worsen heart failure.

Thyroid disorders

The thyroid stimulating hormone (TSH) test is the most common test for thyroid disorders. TSH is elevated in hypothyroidism and low in hyperthyroidism. Testing of T_4 (thyroxine) and T_3 (triiodothyronine) can further differentiate thyroid disorders. Hypothyroidism is far more common than hyperthyroidism and is treated with thyroid hormones (e.g., levothyroxine) titrated to effect.

Glucocorticoid use

Many glucocorticoids are available for systemic or topical use (e.g., prednisone, hydrocortisone). Systemic glucocorticoids are used for a wide range of indications including severe asthma, adrenal insufficiency, and immune and inflammatory disorders. Chronic use carries the risk of a wide variety of adverse effects, many of which can be severe. These adverse effects include mental status changes, impaired wound healing, increased infection risk, osteoporosis, and fluid and electrolyte abnormalities. Patients on chronic therapy should not be stopped abruptly because of acute risk of adrenal insufficiency.

Infectious Diseases

Upper respiratory infections (sinusitis, pharyngitis, otitis media)

Most upper respiratory infections are viral and do not require antibiotics. When caused by bacteria, *Streptococcus* species and *Haemophilus influenzae* are common pathogens. Treatment of otitis media depends on patient age, presentation, and illness severity. In general, antibiotics are reserved for patients with severe or bilateral disease, or both. Ten days of high-dose amoxicillin is first line, with high-dose amoxicillin-clavulanate used for recurrences. Oral cephalosporins, macrolides, or clindamycin are used for penicillin allergy. The use of antibiotics for sinusitis is determined by the duration and severity of symptoms. If used, recommended first-line antibiotics are amoxicillin (with or without clavulanate) or doxycycline (adults only). More intensive therapy is needed for patients with risk factors for resistant organisms (e.g., day care attendance) and includes high-dose amoxicillin-clavulanate, respiratory quinolone (levofloxacin or moxifloxacin), or clindamycin plus cefixime. Pharyngitis should be treated with antibiotics only if the infection is confirmed to be bacterial. Antibiotics include antistreptococcal agents such as penicillin V, amoxicillin, cephalosporins, azithromycin, and clindamycin.

Pneumonia

Treatment of community-acquired pneumonia (CAP) depends on patient age, comorbid conditions (e.g., heart, lung, liver, or kidney disease; diabetes), and severity (outpatient, inpatient, or intensive care unit [ICU]). *S. pneumoniae* (pneumococcus), *H. influenzae*, and atypical organisms such as *Mycoplasma pneumoniae* are common. Adult outpatient CAP is treated with doxycycline or newer macrolides (azithromycin, clarithromycin). Patients with comorbidities are treated with a respiratory quinolone or have high-dose amoxicillin (+/– clavulanate) added to the first-line agents. Adult inpatient CAP is treated with a respiratory quinolone or a combination of a cephalosporin with expanded pneumococcal activity (commonly ceftriaxone) plus azithromycin, clarithromycin, or doxycycline. Patients in the ICU require antipseudomonal coverage (e.g., cefepime, piperacillin–tazobactam, meropenem) and possibly methicillin-resistant *Staphylococcus aureus* (MRSA) coverage (e.g., vancomycin).

Skin and skin structure infections

Treatment for skin infections varies widely depending on the site, severity, and presentation of infection (e.g., purulence). Broadly, nonpurulent infections are cellulitis and purulent infections are abscesses. Many less severe infections can be drained or treated with topical antibiotics alone. For infections that require systemic treatment, general recommendations for nonpurulent infections include targeting *Streptococcus* species with agents such as penicillin, cephalexin, or clindamycin. If an infection is severe, treat with vancomycin plus piperacillin–tazobactam. Purulent infections should target MRSA. Doxycycline or trimethoprim–sulfamethoxazole (TMP–SMX) is used for moderate infections, and IV therapy (e.g., vancomycin, linezolid, daptomycin, ceftaroline) is used for severe infections. Diabetic foot infections require additional coverage for pseudomonas and anaerobes.

Clostridium difficile–associated diarrhea

Clostridium difficile–associated diarrhea (CDAD) is treated for 10–14 days with oral or IV metronidazole if less severe, or oral vancomycin if more severe. The most severe cases are treated with metronidazole and oral vancomycin. Recurrence is common and is treated with the same agent (or vancomycin if severe), or fidaxomicin (expensive). Multiple recurrences are treated with long-term vancomycin (4–6 weeks), fidaxomicin, or fecal microbiota transplant (selected centers).

Urinary tract infection

Treatment of a urinary tract infection (UTI) depends on severity and other risk factors (e.g., male sex, catheterization, recurrences). Uncomplicated infections are most commonly caused by *Escherichia coli*. Uncomplicated cystitis can be treated with nitrofurantoin for 5 days or TMP–SMX for 3 days. Alternatives include (1) a quinolone for 3 days, or (2) the somewhat less effective options of fosfomycin × 1 day or various β-lactams with activity against *E. coli* for 3–7 days. Outpatient pyelonephritis is treated with a quinolone for 7 days or TMP–SMX for 14 days. Patients hospitalized because of their UTI require a quinolone, an antipseudomonal β-lactam, or both depending on risk factors. Aminoglycosides are added in some cases but carry a risk of nephrotoxicity.

Endocarditis

Streptococcus viridans, staphylococci, and enterococci are the most common pathogens with definitive treatment determined by the organism isolated from blood cultures. Susceptible streptococci can be treated with penicillin G or ceftriaxone for 2–4 weeks. Vancomycin is an alternative for β-lactam allergy for all Gram-positive bacteria. Some general concepts for treating more difficult cases are that (1) staphylococci require 6 weeks of therapy, perhaps with a short course of aminoglycosides for 3–5 days; (2) enterococci require 4–6 weeks of therapy; and (3) prosthetic valve endocarditis requires combination therapy with an aminoglycoside and perhaps rifampin added to the regimen for 2–6 weeks.

Meningitis

Drug selection depends on patient age and other factors. The most common organisms are pneumococcus and *Neisseria meningitides* (meningococcus). *H. influenzae* is less common because of vaccination. Empiric therapy is ceftriaxone plus vancomycin for children greater than 3 months old and adults. Ampicillin is added for *Listeria* coverage in adults greater than 60 years old. Infants less than 3 months old receive ampicillin plus either cefotaxime or an aminoglycoside. Surgical, shunt, or post-traumatic infections involve MRSA coverage (e.g., vancomycin) plus an antipseudomonal β-lactam. Dexamethasone may be started immediately before antibiotics and continued for 2–4 days. Definitive therapy can be narrowed per the CSF fluid culture results.

Surgical prophylaxis

Antibiotic dosing should start within 60 minutes of incision (120 minutes for quinolones and vancomycin). Drugs should be redosed every 2 half-lives during surgery (e.g., every 4 hours for cefazolin). Duration of prophylaxis should not exceed 24 hours except in selected cases. For most procedures, cefazolin is the drug of choice with clindamycin or vancomycin as alternatives for β-lactam allergy. When extra anaerobic coverage is needed (e.g., colorectal surgery), metronidazole can be added or a β-lactam with coverage against *Bacteroides fragilis* can be used (e.g., cefotetan, ertapenem).

Sepsis management

The Surviving Sepsis Guidelines provide detail on sepsis management. A key concept is to use rapid, aggressive crystalloid (e.g., normal saline, lactated Ringer's) fluid resuscitation to maintain MAP (mean arterial pressure) greater than 65 mmHg and normalize hyperlactatemia. Albumin can be used in patients with high fluid requirements. Other colloids (e.g., hetastarch products) are not recommended. For persistent shock, norepinephrine infusion is the vasopressor of choice, with the addition of vasopressin or another catecholamine based on hemodynamic needs. Last, low-dose corticosteroid therapy can be considered for patients failing vasopressors.

Fungal infections

The Infectious Diseases Society of America provides several guidelines on fungal infections. Less serious infections such as *Candida* vaginitis can be treated topically or with short courses of fluconazole. Treatment of invasive infections depends on a number factors including immune system status, site of infection, and expected pathogens. Fluconazole-sensitive *Candida* species (e.g., *C. albicans, C. tropicalis, C. parapsilosis*) can be treated with that agent. Fluconazole-resistant *Candida* species (e.g., *C. glabrata, C. krusei*) are treated with echinocandins (e.g., caspofungin), amphotericin B products, or newer azoles (e.g., voriconazole). The drug of choice for aspergillus is voriconazole. Endemic, soil-based organisms (e.g., *Histoplasma, Blastomyces, Coccidioides*) or *Cryptococcus* are treated with fluconazole or itraconazole for milder infections and amphotericin B (+/–flucytosine) for more serious infections. *Mucorales* (*Zygomycetes, Rhizopus*) are treated with amphotericin B products or the new azole, isavuconazole (Cresemba).

Notable adverse effects

Essentially all antibiotics have the potential to cause GI upset and increased risk for CDAD. β-lactams have a generally good risk profile, but all agents have the potential to cause seizures (worse with imipenem) or liver or renal dysfunction, and allergies are commonly reported. Quinolones can cause tendon rupture, peripheral neuropathies, QT-interval prolongation, and dysglycemia. Aminoglycosides and vancomycin can be nephrotoxic. Linezolid can cause anemias (particularly thrombocytopenia) and neuropathies and should not be given with serotonergic drugs. Daptomycin can cause myopathies. TMP–SMX can cause mild to severe skin reactions (e.g., Stevens–Johnson syndrome [SJS], toxic epidermal necrolysis [TEN]), anemias, and hyperkalemia. Among the antifungals, amphotericin products can cause nephrotoxicity, infusion reactions, and electrolyte disturbances. Lipid-based products are better tolerated.

Key points regarding diagnostic tests

- *White blood cell count* is a nonspecific indicator of infection if elevated (or rarely below normal).
- *Serum creatinine* can be used to estimate the renal function via equations (e.g., Cockcroft-Gault, several others). It is critical for optimal dosing of renally cleared antimicrobials.

Renal Function

Attention to renal function is critical to avoid toxicity with renally eliminated drugs. In addition, a number of drugs are potentially nephrotoxic including aminoglycoside antibiotics, vancomycin, amphotericin B,

IV contrast dye, NSAIDs, ACEIs and ARBs, β-lactams (notably piperacillin–tazobactam), and loop diuretics. Clinicians should also be mindful to search for appropriate drug dosing for patients on renal replacement therapy and be aware that dosing can be different for various modalities (e.g., intermittent hemodialysis versus continuous renal replacement therapy [CRRT]). Note that there are several modes of CRRT and that dosing recommendations can vary among them. Some general management issues in acute and chronic renal failure include controlling volume status with diuretics, controlling electrolyte abnormalities (e.g., hyperphosphatemia, hyperkalemia), and avoiding nephrotoxins when possible.

29-7 Narrow Therapeutic Index Drugs

Narrow therapeutic index drugs have a relatively small span of levels in the body that range from subtherapeutic (i.e., ineffective) to supratherapeutic (i.e., a large increase in adverse effects). Some of the most common drugs with a narrow therapeutic index are renally cleared; thus, monitoring renal function (serum creatinine) and adjusting doses when appropriate to avoid accumulation and adverse effects are important. In addition, serum creatinine should be monitored for some agents because they cause nephrotoxicity. A number of agents can cause anemias, which is monitored via the complete blood count (CBC). Some agents cause liver damage, which necessitates monitoring liver function tests (LFTs). Some of the most common drugs are as follows:

- ***Phenytoin:*** Monitor serum drug concentrations and serum albumin (to properly assess levels in hypoalbuminemia). Alternatively, monitor free concentrations if available. Monitor CBC and LFTs. Other toxicities include CNS changes (ataxia, nystagmus, seizures), as well as rashes that can be severe (e.g., SJS, TEN).
- ***Carbamazepine:*** Monitor serum drug concentrations, CBC, LFTs, and sodium (can cause hyponatremia). Rashes similar to those with phenytoin can result.
- ***Warfarin:*** Monitor INR at least monthly (more often when starting or titrating dose). Monitor hematocrit and clinical signs and symptoms for bleeding. Many drug interactions can affect warfarin metabolism and subsequently the INR (e.g., TMP–SMX, amiodarone), or they can directly increase the risk of bleeding (e.g., antiplatelet agents).
- ***Digoxin:*** Monitor serum drug concentrations, creatinine, potassium, magnesium, and calcium; perform periodic ECG for arrhythmias.
- ***Aminoglycosides:*** Monitor serum drug concentrations, creatinine (renally cleared and nephrotoxic), potassium, magnesium, and urine output; monitor hearing if warranted.
- ***Thyroid supplements (e.g., levothyroxine):*** Monitor TSH and other thyroid levels if appropriate.
- ***Immunosuppressants (e.g., cyclosporine, tacrolimus):*** Monitor serum drug concentrations, creatinine (some are renally cleared; some nephrotoxic), and CBC.
- ***Theophylline:*** Monitor serum drug concentrations. Adverse effects include CNS excitation and tachycardia or arrhythmias.
- ***Lithium:*** Monitor serum drug concentrations, creatinine, sodium, CBC, and TSH.

29-8 Dietary Drug Therapies

Fat-Soluble Vitamins

Vitamin A

Vitamin A describes a group of compounds including retinol and beta-carotene that affect growth and development and the visual and immune systems. Deficiency can cause night blindness. Toxicity can cause various GI, liver, CNS, and dermatologic effects including orange skin discoloration.

Vitamin D

Vitamin D describes a group of compounds (D_2 is ergocalciferol, D_3 is cholecalciferol) that affects bone development and calcium homeostasis. Deficiency can cause bone-related diseases. Its primary use is for preventing fractures in selected patients.

Vitamin E

Vitamin E describes a group of compounds including tocopherols that have a number of effects, including acting as antioxidants. Deficiency can cause neuromuscular impairments among other effects. Toxicity can cause bleeding by interfering with vitamin K and platelet function.

Vitamin K (phytonadione)

Vitamin K is an important cofactor in the production of clotting factors II, VII, IX, and X. Vitamin K is found in high amounts in green, leafy vegetables and can antagonize the effect of warfarin. In selected situations, it can be administered to counteract the effect of warfarin.

Water-Soluble Vitamins

Note: Unless noted, toxicity is rare from water-soluble vitamins because they are not stored in large amounts in the body and they can be rapidly cleared by the kidneys.

Vitamin B_1 (thiamine)

Vitamin B_1 is important in carbohydrate metabolism and neurologic function. Common causes of deficiency include alcoholism, malabsorptive states, and poor diet. Deficiency can cause a number of cardiac and neuromuscular effects, including death from Wernicke–Korsakoff syndrome in patients with alcoholism. Thiamine is often administered to such patients to prevent that syndrome.

Vitamin B_6 (pyridoxine)

Vitamin B_6 is a cofactor for many enzymes and is used in heme production. Deficiency may result from alcoholism, malabsorptive states, medications (e.g., isoniazid, hydralazine), or genetic disorders. Effects of deficiency can include neuropathies, dermatitis, oral lesions, and anemia. Pyridoxine is given with isoniazid to avoid neuropathies.

Vitamin B_{12} (cyanocobalamin)

Vitamin B_{12} is important for red blood cell development and neurologic function.

Deficiency may be caused by malabsorptive states, strict vegetarian diets, or increased gastric pH (e.g., H2RAs, PPIs). Deficiency causes pernicious anemia, which is treated with oral supplements or, in severe cases, IM injections.

Vitamin C (ascorbic acid)

Vitamin C is an antioxidant and is involved in tissue repair and immune function. Deficiency (scurvy) is very rare but may include bleeding gums and impaired wound healing. High doses are taken by some patients to prevent or treat the common cold, but this is not supported by data and may cause kidney stones.

Folic acid (folate)

Folic acid is important for normal cellular development including DNA (deoxyribonucleic acid) and RNA (ribonucleic acid) synthesis. Most notably, folate deficiency can cause neural tube defects in children. As such, folate is added to some foods. Deficiency may be due to vitamin B_{12} deficiency, alcoholism, malabsorptive states, malnutrition, hepatic disease, or drugs that inhibit folate metabolism (e.g., TMP–SMX, phenytoin). Symptoms include macrocytic anemia and are similar to vitamin B_{12} deficiency.

Niacin (nicotinic acid)

Niacin is important in cellular metabolism. Deficiency is rare and occurs primarily in individuals with alcoholism, malnourished elderly adults, and people with unusual diets. Deficiency may result in pellagra, characterized by dermatitis, diarrhea, dementia, and neuropathies. Niacin has been used to treat hyperlipidemia, but it has fallen out of favor because of adverse effects (e.g., flushing) and a lack of long-term benefits.

Electrolytes

Calcium

Calcium is the primary mineral in bone and is important for the cardiac and neuromuscular systems. Causes of deficiency include malabsorptive states, malnutrition, hypoparathyroidism, and renal failure. Supplementation is recommended in some patient groups to prevent osteoporosis. Calcium supplements are available in several forms. The carbonate form is widely used, but absorption may be impaired with PPI use. Constipation is a common adverse effect. Toxicity can result in kidney stones, GI distress, and arrhythmias.

Iron

Iron is an important component of hemoglobin. Deficiency most commonly causes microcytic anemia and fatigue. Deficiency may be caused by malnutrition, malabsorptive states, pregnancy or lactation, or bleeding (including heavy menstruation). Common adverse effects include nausea, abdominal pain, constipation, and dark stools. Enteric-coated and delayed-release products may cause fewer GI effects. Iron overdose is life threatening (particularly in children) and requires treatment in an emergency department.

Magnesium

Magnesium is needed for proper bone formation and neurologic and cardiac function. Deficiency may be due to malabsorptive states, malnutrition, alcoholism, excessive vomiting or diarrhea, and medications (e.g., diuretics, amphotericin B). Hypomagnesemia may result in hypokalemia, hypocalcemia, muscle weakness, and CNS changes. Oral magnesium supplements can cause diarrhea, and doses should be reduced in renal dysfunction. Hypermagnesemia can cause muscle weakness and arrhythmias.

29-9 Questions

1. Which of the following blood tests is most appropriate to monitor when patients receive medications known to cause hepatic injury?

A. Hematocrit
B. AST and ALT
C. Creatinine
D. INR

2. Which of the following commonly used analgesia agents has the highest risk of causing liver toxicity?

A. Acetaminophen
B. Aspirin
C. Ibuprofen
D. Naproxen

3. Which of the following analgesia agents is most appropriate for treating neuropathic pain?

A. Morphine
B. Pregabalin
C. Celecoxib
D. Fentanyl

4. Which of the following agents is most appropriate to treat hypertension and also prevent renal dysfunction (i.e., provide renal protection) in patients with diabetes?

A. Hydrochlorothiazide
B. Metoprolol
C. Lisinopril
D. Amlodipine

5. Which of the following agents is most appropriate to treat hypertension and also provide heart rate control in a patient with atrial fibrillation?

A. Spironolactone
B. Amlodipine
C. Valsartan
D. Atenolol

6. Which of the following is most commonly a first-line agent for treating congestive heart failure?

A. Hydralazine
B. Digoxin
C. Diltiazem
D. Carvedilol

7. Which of the following agents is the most appropriate first-line option for treating hyperlipidemia in most cases?

A. Atorvastatin
B. Niacin
C. Ezetimibe
D. Fenofibrate

8. A patient's asthma is not well controlled with inhaled albuterol prn. Which of the following is the most appropriate escalation in therapy at this time?

A. Change inhaled albuterol to scheduled dosing every 6 hours.
B. Add a low-dose inhaled corticosteroid.
C. Add a long-acting inhaled β_2-agonist.
D. Add an oral corticosteroid.

9. Which of the following is the most appropriate initial therapy for a patient with chronic obstructive pulmonary disease in addition to a prn short-acting inhaled β_2-agonist?

A. Inhaled corticosteroid
B. Theophylline
C. Long-acting inhaled anticholinergic
D. Short-acting inhaled anticholinergic

10. A patient with a cold wants a recommendation for an OTC drug to relieve her coughing so she can sleep at night. Which of the following is most appropriate?

A. Nasal corticosteroid
B. Loratadine
C. Pseudoephedrine
D. Dextromethorphan

11. A patient is interested in an OTC nasal corticosteroid spray for her seasonal allergies. Which of the following is an important counseling point regarding the drawbacks of this medication?

A. It can cause sedation.
B. It can cause anticholinergic effects such as dry mouth.
C. It can be used for a maximum of 72 hours only.
D. Effects will not occur immediately.

12. Which of the following is generally the most appropriate agent to treat mild diarrhea in most situations?

A. Bismuth subsalicylate
B. Diphenoxylate–atropine
C. Loperamide
D. Psyllium

13. Which of the following is the most appropriate first-line drug therapy for type 2 diabetes in most patients?

A. Insulin
B. Metformin
C. Glyburide
D. Pioglitazone

14. Which of the following tests is best for assessing overall glycemic control over the past several months in patients with diabetes?

A. Hemoglobin A1c test
B. Hematocrit and hemoglobin
C. Serum creatinine
D. AST and ALT

15. A health care provider determines that an adult patient with sinusitis needs antibiotics. The patient has no drug allergies or comorbidities. Which of the following is the most appropriate treatment?

A. Azithromycin
B. Amoxicillin
C. Cephalexin
D. Clindamycin

16. An adult patient presents to your clinic with community-acquired pneumonia. She does not require hospital admission and has no drug allergies or significant comorbidities. Which of the following is the most appropriate treatment?

A. Amoxicillin
B. Clindamycin
C. Doxycycline
D. Levofloxacin

17. Which of the following is the most appropriate treatment for a severe case of *Clostridium difficile*–associated diarrhea in a hospitalized patient?

A. Oral metronidazole
B. IV metronidazole
C. Oral vancomycin
D. IV vancomycin

18. Which of the following vitamins is found in green, leafy vegetables and can counteract the effect of warfarin?

A. Vitamin A
B. Vitamin D
C. Vitamin E
D. Vitamin K

19. Which of the following vitamins should be given to prevent Wernicke–Korsakoff syndrome in patients with alcoholism?

A. Thiamine
B. Niacin
C. Pyridoxine
D. Folic acid

20. Which of the following drugs with a narrow therapeutic index is most likely to cause severe rashes and CNS changes?

A. Aminoglycoside antibiotics
B. Digoxin
C. Phenytoin
D. Warfarin

29-10 Answers

1. B. AST and ALT are common markers of drug-induced hepatocellular damage. Hematocrit is used to assess bleeding and anemias. Creatinine is used to assess renal function. INR is used to assess blood coagulation and can be increased in liver failure, but it is less commonly used for monitoring drug-induced hepatocellular damage.

2. A. Acetaminophen is a common hepatotoxic drug when taken at high doses (greater than 4,000 mg/day). Aspirin, ibuprofen, and naproxen are proper NSAID drugs whose common adverse effects include GI bleeding and renal dysfunction.

3. B. Pregabalin is one of the primary drugs used for neuropathic pain. Morphine and fentanyl are opiates used for other types of acute and chronic pain (e.g., somatic, visceral, musculoskeletal). Celecoxib is an NSAID agent used for inflammatory and musculoskeletal pain.

4. C. Lisinopril is an ACEI. ACEIs and ARBs treat hypertension and provide renal protection in patients with diabetes. Hydrochlorothiazide (diuretic), metoprolol (β-blocker), and amlodipine (CCB) are also antihypertensive agents, but they do not provide additional renal protection in patients with diabetes.

5. D. Atenolol is a β-blocker agent that provides heart rate control (i.e., lowers heart rate) in addition to blood pressure control. Spironolactone is a diuretic primarily used in CHF but can be used for hypertension. It does not control heart rate. Amlodipine (CCB) and valsartan (ARB) are antihypertensive agents but neither provides heart rate control.

6. D. Carvedilol is a β- and alpha-blocking agent commonly used for CHF. Hydralazine can be used in CHF (especially in African American patients) but is not a first-line agent. Similarly, digoxin can be used in CHF but is not a first-line agent. Diltiazem is not used in CHF because of negative inotropic effects.

7. A. Atorvastatin or other statin drugs have become the dominant first-line agents for hyperlipidemia. Niacin and fenofibrate have fallen out of favor in most cases because of adverse effects and a lack of long-term benefits. Ezetimibe is a second-line agent that is either added to statin therapy or added as an alternative to statins in patients who cannot tolerate those drugs.

8. **B.** In the standard stepwise approach to asthma treatment, the recommended treatment in patients not controlled with a prn SABA is to add a low-dose ICS. Scheduled albuterol is not generally recommended. Adding a LABA or an oral corticosteroid are recommended in various later steps after adding an ICS.

9. **C.** A long-acting anticholinergic (or a LABA) should be started with a prn SABA. Short-acting anticholinergics have been replaced by long-acting agents. Theophylline and ICS are reserved for more refractory patients.

10. **D.** Dextromethorphan is the only cough suppressant available OTC. Loratadine is a nonsedating antihistamine that could help with cough in selected patients with cough caused by allergies, but not with a cough caused by a cold. Pseudoephedrine and nasal corticosteroids are decongestants and would not be expected to relieve coughing.

11. **D.** A primary drawback of nasal corticosteroids is that they have a long onset of action (from days to weeks). Patients may get frustrated if they expect an immediate effect. They do not cause sedation or anticholinergic effects like first-generation antihistamines. The 72-hour limitation on therapy is for direct nasal decongestants such as oxymetazoline.

12. **C.** Loperamide has become the primary first agent for diarrhea in most cases. It is available over the counter, highly effective, and well tolerated. Bismuth subsalicylate is preferred only when diarrhea is caused by a bacterial infection. Diphenoxylate–atropine is not available over the counter, and psyllium is a secondary option.

13. **B.** Metformin is widely recognized as the first-line treatment for type 2 diabetes. Insulin, glyburide, and pioglitazone are some of the many options that can be added to metformin on the basis of a number of patient factors.

14. **A.** Hemoglobin A1c measures average glucose control over the past several months and is the long-term glucose management marker in diabetes. Hematocrit and hemoglobin assess anemias and bleeding. Serum creatinine assesses renal function, and AST and ALT assess liver function.

15. **B.** Amoxicillin (with or without clavulanate) is a first-line option for adults with sinusitis who require antibiotics. Doxycycline is also acceptable and would be used if a β-lactam could not be used (i.e., penicillin allergy). Azithromycin, cephalexin, and clindamycin are used in pharyngitis but are not first-line choices for sinusitis.

16. **C.** Doxycycline is a first-line agent for treating outpatient CAP in adults without comorbidities. Azithromycin or clarithromycin would also be acceptable. Neither amoxicillin nor clindamycin has a broad enough spectrum for empiric CAP treatment. Levofloxacin is reserved for patients with comorbidities or other special situations (e.g., relapses, resistant pneumococcus).

17. **C.** The therapy of choice for severe CDAD is po vancomycin. IV vancomycin is not used in CDAD because it does not generate significant vancomycin levels in the lumen of the GI tract. IV or po metronidazole is used for nonsevere cases of CDAD.

18. **D.** Vitamin K is found in green, leafy vegetables and can counteract warfarin. Warfarin inhibits the vitamin K–dependent clotting factors, so providing more vitamin K counters that effect. Vitamins A, D, and E are the other fat-soluble vitamins, but they do not interact with warfarin as does vitamin K.

19. **A.** Thiamine (vitamin B_1) is given to prevent Wernicke–Korsakoff syndrome in patients with a history of alcohol abuse. Niacin and folic-acid deficiency can occur in patients with alcohol abuse, but they are not routinely supplemented unless there are signs of deficiency (e.g., pellagra, macrocytic anemia). Pyridoxine is used to prevent isoniazid-induced neuropathies.

20. **C.** Phenytoin can cause a number of adverse effects including skin rashes (sometimes severe) and CNS changes when serum levels are supratherapeutic. The primary adverse effect for aminoglycosides is nephrotoxicity, and for warfarin, it is bleeding. Digoxin toxicity can cause CNS changes but more commonly causes arrhythmias; it does not cause severe rashes.

29-11 Additional Resources

AHRQ National Guideline Clearinghouse Web site. https://guidelines.gov. Accessed December 17, 2017.

Chisholm-Burns MA, Schwinghammer TL, Wells BG, et al., eds. *Pharmacotherapy Principles and Practice.* 4th ed. New York, NY: McGraw-Hill Education; 2016.

DiPiro JT, Talbert RL, Yee GC, et al., eds. *Pharmacotherapy: A Pathophysiologic Approach.* 10th ed. New York, NY: McGraw-Hill Education; 2017.

Krinsky DL, Ferrari SP, Hemstreet BA, et al., eds. *Handbook of Nonprescription Drugs.* 19th ed. Washington, DC: American Pharmacists Association; 2017.

Lee M, ed. *Basic Skills in Interpreting Laboratory Data.* 6th ed. Washington, DC: American Society of Health-Systems Pharmacists; 2017.

O'Connell MB, Korner EJ, Rickles NM, Sias JJ. Cultural competence in health care and its implications for pharmacy: part 2—overview of key concepts in multicultural health care. *Pharmacotherapy.* 2007;27(7):1062–1079.

O'Connell MB, Rickles NM, Sias JJ, Korner EJ. Cultural competency in health care and its implications for pharmacy: part 2—emphasis on pharmacy systems and practice. *Pharmacotherapy.* 2009;29(2):14e–34e.

Pharmacists' Patient Care Process. The Joint Commission of Pharmacy Practitioners' Web site. Available at: https://jcpp.net/patient-care-process/. Accessed December 17, 2017.

Toxicology

30

PETER A. CHYKA

30-1 KEY POINTS

- Medications are the most common cause of poisoning morbidity and mortality. Any chemical can become toxic if too much is taken in relation to body weight and physiologic capacity.
- Immediate first aid for a poison exposure can minimize potential toxic effects and involves water and fresh air, depending on the route of exposure. Contact a poison control center immediately through the nationwide access number (1-800-222-1222) to determine whether first aid should be administered or whether a poisoning emergency exists.
- Hospital-based therapies include supportive and symptomatic care, single or multiple doses of activated charcoal (to reduce absorption or to enhance systemic elimination, respectively), whole bowel irrigation (to evacuate the intestinal tract), hemodialysis (to enhance systemic elimination), and use of antidotes (to antagonize or reverse toxic effects).
- Few antidotes are available relative to the large number of potential poisons. The use of an antidote is usually an adjunct to conventional and supportive therapies. Commonly used antidotes include activated charcoal, acetylcysteine, atropine, pralidoxime, digoxin immune Fab, and naloxone.
- Substance abuse often leads to acute and chronic toxicity from a variety of medications, commercial products, and illicit agents. The management of acute toxicity from substance abuse typically follows the same general approaches as those for poisoning and overdose. Chronic abuse can lead to dependence, tolerance, withdrawal, and addiction.
- Substance use disorder is a disease that typically starts with drug experimentation and escalates to maladaptive patterns of substance use to produce physiologic, behavioral, and mental changes.
- A comprehensive treatment plan for substance use disorder involves a variety of approaches including medication-assisted therapy with long-term use of drug-substitution, drug-aversion, and drug-antagonist therapy.
- Pharmacists need to have an awareness of the potential for terrorism, an appreciation for epidemiologic clues of a chemical or biological terrorism event, and a basic understanding of the classes of agents that can be weaponized and their effects.

30-2 STUDY GUIDE CHECKLIST

The following topics may guide your study of this subject area:

- ☐ Basic first-aid and general treatment measures for a poison exposure
- ☐ Poison prevention measures for patient counseling
- ☐ Matching of antidotes for poisonings or the medication-assisted therapy for substance abuse with the offending agent
- ☐ The mechanism of action of common antidotes for poisonings and medication-assisted therapy for substance abuse
- ☐ The route of administration of common antidotes for poisonings and medication-assisted therapy for substance abuse
- ☐ Approaches to reducing drug-related overdose deaths
- ☐ General categories of potential chemical and biological terrorist threats

30-3 Overview of Poisoning and Toxicology

Poisoning in America

Poison exposures and drug overdoses affect more than 2.2 million people annually, resulting in 68,995 deaths in 2016. Of those, 63,632 (92%) were related to drugs. A large number of poisonings occur in young children, but most fatalities occur in adults (less than 1% of deaths are in preschool-age children). Most poisonings in preschool-age children are unintentional or accidental. Unintentional poisonings can also occur in adolescents and adults. Intentional (suicide and drug abuse) poisonings and overdoses are common (Box 30-1). Since 2008, poisoning has become the leading cause of injury-related death in the United States. Medications are the most common cause of poisoning morbidity and mortality.

Any chemical can become toxic if the exposure is too great in relation to body weight and physiologic capacity. In general, toxicity occurs when too much of a substance is taken in relation to a normally tolerable dose. Different mechanisms by which a chemical can produce toxicity include the following:

- Exaggeration of pharmacologic effects
- Formation of reactive toxic metabolites
- Formation of intracellular free radicals
- Interference with enzyme action
- Interference with DNA (deoxyribonucleic acid) or RNA (ribonucleic acid) synthesis
- Inactivation of biochemical cofactors
- Initiation of premature cell aging (apoptosis)
- Tissue destruction on contact

Toxicology is the study of the adverse effects of chemicals and other xenobiotics (substances that are foreign to the body) on living organisms. Toxicology has several specialized areas, including basic science and clinical, analytical, forensic, regulatory, and occupational settings, that have a unique focus and purpose. Toxicology studies are part of preclinical drug development to assess several toxic risks (see Chapter 7, Section 7).

30-4 Acute and Chronic Toxic Effects

Acute Toxicity

Acute toxicity typically occurs within minutes to hours of a single exposure episode of a toxin. Typically, unintentional poisonings in children and intentional drug overdoses in adolescents or adults (suicide attempts or drug abuse) are acute episodes.

BOX 30-1. Common Circumstances of Poison Exposures

Unintentional

- General "accident"
- Misuse (error in use)
- Venomous bite or sting
- Environmental
- Occupational
- Food poisoning
- Adverse reaction

Intentional

- Suicide
- Misuse (disregard directions)
- Substance abuse
- Abuse of others
- Homicide
- Product tampering

Unknown

Chronic Toxicity

Chronic toxicity typically occurs from multiple or long-term exposure to toxins. The amount may not be toxic with an acute exposure, but the chronic exposure may lead to accumulation or toxin-induced conditions that decrease elimination. Exposures in the occupational setting, from environmental contamination, or from long-term substance abuse can lead to chronic toxicity.

Substance Abuse

Substance abuse can produce acute and chronic toxicity. In acute conditions, management of substance abuse cases generally follows the same guidelines as management of poisonings and overdoses. Chronic abuse can foster dependence, which often leads to withdrawal symptoms on stopping use and the need for detoxification programs, long-term behavioral counseling, and drugs to produce aversion to or substitution for drug-taking behaviors.

30-5 Poison Prevention Approaches and Pharmacy

Poison Prevention Packaging Act of 1970: Safety Caps

The Poison Prevention Packaging Act of 1970 was enacted to prevent preschool-age children from opening packaging and ingesting harmful substances or to delay the opening of packaging containing such substances (to limit the amount of harmful substance that may be ingested within a reasonable amount of time).

Drugs requiring safety caps include aspirin, ibuprofen, acetaminophen, and all oral prescription drugs with certain exceptions (e.g., birth control pills and nitroglycerin).

Use of poison control centers

A poison control center determines if a true poisoning exists, recommends first aid, refers poisoning victims to health care facilities for further evaluation and treatment, monitors the progress and outcome of each poisoning case, and documents poisoning experiences. Programs and materials on poison prevention are also available.

Nationwide access is available by calling 1-800-222-1222 for 24-hour poison control center services for the area from which the call is placed in the United States. Calls are accepted from any person, typically the general public and health care professionals, 24 hours a day every day of the year.

Poison prevention tips for consumers include the following:

- Store all drugs and chemicals out of the reach of children.
- Never put chemicals in food containers.
- Choose products with safety caps when there is a choice, and use them properly.
- Read and follow all label directions carefully.
- Never call medication "candy."
- Use safety latches for cabinets where medications or chemicals are stored.

30-6 General Treatment of Poisonings

Emergency Actions

First aid for poisoning emergencies should be administered, if applicable. Table 30-1 describes first-aid techniques.

TABLE 30-1. First Aid for Poisoning Emergencies

Type of emergency	First-aid response
Inhaled poison	Immediately get the person to fresh air. Avoid breathing fumes. Open doors and windows wide.
Poison on the skin	Remove any contaminated clothing. Flood skin with water for at least 15 minutes.
Poison in the eye	Remove contact lenses. Flood the eye with water, pouring it from a large glass 2–3 inches from the eye. Repeat for a total of 15–30 minutes. Do not force the eyelid open.
Swallowed poison	Unless the victim is unconscious, is having convulsions, or cannot swallow, give a small glassful (2–4 oz) of water immediately. Call a poison control center for advice about whether other actions are needed.

Other considerations include the following:

- Avoid wasting time looking for an antidote at home.
- Do not use home remedies such as saltwater, mustard powder, raw eggs, hydrogen peroxide, cooking grease, or gagging.
- Immediately call 911 or an ambulance if the person is not breathing, has had a seizure, or is unresponsive.
- For other situations, contact a poison control center immediately to determine whether first aid should be used or whether a poisoning emergency exists.

Decontamination of the Gastrointestinal Tract

During the past three decades, the practice of using drugs to decrease the absorption of other drugs from the gastrointestinal tract has declined in the United States. Current recommendations, as well as basic information about the drugs and procedures used to decontaminate the gastrointestinal tract, are described in this section.

Current recommendations

Ipecac syrup (an emetic) has questionable effectiveness, and its use is generally avoided.

Gastric lavage involves placing a tube into the stomach through a nostril or the mouth and repetitively washing out the stomach contents with water or a saline solution. This method of gastric decontamination is of questionable effectiveness, particularly if it is performed more than 1 hour after ingestion of the toxin.

Cathartics such as magnesium citrate are no longer routinely used.

Activated charcoal given orally is often the only treatment necessary if the toxin is adsorbed to it. The activated charcoal is most effective when used within 1–2 hours of ingestion of the toxin.

Whole bowel irrigation with aqueous solutions of polyethylene glycol and electrolytes can be considered if the toxin is poorly adsorbed to activated charcoal or slowly absorbed and its presence in the gastrointestinal tract is likely.

Activated charcoal

Indications and dosage

This drug adsorbs poisons in the gastrointestinal tract and reduces the extent of absorption. It is administered as a slurry by mouth in alert patients or through a lavage tube as a single dose:

- ***Children:*** 25–50 g
- ***Adults:*** 25–100 g

Contraindications

- Ingestion of aliphatic hydrocarbons and caustics
- Absence of patient's bowel sounds
- Ingestion of heavy metals (lithium, iron, or lead) or simple alcohols

Adverse effects

- ***Uncommon:*** Tracheal aspiration, pneumonitis
- ***Common:*** Emesis, soiling of clothes and furnishings
- ***Note:*** Saline cathartics were previously used with activated charcoal to decrease gastrointestinal transit time, but their efficacy is unproved. Cathartics may contribute to emesis following activated charcoal use. Fluid and electrolyte disturbances are possible with repeated doses of cathartics.

Advantages and disadvantages

- ***Advantages:*** Rapid onset of action, nonspecific action for a wide variety of chemicals, reasonable effectiveness within 1–2 hours of ingestion of the toxin; beneficial 4–8 hours after ingestion in some cases
- ***Disadvantages:*** Messy and difficult administration, possible removal of beneficial drugs together with the toxin

Whole bowel irrigation

Indications and technique

Whole bowel irrigation is generally used to wash out the gastrointestinal tract when use of charcoal may be inappropriate (e.g., if iron or lithium was ingested) and when the toxin is suspected to be present in the gastrointestinal tract (e.g., when drugs are sustained-release formulations or when the patient ingested illicit drugs packed in condoms). It is not routinely used to treat poisonings except in these unique circumstances.

Larger volumes of polyethylene glycol electrolyte solutions (e.g., CoLyte, GoLYTELY) are used than the amounts conventionally used for bowel preparation for colonoscopy. Administer by mouth or through a gastric or duodenal tube for the treatment of poisoning:

- ***Children:*** 25 mL/kg/h (approximately 500 mL/h) up to 2–5 L
- ***Adults:*** 2 L/h up to 5–10 L

Contraindications

- Ingestion of caustics or aliphatic hydrocarbons
- Patients with absent bowel sounds or gastrointestinal tract obstruction

Adverse effects

Few adverse effects have been reported, but limited results are available from which to draw conclusions. Nausea, vomiting, and abdominal cramping have been reported.

Advantages and disadvantages

- ***Advantages:*** Prompt whole bowel evacuation within 2–4 hours
- ***Disadvantages:*** Messy procedure because of rectal effluent

Other hospital-based therapies

These therapies include supportive and symptomatic care, multiple doses of activated charcoal (to enhance systemic elimination when appropriate), hemodialysis (to enhance systemic elimination when appropriate), and use of antidotes (to antagonize or reverse toxic effects when indicated).

30-7 Antidotes

An antidote counteracts or changes the nature of a poison. Few antidotes are available relative to the large number of potential poisons (Table 30-2). Antidotes have special characteristics compared to drugs used for other therapeutic uses, including the following:

Most antidotes are used only in life-threatening situations.

- Most therapy is single dose or short course (1–3 days).
- Most antidotes are administered parenterally.

TABLE 30-2. Commonly Used Antidotes in the United States

Antidote	Toxic substance	Route
Acetylcysteine	Acetaminophen	IV, oral
Activated charcoal	Nearly all organic chemicals	Oral
Atropine	Anticholinesterase agents	IV, IM
Crotalidae polyvalent immune Fab (ovine) (CroFab)	*Crotalidae* snake envenomation (rattlesnake, copperhead, cottonmouth)	IV
Deferoxamine	Iron	IV, IM
Digoxin immune Fab (DigiFab)	Digoxin	IV
Dimercaprol	Heavy metals	IM
Edetate calcium disodium	Lead	IV, IM
Ethanol	Ethylene glycol, methanol[a]	IV, oral
Flumazenil (Romazicon)	Benzodiazepines	IV, IM
Fomepizole (Antizol)	Ethylene glycol, methanol	IV
Glucagon (GlucaGen)	β-adrenergic blockers[a]	IV
Hydroxocobalamin (CyanoKit)	Cyanide	IV
Idarucizumab (Praxbind)	Dabigatran (Pradaxa)	IV
Insulin/dextrose	Calcium channel blockers, β-adrenergic blockers[a]	IV
Methylene blue	Methemoglobinemia-forming toxins	IV
Naloxone	Opioids	IV, IM, nasal
Octreotide (Sandostatin)	Oral sulfonylurea drugs[a]	IV
Oxygen	Carbon monoxide	Inhalation
Penicillamine	Heavy metal poisoning	Oral
Physostigmine	Anticholinergic toxins	IV, IM
Phytonadione (vitamin K_1)	Anticoagulants (warfarin)	IV
Pralidoxime	Anticholinesterase agents	IV, IM
Pyridoxine (vitamin B_6)	Isoniazid[a]	IV
Sodium bicarbonate	Tricyclic antidepressants[a,b]	IV
Sodium nitrite, sodium thiosulfate (Nithiodote)	Cyanide	IV
Succimer (Chemet)	Lead	Oral

IM, intramuscular; IV, intravenous.
a. "Off-label" use.
b. Includes overdoses of tricyclic antidepressants and other drugs that inhibit the myocardial sodium fast channel to cause widening of the QRS complex such as cocaine, antihistamines (diphenhydramine, chlorpheniramine), and class I antiarrhythmics (flecainide, procainamide, quinidine).

- Most antidotes have a rapid onset of action.
- Some antidotes are adaptations of "off-the-shelf" drugs with other indications, are not approved by the U.S. Food and Drug Administration (FDA) for the antidotal indication, and are considered to be acceptable practice as "off-label uses."
- Randomized controlled clinical trials are not possible because of ethical concerns regarding risks to human subjects.
- Clinical studies in poisoned patients are problematic because details of the toxin and exposure are often unverified or unknown.

The pharmacy and therapeutics committee of a hospital should regularly review the inventory of antidotes that are stocked at the hospital and ensure sufficient quantities are available when needed. Functional categories of antidote action (Box 30-2) are described with examples below.

Chemical Action

Antidotes that act chemically have a direct chemical reaction between an antidote and toxin to form a product that is less toxic and may be more rapidly excreted.

Adsorbents

Activated charcoal acts by nonspecific adsorption of many drugs and toxins by chemical binding to the inner and outer surfaces of the charcoal particle. It is administered orally as a single dose to prevent toxin absorption from the gastrointestinal tract. Some chemicals (e.g., iron, lithium, lead) are poorly adsorbed. Multiple doses of activated charcoal given over 24–48 hours can also enhance the systemic elimination of some toxins (e.g., phenobarbital, carbamazepine, theophylline, dapsone).

Chelating agents

Succimer (Chemet) is a chelating agent that is used in the treatment of poisoning from several heavy metals, principally lead. It is administered orally. Chelators form a coordinating compound to enhance the urinary excretion of lead and other heavy metals and thereby decrease the body burden and toxicity of the heavy metal. Other chelating agents include the following:

- Edetate calcium disodium (Calcium Disodium Versenate) intravenous (IV) or intramuscular (IM); chelates lead and other metals.
- Dimercaprol (British anti-Lewisite, BAL in Oil) IM only; chelates arsenic, gold, lead, mercury.
- Penicillamine (Cuprimine) oral; chelates copper, arsenic, and lead.
- Deferoxamine (Desferal) IV or IM; chelates iron.

BOX 30-2. Functional Categories of Antidote Actions[a]

Chemical action
- Adsorbents
- Chelating agents
- Antibodies
- Chemical group exchange

Formation of a detoxifying substance

Detoxification of enzymatic systems
- Action as co-substrates
- Prevention of toxic metabolite formation

Pharmacological action on receptors

Reaction with an enzyme-toxin complex

Reaction with a toxic metabolite

a. Several antidotes act by multiple or other mechanisms.

Drug-specific antibodies

Digoxin-specific Fab fragment antibodies (DigiFab) have a high binding affinity for digoxin and several other digoxin-like cardiac glycosides. The Fab fragment of IgG (immunoglobulin G) antibody is derived from sheep (ovine). The digoxin-Fab complex is no longer pharmacologically active and is excreted in urine. It is administered intravenously.

Other toxin-specific antibodies include Centruroides immune F(ab')$_2$ (equine) injection (Anascorp) for treatment of scorpion envenomation. Crotalidae polyvalent immune Fab ovine (CroFab) and Crotalidae immune F(ab')$_2$ equine (Anavip) are used for the treatment of envenomation from *Crotalidae* (also known as *Crotalinae*) species of North American snakes (rattlesnakes, cottonmouth, copperhead).

Chemical group exchange

Hydroxocobalamin (Cyanokit) is an antidote for cyanide poisoning. It rapidly exchanges its hydroxyl group with free cyanide to produce nontoxic, stable cyanocobalamin (vitamin B_{12}), which is eliminated in the urine. It is administered intravenously.

Formation of a Detoxifying Substance

These agents do not act chemically to bind a toxin, but instead produce a substance that binds the toxin.

Sodium nitrite is a cyanide antidote that oxidizes hemoglobin (Fe^{2+}) to methemoglobin (Fe^{3+}) to bind cyanide (CN^{3-}). With administration of thiosulfate, thiocyanate is formed and it is excreted in the urine. Both are administered intravenously (Nithiodote).

Detoxification of Enzymatic Systems

Several antidotes act as co-substrates or prevent formation of toxic metabolites. These drugs act on an enzyme(s) that can enhance detoxification by increasing activity or prevent toxin formation by inhibiting activity.

Sodium thiosulfate (administered after sodium nitrite) is a sulfur donor to rhodanase that promotes the conversion of cyanide to the less toxic thiocyanate, which is excreted in the urine. It is administered intravenously (Nithiodote).

Fomepizole (Antizol) is a competitive inhibitor of alcohol dehydrogenase, the first enzyme in the metabolism of ethanol and other alcohols. It prevents formation of the toxic metabolites of methanol or ethylene glycol. It is administered intravenously.

Ethanol is another antidote for methanol or ethylene glycol. It is a competitive substrate for alcohol dehydrogenase that preferentially metabolizes ethanol compared to methanol or ethylene glycol and thereby prevents formation of toxic metabolites. It can be administered intravenously or orally.

Pharmacological Action on Receptors

Several antidotes act on characterized receptors or other macromolecules. The interaction of the antidote with pharmacologic or physiologic receptors antagonizes the action of the toxin.

Naloxone is an opioid antagonist that competitively blocks principally mu-, kappa-, and delta-opioid receptors to reverse the life-threatening effects of opioid overdose. It is administered by IV or IM routes, IM autoinjector (Evzio), and nasal spray (Narcan Nasal Spray).

Atropine IV treats many of the life-threatening effects from cholinesterase inhibitors (anticholinesterase agents) after exposure to organophosphate insecticides, "nerve agent" chemical warfare agents, and carbamate insecticides. It competitively blocks the action of acetylcholine at muscarinic receptors and is administered intravenously.

Reaction with Enzyme-Toxin Complex

The interaction of the antidote and an enzyme-toxin complex forms a product that is less toxic and more excretable.

Pralidoxime (Protopam) treats poisonings from anticholinesterase insecticides and "nerve agent" chemical warfare agents. It reverses acetylcholinesterase inhibition by reactivating the phosphorylated acetylcholinesterase and protects the enzyme from further inhibition, thereby reducing cholinergic excess. The pralidoxime-anticholinesterase compound is excreted in the urine. It is administered intravenously and intramuscularly in conjunction with atropine therapy.

Reaction with Toxic Metabolite

The interaction of the antidote with a toxic metabolite prevents formation of a toxic metabolite or forms a product that is less toxic.

Acetylcysteine prevents and treats toxicity of acetaminophen overdose from supratherapeutic and acute overdose exposures. It principally serves as a sulfhydryl (-SH) surrogate for intracellular glutathione to rapidly bind and detoxify a highly reactive toxic intermediary metabolite of acetaminophen in liver cells. It is administered intravenously (Acetadote) or orally (Mucomyst).

30-8 Substance Abuse

During 2016, 44.6 million Americans 12 years of age and older (18% of the population) admitted in a national survey on drug use and health to use of an illicit drug in the past year. Within that group, 4.5 million adults (18 years of age and older) also reported having a co-occurring serious mental illness. In that same year, 20.1 million Americans (7.5% of the population) had a substance use disorder related to alcohol or illicit drug use. Substance abuse often leads to acute and chronic toxicity. Management of the acute condition generally follows the same guidelines as those for management of poisonings and overdoses as described earlier. A challenge in treating patients with an acute drug overdose is determining the possible substances taken and the possible adulterants or contaminants (e.g., talc, other drugs, illicitly manufactured substances, bacteria, viruses, fungi).

Nature of Substance Abuse

Substance use disorder is a maladaptive pattern of substance use leading to clinically significant impairment or distress within a 12-month period. It is a disease that typically starts with life-style choices that lead to physiologic, behavioral, and mental changes. The spectrum of substance use disorder generally follows an order of stages: initiation of substance misuse by experimentation, regular substance abuse, addiction, and recovery. The first three stages produce harmful health, behavioral, and societal effects with increasing intensity.

The following terms are related to substance abuse:

- ***Drug abuse:*** Use of a drug for a nontherapeutic effect to alter mood, emotion, or state of consciousness
- ***Addiction:*** A primary, chronic, neurobiological disease with genetic, psychosocial, and environmental factors influencing its development and manifestations; characterized by impaired control over substance use, compulsive use, craving, and continued use despite adverse social, psychological, and physical consequences
- ***Tolerance:*** The body's physical adaptation to a drug where greater amounts are required over time to achieve the initial desired effect or continued use of the same amount produces markedly diminished effect

- ***Dependence:*** A physical state that develops during regular drug use in which a withdrawal syndrome results upon drug cessation or tolerance
- ***Withdrawal:*** Unpleasant symptoms after abrupt cessation, rapid dose reduction, decreasing drug concentrations, or administration of an antagonist (also known as abstinence syndrome)
- ***Drug overdose:*** Intentional or unintentional acute consumption of an excessive (supratherapeutic) amount of a drug (similar to the definition of poisoning)
- ***Unintentional drug overdose death:*** One or more drugs taken or given without awareness of the potential risk of death

Treatment Options for Substance Use Disorders

The choice of treatment depends on the assessment, urgency, resources, substances abused, presence of co-occurring mental disorders, and a variety of other individual circumstances. A comprehensive treatment plan includes several of the following options:

- Screening, assessment, and diagnosis of substance use disorder
- Individual counseling and monitoring
- Acute detoxification, withdrawal, and stabilization
- Residential and outpatient rehabilitation programs
- Support groups and recovery programs
- Long-term drug-substitution, -aversion, and -antagonist therapy (medication-assisted therapy)

30-9 Selected Medication-Assisted Therapies for Substance Use Disorders

Medication-assisted therapy (MAT) for substance use disorder is generally indicated for patients who are motivated to adhere to a treatment plan and who have no contraindications to the drug therapy. It should be part of a comprehensive management program that includes psychosocial support. The phases of treatment typically include the following:

- The person has abstained from using the problem substance (e.g., 12 to 24 hours for many opioids) and is in the early stages of withdrawal (induction).
- The person has discontinued or greatly reduced misuse of the problem substance, no longer has cravings, and experiences few side effects so that the dose of the MAT drug can be adjusted (stabilization).
- The patient is doing well on a steady dose of the MAT drug (maintenance).

Buprenorphine

Buprenorphine is a partial opioid antagonist used to treat opioid dependence by lowering the potential for misuse and diminishing the effects of physical dependency to opioids, such as withdrawal symptoms and craving. Buprenorphine is indicated for treatment of opioid use disorder.

It is available in several forms such as sublingual (SL) tablets and buccal films without naloxone (Subutex and generic) and SL tablets and buccal films with naloxone (Suboxone, Zubsolv, Bunavail). It is also available as an intradermal implant (Probuphine). Buprenorphine is a schedule III (C-III) drug under the drug classification schedules of the Controlled Substances Act. Qualified prescribers trained and certified in its use can prescribe buprenorphine for office- or clinic-based treatment. It can be dispensed by any pharmacy. Probuphine is available only through a restricted program called the Probuphine REMS Program.

Methadone

Methadone is an opioid agonist that acts to detoxify and serve as a maintenance treatment of opioid addiction. By serving as an opioid substitute, methadone lessens the distressing symptoms of opioid withdrawal, blocks the euphoric effects of opioids, and allows patients to manage their addiction.

Methadone is available as a liquid, tablet, or wafer diskette. It is a schedule II (C-II) drug under the drug classification schedules of the Controlled Substances Act.

Methadone can be prescribed only by authorized physicians and dispensed through a federally certified opioid treatment program (methadone clinic).

Naltrexone

Naltrexone is an opioid receptor antagonist that blocks the actions of opioids and may reduce craving in patients with opioid use disorders who typically receive an extended-release injectable form. Its action for alcohol use disorder is not well understood, but it appears to reduce the rewarding, pleasurable effects of alcohol (reduces heavy drinking) and the craving for it (helps abstinence).

It is available as a tablet (ReVia, Depade) and in an IM injectable extended-release form (Vivitrol). It is not a controlled substance. Any licensed prescriber can prescribe naltrexone. The injectable form is administered by a health care provider and is available through specialty pharmacies.

Acamprosate

Acamprosate (Campral) is FDA approved for the treatment of alcohol use disorder. This drug is not covered by the Controlled Substances Act. Acamprosate's mechanism of action has not been clearly established, but it may restore the balance of neuronal excitation and inhibition compromised from chronic alcohol use by acting on the glutamate neurotransmitter system. Acamprosate is most effective for patients who are motivated to achieve complete abstinence from alcohol rather than decrease drinking.

It is available as a delayed-release tablet and can be prescribed by any licensed prescriber and dispensed by any pharmacy.

Disulfiram

Disulfiram (Antabuse) is FDA approved for the treatment of alcohol use disorder. This drug is not covered by the Controlled Substances Act. Disulfiram is an alcohol-aversive agent and causes acute, unpleasant to serious physical reactions when a patient drinks or applies alcohol. Disulfiram may not reduce the urge to drink alcohol, but the severe reaction after drinking alcohol may motivate patients to remain abstinent. The disulfiram-ethanol reaction increases serum acetaldehyde concentrations, a metabolite of ethanol, and causes the unpleasant symptoms. Disulfiram inhibits the action of aldehyde dehydrogenase on acetaldehyde in the liver and thereby increases acetaldehyde in the blood after consuming ethanol.

It is available as a tablet and can be prescribed by any licensed prescriber and dispensed by any pharmacy.

30-10 Reducing Drug-Related Overdose Deaths

In 2018, the United States is in the midst of a public health crisis of overdose deaths from prescription and illicit drugs. The number of drug-related deaths has risen every year since 1999. To reduce deaths from drug overdose, several approaches have been initiated that pharmacists should promote, incorporate in their practice, and include in patient counseling:

- Drug take-back, drop-box, and disposal programs (see Chapter 13, Section 13-8)
- Naloxone rescue by family, friends, active bystanders, emergency medical services, and police

- Co-prescriptions for naloxone when opioids are dispensed to patients at high risk for overdose
- Innovative drug products with deterrents to abuse
- Prescription drug monitoring programs (also known as controlled substances monitoring databases)
- Risk evaluation and mitigation strategies (see Chapter 13, Section 13-6)
- Diversion safeguards in health care facilities, warehouses, and shipments
- Improved health and behavioral care for substance use disorders, rehabilitation, and co-occurring mental illness

30-11 Terrorism and Disaster Preparedness

The world continues to face the threat of attacks with biological, chemical, explosive, and radiological weapons. Health care professionals should have an awareness of the potential for biological terrorism, an appreciation for epidemiologic clues of a chemical or biological terrorism event, and a basic understanding of the classes of agents that can be weaponized and their effects.

Biological Threats

Bioterrorism is the deliberate use of infectious biological agents to cause illness and is categorized for risk by the U.S. Centers for Disease Control and Prevention (CDC) as follows:

- *Category A* agents are high-priority agents that can be easily transmitted, can result in high mortality rates, and have the potential for major public health impact. They include smallpox, anthrax, plague, botulism, tularemia, and viral hemorrhagic fevers (filoviruses [e.g., Ebola, Marburg] and arenaviruses [e.g., Lassa, Machupo]).
- *Category B* agents include brucellosis; epsilon toxin of *Clostridium perfringens;* food safety threats (e.g., *Salmonella* species, *Escherichia coli* O157:H7, *Shigella*); glanders (*Burkholderia mallei*); melioidosis (*B. pseudomallei*); psittacosis (*Chlamydia psittaci*); Q fever (*Coxiella burnetii*); ricin; staphylococcal enterotoxin B; typhus fever; viral encephalitis (alphaviruses such as Venezuelan equine encephalitis, eastern equine encephalitis, and western equine encephalitis); and water safety threats (e.g., *Vibrio cholerae, Cryptosporidium parvum*).
- *Category C* agents include emerging infectious disease threats such as Nipah virus and hantavirus.

The mode of transmission for many biological agents is similar to that of other infectious diseases such as aerosol (most common form for biological weapons), dermal contact, injection, food, and water.

The management of exposures to biological agents involves the administration of specific antimicrobial agents or antitoxin and supportive and symptomatic care or, in some cases, only supportive and symptomatic care.

Chemical Threats

Toxic chemicals used in warfare and in a chemical terrorism attack typically act quickly and disable, maim, or kill people. The following chemicals have been used in warfare and in terrorist attacks:

- Nerve agents (e.g., anticholinesterase agents such as sarin)
- Blistering or vesicant agents (e.g., mustard agents, lewisites)
- Blood toxins (e.g., arsine, cyanide)
- Pulmonary system caustics (e.g., phosgene, chlorine, ammonia)
- Incapacitating agents (e.g., fast-acting and potent opioids, central nervous system depressants, hallucinogens)

- Riot control agents (e.g., lacrimating agents such as chloroacetophenone and vomiting agents such as adamsite)

Chemicals used for these purposes are liquids, gases, or solids. Often they are dispersed in the air as aerosols or delivered by bombs or missiles.

The management of exposures to chemical agents involves evacuation from the scene of the attack; use of specific antidotes; rapid decontamination of the skin; and supportive and symptomatic care; or, in some cases, only evacuation, decontamination, and supportive and symptomatic care.

Radiological Threats

Radiological weapons involve nuclear radiation or radioactive materials with various radionucleotides. Radionucleotides can produce topical and systemic effects that may be immediate or delayed, depending on the agent, route of exposure, and extent of exposure. Medical management of radiological emergencies is specific for the radionucleotide involved or suspected.

Emergency Preparedness

Pharmacists are in a unique position to quickly recognize communitywide patterns of symptoms, illness, and mortality in humans and animals that can be important clues to terrorist events.

The CDC advises that if citizens believe that they have been exposed to a biological or chemical agent, or if they believe an intentional biological threat will occur or is occurring, they should contact their local health or police department or another law enforcement agency (e.g., the Federal Bureau of Investigation). These agencies will notify the state health department and other response partners through a pre-established notification list that channels to the CDC.

The CDC maintains the Strategic National Stockpile (SNS) to ensure the availability and rapid deployment of life-saving pharmaceuticals, antidotes, and other medical supplies and equipment necessary to counter nerve agents, biological pathogens, and chemical agents. The SNS program stands ready for immediate deployment to any U.S. location in the event of a terrorist attack using a biological toxin or chemical agent directed against a civilian population. A limited stock of drugs to treat nerve agents (CHEMPACK) has been deployed to emergency medical services and hospital sites throughout the United States and is maintained by the CDC.

Pharmacists should consider volunteering in their communities to assist with emergency preparedness. Roles in mass dispensing and vaccination clinics, SNS deployment, and general disaster medical relief are possible opportunities. Contact the local health department or emergency medical services agency.

Essential steps to volunteering for emergency preparedness include reaching an understanding with one's family and employer, registering as a volunteer and identifying skills to contribute, obtaining security credentials, participating in training, and doing whatever it takes when needed.

30-12 Questions

1. Which of the following situations is an example of acute toxicity?

A. Abusing amphetamines during college years
B. Spilling a corrosive cleaner on the skin
C. Smoking crack cocaine during a 2-week vacation
D. Inhaling solvents on weekends

2. Which of the following toxin antidotes and toxins are correctly matched? (Mark all that apply.)

A. Atropine and anticholinesterase insecticides
B. Hydroxocobalamin and cyanide
C. Succimer and digoxin
D. Activated charcoal and lead

3. Which of the following antidotes can be administered orally? (Mark all that apply.)

A. Acetylcysteine
B. Activated charcoal
C. Naloxone
D. Pralidoxime

4. If a person's eye is splashed with a household cleaner, what is the best first action to take?

A. Flush immediately for 30 minutes with water, and instill vasoconstrictor eye drops if redness persists.
B. Remove any contact lenses, and irrigate eyes with 10–15 mL of contact lens saline solution.
C. Remove any contact lenses, irrigate eyes for 15–30 continuous minutes with water, and evaluate need for further care.
D. Manage pain with acetaminophen tablets and an eye patch.

5. How does single-dose activated charcoal act as a treatment for an ingestion of a poison?

A. Adsorbs the poison in the gastrointestinal tract
B. Blocks gastrointestinal p-glycoproteins
C. Decreases gastrointestinal motility
D. Suppresses secretion of gastrointestinal fluids

6. Which mechanism of action best describes the action of atropine for an anticholinesterase insecticide poisoning?

A. Chelates the anticholinesterase insecticide
B. Blocks muscarinic-type cholinergic (parasympathetic) receptors competitively
C. Inhibits sodium-potassium ATPase activity
D. Phosphorylates acetylcholinesterase

7. Which of the following statements best describes the services or operations of a poison control center in the United States?

A. A poison control center provides advice on suspected poisonings and monitors the progress and outcome of a patient through follow-up contacts.
B. It is available 24 hours a day for health care professionals, but it is available only during regular business hours for the public.
C. It dispatches an ambulance with poison center personnel.
D. It performs chemical analysis on unknown substances.

8. Which of the following treatments is no longer used to decontaminate the gastrointestinal tract for an acute poisoning in an alert adult? (Mark all that apply.)

A. Ipecac syrup
B. Saline cathartics (laxatives)
C. Activated charcoal
D. Whole bowel irrigation

9. Which of the following medications are not required to be packaged or dispensed in a child-resistant container (safety cap)? (Mark all that apply.)

A. Acetaminophen with hydrocodone tablets
B. Nitroglycerin tablets
C. Aspirin tablets
D. Corticosteroid ointment

10. Which of the following antidotes would be categorized as one that reacts with a toxic metabolite of a drug?

A. Acetylcysteine
B. Activated charcoal
C. Naloxone
D. Pralidoxime

11. Which route of administration of naloxone is not effective to treat an opioid poisoning?

A. Intramuscular
B. Intranasal
C. Oral
D. Intravenous

12. When multiple doses of activated charcoal are indicated, what is the expected outcome of its use on the toxin?

A. Enhance systemic elimination
B. Increase renal excretion
C. Increase protein binding
D. Increase intestinal peristalsis

13. Which of the following medication-assisted therapies is used for opioid use disorder? (Mark all that apply.)

A. Buprenorphine, oral
B. Disulfiram, oral
C. Naloxone, injection
D. Methadone, oral

14. "Addiction" is best described by which of the following statements?

A. Use of a drug for a nontherapeutic effect to alter mood, emotion, or state of consciousness
B. The body's physical adaptation to a drug whereby greater amounts are required over time to achieve the initial desired effect or continued use of the same amount produces markedly diminished effect
C. Unpleasant symptoms after abrupt cessation, rapid dose reduction, decreasing drug concentrations, or administration of an antagonist
D. A primary, chronic, neurobiological disease characterized by impaired control over substance use, compulsive use, craving, and continued use despite adverse social, psychological, and physical consequences

15. Which of the following drugs for substance use disorder is an extended-release IM injection or an intradermal implant? (Mark all that apply.)

A. Naltrexone
B. Buprenorphine
C. Methadone
D. Acamprosate

16. Which of the following drugs should not be given or taken when alcohol is present in the body?

A. Disulfiram
B. Naloxone
C. Naltrexone
D. Acetylcysteine

17. Which of the following drugs is indicated for the initial management of muscarinic symptoms from an organophosphate poisoning?

A. Sodium bicarbonate
B. Atropine
C. Succimer
D. Pralidoxime

18. Which of the following is a treatment option for exposures to infectious biological terrorist substances? (Mark all that apply.)

A. Administration of the appropriate antibiotic
B. Hyperbaric oxygen therapy
C. Decontamination of exposed skin with soap and water
D. Hemodialysis

19. Which of the following categories of chemical warfare agents includes anticholinesterase toxins?

A. Blistering chemicals
B. Blood toxins
C. Riot control agents
D. Nerve agents

20. Which of the following categories of chemical warfare agents applies to super-potent analogs of fentanyl?

A. Blistering chemicals
B. Blood toxins
C. Incapacitating substances
D. Nerve agents

30-13 Answers

1. **B.** A corrosive will burn on contact. The other situations have acute episodes at the time of use, but the choices imply more than one short-term exposure and not every use leads to toxicity. These other situations may produce toxicity from chronic exposure, which is different from toxicity caused by acute exposure.

2. **A, B.** Atropine and hydroxocobalamin are correctly matched. Succimer is used for lead poisoning, and activated charcoal does not significantly adsorb heavy metals like lead.

3. **A, B.** Acetylcysteine can be given orally (Mucomyst) and intravenously (Acetadote). Naloxone is not active when ingested, and pralidoxime is given only parenterally.

4. **C.** Irrigating eyes with water for 15–30 minutes is the best choice. A vasoconstrictor will reduce conjunctivitis, which serves as an important marker of continuing ocular irritation. Finding contact lens saline solution—if any is available at the scene—wastes time, and 10–15 mL is insufficient. Taking acetaminophen and wearing an eye patch are not first actions.

5. **A.** Single-dose activated charcoal adsorbs poisons in the gastrointestinal tract to prevent absorption into the bloodstream. The other options are not actions of activated charcoal.

6. **B.** Blocking muscarinic receptors is the principal action of atropine and can reduce the cholinergic

effects of anticholinesterase insecticides. Answers A and D are not actions of atropine. Phosphorylating anticholinesterase is the action of anticholinesterase insecticides.

7. **A.** Option A describes the fundamental function of a poison control center. Centers are available 24 hours a day for anyone who calls. Poison center personnel do not travel to the scene of a poisoning nor do they perform analytical analysis.

8. **A, B.** Ipecac syrup and cathartics are no longer routinely used to treat ingestions. Activated charcoal and whole bowel irrigation are used when indicated.

9. **B, D.** Child-resistant containers, also known as safety caps, are required for all oral prescription drugs with the exception of drugs such as nitroglycerin. Ointments do not require caps.

10. **A.** One of the major actions of acetylcysteine is to provide sulfhydryl groups in the liver to detoxify an intermediary toxic metabolite of acetaminophen, N-acetyl-p-benzoquinoneimine.

11. **C.** Naloxone is effective by IV, IM, and intranasal routes of administration, but it is not active when taken orally.

12. **A.** Multiple doses of activated charcoal given over 24–48 hours can enhance systemic elimination of some toxins by interrupting enterohepatic recirculation or by attracting the drug across the mesenteric capillary bed into the lumen of gastrointestinal tract, thereby adsorbing it to activated charcoal and evacuating the complex in the stool.

13. **A, D.** Buprenorphine with or without naloxone in oral preparations and methadone are used to treat opioid use disorder. Disulfiram is for alcohol use disorder, and naloxone injection is used for treatment of acute opioid overdoses as a rescue drug.

14. **D.** Addiction is a disease state. The other answer choices are characteristics that typically constitute or lead to addiction.

15. **A, B.** Naltrexone can be given as an IM injection monthly, and buprenorphine is available as an implantable pellet that lasts for 6 months. The other drugs are available in oral forms.

16. **A.** Disulfiram will cause aversive, unpleasant effects when alcohol is in the body and can lead to life-threatening reactions. The other drugs can be taken with alcohol present in the body, but alcohol use should be discouraged in a comprehensive plan to treat substance use disorder.

17. **B.** Atropine is used to treat the organophosphate-induced muscarinic symptoms (miosis; nausea and vomiting; diarrhea; urination; bradycardia; excessive bronchial, lacrimal, dermal, nasal, and salivary secretions). Pralidoxime is used with atropine to resolve severe organophosphate symptoms (such as those from exposure to nerve agents), including nicotinic symptoms of muscle weakness and cramps, fasciculations, and tachycardia and CNS symptoms such as coma and seizures. Succimer is used for lead poisoning. Sodium bicarbonate has several uses including the treatment of tricyclic antidepressant toxicity. Neither succimer nor sodium bicarbonate has a role for the muscarinic effects.

18. **A, C.** The appropriate antibiotic, if one is available for the infectious agent, is the best choice. If the person's skin has been exposed to the infectious agent, decontaminating the skin is also important to prevent further absorption and to protect health care personnel. Methods of decontamination in addition to soap and water may be needed. The other answer choices are not relevant for this type of exposure unless other toxins or conditions exist.

19. **D.** Anticholinesterase agents are categorized as nerve agents in that they act on the autonomic, neuromuscular, and central nervous systems.

20. **C.** Super-potent fentanyl analogs have been used to incapacitate victims by dispersion through ventilation systems in enclosed spaces such as auditoriums or meeting rooms. If the doses are not carefully controlled and monitored, incapacitation can lead to death by opioid overdose.

30-14 Additional Resources

Antidotes. March 2017. California Poison Control System Web site. https://calpoison.org/topics/antidotes. Accessed February 22, 2018.

Bradberry S, Vale A. Management of poisoning: antidotes. *Medicine*. 2015;44(2):101–102. Available at: https://www.sciencedirect.com/science/article/pii/S1357303915003138. Accessed February 23, 2018. Note: This is a European publication with some drug names spelled differently than those in the United States.

Dart RC, Goldfrank LR, Erstad BL, et al. Expert consensus guidelines for stocking of antidotes in hospitals that provide emergency care. *Ann Emerg Med*. 2018;71(3):314–325.

Medication-assisted treatment (MAT). U.S. Department of Health and Human Services, Substance Abuse and Mental Health Services Administration Web site. https://www.samhsa.gov/medication-assisted-treatment. Accessed February 23, 2018.

Reus VI, Fochtmann J, Bukstein O, et al. The American Psychiatric Association practice guideline for the pharmacological treatment of patients with alcohol use disorder. *Am J Psychiatry*. 2018;175(1):86–90.

U.S. Department of Health and Human Services, Substance Abuse and Mental Health Services Administration. *Medications for Opioid Use Disorder: For Healthcare and Addiction Professionals, Policymakers, Patients, and Families*. Rockville, MD: Substance Abuse and Mental Health Services Administration; 2018. HHS Publication No. (SMA) 18-5063. Available at: https://store.samhsa.gov/shin/content//SMA18-5063FULLDOC/SMA18-5063FULLDOC.pdf. Accessed February 7, 2018.

U.S. Department of Health and Human Services, Substance Abuse and Mental Health Services Administration. *SAMHSA Opioid Overdose Prevention Toolkit*. Rockville, MD: U.S. Department of Health and Human Services, Substance Abuse and Mental Health Services Administration; 2016. HHS Publication No. (SMA) 16-4742. Available at: https://www.samhsa.gov/capt/tools-learning-resources/opioid-overdose-prevention-toolkit. Accessed February 23, 2018.

U.S. Department of Justice, Drug Enforcement Administration. *Drugs of Abuse: A DEA Resource Guide*. Washington, DC: U.S. Department of Justice, Drug Enforcement Administration; 2017. Available at: https://www.dea.gov/pr/multimedia-library/publications/drug_of_abuse.pdf. Accessed February 23, 2018.

Index

Page numbers followed by *b*, *f*, or *t* indicate material in boxes, figures, or tables, respectively.

G